Arachnoid Cysts

Mehmet Turgut • Ali Akhaddar
Ahmet T. Turgut • Walter A. Hall
Editors

Arachnoid Cysts

State-of-the-Art

Springer

Editors
Mehmet Turgut
Department of Neurosurgery
Aydın Adnan Menderes University
Aydın, Turkey

Ali Akhaddar
Department of Neurosurgery
Mohammed V University in Rabat
Rabat, Morocco

Ahmet T. Turgut
Department of Radiology
Ankara Medipol University
Ankara, Turkey

Walter A. Hall
Department of Neurosurgery
SUNY Upstate Medical University
Syracuse, NY, USA

ISBN 978-3-031-22700-4 ISBN 978-3-031-22701-1 (eBook)
https://doi.org/10.1007/978-3-031-22701-1

This Springer imprint is published by the registered company Springer Nature Switzerland AG
The registered company address is: Gewerbestrasse 11, 6330 Cham, Switzerland

Foreword

Very few nosographic entities have attracted the attention of pediatric and adult neurosurgeons like arachnoid cysts (ACs). There are several reasons for such an interest, namely the heterogeneous nature of these lesions due to their different locations, their variable impact on the neurocognitive development, the possible association with disturbances of the cerebrospinal fluid (CSF) dynamics, the induced endocrinological alterations, and seizure disorders.

The treatment of an AC can be challenging. Indeed, a conservative management can be adopted in some specific cases; in others the surgical indication depends not only on the mere presence of the malformation but also on the age of the patient at the time of its diagnosis. A typical example is provided by the quite common temporal ACs that interfere with the cerebral development in early life, thus requiring a prompt surgical excision if recognized. However, these cysts often reach a stable spatial equilibrium with the brain and tend to remain unchanged after childhood and adolescence. Consequently, in the case of accidental late recognition a wait-and-see policy should be taken into account. A similar consideration could be made for asymptomatic and accidentally discovered interhemispheric ACs diagnosed at a late age. On the other hand, the surgical indications cannot be ignored in cases of chiasmatic region or posterior cranial fossa ACs because of their obvious role in causing severe endocrinological and CSF dynamics disturbances.

A further limitation on the correct surgical indications can be in some cases due to the difficulty in the interpretation of the clinical manifestations attributed to the presence of the cyst. Once more, this limit concerns the temporal ACs when associated with seizure disorders. Often, the epilepsy does not resolve even after the complete surgical excision of the lesion, thereby demonstrating that the cyst was not the cause of the seizures but rather a manifestation of an underlying developmental malformative process of the temporal lobe. Also, those cases of surprising re-bleeding of ACs operated on because of intracystic hemorrhage can be interpreted on the grounds of the abovementioned consideration.

For several years the debate on the most appropriate surgical modality has been centered on the choice between the craniotomic direct approach for the surgical excision of the lining membranes or for the diversion of the cyst fluid content into the ventricular system and subarachnoid spaces or an indirect approach, in most cases a cysto-peritoneal shunt. The advent of endoscopy has deeply modified the surgical management of ACs providing a further and effective management tool that is apt to reduce the surgical risk for several patients.

On the grounds of these considerations and the still ongoing discussion of the more appropriate management of ACs, the editors should be congratulated for the timely chosen subject, still open to research, of their well-organized book as well as for the numerous and widely respected coauthors that they were able to gather.

I wish them and the book the deserved success.

Concezio Di Rocco

Pediatric Neurosurgery
International Neuroscience Institute
Hannover, Germany

Contents

Part I

General Information About Arachnoid Cysts

Editor's Summary

In this "Part I: General Information About Arachnoid Cysts," there are a total of six chapters describing the general aspects of the arachnoid cysts (ACs), noncancerous collections of cerebrospinal fluid (CSF) localized by the arachnoid membranes of the brain or spinal cord. Even today, unlike many other space-occupying lesions, they are usually asymptomatic and their management can be challenging for neurologists, neuroradiologists, and neurosurgeons due to the heterogeneous nature of these lesions. The first of the chapters in this section compiles the historical and etymological aspects of ACs in light of the current literature. In the second chapter, the authors review both the gender distribution and lateralization of ACs, which can present in many different locations within the central nervous system. In the subsequent two chapters, the embryological and histological features of ACs that influence their cerebral development in early life, the authors illustrate this process with demonstrative histological figures and special drawings. Interestingly, these cysts usually reach a stable spatial equilibrium with the brain or spinal cord, and they tend to remain unchanged all throughout life. The fifth chapter addresses a variety of pathophysiological mechanisms for their formation and their possible association with disturbances of the CSF dynamics, such as fluid secretion and slit-valve mechanism. The last remaining chapter provides the biochemical findings of the AC fluid in detail for the readers of the book.

History and Etymology of Arachnoid Cysts

Timothy Beutler

1 Introduction

The history of arachnoid cysts (ACs) is difficult to trace through the literature. The nomenclature has changed over time, and some of the earliest reports likely mixed in with different pathologies including resolving subdural hematoma and infections. Early descriptions of ACs associate the entity with a variety of conditions ranging from spontaneous and seemingly incidental to posthemorrhagic and inflammatory conditions.

The history of ACs begins in the early nineteenth century with postmortem autopsy studies. ACs in most of these patients were incidental findings and not related to the cause of death. In the early twentieth century, we begin to see the earliest operative reports of patients with symptomatic ACs. By the mid-twentieth to late twentieth century, new imaging technology led to the increased discovery of asymptomatic ACs and the emergence of modern management practices.

2 Early History

The early history of ACs is derived primarily from postmortem pathology studies which became more prevalent in the nineteenth century. Many of these studies were unfortunately performed in asylum populations, so some of the literature has bias toward an association with mental illness. Additionally, early studies also tended to describe any cyst or collection located beneath the dura as an AC and most likely included additional pathologies such as resolving hemorrhages and infections.

One of earliest attempts to characterize the prevalence of ACs was completed by Crichton Brown in 1875 and estimated a 5% prevalence in his asylum population after reviewing over 1000 autopsies [7]. However, this study likely overestimated the true prevalence of the condition as some descriptions appeared to describe a variety of hemorrhagic, infectious, and inflammatory pathologies.

3 Serous Cysts in the Arachnoid

The earliest description of an AC is attributed to the English physician Richard Bright who practiced at Guy's Hospital in London in the early nineteenth century. He utilized autopsies to understand a variety of diseases and published two large volumes of medical cases with accompanying illustrations in 1831 [6]. In the section on diseases of the brain and nervous system, he reports two cases of ACs that were discovered on autopsy and publishes what is considered the first two medical illustrations of the condition. The

T. Beutler (✉)
Department of Neurosurgery, SUNY Upstate Medical University, Syracuse, NY, USA
e-mail: beutlert@upstate.edu

M. Turgut et al. (eds.), *Arachnoid Cysts*, https://doi.org/10.1007/978-3-031-22701-1_1

first illustration shows what appears to be a large middle cranial fossa AC (Fig. 1), while the second illustration shows two smaller ACs located over the convexity (Fig. 2).

Bright observed that the cysts were apparently asymptomatic and discovered incidentally at autopsy. They are described as being located between the layers of the arachnoid or attached to the arachnoid by thin adventitious membranes. Their sizes varied from the "size of a pea to that of a large orange" [6]. Notably, he postulated that the condition was likely chronic and observed that the "bone of the skull is molded to their form" [6].

As early as the 1860s, it was recognized that cysts in the arachnoid space were not uncommon [25]. At that point, there were two prevailing theories regarding their pathophysiology that lead to occasionally confusing nomenclature in the early literature. The first theory was that they were a result of an accumulation of lymph that occurs secondary to arachnoiditis. The second theory was that they are the result of chronic changes from previous hemorrhage.

CHRONIC SEROUS CYST.

FIG. 1. A cyst, containing half a pint of serous fluid, discovered in the fissura Sylvii of the left hemisphere, in a man who died of fever. This cyst appeared to be composed of layers of the arachnoid, or of thin adventitious structures, closely attached to that membrane. It had left a deep and permanent depression on the anterior lobe of the cerebrum, and the large vessels appeared to continue their course behind it, on the brain, without suffering any interruption. (Page 438.) A smaller cyst of the same description is represented, Plate XXI. Fig. 4., together with the permanent depressiou corresponding to it in the bone of the skull. (Fig.1.)

a, the anterior lobe of the left hemisphere.
b, slight sketch of the medulla oblongata.
c, ———————— pons Varolii.
d, optic nerves.
ee, external surface of the cyst.
ff, a portion of the external layer of the cyst thrown back.
gg, a portion of the internal layer.
h, a large vessel passing behind the cyst and covered by a membrane.

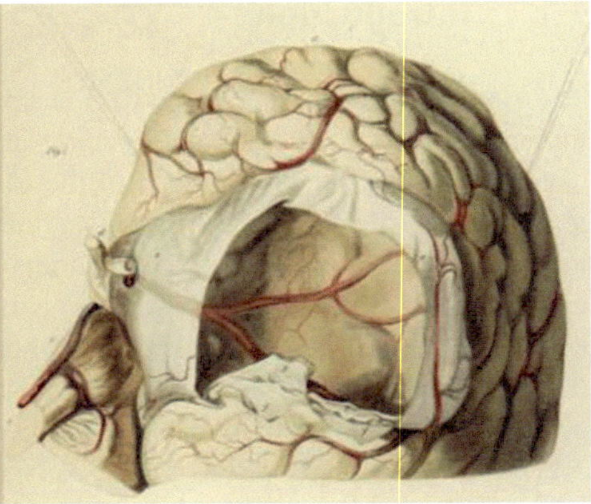

Fig. 1 Large middle cranial fossa cyst. (Depicted by Richard Bright in "Reports of Medical Cases, Selected with a View of Illustrating the Symptoms and Cure of Diseases by a Reference to Morbid Anatomy." Volume II "Diseases of the Brain and Nervous System: Part I": Fig. 1 on plate II and corresponding legend description. Originally published in 1831)

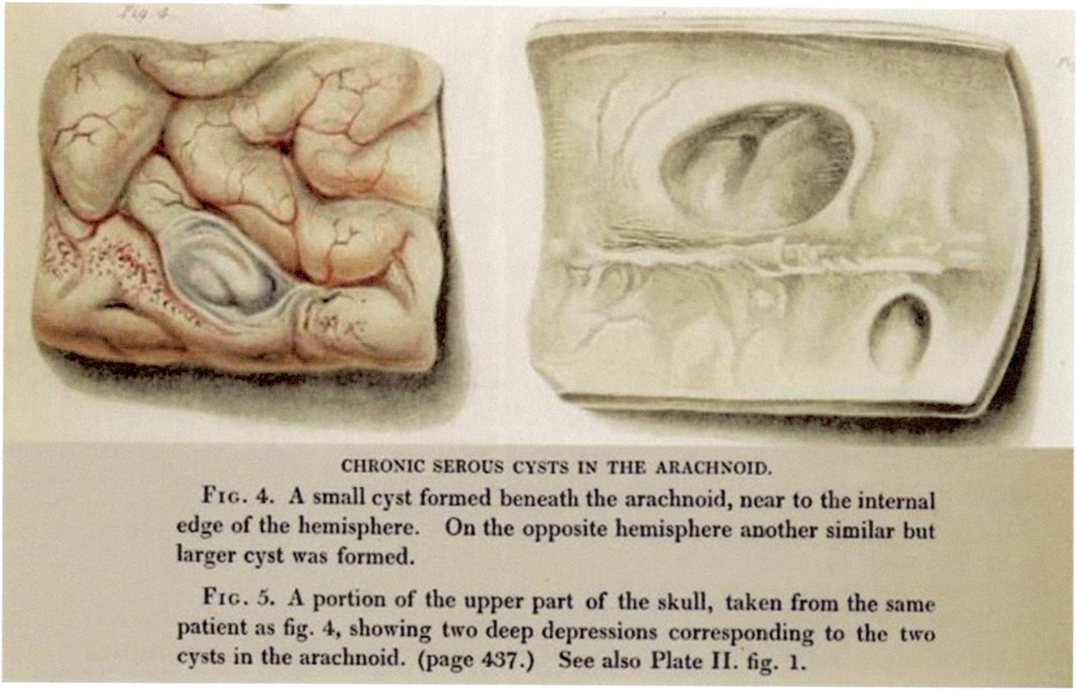

Fig. 2 Small AC and corresponding portion of the skull. (Depicted by Richard Bright in "Reports of Medical Cases, Selected with a View of Illustrating the Symptoms and Cure of Diseases by a Reference to Morbid Anatomy." Volume II "Diseases of the Brain and Nervous System: Part II": Figs. 4 and 5 on plate XXI and corresponding legend description. Originally published in 1831)

4 Organization of Lymph

The organization of lymph is perhaps the earliest theory regarding the pathophysiology of ACs. It is unclear from where the lymph theory originated; however, in an 1865 paper by Samuel Wilks entitled "Cyst in the Cavity of the Arachnoid," he described an AC specimen in Guy's Hospital that Thomas Hodgkin attributed to the organization of lymph [25].

Arachnoiditis was thought to lead to a spontaneous accumulation of lymph between the layers of the arachnoid leading to the formation of ACs. However, this theory was supplanted by the belief that ACs were formed as a result of an effusion of blood. While ACs were found in patients with no history of either trauma or infection, apoplexy had been commonly observed, whereas spontaneous arachnoiditis had not been seen. Even French physician Achille-Louis Foville, while classifying ACs under his "Meningite parietale," admitted that "their inflammatory nature" [was] not sufficiently well established [25].

5 Extravasation of Blood into the Cavity of the Arachnoid

In 1845, Prescott Hewett attempted to outline the pathophysiology of ACs in a paper entitled "Extravasations of Blood into the Cavity of the Arachnoid" [13]. He described four divisions of hemorrhage in the subarachnoid space ranging from simple to complex collections.

At first glance, to a modern reader, the work of Hewett appears to be unrelated to ACs and seems to better describe the pathophysiology that we commonly encounter with resolving intraparenchymal and subdural hemorrhages. However, careful examination of the manuscript reveals references to AC case descriptions provided by Hodgkin and Bright from Guy's Hospital [13].

Hewett describes the pathology of ACs in the following excerpt:

> Thus organized, these cysts possess all the physiological characters of an original serous membrane; they secrete, they absorb; they have been found filed with clots of fibrine and blood-tinged serum; sometimes they contain serum alone, of various colours, and often times, in the cavity of the same cyst, are found coagula of blood of various hues, some recently effused, and others of long standing [13].

By 1865, Samuel Wilks wrote that the work of Hewett was generally accepted as the correct explanation for the origin of ACs. He further describes the end result of the cyst after all the blood had been reabsorbed:

> The interior of the cyst, if it be old, has generally lost all traces of blood, and contains merely shreds of fibrous material of the same structure as the walls, together with a limpid fluid and cholesterine [25].

6 Chronic and Asymptomatic

Even from the earliest descriptions by Richard Bright in 1831, there was the belief that ACs were generally chronic and asymptomatic entities. The earliest cysts were discovered incidentally on autopsy studies, and so they were associated with a benign and indolent course. During the early pre-surgical era, even large supratentorial ACs were discovered. One case report from 1879 by D.J. Cunningham described discovering a cystic cavitation in the right parietal lobe "large enough to hold a hen's egg" in a patient who passed away from diabetes [9]. What was remarkable at the time was that the cyst extended posteriorly to the Rolandic fissure and the patient was not known to have any weakness (Fig. 3). Observations such as this one reinforced the belief that ACs were asymptomatic and chronic entities. However, our understanding of the etiology of ACs changed again in the early twentieth century with the emergence of neurosurgery as a surgically discipline.

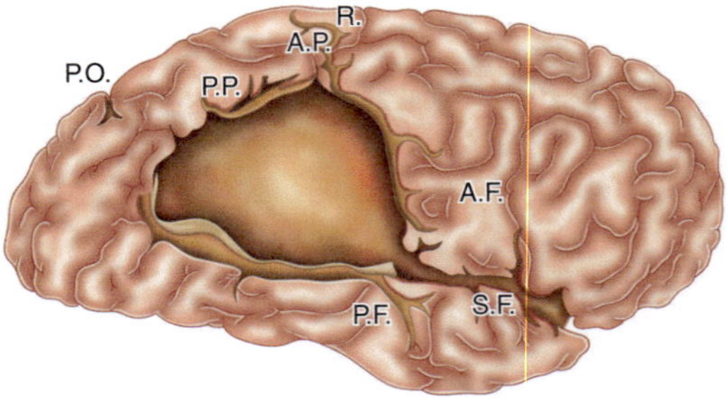

Profile of right hemisphere to show position of cyst (reduced to a little more than half size). SF, Sylvian fissure; R, Fissure of Rolando; PO, Parieto-occipital fissure; PF, Parallel fissure; AF, Ascending frontal convolution; PP, Postero-parietal convolution; AP, Ascending parietal convolution.

Fig. 3 Large right middle fossa AC. (Depicted by D.J. Cunningham in "A large sub-arachnoid cyst involving the greater part of the parietal lobe of the brain." Journal of anatomy and physiology originally published in 1879)

7 Early Surgical Experience

In the early twentieth century, due largely in part to advancements in anesthesia and the localization of neurologic disease, case reports of successful surgery for symptomatic ACs begins to emerge in the literature. X-rays were only invented by Wilhelm Rontgen in 1895, so localization of symptoms based on a detailed neurologic exam was paramount for the successful surgical treatment of a patient with neurologic disease.

8 Spinal Arachnoid Cysts

Some of the earliest reports of successful surgery for ACs were for spinal ACs [5, 21, 23]. The earliest American report of a spinal AC was written by Spiller, Musser, and Martin in 1903 [23]. They presented a case of a lumbar AC in a young woman who presented with progressive left leg pain, weakness, and paresthesias. They describe treatment with an L2–L4 laminectomy and report encountering a cyst measuring approximately an inch and a half in length after opening the dura. The walls of the cyst were described as of a "flimsy consistency" and filled with clear fluid which they reported was under "unusual intradural pressure" [23]. After surgery, they reported the gradual improvement in the patient's preoperative symptoms with near complete recovery after 6 years. Their description is unique from many other craniospinal cysts described during this era which were secondary to parasitic infections from cysticercus and echinococcus.

By 1915, there were at least six spinal ACs that had been described in the surgical literature [21]. These cysts ranged in location throughout the cervical, thoracic, and lumbar spine. Diagnostic tools were limited at this time, and much emphasis was placed on thoroughly documenting a neurologic exam for localization of spinal symptoms. Rachiocentesis was also recommended as part of the workup and sometime completed at levels above and below where the suspected lesion was located. Outcomes for these early patients were often reported as good as long as the surgery was completed early in course of the patient's symptoms. Those who presented with severe symptoms such as paraplegia did not have outcomes as good as those who presented with only pain and sensory changes.

In a review of the first six cases of spinal ACs, Skoog describes all the cases having been found in women aged 17 to 50 years [21]. Histological reports are limited from the early literature as the thin walls of the cysts were difficult to preserve during surgery. Trauma and infectious etiologies were still thought to be the most likely provocative factors contributing to cyst formation. Skoog writes regarding their pathogenesis:

> I believe that there may be several provocative agents in the different cases and that from one of the irritating factors there are formed adhesions with the endothelial cells and fibers of the arachnoid. This is followed by an exudate or secretion from the delicate endothelial cells lining the fibrils or covering the interior of the cyst. Thus there is a very slow accumulation of fluid followed by the gradual development of the cord compression [21].

9 Posterior Fossa Cysts

In 1893, William Krause presented a case of a 36-year-old man with worsening posterior headaches, nausea, vomiting, vertigo, and an unsteady gait [16]. While the patient's symptoms were correctly localized to the cerebellum, he unfortunately passed away before any treatment. Upon autopsy, a large cystic cavity was found in the right cerebellum filled with an amber-colored fluid. While this cyst was likely not a primary AC, Krause wrote his article to show that the constellation of symptoms for posterior fossa lesions was specific and distinct enough to support surgical intervention.

By the 1930s, a series of cases had been described by multiple surgeons of ACs in the posterior fossa [3, 10, 14]. At this time, theories of infection and hemorrhage still remained common despite little evidence to support either consideration. Most of the cysts in the posterior fossa were reported either in a midline location or in the cerebellopontine angle (CPA). Posterior fossa cysts would often present with findings consistent with elevated intracranial pressure and obstructive hydrocephalus. Those cysts in the CPA were often associated with inflammation and otitis media. Many of the midline cerebellar cysts, including some of Cushing's cases described by Horrax, appear more consistent with arachnoiditis or dilation of the cisterna magna than with well-circumscribed cysts [14].

10 Primary Arachnoid Cysts

While ACs were described in earlier literature, there was little distinction between what a modern reader would recognize as an AC and any other kind of cystic pathology. The early literature was often limited to gross anatomic descriptions of lesions, and histologic reports of the lesions are more difficult to find because the walls of many cysts were thin and difficult to preserve. The histologic descriptions that were available varied greatly with some reporting structures similar to normal arachnoid, some reporting resolving hemorrhage, and others describing nonspecific inflammatory changes.

Throughout the first half of the twentieth century, diagnostic imaging techniques continued to advance. As a result, preoperative workup progressed to include a number of techniques including cerebral angiography, air encephalography, and electroencephalography [20].

For example, in the case of large middle cranial fossa cyst, plain X-rays may show thinning and expansion of the temporal squama and surrounding frontal and parietal bone enlarging the middle cranial fossa and elevating the lesser wing of the sphenoid. Cerebral angiography may show displacement of the arteries on the ipsilateral side with the middle cerebral arteries being shifted upward and medially and the anterior cerebral artery shifted contralaterally. Air encephalography could show some contralateral shift of the lateral ventricles as well as a truncated or dorsally displaced ipsilateral temporal horn. Electroencephalogram may be unremarkable or show some generalized slowing in the region of the cyst.

Advancements in imaging as well as greater attention to the histology of ACs ultimately led to the development of one of the earliest classifications of ACs.

In a case reported by Leslie Oliver in 1958, he described a 21-year-old man who presented with worsening headaches, vomiting, and diplopia 10 weeks after sustaining a traumatic sports injury to the chest [19]. On physical exam, he experienced diplopia when looking to the right and was noted to have left upper facial weakness. Fundoscopic exam revealed bilateral papilledema, and the lumbar puncture showed an opening pressure of 30 cm of H_2O. Ventriculography showed that the ventricles were displaced to the left. The patient underwent a right-sided craniotomy, and a large AC was discovered filled with yellow fluid. The cyst separated the Sylvian fissure and extended well into the anterior and middle fossa.

Histologic examination of the cyst wall showed "arachnoid membrane thickened by fibrosis, and showing (a) considerable recent focal haemorrhage, and (b) areas of greatly increased vascularity associated with chronic inflammatory infiltration and considerable numbers of macrophages containing iron pigment" [19].

Because of the patient's recent trauma and histologic description, the etiology of the cyst was originally attributed to trauma. However, air encephalography completed 8 weeks after surgery revealed a persistent empty space in the area formerly occupied by the cyst, which raised the question of whether the cyst had been present for much longer.

Oliver's discussion of the AC is significant because he proposed classifying ACs as either primary or secondary. Primary ACs were defined as congenital lesions that were formed by the absence rather than displacement of nervous tissue, whereas secondary ACs were those lesions that formed due to injury, inflammation, or tumors.

The same year that Oliver's paper was published, an autopsy series of four cases of ACs was published by Starkman, Brown, and Linell [22]. In this report, they described how these idiopathic cysts differed in their anatomic relationships from those cysts that are associated with inflammation and other secondary causes. They concluded that idiopathic or primary ACs likely result from a focal derangement in the normal development of the leptomeninges.

11 Temporal Lobe Agenesis

Congenital and developmental theories concerning AC formation varied in the lateral half of the twentieth century. While Starkman, Brown, and Linell thought these cysts formed due to aberrant development of the leptomeninges, others such as Robinson thought that cyst formation was due to a defect in brain formation. Robinson referred to this process as temporal lobe agenesis [20].

Patients with temporal lobe agenesis usually presented at a young age with local bulging of the skull with underlying large intracranial collections of fluid. These lesions were described as "bluish transparent cyst[s]" containing clear fluid [20]. They often were so large that upon opening the outer cyst wall, the tentorium, optic nerve, and carotid artery were visible without any retraction of the brain. In a literature review by Robinson, he found that these lesions were often described as subdural hygromas by previous authors and thought to be secondary to minor head injuries [20]. The problem with the trauma theory was that the brain tissue often appeared normal without displacement or compression. Robinson's impression of these cases was that the temporal pole was congenitally absent and called this developmental abnormality temporal lobe agenesis.

The theory of temporal lobe agenesis framed the pathophysiology of ACs as an underdevelopment of the temporal lobe as opposed to an abnormal development of the leptomeninges. Because many of these patients presented only with misshaped heads and nonspecific headaches, this theory ultimately contributed to decreasing the rates of surgery for the condition because there was no role for decompressive surgery if there was no compression of the brain. However, opponents to this theory argued that it could not easily account for the expansion of the skull. Other variants of agenesis of the brain were typically associated with a corresponding lack of skull development. Temporal lobe agenesis also could not easily explain the elevated intracranial pressure that was associated with some ACs. Today, the primary agenesis hypothesis has been largely abandoned, in favor of more widely accepted congenital leptomeningeal developmental theories.

12 Arachnoid Cysts in the Age of Modern Imaging

The 1970s revolutionized the treatment of neurologic conditions. In 1971, Hounsfield obtained the first images of the brain with a computed tomography (CT) scanner. Later in 1978, clinical teams at EMI laboratories lead by Ian Robert Young and Hugh Clow developed magnetic resonance imaging (MRI) imaging. These new imaging techniques allowed for the structure of the brain to be imaged for the first time. With the development and widespread adoption of these imaging techniques, ACs could be identified and diagnosed much more easily.

Modern imaging techniques have allowed for the distinct diagnosis of primary ACs from a variety of other pathologies with which they had historically been associated such as hemorrhages, hygromas, infection, tumors, and arachnoiditis.

Imaging also made it possible to start classifying ACs beyond just describing their anatomic location. In 1982, Galassi published his classification of middle cranial fossa ACs [12]. Middle cranial fossa ACs are thought to represent approximately half of all cranial ACs. Galassi classified these lesions into three types. Type I cysts were small, spindle-shaped lesions that were limited to the anterior portion of the middle cranial fossa, typically below the sphenoid ridge. These lesions were typically asymptomatic and did not require surgical intervention. Type II cysts extended superiorly to the Sylvian fissure and displaced the temporal lobe resulting in slowed flow of cerebrospinal fluid (CSF) in the subarachnoid space. Type III cysts filled the entire middle cranial fossa and often displaced not just the temporal lobe but also the frontal and parietal lobes. Type III cysts could present with midline shift and were associated with impaired CSF flow.

Modern imaging techniques and access to imaging led to easier diagnosis and the re-emergence of incidental asymptomatic ACs. Similar to the early literature, where postmortem studies first identified ACs, CT and MRI led to the discovery of a wide variety of small asymptomatic ACs located throughout the neuroaxis. Modern retrospective reviews of imaging have estimated the prevalence of ACs being found on brain imaging as 1.4% in adults and 2.6% in children [1, 2]. While this is a lower prevalence than reported in older autopsy studies, it likely represents a more homogenous group of pathologies.

13 Modern Presentation, Management, and Pathogenesis

Today, ACs are found throughout the brain and spine. They can still be classified as primary cysts which form due to congenital splitting of the arachnoid or as secondary cysts which form as a result of trauma, surgery, infection, hemorrhage, or inflammation [11]. Due to prevalence and availability of imaging, over 90% of ACs that are discovered are asymptomatic and do not require any surgery [15].

ACs that are symptomatic can present with diverse symptoms depending on their size and anatomic location. Cranial lesions have been described presenting with obstructive hydrocephalus, headaches, elevated intracranial pressure, endocrinopathies from compression of the hypothalamic-pituitary axis, seizures, remodeling/deformity of the temporal bone and/or orbit, as well as cranial nerve and brain stem symptoms such as tinnitus, hearing loss, facial palsy, nystagmus, and vertigo. Some middle fossa ACs have also have been associated with acute and/or recurrent subdural hematomas and may present with focal neurologic weakness. Spinal ACs may be associated with pain or progressive neurologic symptoms such as weakness or paresthesias.

Treatment is typically recommended for symptomatic ACs. Although, on occasion, it may be difficult to determine if patients are symptomatic from their AC, there are three primary treatment options that are available: open microsurgical cyst resection and fenestration, endoscopic cyst fenestration, and cyst shunting. The optimal choice of treatment depends on a patient's symptoms and the location of the cyst. Subsequent chapters of this book will explore the various presentations of ACs as well as their treatment options in more details.

Modern pathogenesis of ACs remains quite similar to many of the early prevailing theories. Most common explanations given for ACs involve congenital, traumatic, and infectious/inflammatory etiologies. Given the diverse pathology of ACs in the nervous system, there are likely multiple pathways through which they can form. In large part due to modern imaging, we now have documented reports in the literature of ACs forming after traumatic injuries, infections, and inflammatory conditions as well as by spontaneous formation during early childhood development without any obvious inciting events [8, 24].

There is much that is still not understood of about the development of ACs. While there have been some studies that have linked different genetic polymorphisms to the development of both cranial and spinal ACs, more research is needed to understand how these lesions develop [4, 17, 18].

14 Conclusion

ACs represent a diverse pathology of lesions that can be found throughout the central nervous system. Throughout the years, a variety of pathophysiologic mechanisms have been associated with these lesions including congenital, developmental, traumatic, infectious, and inflammatory etiologies. Most of these theories have been present in some form or another since shortly after ACs were first described in the early nineteenth century.

The history of ACs can be divided into three primary eras: pre-surgical history, early surgical history, and the modern era (Fig. 4). While some of the nomenclature and terminology may have changed, many early observations of ACs still hold true. ACs can vary greatly in size and location. Most ACs are incidental findings and do not require any intervention. Decompression of symptomatic lesions can provide symptomatic relief. Future study into the imaging characteristics, pathology, and genetic expression of these lesions may help us understand more about their diverse pathology.

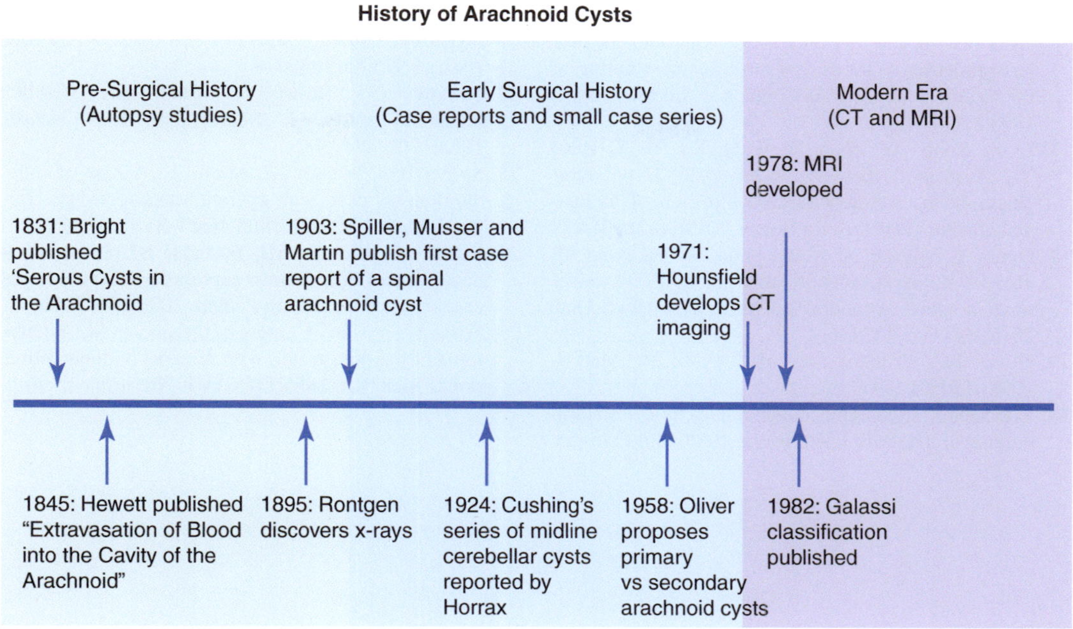

Fig. 4 History of ACs. Three distinct eras of literature can be found. Pre-surgical history primarily consists of autopsy studies of asymptomatic patients. Early surgical history consists of small case series of symptomatic patients. The emergence of computed tomography and magnetic resonance imaging marks the beginning of the modern era of management and classification of ACs

References

1. Al-Holou WN, Terman S, Kilburg C, Garton HJ, Muraszko KM, Maher CO. Prevalence and natural history of arachnoid cysts in adults. J Neurosurg. 2013;118(2):222–31.
2. Al-Holou WN, Yew AY, Boomsaad ZE, Garton HJ, Muraszko KM, Maher CO. Prevalence and natural history of arachnoid cysts in children. J Neurosurg Pediatr. 2010;5(6):578–85.
3. Allen I, Corkill H. Arachnoid cysts involving the cisterna magna. NZ Med J. 1937;36:291–307.
4. Bayrakli F, Okten AI, Kartal U, Menekse G, Guzel A, Oztoprak I, et al. Intracranial arachnoid cyst family with autosomal recessive trait mapped to chromosome 6q22. 31-23.2. Acta Neurochir. 2012;154(7):1287–92.
5. Bliss M. Cysts within the spinal canal. J Am Med Assoc. 1909;52(11):885–6.
6. Bright R. Serous cysts in the arachnoid. Reports of medical cases selected with a view of illustrating the symptoms and cure of diseases by a reference to morbid anatomy. In: Part I. Diseases of the Brain and Nervous System, vol. 2. London: Richard Taylor; 1831. p. 437–9.
7. Browne JC. Arachnoid cysts. J Psychol Med Ment Pathol (Lond). 1875;1(2):167.
8. Choi J-U, Kim D-S. Pathogenesis of arachnoid cyst: congenital or traumatic? Pediatr Neurosurg. 1998;29(5):260–6.
9. Cunningham DJ. A large sub-arachnoid cyst involving the greater part of the parietal lobe of the brain. J Anat Physiol. 1879;13(Pt 4):508.
10. de Martel T, Guillaume J. Sept cas de neoformations de la fosse occipitale optrhs et gueris. Rev Neurol. 1930;2:537–45.
11. Fatima M, Sanaullah B, Aneela D. Management of Arachnoid Cysts: a comprehensive review. Cureus. 2018;10(4):e2458.
12. Galassi E, Tognetti F, Gaist G, Fagioli L, Frank F, Frank G. CT scan and metrizamide CT cisternography in arachnoid cysts of the middle cranial fossa: classification and pathophysiological aspects. Surg Neurol. 1982;17(5):363–9.
13. Hewett P. On extravasations of blood into the cavity of the arachnoid, and on the formation of the false membrane which sometimes envelops these extravasations. Med Chir Trans. 1845;28:45.
14. Horrax G. Generalized cisternal arachnoiditis simulating cerebellar tumor: its surgical treatment and end-results. Arch Surg. 1924;9(1):95–112.
15. Jafrani R, Raskin JS, Kaufman A, Lam S. Intracranial arachnoid cysts: Pediatric neurosurgery update. Surg Neurol Int. 2019;10:15.

16. Krause WC. Cerebellum cyst—ante-mortem diagnosis read in the section of neurology and medical jurisprudence, at the forty-fourth annual meeting of the American Medical Association. J Am Med Assoc. 1893;21(14):481–2.
17. Li K, Kong DS, Zhang J, Wang XS, Ye X, Zhao YL. Association between ELP4 rs986527 polymorphism and the occurrence and development of intracranial arachnoid cyst. Brain Behav. 2019;9(12):e01480.
18. Ogura Y, Miyake N, Kou I, Iida A, Nakajima M, Takeda K, et al. Identification of HOXD4 mutations in spinal extradural arachnoid cyst. PLoS One. 2015;10(11):e0142126.
19. Oliver LC. Primary arachnoid cysts. Br Med J. 1958;1(5080):1147.
20. Robinson R. Intracranial collections of fluid with local bulging of the skull. J Neurosurg. 1955;12(4):345–53.
21. Skoog A. Spinal cord compression from leptomeningeal cysts: with a report of two cases. J Am Med Assoc. 1915;65(5):394–8.
22. Starkman SP, Brown TC, Linell EA. Cerebral arachnoid cysts. J Neuropathol Exp Neurol. 1958;17(3):484–500.
23. Spiller WG, Musser JH, Martin E. A case of intradural spinal cyst, with operation and recovery. Univ Pennsylvania M Bull. 1903;16:27–31.
24. Struck AF, Murphy MJ, Iskandar BJ. Spontaneous development of a de novo suprasellar arachnoid cyst: case report. J Neurosurg Pediatr. 2006;104(6):426–8.
25. Wilks S. Cysts in the cavity of the arachnoid, or hematoma of the dura mater, with remarks on their formation. J Ment Sci. 1865;11(53):94–101.

Gender Distribution and Lateralization of Arachnoid Cysts

Robert Shumkovski, Ivica Kocevski, and Mikjun Mikjunovikj

1 Introduction

Cerebrospinal fluid (CSF) is a transparent serous liquid/fluid that provides essential mechanical hydrostatic and hydrodynamic medium for the central nervous system. Produced by the intraventricular choroid plexus, infilles the ventricular system, flows from the lateral ventricles, through Monroe foramina into the third ventricle, continues through the aqueduct towards the fourth ventricle and fluxes through the aperture mediana Magendy and lateral foramina Lushka, into the subarachnoid compartment spreaded on the skullbase, convexity of the brain and cerebellum and spinal canal, finalyresorpted in parasagitalPaccioni granules/bodies. The CSF fluxes through naturally creating a space formatted in subarachnoid cisterns and canals, comprising the subarachnoid compartment. Evolutionarily, it is created by the mesenchymal arachnoid—leptomeninga, carring the blood vesels. Physiologically, no nutritive, but hydrostatic, mechanical, gravity balancing role of CSF is defined.

R. Shumkovski (✉) · I. Kocevski
University Clinic for Neurosurgery, Clinical Center Mother Teresa, School of Medicine, University St. Cyril & Methodius, Skopje, Republic of North Macedonia

M. Mikjunovikj
Specialized Hospital for Orthopedic Surgery and Traumatology, St. Erazmo, Ohrid, Republic of North Macedonia

On that pathway, from the origin up to resorption, the CSF circulates through the subarachnoid compartment, driven by the capillarity and flow pressure gradient and provided by the pulsatile brain activity, providing medium for the blood vessels and neurologic elements, without direct/intimate encounter with the neurons of the brain, cerebellum, brain stem, and medulla. The separation/distinction is provided by the visceral arachnoid and pia mater, most deep intimate to the cortex leptomeninga.

By numerous, diverse influences, and etiological factors, as genetics, idiopathic, mechanical/physical, biological infectious, and chemical noxes, the normal CSF flux can be disturbed and compromised. This story is to depict the abnormal arachnoid collection defined as arachnoid cyst (ACs). The supreme delicate system of the subarachnoid compartment and CSF flux can be interrupted most frequently by mechanical means, aggravating, obstructing, and compromising the flux and finally accumulating similar to CSF, creating the morphologic issue, i.e., AC. The basic content is similar but not the same with CSF. Most likely, it is CSF plus protein, peptide, crystalloids, micro-blood pigment residua, or detritus of arachnoid desquamation. Mostly, they are occasional/incidental findings in the skull and spinal canal during neuroimaging studies. Thus, they can be primary, congenital idiopathic, or secondary provoked by trauma, i.e., mechanical rupture of the arachnoid, infection, and vascular and oncologic lesion, as well as a result of sur-

M. Turgut et al. (eds.), *Arachnoid Cysts*, https://doi.org/10.1007/978-3-031-22701-1_2

gery, provoking stasis and accumulation of the CSF synergically with the pulsatile brain activity, locally creating valve mechanism obstruction, leading to the accumulation of the CSF-like content, defined as AC.

The natural evolution of the ACs as benign lesion is still not clear, with variety of dimension, location, distribution and variable degree of communication with the subarachnoid compartment.

Clinically, they can present with local compressive phenomenon, focal neurologic deficit, or more often symptoms of generally increased intracranial pressure (headache, nausea and vomiting, dizziness) or clinical signs of suboptimal cerebral function, i.e., epilepsy, mental disturbances, psychiatric disorders, dementia, impaired cognition, etc.

With the evolution of the diagnostic technologies, e.g., magnetic resonance imaging (MRI), certainly, the evidence-based knowledge concerning the predilection of AC location, side, and sex distribution emerged more unveiled and clear.

Definitely, the recent static and dynamic diagnostic high-technology procedures are essential tool for diagnosis, estimation, and evaluation of the ACs.

Furthermore, accurate analysis of the patient series, based on "double individual concept" comprising of the factors of the patient and factor of the therapist, has the mission of the most important conclusive prediction of the natural evolution, with or without active neurosurgical treatment of this phenomenon.

The basic neurosurgical questions—"what, when, and how"—should be answered by a high pool of accumulated direct and collateral systematized information comprising knowledge for the ACs.

Certainly, the statistical analysis of the gender distribution, location, and lateralization of the ACs should contribute to their surgical or not surgical solution, accomplishing the patient's well-being as our duty, which requires all of our commitment without distraction.

ACs represent fluid-filled duplications of the arachnoid membrane with a content which is similar but not equal to the CSF [45]. Another definition states that the ACs are loculated cavities within the arachnoid mater without discrimination of the wall or cyst content, meaning that the wall is composed by arachnoid cells connected with a normal arachnoid membrane [12, 14]. They do not communicate with the ventricles or subarachnoid space and may be unloculated or may have septations.

On the basis of their origin, the ACs can be primary (also known as "true") and secondary ACs. The primary ACs are considered to be congenital in nature, [4] nontumoral, extra-axial, intradural masses, characterized by a single layer of arachnoid cells covered by a vascularized collagen membrane in continuity with the arachnoid [11], while the secondary or acquired ACs result from a primary traumatic, hemorrhagic, tumoral infection (meningitis) or iatrogenic event that causes a prevalent inflammatory process leading to a loculation of the subarachnoid space [29, 30, 31, 38, 46].

ACs usually occur as sporadic and single malformations. However, the occurrence of bilateral or multiple ACs is not exceptional, especially in patients with metabolic disorders or syndromes [12, 28]. In particular, the occurrence of bilateral Sylvian ACs combined with macrocrania and cerebral palsy-like dystonia may suggest a condition known as glutaric aciduria type I (GAT1) [25, 26]. A recently identified gene located on the sixth chromosome (6q22.31-23.2), with an autosomal recessive pattern of inheritance, has been linked to the formation of congenital ACs. The gene was identified in a consanguineous family, and there did not appear to be a pattern in the location or size of the cysts [5]. Certain hereditary syndromes, such as Marfan syndrome [21], neurofibromatosis [27, 41, 47], glutamic aciduria type I [19], autosomal dominant polycystic kidney disease [3], and tuberous sclerosis [7], have demonstrated a higher incidence of ACs than the general population.

Population studies estimate that ACs make up approximately 1% of intracranial space-occupying lesions [9, 10, 36] and are found in approximately 1.7% of the adult population [1] but also represent the most common type of intracranial cyst in the clinical practice [8].

2 Lateralization and Frequency

There have been quite a few studies in the last two decades trying to estimate the prevalence of the ACs. Some large, hospital-based, and population-based studies have demonstrated a prevalence of ACs among the population of about 2%, varying from 0.23% to 2.6% [1, 2, 15, 34, 39, 40]. Some autopsy studies demonstrated a lower prevalence of ACs at 0.1% of individuals [37]. Two peaks in prevalence at 1 and 5 years (3.8% and 4.6% of pediatric cases, respectively) have been reported [2, 29]. Males are affected twice than females (M/F ratio: 2/1) [28]. It is more frequently diagnosed in the pediatric population where the prevalence of ACs is 2.6% [2].

The true incidence of ACs in the population can hardly be known, due to the possible asymptomatic course throughout life, which makes them hardly detectible, but also the different availability of radiodiagnostic tools in the different countries, which likely account for the different rates of their incidental recognition and the difficulty in obtaining specimens for the histological diagnosis, which may result in their underreporting [28].

3 Gender Distribution

A male predominance (2:1 males to females) is noted in both adults and children [1, 2, 29]. As described in a paper by Wester, ACs seemed to occur more frequently in males and on the left side. According to the author, this latter phenomenon could be explained by a greater significance attributed to symptoms from the dominant hemisphere as a justification for invasive procedures in the pre-computed tomography (CT) era. Based on CT studies, it has been determent there is a significant tendency for these cysts to occur in males, with a male/female ratio of nearly 3:1. This preponderance toward males could not be explained by the somewhat higher frequency of associated subdural hematomas that was found in male patients. The survey also showed that middle fossa ACs occur or are detected significantly more frequently on the left side than on the right, with a ratio of 1.8:1 [42].

However, in one of the largest cohorts, Al-Holou et al. studied a total of 48,417 patients who underwent brain MRI. ACs were identified in 661 patients (1.4%). Men had a higher prevalence than women ($p < 0.0001$). Multiple ACs occurred in 30 patients. The most common locations were middle fossa (34%), retrocerebellar (33%), and convexity (14%). Middle fossa cysts were predominantly left-sided (70%, $p < 0.001$). Thirty-five patients were considered symptomatic and 24 underwent surgical treatment. Sellar and suprasellar cysts were more likely to be considered symptomatic ($p < 0.0001$). Middle fossa cysts were less likely to be considered symptomatic ($p = 0.01$) [1].

In a study of pediatric ACs, Al-Holou et al. reviewed a consecutive series of 11,738 patients who were 18 years of age or younger during an 11-year period. In their study, 309 ACs (2.6% prevalence rate) were identified with an increased prevalence of ACs in males ($p < 0.000001$). Of those, 111 patients met all criteria for inclusion in the natural history analysis. The patients were followed for 3.5 years, after which 11 ACs increased in size, 13 decreased, and 87 remained stable. The authors concluded that younger age at presentation was significantly associated with cyst enlargement ($p = 0.001$) and the need for surgery ($p = 0.05$). No patient older than 4 years of age at the time of initial diagnosis had cyst enlargement, demonstrated new symptoms, or underwent surgical treatment, meaning that an older age at the time of presentation is associated with a lack of clinical or imaging changes over time [2].

4 Gender Distribution and Lateralization According to Location

On the basis of their location, the ACs can simply be divided into intracranial and spinal ACs. The intracranial ACs can further be subdivided into supratentorial and infratentorial, whereas the spinal ACs can be divided into extraspinal and intraspinal cysts and may also be both intradural and extradural masses [11, 24]. A previous study on spinal ACs in the pediatric age group has demonstrated an association with neural tube defects, such as myelomeningocele and diastematomyelia [35].

In the era before CT and MRI, a literature review demonstrated 49% of cysts in the middle fossa or Sylvian fissure; in the cerebellopontine angle (CPA), 11%; quadrigeminal plate area, 10%; vermis, 9%; suprasellar area, 9%; interhemispheric fissure, 5%; cerebral convexity, 4%; and interpeduncular area, 3% [34].

About 80–90% of the ACs are located in the supratentorial space, including the quadrigeminal plate region [2, 12, 9] (see Table 1).

The great majority of them originates from the Sylvian fissure (50–60% of all intracranial ACs) and occupies the temporal fossa, followed by those arising from the chiasmatic and the quadrigeminal plate cistern. The interhemispheric fissure and the subarachnoid spaces of the convexity represent less common sites of origin. With regard to the infratentorial space, the lateral (CPA) and the midline retrocerebellar locations are quite equivalent, while the interpeduncular and prepontine cisterns are a rare site of origin of ACs [28].

Different from children, the retrocerebellar location is often found to be as common as the middle fossa location in adults [1]. While ACs of the middle cranial fossa are often discovered incidentally and tend to remain asymptomatic, those arising from other regions are more frequently associated with clinical signs and symptoms and are often associated with hydrocephalus [23]. Indeed, some ACs, namely, the suprasellar and the quadrigeminal plate ACs, may grow toward and even within the cerebral ventricles.

Wester et al. investigated 123 patients with 129 intracranial cysts, consecutively admitted to the Department of Neurosurgery in Bergen 1988–1997. Data were analyzed with regard to intracranial location and gender distribution. Cysts were much more commonly located in the temporal fossae than one would expect if the distribution were random; 68.1% of patients had temporal cysts. Temporal cysts were significantly more frequent in males than in females (3.9:1), while cysts of other locations did not show preponderance for a specific gender. The authors of this study described a connection between gender distribution and sidedness: the significant predominance of left-sided temporal cysts was found only in males. In patients with a unilateral temporal cyst, the left/right ratio was 2.0:1 (males 44 left and 20 right, females 8 left and 6 right) [44].

Table 1 Synopsis of the distribution of ACs and their related clinical findings

Location	Rate	Main clinical features
Supratentorial space	67–80%	Mainly asymptomatic, rupture, headache, seizures,
Sylvian fissure/middle fossa	50%	developmental delay, bone scalloping
Sellar/suprasellar region	10%	Hydrocephalus, headache, vomiting, macrocrania, hormonal deficit, bobble-head doll syndrome, visual loss
Interhemispheric fissure	5%	Macrocrania, headache, seizures, focal deficits
Convexity	5%	Headache, seizures, bone scalloping
Tentorial space	10%	Hydrocephalus, headache, vomiting, macrocrania,
Quadrigeminal plate	10%	precocious puberty, Parinaud' syndrome
Infratentorial space	10–23%	Cerebellar signs, hydrocephalus
Midline	8%	Vertigo, tinnitus, hearing loss, facial sensory loss or
CP angle	10%	weakening, cerebellar signs
Other (e.g., intraventricular, clival region/interpeduncular cistern)	2%	Hydrocephalus, brain stem signs, cranial nerve deficits

Massimi L, Caldarelli M, Di Rocco C. (2020) Intracranial Congenital Arachnoid Cysts. In: Di Rocco C., Pang D., Rutka J. (eds) Textbook of Pediatric Neurosurgery. Springer, Cham

In another study by Wester, 126 patients with 132 ACs were studied. The cysts had a strong predilection for the middle cranial fossa; 86 patients (65.2%) had cysts in this location. Of 106 cysts with clearly unilateral distribution, 64 were located on the left side and 42 on the right side. This significant difference resulted solely from the marked preponderance of middle fossa cysts for the left (left-to-right ratio, 2.1:1). There were significantly more males than females (92 males/34 females). This difference was exclusively due to male preponderance of unilateral middle fossa cysts (66 males/14 females, ratio, 4.7:1). For all other cyst locations, there was no difference between the two sexes (26 males/20 females) or the two sides (10 left, 16 rights). The marked left-sidedness for middle fossa cysts was found only in males. Females had an even distribution between the two sides. The author concludes that the strong predilection of ACs for the middle cranial fossa may be explained by a meningeal maldevelopment theory: the arachnoid coverings of the temporal and frontal lobes fail to merge when the Sylvian fissure is formed in early fetal life, thereby creating a noncommunicating fluid compartment entirely surrounded by arachnoid membranes. Why males develop more middle fossa cysts on the left side remains a mystery (Neurosurgery 45:775–779, 1999) [43].

A case series from The Johns Hopkins Hospital analyzed a group of 20 patients with ACs that underwent surgery. Of the patients enrolled in the study, 20% had supratentorial ACs, 5% infratentorial, and 25% spinal. Gender and age of the patients enrolled in the study were as follows: 12 male (60%) and 8 female (40%) patients, ranging in age from 2 weeks to 39 years (mean age of 10.9 years) at the time of surgery. Twenty-five percent of the cysts were Sylvian, 20% intraventricular, and 20% suprasellar. Supratentorial cysts were treated endoscopically in 73% of patients and with open resection in the remaining 27%. Symptoms at presentation included headache (41%), weakness (23%), seizure (14%), hydrocephalus (9%), scoliosis (4%), cognitive decline (4%), and visual loss (4%) [32].

4.1 Supratentorial ACs

Sylvian fissure ACs (also referred to as middle or temporal fossa cysts) are the most common type of intracranial cysts. Roughly, half of pediatric cysts are located in the middle fossa, and they tend to occur more frequently in males and on the left side (66%) [2]. Although slightly less prevalent in adults (34% of cases), the distribution between left and right is similar to children [1]. Helland and colleagues described a similar prevalence, sex, and side distribution but added that sex differences did not demonstrate statistical significance outside of the temporal fossa [20].

In a study performed by Helland et al., there was a strong predilection (198 patients [66.2%]) for intracranial ACs in the temporal fossa. Forty-two patients had cysts overlying the frontal convexity, 36 had cysts in the posterior fossa, and 23 patients had cysts in other different locations. Of 269 cysts with clearly unilateral distribution, 163 were located on the left side and 106 on the right side. This difference resulted from the marked preponderance of temporal fossa cysts on the left side (left-to-right ratio, 2.5:1; $p < 0.0001$ [adjusted <0.0005]). For cysts in the CPA, there was preponderance on the right side ($p = 0.001$ [adjusted $= 0.005$]). Significantly more males than females had cysts in the temporal fossa ($p = 0.002$ [adjusted $= 0.004$]), whereas in the CPA a significant female preponderance was found ($p = 0.016$ [adjusted $= 0.032$]). For all other cyst locations, there was no difference between the two sexes. The authors also conclude that there is a sex dependency for some intracranial locations of ACs, with temporal cysts occurring more frequently in men, and CPA cysts found more frequently in women. Furthermore, there is a strong location-related sidedness for ACs, independent of patient sex. These findings and reports from the literature suggest a possible genetic component in the development of some ACs [20].

In a landmark paper from 1988 by Galassi et al., ACs of the middle cranial fossa (also known as Sylvian cysts) were shown to represent the most common type of intracranial leptomeningeal malformation. Among the 102 intracranial ACs that underwent surgery, 77 cases (75%) were located in the middle cranial fossa. The ACs reviewed in Galassi's paper had higher incidence in the first two decades of life (51 cases) as well as marked predilection for male sex (60 cases) and the left hemispheric location (55 cases). As for clinical presentation, cranial deformities, symptoms of raised intracranial pressure, and epilepsy constituted the most frequent features. In 13 patients, a complicating lesion was associated: subdural or intracystic hematomas in 7 cases, subdural hygromas in 4 cases, and extradural hematomas in 2 cases. Based on the appearance of the CT scan and the results of the CT cisternography, the authors proposed a classification into three basic types of increasing severity and different pathophysiologic conditions. All of the patients underwent craniotomy, excision of the cyst walls, and perforation into the basal cisterns. There was one postoperative death (mortality rate of 1.3%) due to meningitis. The remaining clinical results were gratifying in all three types of lesion; on follow-up CT scans, the cysts of type I and II exhibited a steady tendency to reduction or obliteration, while cerebral reexpansion seemed less evident in the third, most severe, type [17].

Although middle fossa or Sylvian fissure cysts remain the most common in all age groups, it is possible that some of the differences in prevalence reflect the likelihood of cysts in each location to cause symptoms. In their study of adults with radiographically diagnosed ACs, Al-Holou and colleagues found a statistically significant increased rate of symptomatic cysts for cysts located in the CPA, quadrigeminal cistern, sella, and ambient cisterns [1]. Middle fossa cysts in adults were associated with a significantly lower rate of symptoms [1].

4.2 Infratentorial ACs

The infratentorial compartment represents the second most common location of arachnoid malformations [18] and is often associated with hydrocephalus [22]. When evaluating ACs in the posterior fossa, it is often advised to first rule out a Dandy-Walker syndrome in doubtful cases and to obtain information about the CSF circulation, especially before undertaking more invasive diagnostic or therapeutic measures. It is particularly important to establish the presence and type of communication of cysts with the CSF pathways. Although infratentorial cysts often communicate, they can be space-occupying masses because of increasing CSF retention, which may be due to a ball-valve mechanism or to inadequate communication. The frequently associated hydrocephalus seemed to be dependent mainly upon mechanical factors [18]. A case series by di Rocco et al. evaluating eight children who have been surgically treated for posterior fossa AC have shown that intracranial hypertension was evident in six patients; two children were clinically regarded as being affected by "arrested" hydrocephalus [13].

In a retrospective study of 26 patients with posterior fossa cysts, Arai and Sato came up with four major findings: First, posterior fossa intra-arachnoid cysts were encountered more frequently than expected and were found to be surgically treatable. Second, although IV ventricular cysts were categorized as Dandy-Walker malformation, Dandy-Walker variant, and persistent Blake's pouch in this study, the distinctions of neuroimaging findings between these three types are uncertain. Third, the diagnostic criteria for mega cisterna magna were established, and it was found to be a surgically untreatable condition. Finally, in cases with the following neuroimaging findings, surgery appears to be indicated: (1) occipital bossing or petrosal scalloping with distortion or obliteration of CSF cisterns of the posterior fossa, (2) compression and deformity of the brain surrounding the cyst, (3) radioisotope and/or computed tomography cisternography findings suggestive of disturbance of intracystic CSF circulation, (4) a noncommunicating cyst [4].

Literature review revealed no recent and/or significant study evaluating lateralization and gender distribution of posterior fossa cysts.

4.3 Spinal ACs

The spinal ACs are quite uncommon compared to the intracranial ACs. A paper by Robb et al. reviews the spinal ACs in series of 11 pediatric patients. According to the same paper, the distribution of lesions was as follows: cervicomedullary (one patient), cervical (one), cervicothoracic (two), thoracic (four), lumbar (two), and sacral (one). Four of the 11 ACs (all intradural) were located anterior to the spinal cord, 3 of which were in children with a myelomeningocele. Only two of the cysts were extradural; both were found in the lumbosacral region, and one was associated with diastematomyelia [33].

In a study of 31 pediatric patients (median age 6.9 years) who underwent operative intervention for spinal ACs between 1992 and 2008, there were 17 female patients (55%) and 14 male patients (45%). Twenty-one patients (68%) presented with symptoms of radiculopathy or myelopathy. The most common presenting symptoms were pain (42%), lower-extremity weakness (39%), gait instability (32%), spasticity (19%), sensory loss (10%), and bladder dysfunction (7%). In three patients (10%), spinal ACs were incidental findings. Intradural spinal ACs were more common (18 patients, 58%) than extradural spinal ACs (11 patients, 36%). One patient (3%) had extradural and intradural components. One patient (3%) had a purely intramedullary cyst, and one patient (3%) had both an intradural and an intramedullary component. Of the 18 intradural spinal ACs, 9 (50%) were located ventral to the spinal cord, and 9 (50%) were dorsally situated. One dorsal intradural spinal AC had an intramedullary component. All extradural spinal ACs were located dorsal to the spinal cord. Intradural spinal ACs were primarily concentrated in the cervical and thoracic regions (67%), whereas extradural cysts were more evenly distributed between thoracic, lumbar, and sacral regions. Of the 18 patients with intradural spinal ACs, 13 (72%) had significant previous CNS abnormalities, compared with 3 (27%) of 11 patients with extradural spinal ACs [6].

In a study evaluating spinal ACs, Fam et al. identified 22 patients with spinal ACs with a mean age of at presentation 53.5 years. Of those 22, 17 patients were women, representing an almost 3:1 sex distribution. Symptoms comprised back pain ($n = 16$, 73%), weakness ($n = 10$, 45%), gait ataxia ($n = 11$, 50%), and sphincter dysfunction ($n = 4$, 18%). The mean duration of symptoms was 15 months. Seven patients (32%) exhibited signs of myelopathy. The spinal ACs identified in this cohort were located in the thoracic spine ($n = 17$, 77%) and less commonly in the lumbar spine ($n = 3$, 14%) and cervical/cervicothoracolumbar region ($n = 2$, 9%). Based on imaging findings, the cysts were interpreted as intradural spinal ACs ($n = 11$, 50%), extradural spinal ACs ($n = 6$, 27%), or ventral spinal cord herniation ($n = 2$, 9%); findings in three patients (14%) were inconclusive. Nineteen patients underwent surgical treatment consisting of laminoplasty in addition to cyst resection ($n = 13$, 68%), ligation of the connecting pedicle ($n = 4$, 21%), or fenestration/marsupialization ($n = 2$, 11%). Postoperatively, patients were followed up for an average of 8.2 months (range 2–30 months). Postoperative MRI showed complete resolution of the SAC in 14 of 16 patients [16].

5 Conclusion

Numerous evidence, both empirically and clinically tested, have proven that ACs are nearly twice as more common in males and on the left side, almost 50% in the Sylvian fissure.

References

1. Al-Holou WN, Terman S, Kilburg C, et al. Prevalence and natural history of arachnoid cysts in adults. J Neurosurg. 2013;118:222–31.
2. Al-Holou WN, Yew AY, Boomsaad ZE, et al. Prevalence and natural history of arachnoid cysts in children. J Neurosurg Pediatr. 2010;5:578–85.
3. Alehan FK, Gurakan B, Agildere M. Familial arachnoid cysts in association with autosomal dominant polycystic kidney disease. Pediatrics. 2002;110:e13.

4. Arai H, Sato K. Posterior fossa cysts: clinical, neuroradiological and surgical features. Child's Nerv Syst. 1991;7:156–64. https://doi.org/10.1007/BF00776713.
5. Bayrakli F, Okten AI, Kartal U, et al. Intracranial arachnoid cyst family with autosomal recessive trait mapped to chromosome 6q22.31-23.2. Acta Neurochir. 2012;154:1287–92.
6. Bond AE, Zada G, Bowen I, McComb JG, Krieger MD. Spinal arachnoid cysts in the pediatric population: report of 31 cases and a review of the literature. J Neurosurg Pediatr. 2012;9(4):432–41.
7. Boronat S, Caruso P, Auladell M, et al. Arachnoid cysts in tuberous sclerosis complex. Brain and Development. 2014;36:801–6.
8. Choi JU, Kim DS. Pathogenesis of arachnoid cyst: congenital or traumatic. Pediatr Neurosurg. 1998;29:260–6.
9. Cincu R, Agrawal A, Eiras J. Intracranial arachnoid cysts: current concepts and treatment alternatives. Clin Neurol Neurosurg. 2007;109:837–43.
10. Clemenceau S, Carpenter A. Intracranial arachnoid cysts. Rev Neurol. 1999;155:604–8.
11. Conde Sardon R. Arachnoid cysts. Historical evolution of the concept and pathophysiological theories. Neurocirugia. 2015;26:192–5. [Spanish
12. Di Rocco C, Caldarelli M. Cortical cysts. In: Raimondi AJ, Choux M, Di Rocco C, editors. Intracranial cyst lesions. Berlin: Springer; 1993. p. 143–52.
13. Di Rocco C, Caldarelli M, Di Trapani G. Infratentorial arachnoid cysts in children. Childs Brain. 1981;8(2):119–33.
14. Di Trapani G, Di Rocco C, Pocchiari M, Abbamonti AL. Arachnoid cysts in children: ultrastructural findings. Acta Nerupathologica. 1981;7:392–5.
15. Eskandary H, Sabba M, Khajehpour F, Eskandari M. Incidental findings in brain computed tomography scans of 3000 head trauma patients. Surg Neurol. 2005;63:550–3.
16. Fam MD, Woodroffe RW, Helland L, Noeller J, Dahdaleh NS, Menezes AH, Hitchon PW. Spinal arachnoid cysts in adults: diagnosis and management. A single-center experience. J Neurosurg Spine. 2018;29(6):711–9.
17. Galassi E, Gaist G, Giuliani G, Pozzati E. Arachnoid Cysts of the Middle Cranial Fossa: Experience with 77 Cases Treated Surgically. In: Proceedings of the 8th European Congress of Neurosurgery Barcelona, September 6–11, 1987; 1988. p. 201–4.
18. Galassi E, Tognetti F, Frank F, Fagioli L, Nasi MT, Gaist G. Infratentorial arachnoid cysts. J Neurosurg. 1985;63(2):210–7.
19. Hald JK, Nakstad PH, Skjeldal OH, et al. Bilateral arachnoid cysts of the temporal fossa in four children with glutaricaciduria type I. AJNR Am J Neuroradiol. 1991;12:407–9.
20. Helland CA, Lund-Johansen M, Wester K. Location, sidedness, and sex distribution of intracranial arachnoid cysts in a population-based sample. J Neurosurg. 2010;113:934–9.
21. Ikeda M, Tsuchiya K, Kurosawa T, et al. Marfan's syndrome associated with a frontal arachnoid cyst. Rinsho Shinkeigaku. 1988;28:1076–8.
22. Kuratsu J, Matsukado Y, Kodama T. Large infratentorial multilocular arachnoid cyst. Childs Brain. 1983;10:67–72. https://doi.org/10.1159/000120099.
23. Levy ML, Meltzer HS, Hughes S, Aryan HE, Yoo K, Amar AP. Hydrocephalus in children with middle fossa arachnoid cysts. J Neurosurg Pediatr. 2004;101(2):25–31.
24. Liu JK, Cole CD, Kan P, Schmidt MH. Spinal extradural arachnoid cysts: clinical, radiological, and surgical features. Neurosurg Focus. 2007;22(2):1–5.
25. Lütcherath V, Waaler PE, Jellum E, Wester K. Children with bilateral temporal arachnoid cysts may have glutaricaciduria type 1 (GAT1); operation without knowing that may be harmful. Acta Neurochir (Wien). 2000;142:1025–30.
26. Martínez-Lage JF, Casas C, Fernández MA, Puche A, Rodriguez Costa T, Poza M. Macrocephaly, dystonia, and bilateral temporal arachnoid cysts: glutaricaciduria type 1. Childs Nerv Syst. 1994;10:198–203.
27. Martinez-Lage JF, Poza M, Rodriguez CT. Bilateral temporal arachnoid cysts in neurofibromatosis. J Child Neurol. 1993;8:383–5.
28. Massimi L, Caldarelli M, Di Rocco C. Intracranial congenital arachnoid cysts. In: Di Rocco C, Pang D, Rutka J, editors. Textbook of pediatric neurosurgery. Cham: Springer; 2020. https://doi.org/10.1007/978-3-319-72168-2_39.
29. Oberbauer RW, Haase J, Pucher R. Arachnoid cysts in children: a European cooperative study. Child Nerv Syst. 1992;8:281–6.
30. Pascual-Castroviejo I, Roche MC, Martinez Bermejo A, Arcas J, García-Blázquez M. Primary intracranial arachnoidal cysts. A study of 67 childhood cases. Childs Nerv Syst. 1991;7:257–63.
31. Pierre-Kahn A, Hanlo P, Sonigo P, Parisot D, McConnell RS. The contribution of prenatal diagnosis to the understanding of malformative intracranial cysts: state of the art. Childs Nerv Syst. 2000;16:619–26.
32. Pradilla G, Jallo G. Arachnoid cysts: case series and review of the literature. Neurosurg Focus. 2007;22(2):1–4.
33. Rabb CH, McComb JG, Raffel C, Kennedy JG. Spinal arachnoid cysts in the pediatric age group: an association with neural tube defects. J Neurosurg. 1992;77(3):369–72.
34. Rabiei K, Jaraj D, Marlow T, Jensen C, Skoog I, Wikkelsø C. Prevalence and symptoms of intracranial arachnoid cysts: a population-based study. J Neurol. 2016b;263:689–94.
35. Rengachary SS, Watanabe I. Ultrastructure and pathogenesis of intracranial arachnoid cysts. J Neuropathol Exp Neurol. 1981;40:61–83.
36. Robinson RG. Congenital cysts of the brain: arachnoid malformations. Prof Neurol Surg. 1971;4:133–17.

37. Shaw CM, Alford EC Jr. Congenital arachnoid cysts and their differential diagnosis. Amsterdam: North Holland Publishing Company; 1977.
38. Talamonti G, D'Aliberti G, Picano M, Debernardi A, Collice M. Intracranial cysts containing cerebrospinal fluid-like fluid: results of endoscopic 828 L. Massimi et al. Nneurosurgery in a series of 64 consecutive cases. Neurosurgery. 2011;68:788–803.
39. Vernooij MW, Ikram MA, Tanghe HL, Vincent AJ, Hofman A, Krestin GP, Niessen WJ, Breteler MM, van der Lugt A. Incidental findings on brain MRI in the general population. N Engl J Med. 2007;357:1821–8.
40. Weber F, Knopf H. Incidental findings in magnetic resonance imaging of the brains of healthy young men. J Neurol Sci. 2006;240:81–4.
41. Wegener M, Prause JU, Thygesen J, et al. Arachnoid cyst causing an optic neuropathy in neurofibromatosis 1. Acta Ophthalmol (Copenh). 2010;88:497–9.
42. Wester K. Gender distribution and sidedness of middle fossa arachnoid cysts: a review of cases diagnosed with computed imaging. Neurosurgery. 1992;31(5):940–4.
43. Wester K. Peculiarities of intracranial arachnoid cysts: location, sidedness, and sex distribution in 126 consecutive patients. Neurosurgery. 1999;45(4):775–9.
44. Wester K, Svendsen F, Hugdahl K. Intrakranialearaknoidalecyster--lokalisasjon, kjønnogsidefordeling [Intracranial arachnoidal cysts--localization, gender and sidedness]. Tidsskr Nor Laegeforen. 1999;119(28):4162–4.
45. Westermaier T, Schweitzer T, Ernestus R-I. Arachnoid cysts. Neurodegener Dis. 2012;724:37–50.
46. Wilkinson CC, Winston KR. Congenital arachnoid cyst and Dandy-Walker complex. In: Albright AL, Pollack IF, Adelson PD, editors. Principles and practice of pediatric neurosurgery. New York: Thieme; 2008. p. 162–86.
47. Yoshioka H, Iino S, Ishimura K, et al. An arachnoid cyst in an 8-year-old boy with neurofibromatosis. Brain and Development. 1984;6:551–3.

Embryology of Arachnoid Mater

Alpaslan Gökçimen

1 Introduction

Structures in the central nervous system (CNS) are protected by meninges, bone, and cerebrospinal fluid (CSF) [4]. The CNS is covered by two sheaths (meninges), which are layers of connective tissue that differ from each other in structure and function; because the outer sheath is hard, it is called "pachymeninges (dura mater)." Since the inner sheath is soft, it is called "leptomeninges (arachnoid mater and pia mater)" [1].

2 Histology and Location of Meninges Brain Tissue

Brain tissues are covered from the outside inward by three membranes: (1) dura mater (hard mother/coarse mother), (2) arachnoid (cobweb-like), and (3) pia mater (tender mother) (Fig. 1).

Dura mater is the strongest of these meninges. This layer is also called the pachymeninx (thick membrane). Outside the brain, the dura mater is continuous with the periosteum of the skull and has no epidural space. In the spinal cord, it is separated from the periosteum of the spine by the epidural space. This space includes loose connective tissue, adipose tissue, and venous plexuses [4].

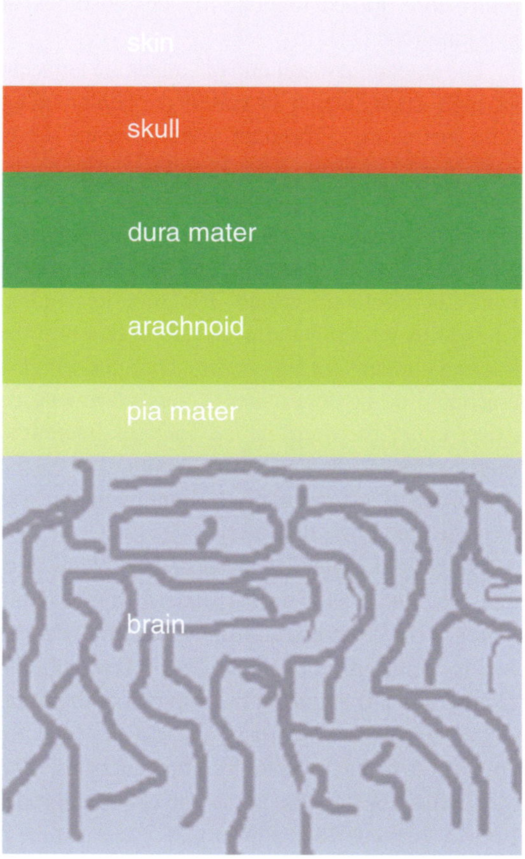

Fig. 1 Structures surrounding the brain: structures surrounding the brain tissue are seen

While covering the cranial cavity, dura mater is observed in two parts as "periosteal dura

A. Gökçimen (✉)
Department of Histology and Embryology, Aydın Adnan Menderes University School of Medicine, Aydın, Turkey

Department of Histology and Embryology, Aydın Adnan Menderes University Health Sciences, Aydın, Turkey

M. Turgut et al. (eds.), *Arachnoid Cysts*, https://doi.org/10.1007/978-3-031-22701-1_3

mater" and "meningeal dura mater." This tissue fuses with the periosteum as a single structure, while the initially extradural veins remain in the dura mater as the "sinus dura mater." The periosteal layer is composed of leaflike layers of thin type I collagen fibers, osteoprogenitor cells, and darkly stained cytoplasm with elongated protrusions, fibroblasts with ovoid nuclei, and blood vessels. The dura mater has extensions called the falx cerebri, cerebelli, and tentorium cerebelli. The inner layer of the meningeal dura mater is called the striated cell layer. This layer is usually composed of flattened fibroblasts exhibiting long protrusions joined together by desmosomes or gap junctions [1].

The arachnoid mater and pia mater are adjacent to each other, which is called the leptomeninx (thin membrane). The dura mater contains blood vessels and sinuses. The best known of these sinuses is the superior sagittal sinus. The inner surface of the sinuses are lined with endothelium, and a muscle layer is absent around the endothelium which is similar for veins. The superior sagittal sinus joins with other sinuses and drains into the internal jugular vein but does not continue with the arachnoid in the dura mater. A very narrow space exists under the dura, which contains interstitial fluid but no CSF. The cavity-facing side of the dura mater is intermittently layered by connective tissue's main cells, fibroblasts [4].

Arachnoid mater is interposed between dura and pia mater with dura mater on top and pia mater on the bottom, and the space between the two is filled with trabeculae. The cell membrane facing outward encircles the gap below the dura. In this layer, there are many fibroblasts which are connected to each other by gap junctions. The trabeculae, located just below the cell membrane, have a cobweb-like appearance (*Arachnoides*) between the upper part and the pia mater. Trabeculae consist of thin cytoplasmic extensions of fibroblasts and their supporting collagen fiber bundles [4]. Fibroblasts are linked together by desmosomes. Trabeculae are filled with CSF as well as fibroblast extensions. CSF protects the CNS structures against physical impact [4].

The arachnoid mater consists of leptomeningeal cells, loose connective tissue, specialized fibroblasts, and a small amount of type III collagen. The leptomeningeal cover of *Arachnoides* is observed as disc-shaped "cellular spots" (maculae cellulares) whose cells are partially arranged concentrically and as villus-shaped "cellular nodes" (nodule cellularis) in which the connective tissue is partially joined. Cellular spots and nodules are completely normal structures found at any age. Maculae cellulares and nodulicellulares are primitive anterior stages of Pacchionian granulations. Granulationes arachnoidales are inserted up to the bone by pushing the thinning dura like a hernia sac, where they form "foveola granularis" on the inner surface of the bone by exerting pressure. The first is a flat, leaflike membrane that contacts the dura mater. The second is a deeper, loosely arranged spider weblike region consisting of "arachnoid trabecular cells" (modified fibroblasts) that lie beneath the pia mater and form trabeculae with several associated collagen fibers. These spiderlike trabeculae bridge the "subarachnoid space" between the pia and the leaflike part of the arachnoid layer [1].

The innermost pia mater covers all the gyri and sulci of the CNS. This layer is a connective tissue consisting of leptomeningeal cells, a single layer of squamous epithelium, type III collagen, elastic fibers, fibroblasts, macrophages, mast cells, basal lamina, and capillaries [4]. Collagen fibers are located between fibroblasts. A thin basal lamina extends on the surface of the fibroblasts facing the brain tissue. In the inner part of this, there are foot processes, where the protoplasmic astrocytes' elephant feet-like appendages terminate. The pia mater is noticeable under the light microscope as a dark layer that is located at the outermost part of the brain tissue and looks like a single layer of squamous epithelium. The pia mater also partially surrounds the blood vessels entering the brain tissue [4].

In addition, there are plenty of nerve fibers in this membrane. Thin nerve bundles partly travel with blood vessels. Thin bundles of axons travel together with blood vessels and form fine networks in their walls and nearby partly separate from blood vessels. These neural propyls form a wide linked plexus that stretches over the entire pia mater and has various sensory axon terminals [1].

3 Development of the Nervous System

In the second embryonal week of development, the bilaminar embryonic disc is formed. The upper part of this disc is composed of primitive ectoderm and the lower part of primitive endoderm. From the beginning of the third week of development, the mesoderm gradually develops between the ectoderm and endoderm. This three-layered embryonic disc is called the trilaminar embryonic disc. The development of all tissues and organs consists of these three layers [6] (Fig. 2).

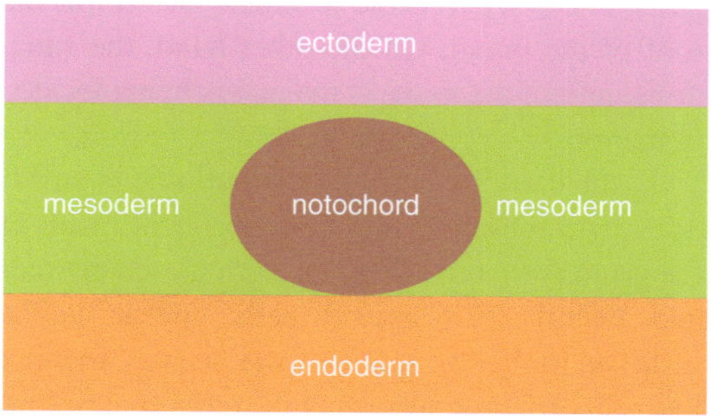

Fig. 2 At the third weekend of development, ectoderm is located above, endoderm below, and mesoderm in the middle. The notochord, which forms the skeletal structure of the embryo, is located in the middle of all structures. The notochord acts as the primary stimulus in the early embryo. The notochord degenerates as it forms the bodies of the vertebrae

Six separate structures develop from the mesoderm: meninges, lateral plate mesoderm, cardiogenic mesoderm, intermediate mesoderm, septum transversum, and paraxial mesoderm. Anterior meninges and posterior meninges develop from the meninges, while splanchnic mesoderm and mesoblastic supporting stroma form from cardiogenic mesoderm [6, 8] (Figs. 3, 4, and 5).

At the end of the third week of development and at the beginning of the fourth week, it forms neural folds by stimulating the primitive ectoderm on the notochord, which determines the axis of the embryo. During this formation, neural crest cells are formed from neuroepithelial cells. The brain develops from the 2/3 proximal part of the neural tube, and the medulla spinalis develops from the distal 1/3 part [3, 5, 6] (Fig. 6).

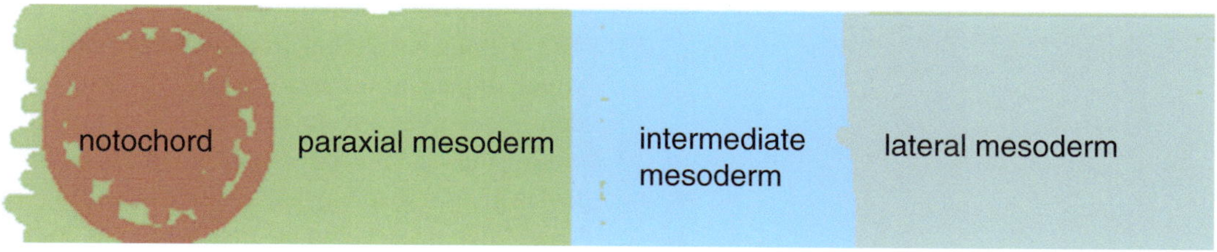

Fig. 3 The paraxial mesoderm is located next to the notochord, the lateral mesoderm is the outermost, and the intermediate mesoderm is located in the middle. Somites develop from the paraxial mesoderm. The origin of the circulatory and urinary system is the intermediate mesoderm

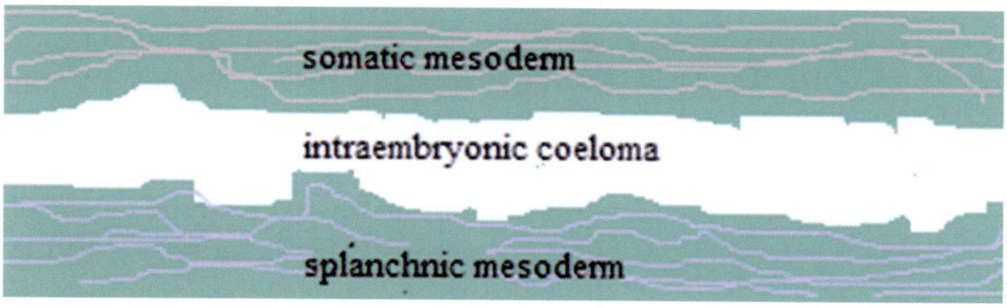

Fig. 4 Occasionally, cavities occur in the lateral mesoderm. These spaces then coalesce to form the intraembryonic coeloma. The structure above the intraembryonic coeloma is called the somatic mesoderm, and the structure below it is called the splanchnic mesoderm

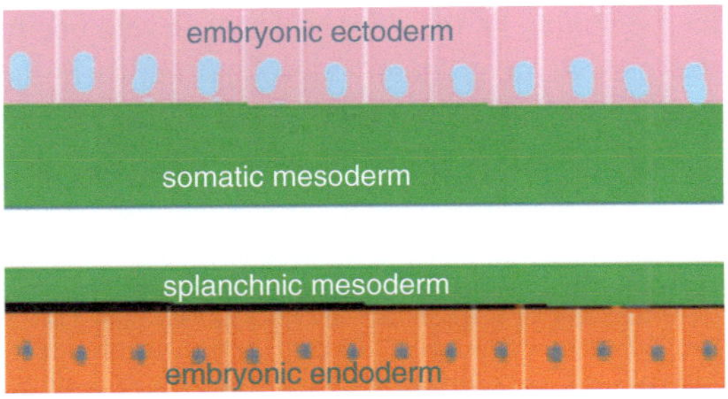

Fig. 5 Somatic mesoderm and embryonic ectoderm together form the somatopleure, and splanchnic mesoderm and embryonic endoderm together form the splanchnopleura. Somatopleure forms the embryonic body wall, and splanchnopleura forms the embryonic intestinal wall

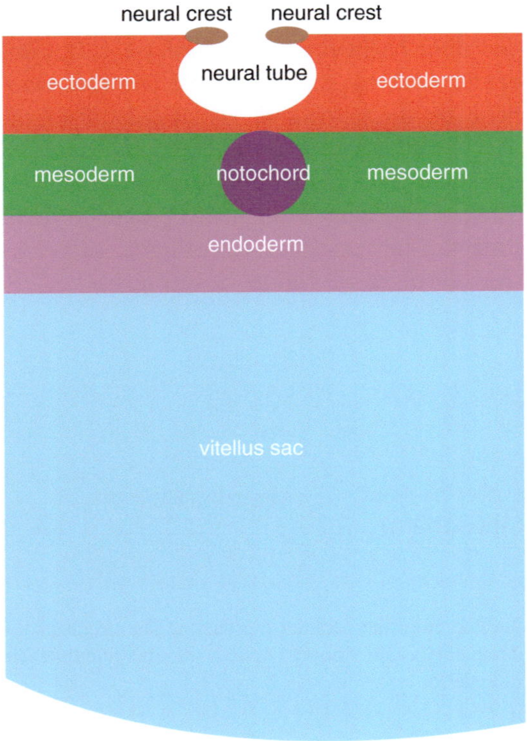

Fig. 6 As the primary stimulus, the notochord stimulates the overlying ectoderm, and the neural fold begins to form. While neural folds are formed, neural crest cells are formed as neuroepithelial cells at the ends of these folds. Sympathetic and parasympathetic ganglia, Schwann cells, melanocytes, medulla of the adrenal gland, and meninges are formed from neural crest cells. The neural folds then fuse to form the neural tube. The brain develops from the 2/3 proximal part of the neural tube, and the spinal cord develops from the distal 1/3 part

4 Emergence of the Meninges

The meninges appear during early development and consist of the pachymeninges or dura mater, and the leptomeninges, which is made up of the arachnoid mater and pia mater; all components show considerable structural and functional heterogeneity. As is known, all tissues consist of two parts. The first part is the stroma, which forms the roof of the organ. On the other hand, the functional unit of the tissue is the parenchyma located in the roof.

In the early embryo, the neural tube is enveloped by a mesenchymal layer that will result in the primary meninx (Fig. 7). Both mesenchymal- and neural crest-derived cells appear to be involved in the formation of the primary meninx that will differentiate during the embryo development and form two different layers: the pachymeninges, or dura mater, and the leptomeninges comprising the arachnoid and the pia mater. The pachymeninges is an external and thick layer of mesenchymal composition, while the leptomeninges is a double and thinner layer that contains both mesenchymal and neural crest cells [2].

Mesenchymal cells together with neural crest cells form the outline of the primary meninges. The meninges develop from two condensations which appear in the head region: the outer condensation gives rise to the skeletogenous layer, while the inner condensation (dural-limiting layer) gives rise to the pia and arachnoid (Fig. 8). These two mesenchymal condensations subsequently differentiate into two different tissue components: the internally located connective tissue (dense in the dura mater and loose in the leptomeninges) and an epithelial component, on the surface of the meninges [2] (Fig. 8).

The meninges are composed of mesenchyme that surrounds the neural tube. As the skull develops, loose tissue forms the subarachnoid space lined by meningeal cells. The meningeal cells form arachnoid between the venous plexus (pia mater) on the brain surface and the dura mater, which covers the inner surface of the skull [8] (Fig. 9).

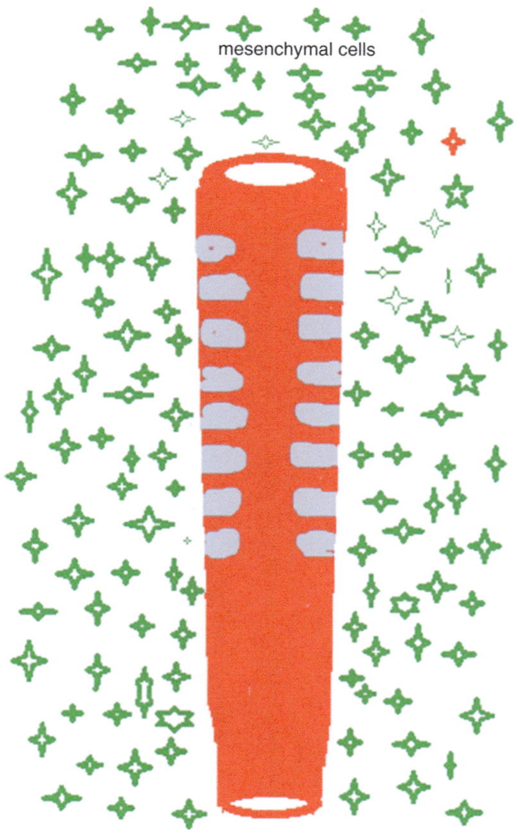

Fig. 7 At the end of the third week of embryonic development, the mesoderm is formed. Mesenchyme cells originating from the mesoderm are very active in terms of mitosis. Mesenchymal cells are widely located around the neural tube. In this way, the primary meningeal layer is formed

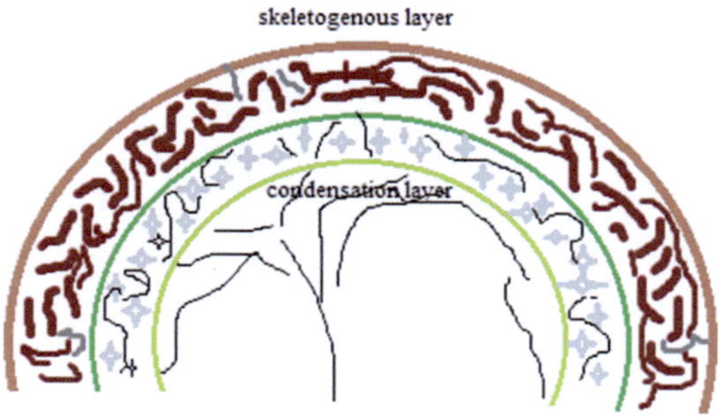

Fig. 8 As a result of the condensation of the mesenchymal tissue, a skeletogenous layer is formed. The dura mater will form from this developing layer. Mesenchymal cell condensation under the developing skeletal tissue is seen as milder. This layer is the part that will later differentiate into the arachnoid and pia mater

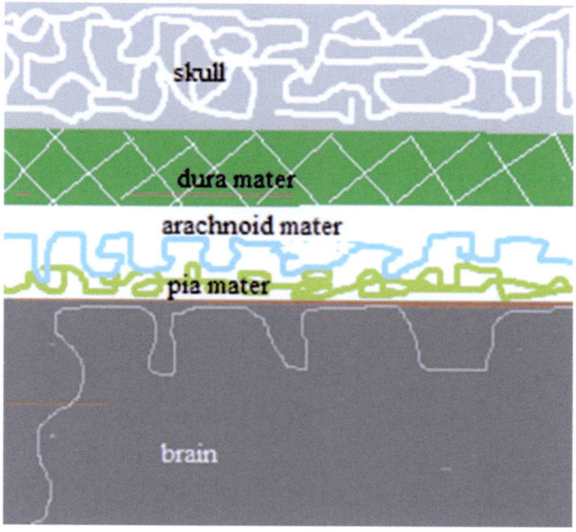

Fig. 9 Mesenchymal cells play an important role in the development of the arachnoid mater. Especially the cytokines and growth factors secreted by these cells are important

Below the dura, the meningeal cells form the outer layer of the arachnoid, a thin epithelial layer that forms the outer boundary of the fluid-filled cavity. Although embedded in the arachnoid dura without a basement membrane, it forms a functional barrier (blood-brain barrier) between the blood and the dura [7] (Fig. 9).

The arachnoid cells spread into the subarachnoid space (arachnoid space), similar to a spider web. These cells form the arachnoid inner layer, which covers the vascular connective tissue (pia mater) on the brain surface and surrounds the bridging veins that drain blood from the cerebral veins in the pia to the venous sinuses [7].

References

1. Baka M. Merkezi sinir sistemi zarları. Nörohistoloji: İzmir Güven Kitapevi; 2012. p. 54–6.
2. Drews U. Serebral venler ve meninksler. Renkli Embriyoloji Atlası: Nobel Tıp Kitabevleri; 2000. p. 354–5.
3. Dudek R. Embriyonik Dönem. Embriyoloji. İstanbul Tıp Kitabevi; 2016. p. 26–32.
4. Gökçimen A. Sinir dokusu. Genel Tıbbi Histoloji: SDÜ Basımevi; 2006. p. 152–3.

5. Joung HL. Meningiomas. London Limited: Springer-Verlag; 2009. p. 25.
6. Moore K, Persaud T. Formation of germs layers and early tissue and organ differentiation: the third week. In: The Developing Human 6th Edition; 1998. p. 63–92.
7. O'Rahilly R, Muller F. The meninges in human development. J Neuropathol Exp Neurol. 1986;45:588–608.
8. Sadler T. Üçüncü ve sekizinci haftalar arası: Embriyonik dönem. Medikal Embriyoloji Palme Yayıncılık; 2011. p. 67–90.

Histological Findings of Arachnoid Cysts

Christine E. Fuller

1 Introduction

Arachnoid cysts (ACs) represent benign fluid-filled cystic lesions that may arise at essentially any site within the central nervous system (CNS) in which arachnoid cap cells reside. Although they frequent the temporal operculum/Sylvian fissure and temporal pole, alternate locations include various posterior fossa sites (cerebellopontine angle, quadrigeminal region [2, 65], cisterna magna), sella/suprasellar regions [36], or along the optic nerves or spinal cord; few intraventricular [23] examples have been described [47, 51, 54, 67]. ACs occur throughout all age groups and may be congenital or acquired secondary to a variety of pathologies that result in inflammation/irritation or hemorrhage involving the leptomeninges.

The majority of ACs are found incidentally on neuroimaging studies, necessitating only conservative management. On both computed tomography (CT) and magnetic resonance imaging (MRI) scan techniques, ACs present a thin wall that lacks enhancement after contrast administration and fluid contents with signal density/intensity typical of cerebrospinal fluid (CSF). On occasion, sizeable and/or strategically situated ACs may become symptomatic, resulting in headaches, dizziness, seizures, weakness, cognitive dysfunction, or focal deficits [67]. Potential surgical options include cystoperitoneal shunting, surgical resection, aspiration, or fenestration. The reader is directed to the respective chapters in this book for a more detailed discussion of the clinical presentation, localization, neuroimaging features, and treatment options related to ACs.

The focus of the current chapter is to outline the spectrum of histological, immunohistochemical, and ultrastructural features of ACs. Comparisons will be drawn with other cystic lesions of the CNS to facilitate a tissue-driven differentiation of ACs from the multitude of potential clinicoradiographic mimics. A brief review of unusual presentations of histologically confirmed ACs is also provided, to include co-occurrence of ACs with a variety of other neoplastic and nonneoplastic pathologies.

2 Microscopic and Immunohistochemical Features of Arachnoid Cysts

Macroscopically, ACs present as fluid-filled cysts with generally delicate walls ranging from thin and translucent to thicker and opaquer. Though fluid contents are often clear and colorless, prior hemorrhage may result in more xanthochromic discoloration.

C. E. Fuller (✉)
Department of Pathology, Upstate Medical University, Syracuse, NY, USA
e-mail: fullerch@upstate.edu

M. Turgut et al. (eds.), *Arachnoid Cysts*, https://doi.org/10.1007/978-3-031-22701-1_4

2.1 Spectrum of Findings by Light Microscopy

The AC lining is composed of two layers. Meningothelial cells, often flattened and/or focally denuded, form the inner layer; the outer layer is collagenous and variable in thickness [9, 17, 25, 31, 33, 39, 70] (Figs. 1 and 2). More opaque-appearing cyst walls tend to be associated with thicker hyalinized collagen components. Foci of meningothelial hyperplasia may be encountered, as can be the occasional sparse inflammatory infiltrate. Ciliated or squamous epithelial cells are absent. The adjacent CNS parenchyma, if sampled, may show reactive astrocytosis.

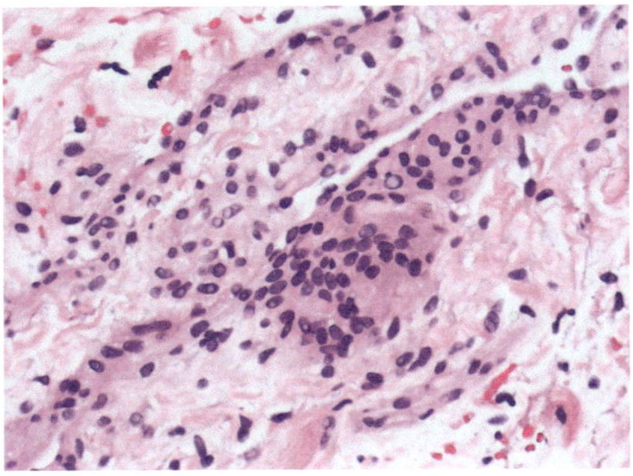

Fig. 1 Microscopic appearance of a typical AC showing bland meningothelial cells upon fibrous tissue (hematoxylin and eosin, ×200)

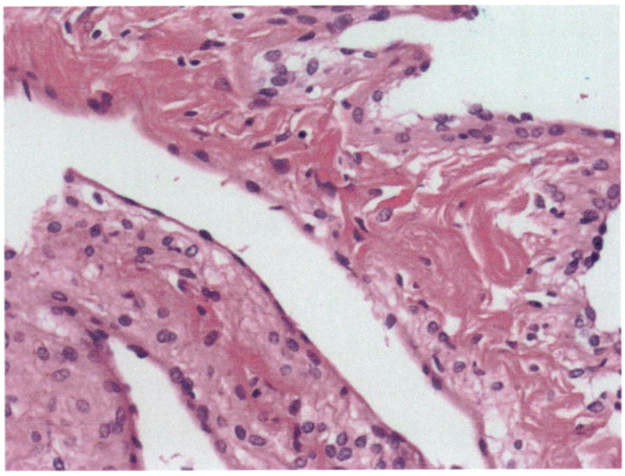

Fig. 2 Some ACs have a more attenuated lining (hematoxylin and eosin, ×200)

On occasion, other histological elements may be encountered within the walls of otherwise typical ACs. For instance, hemosiderin-containing macrophages trapped within AC walls may be seen and imply a prior site of hemorrhage [61]. Morioka et al. described finding nevus cells within a posterior intradural extramedullary thoracic spinal AC that arose in a patient with a large congenital melanocytic nevus involving the skin of his back [41]. ACs with heterotopic neuroglial tissue have been described in multiple instances, mainly in ACs arising in posterior fossa sites [5, 7]. Few ACs containing ectopic choroid plexus have been documented, all within the posterior fossa/cerebellopontine angle region, both in children [24, 55] and adults [59]. Candy et al. report a unique "dual" cyst arising from the cauda equina in a 68-year-old man; this cyst was lined by areas of pseudostratified ciliated columnar epithelium (bronchogenic cyst lining) as well as regions with "pleated fibrovascular tissue lined by monomorphic arachnoid cells" (AC lining). The AC was successfully treated by marsupialization [12].

2.2 Common Patterns of Immunohistochemical Labeling

The meningothelial lining cells of ACs will stain positive for immunohistochemical stains targeting epithelial membrane antigen (EMA) and vimentin [29, 40] (Fig. 3). Unlike a variety of other cystic lesions that may be encountered within the CNS, ACs do not express cytokeratins, glial fibrillary acidic protein (GFAP), S100 protein, transthyretin (prealbumin), or carcinoembryonic antigen (CEA) [40]. That said, immunohistochemistry could be quite helpful in discriminating an AC from other potential diagnostic mimics, as described below.

Several studies for determination of sex hormone status in the lining cells of ACs have been published. Similar to meningiomas, a substantial proportion of ACs will possess progesterone receptor positivity by immunohistochemistry [20, 32, 66]. In contradistinction, ACs have been

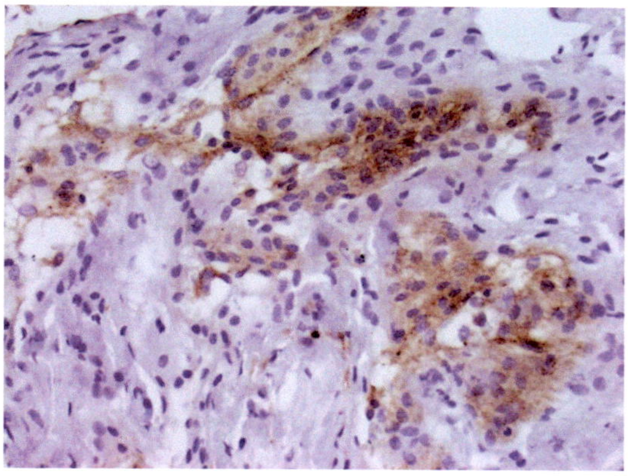

Fig. 3 Meningothelial cells of AC are immunopositive for epithelial membrane antigen (EMA) stain (anti-EMA, ×200)

found to lack both estrogen and androgen receptors (which may be detected in a minor subpopulation of meningiomas), and likewise their lining consistently expresses aromatase, a feature not typical of meningiomas [32]. The clinical relevance of these findings remains unclear.

3 Ultrastructural Features of Arachnoid Cysts

Scanning electron microscope (SEM) examinations of ACs have documented cyst linings rich in microvilli of varying densities. Scattered larger cell surface projections with a filiform or club-like morphology have been encountered [20, 22].

Ultrastructural features observed by transmission electron microscopy (TEM) are those of a single layer of lining cells (meningothelial) that are separated from the surrounding collagen-rich connective tissue by a distinct (though variably discontinuous) basement membrane [20, 22, 38, 42]. Some authors have identified ACs composed of only fibrous tissue walls devoid of a meningothelial cell lining, though in other cases the meningothelial lining was multiple cell layers thick [20, 38]. Splitting of the arachnoid membrane at the cyst margin has been observed [54]. Closer inspection of the lining cells finds surface microvilli often containing vacuoles and sometimes with elongated bulbous formations, but no true cilia [20, 22, 38]. These cells contain irregular-shaped, lobulated nuclei with nucleoli, rough and smooth endoplasmic reticulum, and numerous mitochondria. Multivesicular bodies with coated granules have been demonstrated, as have numerous small intracellular vesicles and pinocytotic pits [20–22]. Where lining cells adjoin, there are often desmosome-like junctional complexes or intercellular interdigitations with sinusoidal dilations containing complex and often tortuous processes [20–22, 38, 42]. Intracytoplasmic tonofilaments have been described, interacting with desmosome-like complexes [21, 22].

More recently, Rabiei et al. conducted a comparative ultrastructural analysis of symptomatic ACs from 24 patients [52]. The diversity of ultrastructural features that they demonstrated led the authors to separate the cysts in their cohort into three groups: (a) cysts lined with arachnoid tissue, (b) fibrous walled cysts, and (c) "cysts with aberrant structure." The first two categories correlate with findings previously described by others above, whereas the "aberrant structure" group had more unusual findings. Although they too were lined by cells with surface microvilli, some also had demonstrable cilia and/or apical secretory-type granules. Subepithelial neuropil and glial components were also seen in this group [52]. From these ultrastructural findings, the authors postulate that these varying cyst wall components provide "different barrier properties and fluid turnover characteristics" [52].

4 Pathologic Differentiation of Arachnoid Cyst from Other Cystic CNS Lesions

ACs need to be differentiated from a wide variety of other lesions that may arise within the CNS. These include neoplastic, infectious, and other nonneoplastic processes that may form (or be associated with) cysts.

4.1 CNS Infections Presenting as Cysts

Several infectious processes may present as cystic lesions within the CNS. Bacterial, fungal, or toxoplasma abscesses all may at least superficially appear "cystic." Their neuroimaging characteristics are typically quite dissimilar from those noted elsewhere for AC in that infectious abscesses contain necrosis and/or fibrinopurulent debris within their central cores and manifest with ring enhancement on post-contrast images. Histological assessment will easily discriminate these necroinflammatory lesions from AC or other CNS cysts.

In contradistinction, parasitic cysts tend to be more truly cystic in architecture, depending on their life stage and region of CNS involvement. Neurocysticercosis, resulting from CNS infection by the pork tapeworm *Taenia solium*, may manifest as intraparenchymal, intraventricular, or subarachnoid/leptomeningeal lesions. Parenchymal cystic lesions are most common and tend to be small and multiple, whereas intraventricular cysts tend to be solitary. Infectious cysts within the subarachnoid space may grow quite large, and some may take on a grapelike "racemose" appearance [60]. It is these subarachnoid and intraventricular infectious cysts that may closely mimic ACs, given that they tend to lack identifiable scolex structures (more typical of the intraparenchymal lesions) and the cyst contents have similar signal characteristic to CSF on MR images. With the eventual death of the encysted parasites, the imaging findings change as well, with surrounding edema and thickening and enhancement of the cyst wall eventually giving way to cyst collapse, retraction, and calcification [64]. Histological examination of the larva cyst wall shows three layers of nonhuman tissue: an outer cuticular, middle cellular, and inner fibrillary layer. A scolex may or may not be present [10, 15].

Neurohydatidosis, resulting from infection with the parasite *Echinococcus granulosus* (or rarely other *Echinococcus* species), is much rarer than parasitic involvement of the liver and lungs. The majority of cerebral hydatid cysts involve cerebral parenchyma supplied by the middle cerebral artery. They may be solitary or multiple. Neuroimaging studies reveal circumscribed nonenhancing intraparenchymal cysts containing fluid isointense with CSF on all MR imaging sequences [11, 49, 50]. Therefore, apart from their typically intraparenchymal location, they show significant neuroimaging overlap with AC. Histological examination of the cyst wall would confirm the diagnosis, as, similar to neurocysticercosis, hydatid cysts have multilayer walls of nonhuman tissue, often with associated brood capsules [10, 45, 63].

4.2 Neuroenteric (Enterogenous/Endodermal) Cysts

Neuroenteric cysts, as their name implies, are benign cysts lined by epithelium that may resemble that typical of the gastrointestinal or respiratory tract. They arise from congenitally displaced elements of the alimentary tract. These cysts most frequently arise in the subarachnoid space anterior to the spinal cord, though they have been encountered in intracranial sites as well, especially within the posterior fossa. Spinal dysraphism may accompany those arising at lumbosacral levels. They typically come to clinical attention due to local mass effect on adjacent structures. By neuroimaging studies, they may resemble a wide variety of CNS cystic lesions, including AC, in that the MRI signal characteristics of their contents are similar to that of CSF. They may closely resemble colloid or Rathke's cleft cysts in neuroimaging characteristics, though location typically gives a strong clue for differentiating between these entities [19]. At surgery, they are mostly small in size, thin-walled, and containing mucinous material. Similar to AC, they do have a thin fibrous wall; however, the lining is that simply of pseudostratified columnar epithelium, variably with cilia, and frequently containing goblet cells [62]. Squamous metaplasia is not uncommon and may sometimes be associated with xanthogranulomatous inflammation [68]. Occasionally, the lining epithelium is more complex and closely resemble gastrointestinal or respiratory-type epithelium; seromucinous glands, ganglia, and lymphoid elements may be present [19]. Given the presence of goblet/mucin-producing cells, the epithelium is typically positive for mucin stains, and the immunohistochemical profile includes positivity for cytokeratin, EMA, CEA, and CA19-9 [1, 19, 40]. S100 may be positive on occasion, but stains targeting GFAP, NSE, and vimentin should be negative [19, 29]. Collagen IV stain decorated basement membrane beneath the epithelial surface.

4.3 Colloid Cyst

Colloid cysts represent mucin-filled benign cysts that arise within the rostral regions of the third ventricle, often near the foramen of Monro. The vast majority occur within young to middle-age adults, presenting with complaints of headache. These cysts may cause intermittent obstruction of CSF flow, and the so-called drop attacks of transient leg paralysis and sudden death may result. Ventriculitis may develop from cyst rupture. Neuroimaging studies typically show a round discrete third ventricular lesion that is bright on T2 and FLAIR images, and does not enhance post-contrast (though there may be a thin rim of enhancement of the capsule itself). Microscopically, though they like AC have a thin fibrous wall, colloid cysts are lined by a ciliated cuboidal to columnar pseudostratified epithelium with variable numbers of interspersed goblet cells. Lining epithelium may also be flattened/attenuated or pseudostratified. Cyst contents are amorphous eosinophilic material, similar to that seen within Rathke's cleft cysts [62]. The epithelial lining cells are immunopositive for both EMA and cytokeratin, the later stain easily differentiating them from AC. The lining is also variably positive for CEA and is negative for GFAP, transthyretin, and S100 [16]. Collagen IV stain decorated subepithelial basement membrane. Periodic acid-Schiff (PAS) stain may decorate cells with mucin production in some cases. Unlike some other CNS cysts (Rathke's cleft or enterogenous cysts), colloid cysts do not develop squamous metaplasia. Long-standing cysts not infrequently incite a surrounding xanthogranulomatous inflammatory reaction.

4.4 Rathke's Cleft Cyst

Similar to neuroenteric cysts, Rathke's cleft cysts are also mucus-containing cysts, in this case arising from Rathke's cleft remnants within the sellar/suprasellar region. Though larger cysts may become symptomatic, oftentimes, these benign cysts appear as incidental findings on neuroimaging studies or at autopsy. Histologically, they are lined by pseudostratified columnar ciliated epithelium with goblet cells [39, 62] (Fig. 4). Squamous metaplasia may be present, as may a xanthogranulomatous reaction in the surrounding tissue. Cyst content itself, when submitted for histological review, is generally an amorphous pink/eosinophilic material. The lining epithelium is consistently immunopositive for both cytokeratin and EMA [16], as well as mucin stains [40]. CEA and S100 expression is more variable [16, 29]. Collagen IV stain highlights basement membrane beneath the epithelium.

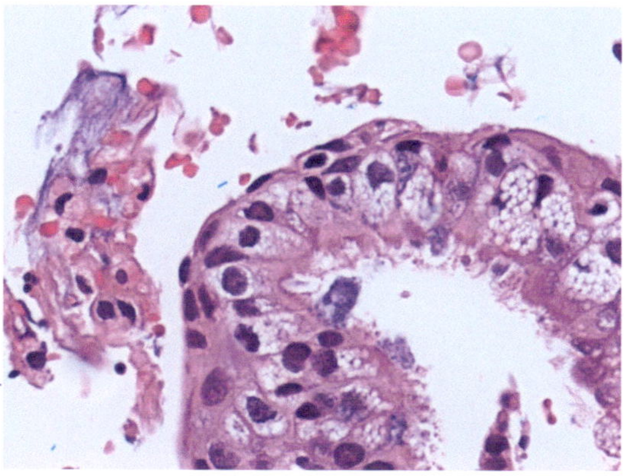

Fig. 4 Rathke's cleft cyst contains a lining of pseudostratified ciliated columnar epithelium with scattered mucin-containing goblet cells (hematoxylin and eosin, ×200)

4.5 Epidermoid and Dermoid Cysts

Epidermoid cysts may arise throughout the neuroaxis, though the cerebellopontine angle is their most favored site. The floor of the fourth ventricle, suprasellar region, and along the spinal cord are other common sites, and they may involve intradiploic calvarium. On neuroimaging studies (both CT and MRI), they may closely mimic AC in that their cyst contents of cellular debris and high cholesterol content can have similar density to CSF. They typically do not enhance after contrast administration, though they may infrequently show focal wall enhancement. Diffusion-weighted imaging (DWI) sequences may help in differentiating epidermoid from ACs, epidermoid cysts being very bright on DWI, which is not a feature of ACs. Often appearing pearly white on gross inspection, epidermoid cysts have fibrous walls lined by mature keratinizing squamous epithelium (Fig. 5). These cysts are filled with anucleated sloughed squames. Lining cells are immunopositive for both cytokeratin and EMA [62].

In contradistinction, dermoid cysts are much less common than epidermoid cysts within the CNS. Dermoid cysts most frequently affect children, and they tend to arise along midline structures, including in association with fontanelles and midline cerebellum/fourth ventricular, or along the spinal canal. Similar to epidermoid cysts, they have fibrous walls and lining of mature keratinizing squamous epithelium; however, they also contain skin adnexa, and their cyst contents contain hair and sebum in addition to anucleated squames [62]. Also, similar to epidermoids, the lining epithelium is immunopositive for cytokeratin and EMA. Cyst rupture may result in a chemical meningitis with foreign body granulomatous inflammatory reaction.

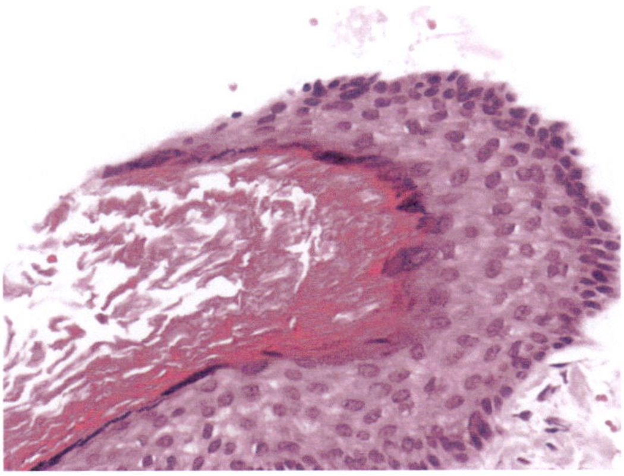

Fig. 5 Epidermoid cyst lining is that of a stratified squamous epithelium (hematoxylin and eosin, ×200)

4.6 Choroid and Ependymal Cysts

Choroid plexus cysts are one of the most common incidental findings detected at brain autopsy. They may be multiple and are generally asymptomatic. On occasion, large choroid plexus cysts might come to clinical attention due to symptoms related to intermittent hydrocephalus due to ball-valve-like mechanical obstruction. Choroid plexus cyst lining, histologically similar to normal choroid plexus epithelium, is immunopositive for cytokeratin, transthyretin, and S100 [16, 29].

Ependymal cysts are uncommon benign cystic lesions that may arise throughout the brain and spinal cord. They are often paraventricular or intraventricular in location and are frequently large with internal septations. Neuroimaging studies show their contents to have signal characteristics typical of CSF, being hypointense on T1-weighted, hyperintense on T2-weighted, and without diffusion restriction on the respective MRI sequences. At surgery, these may closely resemble ACs in gross appearance; however, histologically, they are quite dissimilar. Unlike ACs, ependymal cysts do not have fibrous walls; instead, their simple cuboidal to columnar (and often ciliated) lining epithelium rests upon a surrounding neuroglial wall [62]. Some ependymal cysts alternately have quite gliotic walls, often bearing abundant Rosenthal fibers. Ependymal cysts are immunopositive for S100 and GFAP [16], a testament to their glial lineage. Cytokeratin positivity is lacking, and there is likewise no collagen IV basement membrane staining.

4.7 CNS Neoplasms with Cystic Components

Multiple CNS tumors characteristically have prominent cystic components that might potentially mimic AC. For instance, ACs that arise within the sella/suprasellar region may mimic not only Rathke's cleft cyst as noted above but also craniopharyngioma or cystic teratoma. Both craniopharyngioma and teratoma may present as purely cystic lesions on neuroimaging studies, though they much more frequently exhibit a mixed solid and cystic or purely solid appearance. Calcification (best seen on CT imaging) may also be present, particularly in craniopharyngioma; this would be unexpected for AC [58]. Additional CNS neoplasms that often have a cystic component (which may predominate) include pilocytic astrocytoma, pleomorphic xanthoastrocytoma, ganglion cell tumors (ganglioglioma, gangliocytoma, and desmoplastic infantile ganglioglioma), and hemangioblastoma. Confirmatory histology examination easily discriminates between these lesions and is crucial in guiding patient management and follow-up.

4.8 Miscellaneous Cystic CNS Lesions

Pineal cysts are benign intrapineal cystic lesions that are detectable in approximately 2% of adults, usually encountered as incidental radiographic or autopsy findings. Rarely do they enlarge enough to result in aqueductal compression and resultant clinical symptoms. Although they are well-circumscribed and have CSF-like cyst contents on neuroimaging studies, the similarity with ACs ends there. Pineal cysts characteristically have three detectable layers on histological inspection. The outer layer is leptomeningeal, surrounding a layer of compressed pineal parenchyma, which may show calcification. The innermost layer is essentially a glial scar, often with many Rosenthal fibers and sometimes hemosiderin [39].

Cystic CNS lesions may result from surgical resection of some other process or alternately from traumatic damage, hemorrhage, or brain infarct. All of these give rise to encephalomalacia, regions of parenchymal loss. Though their contents have neuroimaging qualities akin to CSF (similar to ACs), their walls are made up only of the surrounding gliotic brain parenchyma. Similarly, porencephalic cysts result from encephaloclastic insults during early development, producing cystic lesions that communicated with the ventricle and/or subarachnoid space. These pores have smooth walls lacking gliosis, and they contain CSF; however, unlike ACs, they are intraparenchymal and not purely leptomeningeal [28].

Posterior fossa cysts include such developmental abnormalities as Blake's pouch and cysts associated with Dandy-Walker malformation (DWM). Both of these cysts may mimic AC in terms of having a smooth wall and containing CSF; however, the finding of additional anatomic clues on neuroimaging studies will help discriminate between these entities [43]. Blake's pouch and DWM will have an enlarged retrocerebellar space, containing a membranous cyst that is in continuity with the fourth ventricle, and DWM will additionally have evidence of cerebellar vermian hypoplasia or absence [3, 8]. In contradistinction, posterior fossa ACs are distinctly separated from the fourth ventricle, and their fibrous walls are lined only by meningothelial elements; ACs lack ependyma, glia, or neuronal elements that are commonly present in the walls of Blake's pouch or Dandy-Walker cyst [3, 26, 37].

4.9 Unusual Clinicoradiographic Presentations of Arachnoid Cysts for which Histological Confirmation Is Prudent

Although the vast majority of ACs are encountered in locations in which arachnoid cells typically reside (along the surfaces of the brain and spinal cord), on occasion, they may present at unexpected locations. For instance, extradural [4, 14, 27, 34] and intradiploic ACs [6, 30, 69] have been described. Fleck et al. encountered an AC confined to the internal auditory canal [18]. ACs may also rarely present as entirely intraparenchymal cystic lesions, either within the brain [48] or intramedullary spinal cord [46, 57]. In these circumstances, histological examination will be crucial in confirming the definite diagnosis, differentiating ACs from the various entities that would enter into the differential diagnosis as noted above.

ACs may also present concurrently with other unrelated lesions. For example, Rao et al. describe an intrathoracic meningocele pouch found incidentally during evaluation for a dorsal intradural extramedullary AC extending from T1 to T5 spinal levels [53]. Nishio and colleagues describe the co-occurrence of hypothalamic hamartoma with an AC in a pediatric patient [44]. Co-occurrence of intracranial aneurysm and AC has been encountered on multiple occasions. In one case series of nine patients, ACs were mostly within the middle cranial fossa and intracranial aneurysms involving the anterior circulation; these patients present with a mix of signs and symptoms related to aneurysm rupture or mass effect/seizures related to the ACs [13]. Meningioma and AC may also co-occur, sometimes as physically separate lesions [71] or alternately as meningioma arising from the wall of an AC. Of interest, such neoplastic transformations have included examples of higher-grade meningiomas [World Health Organization (WHO) grades II and III] [35, 56]. Histological assessment is clearly crucial in these circumstances for prognostication and appropriate treatment planning, as these higher-grade meningiomas are significantly more biologically aggressive than their WHO grade I counterparts.

5 Conclusion

ACs are benign cystic mass lesions that arise throughout the CNS in areas typically populated by arachnoid cap cells. They occur throughout all age groups and may be congenital or acquired secondary to a variety of pathologies that result in inflammation/irritation or hemorrhage involving leptomeninges. In this chapter, we outlined the typical histological, immunohistochemical, and ultrastructural features of ACs. Some uncommon unusual histological findings of AC were also highlighted. Comparisons were drawn with a wide variety of other cystic lesions of the CNS, highlighting pertinent features to facilitate differentiation of ACs from the multitude of potential clinicoradiographic mimics. Lastly, ACs may be encountered at unusual locations or alongside other unrelated lesions; in these circumstances, histological examination is crucial to determine the ultimate diagnosis.

References

1. Akaishi K, Hongo K, Ito M, Tanaka Y, Tada T, Kobayashi S. Endodermal cyst in the cerebellopontine angle with immunohistochemical reactivity for CA19-9. Clin Neuropathol. 2000;19(6):296–9.
2. Akutagawa K, Tamura G, Tsurubuchi T, Ishikawa E, Matsumura A, Inagaki T. Quadrigeminal arachnoid cyst with perinatal encephalocele. Childs Nerv Syst. 2020;36(7):1393–7. https://doi.org/10.1007/s00381-020-04626-2.
3. Altman NR, Naidich TP, Braffman BH. Posterior fossa malformations. AJNR Am J Neuroradiol. 1992;13(2):691–724.
4. Apel K, Sgouros S. Extradural spinal arachnoid cysts associated with spina bifida occulta. Acta Neurochir. 2006;148(2):221–6. https://doi.org/10.1007/s00701-005-0697-x.
5. Ariai S, Koerbel A, Bornemann A, Morgala M, Tatagiba M. Cerebellopontine angle arachnoid cyst harbouring ectopic neuroglia. Pediatr Neurosurg. 2005;41(4):220–3. https://doi.org/10.1159/000086566.
6. Asahi T, Endo S, Akai T, Takaba M, Takaku A. Nontraumatic convexity intradiploic arachnoid cyst. Neurol Med Chir (Tokyo). 1998;38(6):374–6. https://doi.org/10.2176/nmc.38.374.
7. Aubry K, Wassef M, Guichard JP, Herman P, Tran Ba Huy P. Association of an arachnoid cyst with heterotopic neuroglial tissue in the internal auditory canal. Ann Otolaryngol Chir Cervicofac. 2009;126(3):133–7. https://doi.org/10.1016/j.aorl.2009.03.001.
8. Barkovich AJ, Kjos BO, Norman D, Edwards MS. Revised classification of posterior fossa cysts and cystlike malformations based on the results of multiplanar MR imaging. AJR Am J Roentgenol. 1989;153(6):1289–300. https://doi.org/10.2214/ajr.153.6.1289.
9. Bhandari YS. Non-communicating supratentorial subarachnoid cysts. J Neurol Neurosurg Psychiatry. 1972;35(6):763–70. https://doi.org/10.1136/jnnp.35.6.763.

10. Bhatt AS, Mhatre R, Nadeesh BN, Mahadevan A, Yasha TC, Santosh V. Nonneoplastic cystic lesions of the central nervous system-Histomorphological Spectrum: a study of 538 cases. J Neurosci Rural Pract. 2019;10(3):494–501. https://doi.org/10.1055/s-0039-1698033.
11. Binesh F, Mehrabanian M, Navabii H. Primary brain hydatosis. BMJ Case Rep. 2011;2011:bcr0620103099. https://doi.org/10.1136/bcr.06.2010.3099.
12. Candy N, Young A, Devadass A, Dean A, McMillen J, Trivedi R. Dual lumbar bronchogenic and arachnoid cyst presenting with sciatica and left foot drop. Acta Neurochir. 2017;159(10):2029–32. https://doi.org/10.1007/s00701-017-3284-z.
13. de Oliveira JG, Giudicissi-Filho M, Rassi-Neto A, Borba LA, Rassi MS, Sanchez SL Jr, et al. Intracranial aneurysm and arachnoid cyst: a rare association between two cerebral malformations. Br J Neurosurg. 2007;21(4):406–10. https://doi.org/10.1080/02688690701466313.
14. de Oliveira RS, Amato MC, Santos MV, Simao GN, Machado HR. Extradural arachnoid cysts in children. Childs Nerv Syst. 2007;23(11):1233–8. https://doi.org/10.1007/s00381-007-0414-6.
15. Del Brutto OH. Neurocysticercosis. Semin Neurol. 2005;25(3):243–51. https://doi.org/10.1055/s-2005-917661.
16. Lach B, Scheithauer BW, Gregor A, Wick MR. Colloid cyst of the third ventricle. A comparative immunohistochemical study of neuraxis cysts and choroid plexus epithelium. J Neurosurg. 1993;78(1):101–11.
17. Dyck P, Gruskin P. Supratentorial arachnoid cysts in adults. A discussion of two cases from a pathophysiologic and surgical perspective. Arch Neurol. 1977;34(5):276–9. https://doi.org/10.1001/archneur.1977.00500170030004.
18. Fleck SK, Baldauf J, Langner S, Vogelgesang S, Siegfried Schroeder HW. Arachnoid cyst confined to the internal auditory canal-endoscope-assisted resection: case report and review of the literature. Neurosurgery. 2011;68(1):E267–70. https://doi.org/10.1227/NEU.0b013e3181ff1fb7.
19. Gauden AJ, Khurana VG, Tsui AE, Kaye AH. Intracranial neuroenteric cysts: a concise review including an illustrative patient. J Clin Neurosci. 2012;19(3):352–9. https://doi.org/10.1016/j.jocn.2011.10.005.
20. Go KG, Blankenstein MA, Vroom TM, Blaauw EH, Dijk F, Hollema H, et al. Progesterone receptors in arachnoid cysts. An immunocytochemical study in 2 cases. Acta Neurochir. 1997;139(4):349–54. https://doi.org/10.1007/BF01808832.
21. Go KG, Houthoff HJ, Blaauw EH, Havinga P, Hartsuiker J. Arachnoid cysts of the sylvian fissure. Evidence of fluid secretion. J Neurosurg. 1984;60(4):803–13. https://doi.org/10.3171/jns.1984.60.4.0803.
22. Go KG, Houthoff HJ, Blaauw EH, Stokroos I, Blaauw G. Morphology and origin of arachnoid cysts. Scanning and transmission electron microscopy of three cases. Acta Neuropathol. 1978;44(1):57–62. https://doi.org/10.1007/BF00691640.
23. Guzel A, Tatli M, Kilincer C, Yilmaz F. Posttraumatic intraventricular arachnoid cyst accompanied by pseudomeningoencephalocele in a child. J Clin Neurosci. 2007;14(12):1210–3. https://doi.org/10.1016/j.jocn.2006.04.016.
24. Hamada H, Nonaka Y, Kusaka Y, Nakazaki H, Abdullah SH, Oi S. Huge arachnoid cyst incorporating choroid plexus. Childs Nerv Syst. 2006;22(4):420–3. https://doi.org/10.1007/s00381-005-1174-9.
25. Harrison MJ. Cerebral arachnoid cysts in children. J Neurol Neurosurg Psychiatry. 1971;34(3):316–23. https://doi.org/10.1136/jnnp.34.3.316.
26. Hart MN, Malamud N, Ellis WG. The Dandy-Walker syndrome. A clinicopathological study based on 28 cases. Neurology. 1972;22(8):771–80. https://doi.org/10.1212/wnl.22.8.771.
27. Hayashi Y, Futami K, Munemoto S, Hamada Y, Soma M, Yamashita J, et al. Congenital arachnoid cyst mimicking meningocele. Pediatr Neurosurg. 2002;36(6):324–8. https://doi.org/10.1159/000063537.
28. Hirano A, Hirano M. Benign cystic lesions in the central nervous system. Light and electron microscopic observations of cyst walls. Childs Nerv Syst. 1988;4(6):325–33. https://doi.org/10.1007/BF00270605.
29. Inoue T, Matsushima T, Fukui M, Iwaki T, Takeshita I, Kuromatsu C. Immunohistochemical study of intracranial cysts. Neurosurgery. 1988;23(5):576–81. https://doi.org/10.1227/00006123-198811000-00006.
30. Iplikcioglu AC, Dinc C, Bikmaz K, Bek S, Gokduman CA, Cosar M. Non-traumatic intradiploic arachnoid cyst. Acta Neurochir. 2006;148(6):659–62; discussion 62. https://doi.org/10.1007/s00701-006-0746-0.
31. Krawchenko J, Collins GH. Pathology of an arachnoid cyst. Case report. J Neurosurg. 1979;50(2):224–8. https://doi.org/10.3171/jns.1979.50.2.0224.
32. Leaes CG, Meurer RT, Coutinho LB, Ferreira NP, Pereira-Lima JF, da Costa OM. Immunohistochemical expression of aromatase and estrogen, androgen and progesterone receptors in normal and neoplastic human meningeal cells. Neuropathology. 2010;30(1):44–9. https://doi.org/10.1111/j.1440-1789.2009.01047.x.
33. Little JR, Gomez MR, MacCarty CS. Infratentorial arachnoid cysts. J Neurosurg. 1973;39(3):380–6. https://doi.org/10.3171/jns.1973.39.3.0380.
34. Liu JK, Cole CD, Sherr GT, Kestle JR, Walker ML. Noncommunicating spinal extradural arachnoid cyst causing spinal cord compression in a child. J Neurosurg. 2005;103(3 Suppl):266–9. https://doi.org/10.3171/ped.2005.103.3.0266.
35. Lwu S, Starreveld YP, Branson J, Perry A. Anaplastic meningioma arising from a radiologically diagnosed arachnoid cyst: case report. Neurosurgery.

2010;67(1):212–3. https://doi.org/10.1227/01.NEU.0000370013.55369.92.
36. Mangussi-Gomes J, Gentil AF, Filippi RZ, Momesso RA, Handfas BW, Radvany J, et al. Sellar and suprasellar arachnoid cyst. Einstein (Sao Paulo). 2019;17(1):eAI4269. https://doi.org/10.31744/einstein_journal/2019AI4269.
37. Masuzawa T, Yamamoto H, Sato F. Ultrastructure of the wall of the Dandy-Walker cyst. A case report. Acta Neuropathol. 1984;62(3):225–9. https://doi.org/10.1007/BF00691856.
38. Miyagami M, Kasahara E, Miyazaki S, Tsubokawa T, Kagawa Y. Ultrastructural findings of arachnoid cysts and epithelial cysts. No To Shinkei. 1991;43(6):545–53.
39. Miyagami M, Tsubokawa T. Histological and ultrastructural findings of benign intracranial cysts. Noshuyo Byori. 1993;10(2):151–60.
40. Morimura T, Maeda Y, Tani E, Nishigami T. Immunohistochemical differential diagnosis of benign cysts in the central nervous system. Noshuyo Byori. 1994;11(1):7–13.
41. Morioka M, Hamada J, Ohmori Y, Kageshita T, Ushio Y. Spinal arachnoid cyst containing nevus cells in a patient with a large congenital melanocytic nevus: case report. Neurosurgery. 2004;55(4):983–4. https://doi.org/10.1227/01.neu.0000137280.84648.ce.
42. Nabeshima S, Makita Y, Motomochi M, Itagaki T, Aoyama I, Yamashita S. Electron-microscopic study of the arachnoid cyst (author's transl). No To Shinkei. 1980;32(8):803–9.
43. Nelson MD Jr, Maher K, Gilles FH. A different approach to cysts of the posterior fossa. Pediatr Radiol. 2004;34(9):720–32. https://doi.org/10.1007/s00247-004-1253-1.
44. Nishio S, Morioka T, Hamada Y, Kuromaru R, Fukui M. Hypothalamic hamartoma associated with an arachnoid cyst. J Clin Neurosci. 2001;8(1):46–8. https://doi.org/10.1054/jocn.2000.0771.
45. Nourbakhsh A, Vannemreddy P, Minagar A, Toledo EG, Palacios E, Nanda A. Hydatid disease of the central nervous system: a review of literature with an emphasis on Latin American countries. Neurol Res. 2010;32(3):245–51. https://doi.org/10.1179/016164110X12644252260673.
46. Novegno F, Umana G, Di Muro L, Fraioli B, Fraioli MF. Spinal intramedullary arachnoid cyst: case report and literature review. Spine J. 2014;14(6):e9–15. https://doi.org/10.1016/j.spinee.2013.10.051.
47. Okamura K, Watanabe M, Inoue N, Kanoh M, Ohno T, Mitsui Y, et al. Intraventricular arachnoid cyst--on the origin of intraventricular arachnoid cysts. No To Shinkei. 1996;48(11):1015–21.
48. Park KJ, Kang SH, Chae YS, Chung YG. Supratentorial arachnoid cyst located in the brain parenchyma: case report. Neurosurgery. 2011;68(1):E258–62. https://doi.org/10.1227/NEU.0b013e3181ff355c.
49. Pedrosa I, Saiz A, Arrazola J, Ferreiros J, Pedrosa CS. Hydatid disease: radiologic and pathologic features and complications. Radiographics. 2000;20(3):795–817. https://doi.org/10.1148/radiographics.20.3.g00ma06795.
50. Polat P, Kantarci M, Alper F, Suma S, Koruyucu MB, Okur A. Hydatid disease from head to toe. Radiographics. 2003;23(2):475–94; quiz 536–7. https://doi.org/10.1148/rg.232025704.
51. Pradilla G, Jallo G. Arachnoid cysts: case series and review of the literature. Neurosurg Focus. 2007;22(2):E7. https://doi.org/10.3171/foc.2007.22.2.7.
52. Rabiei K, Tisell M, Wikkelso C, Johansson BR. Diverse arachnoid cyst morphology indicates different pathophysiological origins. Fluids Barriers CNS. 2014;11(1):5. https://doi.org/10.1186/2045-8118-11-5.
53. Rao ZX, Li J, Hang SQ, You C. Congenital spinal intradural arachnoid cyst associated with intrathoracic meningocele in a child. J Zhejiang Univ Sci B. 2010;11(6):429–32. https://doi.org/10.1631/jzus.B0900375.
54. Rengachary SS, Watanabe I. Ultrastructure and pathogenesis of intracranial arachnoid cysts. J Neuropathol Exp Neurol. 1981;40(1):61–83.
55. Schuhmann MU, Tatagiba M, Hader C, Brandis A, Samii M. Ectopic choroid plexus within a juvenile arachnoid cyst of the cerebellopontine angle: cause of cyst formation or reason of cyst growth. Pediatr Neurosurg. 2000;32(2):73–6. https://doi.org/10.1159/000028902.
56. Schul DB, Meier MP, Foldvari Z, Krammer MJ, Lumenta CB. Rare case of convexity meningioma growing into arachnoid cyst. World Neurosurg. 2018;117:199–202. https://doi.org/10.1016/j.wneu.2018.06.040.
57. Sharma A, Sayal P, Badhe P, Pandey A, Diyora B, Ingale H. Spinal intramedullary arachnoid cyst. Indian J Pediatr. 2004;71(12):e65–7.
58. Shin JL, Asa SL, Woodhouse LJ, Smyth HS, Ezzat S. Cystic lesions of the pituitary: clinicopathological features distinguishing craniopharyngioma, Rathke's cleft cyst, and arachnoid cyst. J Clin Endocrinol Metab. 1999;84(11):3972–82. https://doi.org/10.1210/jcem.84.11.6114.
59. Singleton WG, Lawrence T, Green AL, Jeans A, Kerr RS. Cerebellopontine angle arachnoid cyst containing ectopic choroid plexus—case report. Acta Neurochir. 2010;152(5):881–3. https://doi.org/10.1007/s00701-009-0516-x.
60. Sinha S, Sharma BS. Neurocysticercosis: a review of current status and management. J Clin Neurosci. 2009;16(7):867–76. https://doi.org/10.1016/j.jocn.2008.10.030.
61. Spiegelmann R, Rappaport ZH, Sahar A. Spinal arachnoid cyst with unusual presentation. Case

report. J Neurosurg. 1984;60(3):613–6. https://doi.org/10.3171/jns.1984.60.3.0613.
62. Sundaram C, Paul TR, Raju BV, Ramakrishna Murthy T, Sinha AK, Prasad VS, et al. Cysts of the central nervous system : a clinicopathologic study of 145 cases. Neurol India. 2001;49(3):237–42.
63. Taratuto AL, Venturiello SM. Echinococcosis. Brain Pathol. 1997;7(1):673–9. https://doi.org/10.1111/j.1750-3639.1997.tb01082.x.
64. Teitelbaum GP, Otto RJ, Lin M, Watanabe AT, Stull MA, Manz HJ, et al. MR imaging of neurocysticercosis. AJR Am J Roentgenol. 1989;153(4):857–66. https://doi.org/10.2214/ajr.153.4.857.
65. Topsakal C, Kaplan M, Erol F, Cetin H, Ozercan I. Unusual arachnoid cyst of the quadrigeminal cistern in an adult presenting with apneic spells and normal pressure hydrocephalus--case report. Neurol Med Chir (Tokyo). 2002;42(1):44–50. https://doi.org/10.2176/nmc.42.44.
66. Verhagen A, Go KG, Visser GM, Blankenstein MA, Vaalburg W. The presence of progesterone receptors in arachnoid granulations and in the lining of arachnoid cysts: its relevance to expression of progesterone receptors in meningiomas. Br J Neurosurg. 1995;9(1):47–50.
67. Wang Y, Wang F, Yu M, Wang W. Clinical and radiological outcomes of surgical treatment for symptomatic arachnoid cysts in adults. J Clin Neurosci. 2015;22(9):1456–61. https://doi.org/10.1016/j.jocn.2015.03.016.
68. Watanabe N, Akasaki Y, Fujigasaki J, Mori R, Aizawa D, Ikeuchi S, et al. Imaging alterations due to squamous metaplasia in intracranial neurenteric cysts: a report of two cases. Neuroradiol J. 2016;29(3):187–92. https://doi.org/10.1177/1971400916638356.
69. Weinand ME, Rengachary SS, McGregor DH, Watanabe I. Intradiploic arachnoid cysts. Report of two cases. J Neurosurg. 1989;70(6):954–8. https://doi.org/10.3171/jns.1989.70.6.0954.
70. Weinman DF. Arachnoidal cysts in the sylvian fissure of the brain. J Neurosurg. 1965;22:185–7. https://doi.org/10.3171/jns.1965.22.2.0185.
71. Yanaka K, Hyodo A, Fujimori H, Yoshii Y, Nose T. Foramen magnum meningioma and arachnoid cyst coinciding in the lateral cerebellomedullary cistern--case report. Neurol Med Chir (Tokyo). 1992;32(8):581–4. https://doi.org/10.2176/nmc.32.581.

Pathophysiology of Arachnoid Cysts

George W. Koutsouras, Justin Oh, and Satish Krishnamurthy

1 Introduction

Arachnoid cysts (ACs) are collections of cerebrospinal fluid (CSF) contained or walled off by arachnoid membranes. They are either primarily developmental (congenital) or secondarily acquired cysts (Table 1) [9, 17, 34] most often seen within the middle cranial fossa but can be found in the supratentorial or infratentorial compartments and even along the spinal axis. These cysts can develop anywhere in the central nervous system (CNS) given the diffuse existence of the arachnoid meninges. Anatomically, the arachnoid layer sits beneath the dura mater throughout the CNS, and beneath the arachnoid is a layer of pia meninges. Between the arachnoid and pia meninges lies the subarachnoid space. It is within this compartment that CSF is contained. The subarachnoid cisterns lay throughout the brain, and there are larger subarachnoid spaces in which CSF is contained [40].

G. W. Koutsouras (✉) · J. Oh · S. Krishnamurthy
Department of Neurosurgery, SUNY Upstate Medical University, Syracuse, NY, USA
e-mail: koutsoug@upstate.edu; ohj@upstate.edu; krishnsa@upstate.edu

Table 1 Factors contributing to the etiology of AC

Congenital -Most common type [5, 17]
– Splitting of arachnoid membrane [48]
Genetic syndrome [24, 49]
– Autosomal dominant polycystic kidney
– Glutaric aciduria type 1
– Acrocallosal syndrome
– Aicardi syndrome
– Edwards syndrome
– Down syndrome
– Mucopolysaccharidosis
– Schizencephaly
– Neurofibromatosis
Acquired [9]
– Birth head trauma
– Head trauma [9]
– Infection
– Hemorrhage
– Chemical irritation
– Tumors

2 Clinical and Radiographical Features

Patients with ACs present in a variety of ways, often with nonspecific complaints, and most of them are discovered incidentally [1, 2, 17, 19, 44, 49]. Typically, small ACs are asymptomatic and do not typically lead to future neurologic sequelae. Larger ACs, located within the suprasellar or posterior fossa spaces, may lead to signs of intracranial hypertension and hydrocephalus [25]. They may be associated with macrocephaly,

M. Turgut et al. (eds.), *Arachnoid Cysts*, https://doi.org/10.1007/978-3-031-22701-1_5

headaches, cranial nerve palsy, seizures, and rarely unilateral hemiparesthesia or hemiparesis [37, 39]. In a recent report, symptoms seen in children were related to raised intracranial pressure, obstructive hydrocephalus, and rupture of the AC [8, 11]. Subsequent rupture could lead to subdural hematoma or hygroma and intracystic hematoma [3, 31]. Within the spine, spinal cord compression, such a gait disturbance, weakness, or numbness, and pain can be presenting symptoms [13, 29, 30, 35, 42]. Some reports describe hydrocephalus in up to 60% of patients with ACs [17, 33]. This may be in either a communicating or a noncommunicating pattern. If the hydrocephalus is obstructive, the cysts are usually located in the suprasellar region or posterior fossa [10].

In one large-scale review of adults who had undergone an MRI brain, ACs were identified in <2% of the cohort. Of this subgroup, only 5% were symptomatic, and <4% underwent surgical treatment. In this population, sellar and suprasellar cysts were more likely to be symptomatic, and middle cranial fossa ACs were the least likely. This study population was followed for a range of 1 to 6.6 years, in which <2.5% of cysts increased in size and <1% of cysts decreased in size [1]. A similar study was performed in children with brain MRIs. Of over 11,000 children, an AC was identified 2.6% (N = 309) of the time. Males were statistically more likely to have an AC than females. For an average follow-up of 3.5 years, 11 of the 111 ACs followed had grown, with younger age being associated with cyst enlargement. This younger population was more likely to need surgery. They observed that children older than 4 years of age did not have cyst enlargement, develop new symptoms, or need surgery [2]. In another analysis of children, this time in the prenatal population, they discovered 0.2% of fetuses with a prenatally identified AC on ultrasound. Of which, only <10% enlarged and over 80% were not visualized on follow-up imaging. All 81% of nonvisualized ACs on follow-up were previously located within the interhemispheric fissure. Only two children had surgery later in their infant life, and both ACs measured >3 cm in largest diameter [17] In another cohort of patients, Hall demonstrated that younger patients were more likely to be symptomatic and have hydrocephalus than older patients. Of the 485 patients with an AC, 426 were deemed symptomatic. Of the subset of the studied cohort with follow-up of a mean of 2 years with imaging (N = 148), 147 patients either had a stable cyst or reduction in their AC. In this series, 3.6% of cysts in children grew compared to 2.5% in adults [19].

3 Pathophysiological Mechanisms

ACs are separate structures from the subarachnoid cisterns and the rest of the ventricular system [4]. Splitting of the arachnoid meningeal layer may allow for the development of an AC [40]. Choi, Kim, and others postulated that this occurs because of head trauma possibly occurring during birth [9, 26]. Others suggest that this process may occur as early as at 15 weeks of gestation in which the precursor to the arachnoid splits and duplicates, leading to CSF flow into these layers [23]. If a mass structure within the cranium does not fill its nearby space, this may lead to the subsequent formation of an AC as this new compartment fills [10, 16]. Wester described in middle fossa cysts a developmental failure in the conjoining of the arachnoid membranes seen within the frontal and temporal lobe [48]. There are also infectious and post-inflammatory mechanisms that have been discussed. The formation of arachnoiditis may impair CSF flow dynamics and create a process for CSF confinement, as has been described in the spinal intradural AC population [12]. As previously described, these cysts remain stable or regress more likely than they expand [24]. Additionally, they remain asymptomatic more commonly than they yield symptoms in patients.

For when they do grow, there are three main hypotheses behind the growth of ACs: the ball valve hypothesis, fluid secretion from the cellular lining of the AC, and a gradient between intracystic and extracystic compartments (Fig. 1) [4, 33, 38].

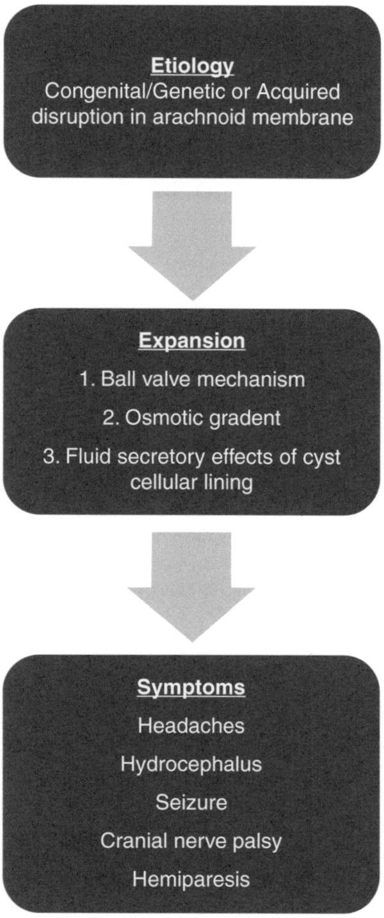

Fig. 1 Pathophysiological process of AC. A suspected disruption in the arachnoid membrane, either congenital or acquired, is the first step in the process of AC. The disruption subsequently leads to the accumulation of AC fluid. Three suspected processes, (1) ball valve mechanism, (2) osmotic gradient, or (3) secretory effects of AC lining, lead to the further development of AC. This formation of AC will lead to a constellation of symptoms

3.1 Ball Valve Mechanism

The ball valve mechanism accounts for communication between the cyst and the subarachnoid space that amounts to a one-way valve. As fluid enters, it subsequently is contained within the cavity and doesn't leave by the way it entered [7, 18, 40]. This mechanism is based on the identification of a small opening, or diaphragm, seen in the arachnoid wall. This valve mechanism is based on the flow of CSF during a cardiac cycle and the relationship to the cranial and spinal compartments [6]. As mentioned by Schroeder and by Halani, there is a preponderance of inflow during the cardiac cycle but a blockage of backflow by certain neurovascular structures [45]. Magnetic resonance and endoscopic evidence of a pressure gradient have highlighted this key mechanistic pathway of cyst expansion [44]. Rohrer characterized the ball valve mechanism in the formation of an intraspinal AC [41, 42]. There are limitations to this hypothesis. First, the evidence behind the mechanism is weak. This hypothesis is refuted in cases of cyst stability and regression. The strength of this mechanistic hypothesis was built based on suprasellar ACs. The arachnoid membrane seen above the basilar artery was responsible for the limited backflow of CSF from exiting a suprasellar cyst by that membrane. This mechanism has not been universally accepted or demonstrated, which brings upon the other hypothesis of mention.

3.2 Secretory Effect of Arachnoid Lining and Presence of Choroid Plexus in some Cysts

In a 1984 analysis, Go studied middle fossa ACs where they observed a stark similarity to normal meningeal epithelium such as those found in subdural and arachnoid granulations [14]. In 1986, the same group described sodium-potassium ATPase activity within the lining of AC epithelium that would suggest an indication of secretory action [15]. Helland analyzed the cellular lining of surgically excised ACs. They detected elevated levels of Na-K-Cl present on the AC cells, emphasizing that a secretory pathway was a key component of AC expansion [21, 22]. There are inherent limitations to this hypothesis. The major argument against this hypothesis is that cysts are most commonly stable in size and do not expand. Also, Basaldella et al. studied to determine if there were aquaporin channels within the lining of the arachnoid membrane that would enhance the fluid shifts through the arachnoid lining; however, they did not find aquaporin-1 channels were within the cystic wall [4].

On occasion in support of the presence of secretion as a source of AC expansion, there are several case reports of choroid plexus being present in the AC during surgery [20, 46].

3.3 The Osmotic Gradient Between Intracystic and Extracystic Spaces

Although similar in much of its composition to CSF, AC cavity fluid may contain greater levels of protein. Sandberg described fluid collected from 54 pediatric patients who underwent craniotomy with fenestration. They compared the composition to expected values typically seen in CSF. Protein levels were significantly different as on average 37 mg/dl were measured compared to the expected 25.6 mg/dl [43]. Some believe there is an osmotic gradient between the extracystic and the intracystic space that leads to the growth of an AC; however, this theory has been refuted by some as there are similarities in the composition to CSF [4]. There is some investigation into the cellular architecture of arachnoid membrane including granu+lation, which may shed light upon this hypothesis further [23]. In support of this hypothesis, there are case reports of fenestration of ACs that have led to the development of hydrocephalus [32, 36, 47]. There is much stronger evidence of osmotic gradients involved in the pathogenesis of hydrocephalus [27, 28].

4 Conclusion

The three pathophysiological mechanisms largely explain the variability in the processes behind AC pathogenesis. Rabiei et al. further emphasized this complexity, as the histopathological study conducted demonstrated diverse characteristics present in the AC lining. Also, etiology may play a role in the pathogenesis and natural history of ACs, as seen by the varied progressions of cysts by patient age and even seen in head trauma patients [10].

References

1. Al-Holou WN, Terman S, Kilburg C, Garton HJ, Muraszko KM, Maher CO. Prevalence and natural history of arachnoid cysts in adults. J Neurosurg. 2013;118(2):222–31.
2. Al-Holou WN, Yew AY, Boomsaad ZE, Garton HJ, Muraszko KM, Maher CO. Prevalence and natural history of arachnoid cysts in children. J Neurosurg Pediatr. 2010;5(6):578–85.
3. Balestrino A, Piatelli G, Consales A, Cama A, Rossi A, Pacetti M, et al. Spontaneous rupture of middle fossa arachnoid cysts: surgical series from a single center pediatric hospital and literature review. Childs Nerv Syst. 2020;36(11):2789–99.
4. Basaldella L, Orvieto E, Dei Tos AP, Della Barbera M, Valente M, Longatti P. Causes of arachnoid cyst development and expansion. Neurosurg Focus. 2007;22(2):E4.
5. Beresford C, Hall S, Smedley A, Mathad N, Waters R, Chakraborty A, et al. Prenatal diagnosis of arachnoid cysts: a case series and systematic review. Childs Nerv Syst. 2020;36(4):729–41.
6. Caemaert J, Abdullah J, Calliauw L, Carton D, Dhooge C, van Coster R. Endoscopic treatment of suprasellar arachnoid cysts. Acta Neurochir. 1992;119(1–4):68–73.
7. Castle-Kirszbaum MD, Uren B, King J, Wang YY, Goldschlager T. Glimpse into pathophysiology of sellar arachnoid cysts. World Neurosurg. 2018;119:381–3.
8. Chan JL, Tan ALJ, Ng LP, Low DCY, Wan Tew S, Low SYY. Paediatric arachnoid cysts: surgical outcomes from a Singapore children's hospital. J Clin Neurosci. 2021;85:122–31.
9. Choi JU, Kim DS. Pathogenesis of arachnoid cyst: congenital or traumatic? Pediatr Neurosurg. 1998;29(5):260–6.
10. Cincu R, Agrawal A, Eiras J. Intracranial arachnoid cysts: current concepts and treatment alternatives. Clin Neurol Neurosurg. 2007;109(10):837–43.
11. Eidlitz-Markus T, Zeharia A, Cohen YH, Konen O. Characteristics and management of arachnoid cyst in the pediatric headache clinic setting. Headache. 2014;54(10):1583–90.
12. Evangelou P, Meixensberger J, Bernhard M, Hirsch W, Kiess W, Merkenschlager A, et al. Operative management of idiopathic spinal intradural arachnoid cysts in children: a systematic review. Childs Nerv Syst. 2013;29(4):657–64.
13. Furtado SV, Thakar S, Murthy GK, Dadlani R, Hegde AS. Management of complex giant spinal arachnoid cysts presenting with myelopathy. J Neurosurg Spine. 2011;15(1):107–12.
14. Go KG, Houthoff HJ, Blaauw EH, Havinga P, Hartsuiker J. Arachnoid cysts of the sylvian fissure. Evidence of fluid secretion. J Neurosurg. 1984;60(4):803–13.

15. Go KG, Houthoff HJ, Hartsuiker J, Blaauw EH, Havinga P. Fluid secretion in arachnoid cysts as a clue to cerebrospinal fluid absorption at the arachnoid granulation. J Neurosurg. 1986;65(5):642–8.
16. Gosalakkal JA. Intracranial arachnoid cysts in children: a review of pathogenesis, clinical features, and management. Pediatr Neurol. 2002;26(2):93–8.
17. Grossman TB, Uribe-Cardenas R, Radwanski RE, Souweidane MM, Hoffman CE. Arachnoid cysts: using prenatal imaging and need for pediatric neurosurgical intervention to better understand their natural history and prognosis. J Matern Fetal Neonatal Med. 2022;35(24):4728–33.
18. Halani SH, Safain MG, Heilman CB. Arachnoid cyst slit valves: the mechanism for arachnoid cyst enlargement. J Neurosurg Pediatr. 2013;12(1):62–6.
19. Hall S, Smedley A, Sparrow O, Mathad N, Waters R, Chakraborty A, et al. Natural history of intracranial arachnoid cysts. World Neurosurg. 2019;126:e1315–e20.
20. Hamada H, Nonaka Y, Kusaka Y, Nakazaki H, Abdullah SH, Oi S. Huge arachnoid cyst incorporating choroid plexus. Childs Nerv Syst. 2006;22(4):420–3.
21. Helland CA, Aarhus M, Knappskog P, Olsson LK, Lund-Johansen M, Amiry-Moghaddam M, et al. Increased NKCC1 expression in arachnoid cysts supports secretory basis for cyst formation. Exp Neurol. 2010;224(2):424–8.
22. Helland CA, Wester K. Arachnoid cysts in adults: long-term follow-up of patients treated with internal shunts to the subdural compartment. Surg Neurol. 2006;66(1):56–61; discussion
23. Holman DW, Grzybowski DM, Mehta BC, Katz SE, Lubow M. Characterization of cytoskeletal and junctional proteins expressed by cells cultured from human arachnoid granulation tissue. Cerebrospinal Fluid Res. 2005;2:9.
24. Jafrani R, Raskin JS, Kaufman A, Lam S. Intracranial arachnoid cysts: pediatric neurosurgery update. Surg Neurol Int. 2019;10:15.
25. Kaliaperumal C, O'Connor B, Marks C. Development of intracranial hypertension after surgical management of intracranial arachnoid cyst: report of three cases and review of the literature. World Neurosurg. 2013;80(1–2):222. e1–4
26. Kim TG, Kim DS, Choi JU. Are arachnoid cysts localized hydrocephali? Pediatr Neurosurg. 2010;46(5):362–7.
27. Krishnamurthy S, Li J. New concepts in the pathogenesis of hydrocephalus. Transl Pediatr. 2014;3(3):185–94.
28. Krishnamurthy S, Li J, Schultz L, Jenrow KA. Increased CSF osmolarity reversibly induces hydrocephalus in the normal rat brain. Fluids Barriers CNS. 2012;9(1):13.
29. Kriss TC, Kriss VM. Symptomatic spinal intradural arachnoid cyst development after lumbar myelography. Case report and review of the literature. Spine. 1997;22(5):568–72.
30. Kumar A, Sakia R, Singh K, Sharma V. Spinal arachnoid cyst. J Clin Neurosci. 2011;18(9):1189–92.
31. Marques IB, Vieira BJ. Arachnoid cyst spontaneous rupture. Acta Medica Port. 2014;27(1):137–41.
32. Martinez-Lage JF, Perez-Espejo MA, Almagro MJ, Lopez-Guerrero AL. Hydrocephalus and arachnoid cysts. Childs Nerv Syst. 2011;27(10):1643–52.
33. Martinez-Lage JF, Ruiz-Macia D, Valenti JA, Poza M. Development of a middle fossa arachnoid cyst. A theory on its pathogenesis. Childs Nerv Syst. 1999;15(2–3):94–7.
34. Matushita H, Cardeal DD, de Andrade FG, Teixeira MJ. Temporal arachnoid cysts: are they congenital? Childs Nerv Syst. 2018;34(2):353–7.
35. Mohindra S, Gupta R, Bal A. Intra-dural spinal arachnoid cysts: a short series of 10 patients. Br J Neurosurg. 2010;24(6):679–83.
36. Ozger O, Kaplan N. Hydrocephalus following surgery of thoracic intradural arachnoid cyst: a case report. Turk Neurosurg. 2020;30(2):307–11.
37. Rabiei K, Jaraj D, Marlow T, Jensen C, Skoog I, Wikkelso C. Prevalence and symptoms of intracranial arachnoid cysts: a population-based study. J Neurol. 2016;263(4):689–94.
38. Rabiei K, Tisell M, Wikkelso C, Johansson BR. Diverse arachnoid cyst morphology indicates different pathophysiological origins. Fluids Barriers CNS. 2014;11(1):5.
39. Raveenthiran V, Reshma KB. Sixth cranial nerve palsy due to arachnoid cyst. J Pediatr Ophthalmol Strabismus. 2014;51:e58–61.
40. Rengachary SS, Watanabe I. Ultrastructure and pathogenesis of intracranial arachnoid cysts. J Neuropathol Exp Neurol. 1981;40(1):61–83.
41. Rohrer DC, Burchiel KJ, Gruber DP. Intraspinal extradural meningeal cyst demonstrating ball-valve mechanism of formation. Case report. J Neurosurg. 1993;78(1):122–5.
42. Sadek AR, Nader-Sepahi A. Spinal arachnoid cysts: presentation, management and pathophysiology. Clin Neurol Neurosurg. 2019;180:87–96.
43. Sandberg DI, McComb JG, Krieger MD. Chemical analysis of fluid obtained from intracranial arachnoid cysts in pediatric patients. J Neurosurg. 2005;103(5 Suppl):427–32.
44. Santamarta D, Aguas J, Ferrer E. The natural history of arachnoid cysts: endoscopic and cine-mode MRI evidence of a slit-valve mechanism. Minim Invasive Neurosurg. 1995;38(4):133–7.
45. Schroeder HW, Gaab MR. Endoscopic observation of a slit-valve mechanism in a suprasellar prepontine arachnoid cyst: case report. Neurosurgery. 1997;40(1):198–200.
46. Singleton WG, Lawrence T, Green AL, Jeans A, Kerr RS. Cerebellopontine angle arachnoid cyst containing

ectopic choroid plexus--case report. Acta Neurochir. 2010;152(5):881–3.
47. Sugimoto T, Uranishi R, Yamada T. Gradually progressive symptoms of Normal pressure hydrocephalus caused by an arachnoid cyst in the fourth ventricle: a case report. World Neurosurg. 2016;85(364):e19–22.
48. Wester K. Peculiarities of intracranial arachnoid cysts: location, sidedness, and sex distribution in 126 consecutive patients. Neurosurgery. 1999;45(4):775–9.
49. Youssef A, D'Antonio F, Khalil A, Papageorghiou AT, Ciardulli A, Lanzone A, et al. Outcome of fetuses with supratentorial extra-axial intracranial cysts: a systematic review. Fetal Diagn Ther. 2016;40(1):1–12.

Arachnoid Cysts: Biochemistry

George W. Koutsouras, Justin Oh, and Satish Krishnamurthy

1 Introduction

Arachnoid cysts (ACs) are relatively common mass lesions, described as 1 to 3% of all mass lesions in the central nervous system [25, 40]. They are typically managed nonsurgically with serial observation. Younger patients with evidence of hydrocephalus and elevated intracranial pressure are most likely to require surgical intervention of these cysts [25]. They have also been hypothesized to be local regions of hydrocephalus or with treatment the potential cause of hydrocephalus [19, 23, 26, 28, 37].

ACs tend to localize to regions of the normal subarachnoid cisterns but can be found within the cerebral ventricles [2, 10, 16]. They have clear relationship to the intra-arachnoid space, with similarities to normal arachnoid morphologically, but with differences compositionally to normal cerebrospinal fluid [11, 32]. Congenital, genetic syndrome and acquired etiologies have been described for ACs with the splitting of the arachnoid membrane as the starting point [4, 9]. Various studies published over the last several decades have aimed to describe the biochemical and structural composition of the AC fluid in a pursuit to uncover a pathophysiological understanding of these lesions. We will aim to describe that existent literature throughout the course of this chapter.

G. W. Koutsouras (✉) · J. Oh · S. Krishnamurthy
Department of Neurosurgery, SUNY Upstate University Hospital, Syracuse, NY, USA
e-mail: koutsoug@upstate.edu; ohj@upstate.edu; krishnsa@upstate.edu

2 Pathophysiology

Slit valve, osmotic gradients, and secretory effect of AC lining are three mechanisms of AC growth and expansion [2]. The slit valve mechanism is exemplary of a one-way valve communication between normal CSF spaces and the AC. The theory is explained by fluid being contained within the cyst, without a reliable outflow system in place [15]. This theory has been identified via radiographic and surgical visualization. However, it has been refuted by others, as many ACs do not expand over time [33, 35]. Another theory is the presence of an osmotic gradient allowing for water transport through the cyst lining. This theory has been supported by morphological studies identifying junctional spaces throughout the cyst lining that allows for water transport through them [16, 17]. Lastly, a secretory effect of the cyst lining has been studied, with expression of genes that are related to transport such as the sodium-potassium-chloride transporter. This is further highlighted in the text below as there is good evidence to support this latter mechanism.

M. Turgut et al. (eds.), *Arachnoid Cysts*, https://doi.org/10.1007/978-3-031-22701-1_6

3 Biochemistry

Several authors have detailed the morphology of these lesions using various techniques, such as electron microscopy [27, 29, 30, 39]. Albeit limited, the current knowledge of AC lining composition and fluid composition highlights the underlying origins and pathogenesis of these lesions. It has been described that the arachnoid lining does not have the expected trabecular processes of normal arachnoid and of hyperplastic arachnoid cells in the AC lining [13, 29]. This hyperplasia may be a result of pressure on the cyst wall as well as the presence of fibrous collagen seen within the AC wall [8].

3.1 Arachnoid Cyst Fluid Composition

Earlier studies by Berle analyzed the composition of AC fluid and compared this to normal expected values of cerebrospinal fluid [7]. Majority of their patient's composition was equivalent, except for the electrolyte phosphate content in the cyst fluid. They identified a significant difference in total quantity of protein and a reduction in ferritin and lactate dehydrogenase (LDH). In a study by Takahashi completed years prior to this last article mentioned, of cystic brain tumors, included at that time as AC, biochemical analyses were performed. Their aim was to analyze LDH and cyclic nucleotides, but also total protein. In their analyses, they identified less protein, less lipid content, and less cyclic nucleotide than other brain tumors and a downward trend in LDH in ACs compared to other brain tumors. In that analysis, LDH quantity correlated well with the degree of malignancy [38]. Similar to Berle, another case report of a tension temporal fossa AC identified on biochemical analysis protein level of 27 mg/dl which is similar to normal CSF quantities [3].

Understanding the chemical properties of AC fluid but in children, Sandberg sampled 54 pediatric patients and identified an increase in total protein levels compared to expected CSF [32]. Electrolyte composition was roughly similar. Regenchary also described similarities in AC fluid protein, electrolyte composition, and glucose composition to CSF [29]. Berle et al. utilized quantitative proteomics and identified a stark similarity of cyst fluid and CSF showing similar protein homogeneity [6]. In another study, further analysis, the same author further quantified a total of 348 proteins within AC fluid from pooled samples and compared this to normal cerebrospinal fluid [5]. They identified 22 proteins that were significantly higher in quantity in AC samples compared to CSF samples. Proteins included carbonic anhydrase 1 (CA-1), alpha-1 antitrypsin, hemoglobin, and fibrinogen. They did identify CA-1 and hemoglobin may be because of a contaminant in sampling [6]. Additional studies support the similarities in composition of AC fluid and CSF by the presence of choroid plexus within ACs [20, 36].

3.2 Arachnoid Cyst Lining

In 2014, Rabiei used electron microscopy to analyze AC lining in 24 patients with symptomatic ACs who had underwent fenestration surgery (Fig. 1). Half of the sampled cyst walls had similar morphology to the normal arachnoid meningeal layer. Other samples had dense fibrous components, and others had numerous microvilli and/or cilia components (Fig. 2) [27]. In earlier studies, Holman obtained AC membranes of in vitro autopsy samples [18]. They used cytochemical methods to understand the expression of cytoskeletal and junctional proteins. Arachnoid cells expressed vimentin, a key cytoskeletal protein, but also had high expression of key junctional proteins such as gap junctions, desmosomes, and tight junctions. Going back to Go's study in 1978 using electron microscopy, they proposed an active transport mechanism through arachnoid cell lining. They identified key organelles and vesicles involved in key transport mechanisms [13]. In later studies, this author demonstrated similar findings, but also microvilli on the arachnoid luminal surface on electron microscopy and sodium potassium ATPase in the

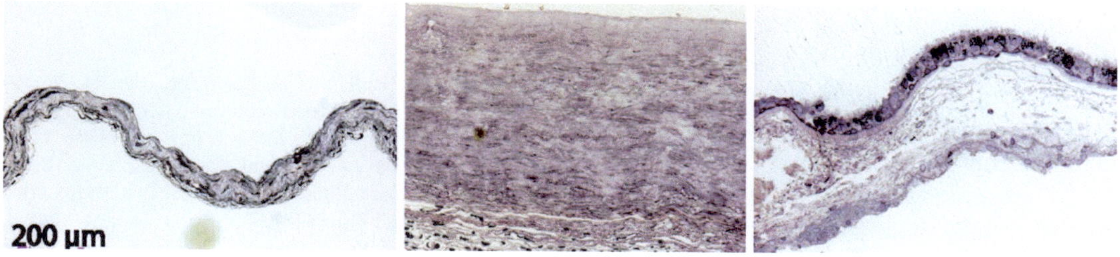

Fig. 1 Light microscopic overviews of 1-µm section of cyst walls. Left to right: arachnoid, fibrous, and aberrant types, the latter with ciliated epithelium. Cyst lumen top, dural side below, Richardson's stain, all scale bars = 200 µm. (Copyright to Rabiel et al. [27] https://www.ncbi.nlm.nih.gov/pmc/articles/PMC4078003/)

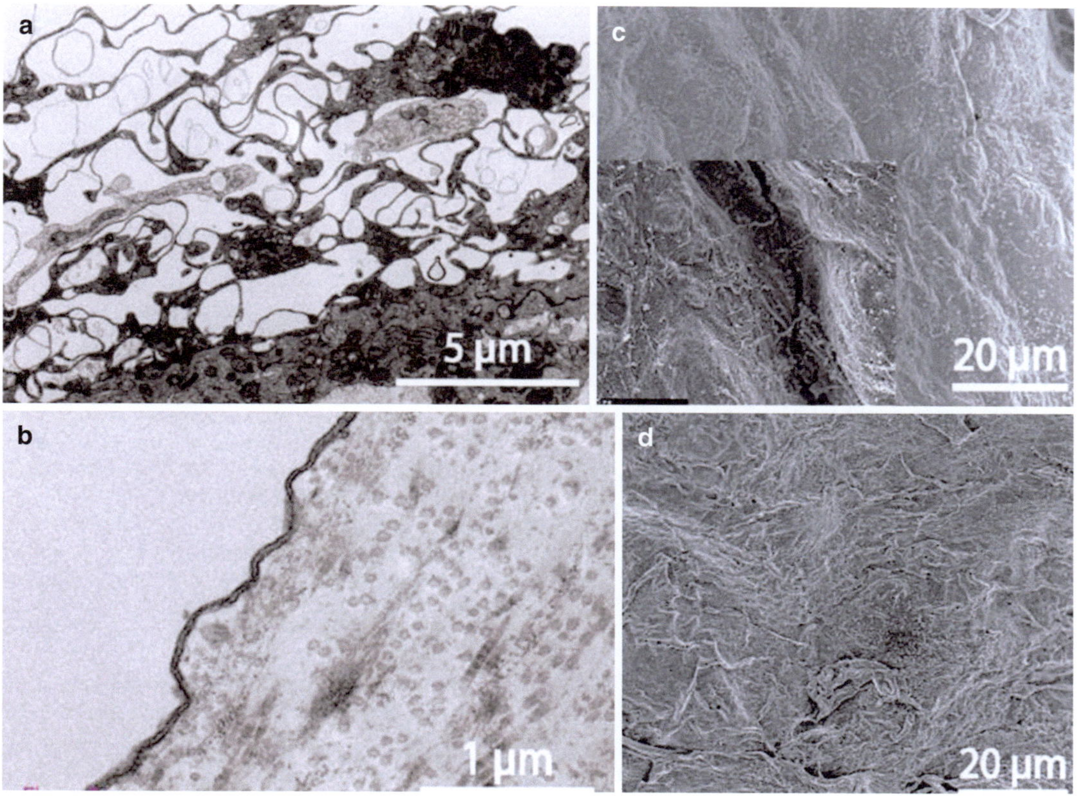

Fig. 2 EM findings on arachnoid and fibrous cysts. TEM of dural aspects of AC (**a**) and fibrous cyst (**b**); SEM of luminal surface of AC (**c**) and of fibrous cyst (**d**). A typical arachnoid organization is seen in (**a**) with highly complex cellular extensions in whorls encircling wide intercellular spaces. In (**b**), only a single extremely attenuated cell covers a matrix rich in collagen and ground substance. In (**c**) and (**d**), scattered microvilli are seen as bright spots. The luminal surface epithelium is smooth in (**c**), more irregular with some overlapping or desquamating cells in (**d**). (Copyright to Rabiel et al. [27] https://www.ncbi.nlm.nih.gov/pmc/articles/PMC4078003/)

AC plasma membranes using cytochemistry [12, 14]. These findings support the secretory role of ACs in the natural history of AC.

Motivated to understand pathogenesis, Helland et al. aimed to study the genomic expression within of AC tissue [17]. Eighteen patients with temporal ACs underwent surgical fenestration, and cyst lining was sampled with DNA/RNA extraction performed. The key finding was the upregulation of NKCC1 gene which expresses sodium-potassium-chloride cotransporter and presence of NKCC on plasma membranes of AC lining using electron microscopy. This gene is known to promote transport of water across membranes. They and others may link NKCC expression with increased prevalence of ACs in patients with autosomal polycystic kidney diseases, which is a known risk factor for AC [21, 24, 31]. For example, one large cohort of patients with ADPKD identified 8% of patients with ACs [34]. The expression of NKCC1 may support original studies by Go et al. that exemplified in the 1980s secretory effects of the cyst lining [12, 14].

Li et al. aimed to characterize the extent a marker of neuronal migration regulation has on the pathophysiology of AC, ELP4, using genomic analysis [22]. They demonstrated an association with ELP4 and development of AC in 85 patients with ACs compared to healthy controls. They concluded that not only did polymorphisms within ELP4 may influence development of an AC but also additionally it increased levels of proinflammatory markers, tumor necrosis factor-a and interleukin-1b. Other studies have aimed to identify several genomic differences within intracranial ACs and arachnoid membrane; however, further evidence is necessary to identify the relationship with the natural history of these lesions [1].

4 Conclusion

The biochemical and physical properties of ACs are key to understanding the pathophysiological mechanisms and natural history of ACs. It is clear from the review that there are differences between the AC fluid and the cerebrospinal fluid with elevated proteins and phosphates. Further studies are imperative to delineate these changes in the AC fluid and how these chemical compositions play a role in their growth and becoming symptomatic. These lesions have variable phenotypes with variable patient tolerance to their presence.

References

1. Aarhus M, Helland CA, Lund-Johansen M, Wester K, Knappskog PM. Microarray-based gene expression profiling and DNA copy number variation analysis of temporal fossa arachnoid cysts. Cerebrospinal Fluid Res. 2010;7:6. https://doi.org/10.1186/1743-8454-7-6.
2. Al-Holou WN, Terman S, Kilburg C, Garton HJ, Muraszko KM, Maher CO. Prevalence and natural history of arachnoid cysts in adults. J Neurosurg. 2013;118(2):222–31. https://doi.org/10.3171/2012.10.JNS12548.
3. Balani A, Kumar AD, Marda SS, Alwala S. Tension arachnoid cyst with transtentorial herniation: a rare entity. Neurol India. 2015;63(5):801–2. https://doi.org/10.4103/0028-3886.166544.
4. Basaldella L, Orvieto E, Dei Tos AP, Della Barbera M, Valente M, Longatti P. Causes of arachnoid cyst development and expansion. Neurosurg Focus. 2007;22(2):E4. https://doi.org/10.3171/foc.2007.22.2.4.
5. Berle M, Kroksveen AC, Garberg H, Aarhus M, Haaland OA, Wester K, et al. Quantitative proteomics comparison of arachnoid cyst fluid and cerebrospinal fluid collected perioperatively from arachnoid cyst patients. Fluids Barriers CNS. 2013;10(1):17. https://doi.org/10.1186/2045-8118-10-17.
6. Berle M, Kroksveen AC, Haaland OA, Aye TT, Opsahl JA, Oveland E, et al. Protein profiling reveals inter-individual protein homogeneity of arachnoid cyst fluid and high qualitative similarity to cerebrospinal fluid. Fluids Barriers CNS. 2011;8:19. https://doi.org/10.1186/2045-8118-8-19.
7. Berle M, Wester KG, Ulvik RJ, Kroksveen AC, Haaland OA, Amiry-Moghaddam M, et al. Arachnoid cysts do not contain cerebrospinal fluid: a comparative chemical analysis of arachnoid cyst fluid and cerebrospinal fluid in adults. Cerebrospinal Fluid Res. 2010;7:8. https://doi.org/10.1186/1743-8454-7-8.
8. Berle MWK. Chapter 7. Biochemistry—composition of and possible mechanisms for production of arachnoid cyst fluid. In: Arachnoid Cysts. Amsterdam: Elsevier; 2018.
9. Cincu R, Agrawal A, Eiras J. Intracranial arachnoid cysts: current concepts and treatment alternatives. Clin Neurol Neurosurg. 2007;109(10):837–43. https://doi.org/10.1016/j.clineuro.2007.07.013.
10. Copley P, Kirkman MA, Thompson D, James G, Aquilina K. Endoscopic surgery for intraventricular arachnoid cysts in children: clinical presentation, radiological features, management, and outcomes over a 12-year period. Childs Nerv Syst. 2018;34(2):257–66. https://doi.org/10.1007/s00381-017-3524-9.
11. Dyck P, Gruskin P. Supratentorial arachnoid cysts in adults. A discussion of two cases from a

pathophysiologic and surgical perspective. Arch Neurol. 1977;34(5):276–9. https://doi.org/10.1001/archneur.1977.00500170030004.
12. Go KG, Houthoff HJ, Blaauw EH, Havinga P, Hartsuiker J. Arachnoid cysts of the sylvian fissure. Evidence of fluid secretion. J Neurosurg. 1984;60(4):803–13. https://doi.org/10.3171/jns.1984.60.4.0803.
13. Go KG, Houthoff HJ, Blaauw EH, Stokroos I, Blaauw G. Morphology and origin of arachnoid cysts. Scanning and transmission electron microscopy of three cases. Acta Neuropathol. 1978;44(1):57–62. https://doi.org/10.1007/BF00691640.
14. Go KG, Houthoff HJ, Hartsuiker J, Blaauw EH, Havinga P. Fluid secretion in arachnoid cysts as a clue to cerebrospinal fluid absorption at the arachnoid granulation. J Neurosurg. 1986;65(5):642–8. https://doi.org/10.3171/jns.1986.65.5.0642.
15. Halani SH, Safain MG, Heilman CB. Arachnoid cyst slit valves: the mechanism for arachnoid cyst enlargement. J Neurosurg Pediatr. 2013;12(1):62–6. https://doi.org/10.3171/2013.4.PEDS12609.
16. Hall S, Smedley A, Sparrow O, Mathad N, Waters R, Chakraborty A, et al. Natural history of intracranial arachnoid cysts. World Neurosurg. 2019;126:e1315–e20. https://doi.org/10.1016/j.wneu.2019.03.087.
17. Helland CA, Aarhus M, Knappskog P, Olsson LK, Lund-Johansen M, Amiry-Moghaddam M, et al. Increased NKCC1 expression in arachnoid cysts supports secretory basis for cyst formation. Exp Neurol. 2010;224(2):424–8. https://doi.org/10.1016/j.expneurol.2010.05.002.
18. Holman DW, Grzybowski DM, Mehta BC, Katz SE, Lubow M. Characterization of cytoskeletal and junctional proteins expressed by cells cultured from human arachnoid granulation tissue. Cerebrospinal Fluid Res. 2005;2:9. https://doi.org/10.1186/1743-8454-2-9.
19. Kim TG, Kim DS, Choi JU. Are arachnoid cysts localized hydrocephali? Pediatr Neurosurg. 2010;46(5):362–7. https://doi.org/10.1159/000321597.
20. Koga H, Mukawa J, Miyagi K, Kinjo T, Okuyama K. Symptomatic intraventricular arachnoid cyst in an elderly man. Acta Neurochir. 1995;137(1–2):113–7. https://doi.org/10.1007/BF02188793.
21. Krauer F, Ahmadli U, Kollias S, Bleisch J, Wuthrich RP, Serra AL, et al. Growth of arachnoid cysts in patients with autosomal dominant polycystic kidney disease: serial imaging and clinical relevance. Clin Kidney J. 2012;5(5):405–11. https://doi.org/10.1093/ckj/sfs111.
22. Li K, Kong DS, Zhang J, Wang XS, Ye X, Zhao YL. Association between ELP4 rs986527 polymorphism and the occurrence and development of intracranial arachnoid cyst. Brain Behav. 2019;9(12):e01480. https://doi.org/10.1002/brb3.1480.
23. Martinez-Lage JF, Perez-Espejo MA, Almagro MJ, Lopez-Guerrero AL. Hydrocephalus and arachnoid cysts. Childs Nerv Syst. 2011;27(10):1643–52. https://doi.org/10.1007/s00381-011-1481-2.
24. Merta M, Rysava R. Brain disorders in autosomal dominant polycystic kidney disease. Sb Lek. 1996;97(4):479–85.
25. Mustansir F, Bashir S, Darbar A. Management of Arachnoid Cysts: a comprehensive review. Cureus. 2018;10(4):e2458. https://doi.org/10.7759/cureus.2458.
26. Ozger O, Kaplan N. Hydrocephalus following surgery of thoracic intradural arachnoid cyst: a case report. Turk Neurosurg. 2020;30(2):307–11. https://doi.org/10.5137/1019-5149.JTN.26870-19.3.
27. Rabiei K, Tisell M, Wikkelso C, Johansson BR. Diverse arachnoid cyst morphology indicates different pathophysiological origins. Fluids Barriers CNS. 2014;11(1):5. https://doi.org/10.1186/2045-8118-11-5.
28. Ramtahal J. Arachnoid cyst mimicking normal pressure hydrocephalus. A case report and review of the literature. J Neurosurg Sci. 2006;50(3):79–81; discussion
29. Rengachary SS, Watanabe I. Ultrastructure and pathogenesis of intracranial arachnoid cysts. J Neuropathol Exp Neurol. 1981;40(1):61–83.
30. Rengachary SS, Watanabe I, Brackett CE. Pathogenesis of intracranial arachnoid cysts. Surg Neurol. 1978;9(2):139–44.
31. Romao EA, Moyses Neto M, Teixeira SR, Muglia VF, Vieira-Neto OM, Dantas M. Renal and extrarenal manifestations of autosomal dominant polycystic kidney disease. Braz J Med Biol Res. 2006;39(4):533–8. https://doi.org/10.1590/s0100-879x2006000400014.
32. Sandberg DI, McComb JG, Krieger MD. Chemical analysis of fluid obtained from intracranial arachnoid cysts in pediatric patients. J Neurosurg. 2005;103(5 Suppl):427–32. https://doi.org/10.3171/ped.2005.103.5.0427.
33. Santamarta D, Aguas J, Ferrer E. The natural history of arachnoid cysts: endoscopic and cine-mode MRI evidence of a slit-valve mechanism. Minim Invasive Neurosurg. 1995;38(4):133–7. https://doi.org/10.1055/s-2008-1053473.
34. Schievink WI, Huston J 3rd, Torres VE, Marsh WR. Intracranial cysts in autosomal dominant polycystic kidney disease. J Neurosurg. 1995;83(6):1004–7. https://doi.org/10.3171/jns.1995.83.6.1004.
35. Schroeder HW, Gaab MR. Endoscopic observation of a slit-valve mechanism in a suprasellar prepontine arachnoid cyst: case report. Neurosurgery. 1997;40(1):198–200. https://doi.org/10.1097/00006123-199701000-00045.
36. Singleton WG, Lawrence T, Green AL, Jeans A, Kerr RS. Cerebellopontine angle arachnoid cyst containing

ectopic choroid plexus--case report. Acta Neurochir. 2010;152(5):881–3. https://doi.org/10.1007/s00701-009-0516-x.

37. Sugimoto T, Uranishi R, Yamada T. Gradually progressive symptoms of Normal pressure hydrocephalus caused by an arachnoid cyst in the fourth ventricle: a case report. World Neurosurg. 2016;85(364):e19–22. https://doi.org/10.1016/j.wneu.2015.08.061.
38. Takahashi H, Nakazawa S. Biochemical analysis of LDH and cyclic nucleotides in the cystic fluid of brain tumors. Nihon Ika Daigaku Zasshi. 1982;49(6):842–5. https://doi.org/10.1272/jnms1923.49.842.
39. Valluru B, Raj R. Images in clinical medicine. Arachnoid Cyst. N Engl J Med. 2015;373(11):e13. https://doi.org/10.1056/NEJMicm1413067.
40. Westermaier T, Schweitzer T, Ernestus RI. Arachnoid cysts. Adv Exp Med Biol. 2012;724:37–50. https://doi.org/10.1007/978-1-4614-0653-2_3.

Part II

Epidemiology of Arachnoid Cysts

Editor's Summary

In this "Part II: Epidemiology of Arachnoid Cysts," there are a total of seven chapters describing the epidemiology of arachnoid cysts (ACs) in depth. Beginning with the incidence of ACs, Part II will then delve into the genetics associated with the development of these neurological entities. A description of the natural history of what happens to these lesions over time will precede a discussion of where they are located within the central nervous system, including the middle cranial fossa and sylvian fissure, interhemispheric fissure, convexity surface, quadrigeminal plate, infratentorial–cerebellopontine angle or retrocerebellar spaces, suprasellar cistern, cavum velum interpositum, and spinal extradural or intradural locations. A manner of classifying the different types of ACs, congenital or acquired, is discussed in Chap. 11. Although usually considered avascular collections, occasionally intracranial hemorrhage (spontaneous subdural or intracystic) can be associated with ACs as is described in the next chapter of the text. The unusual occurrence of spontaneous disappearance of ACs as an interesting phenomenon is discussed in the last chapter of Part II which is devoted to their epidemiology.

Incidence of Arachnoid Cysts

Emrullah Cem Kesilmez and Kasım Zafer Yüksel

1 Introduction

Arachnoid cysts (ACs) are benign, nonneoplastic, and congenital cystic fluid collections that develop within the arachnoid membrane of the cerebral cortex [1, 2, 13, 18]. The contents of these cysts are mostly similar to the clear and colorless nature of the cerebrospinal fluid (CSF). ACs are congenital lesions that typically form in the meninges owing to congenital developmental disorders. In some cases, ACs also present as lesions acquired as a result of post-inflammatory accumulation of CSF in the subarachnoid space after intracranial bleeding or head trauma [6]. Most ACs may not even present with symptoms throughout patients' lives. In some patients, ACs can grow, destroy bones, and lead to parenchymal changes [5, 7, 11, 30].

However, information related to the main developmental anomaly associated with the formation of ACs is lacking. Hypotheses raised to explain how ACs form include the following: they are caused by formative defects in the primitive mesenchyme that forms the outer layer of the arachnoid membrane and the dura, or they are caused by the abnormal flowing of the CSF that forms the subarachnoid space in the early phase during embryogenesis [27]. ACs are also encountered in a wide range of varying locations. A vast majority (i.e., 66%) are detected in the middle fossa, and 17% are encountered in the posterior fossa, followed by the frontal fossa, the cerebral convexity, the suprasellar region, interhemispheric fissure, and the quadrigeminal cistern [40].

ACs may also be encountered with varying clinical presentations. The symptoms that most symptomatic pediatric ACs display are similar to the space-occupying lesions that occur during childhood. Clinical presentations such as macrocephaly, headache, hydrocephalus, intracranial hypertension, and growth retardation indicate that the ACs causing these symptoms require treatment [2, 28].

In adults, the most common symptom in patients with an AC is headache. In addition to headache, ACs might also lead to vertigo, hearing loss, ataxia, seizures, and hydrocephalus [1]. Patients with ACs might also be susceptible to intracranial bleeding after trauma [33]. Computed tomography (CT) and magnetic resonance imaging (MRI) methods can be used for imaging and visualization of the ACs. Additionally, ultrasonography (US) can help easily identify intrauterine or neonatal ACs. Noncontrast CT is usually useful enough to distinguish the AC from other cystic lesions that patients can have. CT ventriculography, CT cisternography, cystography, or ventriculography can be used to evaluate the

E. C. Kesilmez (✉) · K. Z. Yüksel
Department of Neurosurgery, Kahramanmaraş Sütçü İmam University School of Medicine, Kahramanmaraş, Turkey

M. Turgut et al. (eds.), *Arachnoid Cysts*, https://doi.org/10.1007/978-3-031-22701-1_7

connection between the cyst and the basal cisterns and the subarachnoid space [10, 14, 15].

Clinicians often tend to prefer the conservative approach to treat ACs. Owing to the fact that there are asymptomatic patients who are incidentally diagnosed with ACs when undergoing imaging procedures to investigate their central nervous system for other reasons, it is evident that the incidence rate of ACs is much higher than what is currently known. Symptoms are important in deciding the treatment that needs to be administered to manage ACs. In cases that present with the most common symptom, i.e., headache, it is very difficult to confirm that the cause of this headache is the AC, which consequently makes it difficult to decide on the treatment. Since headache is a common medical complaint that patients report, the presence of headache alone will not make it less complicated to treat such patients for symptomatic ACs. Therefore, it is exceedingly important to thoroughly examine and evaluate the patients for their neurological and psychiatric history when diagnosing and examining patients with ACs [23, 32].

Clinicians tend to opt for surgical treatment of the ACs owing to the fact that they have observed postoperative improvement in a number of symptoms such as intracranial hypertension [8, 25]. The common surgical approaches employed include microsurgical resection, cystoperitoneal shunting, and endoscopic fenestration. Studies in pediatric patients show that the outcomes of all of these three surgical techniques are quite similar to each other in terms of quality of life [3].

This section provides information in reference to the studies focusing on the incidence and prevalence of ACs.

2 Incidence of Arachnoid Cysts

The prevalence and natural course of ACs are not well defined in children and adults. Owing to the increased use of MRI and CT, there has been an increase in the number of cases of ACs that are incidentally diagnosed [20, 21, 25, 37, 38]. In addition, the presence of an AC can be detected with prenatal US imaging [12, 22]. In some studies, there are also reports of newly formed ACs that shrink or disappear [26, 29, 31, 32, 34, 36, 39]. Some authors conducted their studies to reveal the prevalence of ACs. Such studies report varying rates for children and adults. The prevalence of ACs in adults is reportedly between 0.2% and 1.7% [4, 9, 20, 21, 38]. As an example of the studies focusing on children, the study where Kim et al. studied 225 MRI images reported that 3 cases were diagnosed with ACs (1.3%) [21]. In a study by Katzman et al., a group of 1600 asymptomatic patients including pediatric and adult cases were evaluated based on their MRIs, and only 3 ACs (0.3%) were detected [20]. Furthermore, in other studies, the prevalence of ACs appeared to be higher in men [17, 19, 28, 35, 40]. Additionally, these studies have revealed that ACs are mostly encountered in the middle fossa [10, 16, 19, 24, 28, 38, 40]. In their study, Al-Holou et al. studied the MRI images of 11,738 pediatric patients and detected 309 ACs. The prevalence in the referred study was calculated as 2.6% [2]. According to the same study, with an incidence rate of 1.8%, men have a higher incidence of ACs. Additionally, ACs were found to have been localized to the middle fossa and the left side, again in the same study by Al-Holou et al. In another study wherein Al-Holou et al. studied a patient group aged ≥19 years, 48,417 MRIs were evaluated, and 696 ACs were detected. According to this study, the reported prevalence of the ACs was 1.4% [1].

In smaller-scale studies, the prevalence of ACs was reported to be between 0.3% and 1% [20, 37]. In a study wherein Weber et al. included soldiers aged ≥17, the researchers investigated 2536 MRIs and detected 43 ACs; the prevalence rate reported was 1.7% [38].

3 Conclusion

It is a well-known fact that the number of cases diagnosed with ACs increases with the increased variety of the current imaging methods. However, it should also be emphasized that each patient is particular as to the nature of the cyst detected and whether the case is symptomatic or asymptomatic and therefore should be evaluated individually while deciding on the follow-up and treatment procedures to be administered for that specific patient. Therefore, further studies with larger populations that focus on the incidence rates of ACs are needed.

References

1. Al-Holou WN, Terman S, Kilburg C, Garton HJ, Muraszko KM, Maher CO. Prevalence and natural history of arachnoid cysts in adults. J Neurosurg. 2013;118(2):222–31.
2. Al-Holou WN, Yew AY, Boomsaad ZE, Garton HJ, Muraszko KM, Maher CO. Prevalence and natural history of arachnoid cysts in children. J Neurosurg Pediatr. 2010;5(6):578–85.
3. Ali ZS, Lang SS, Bakar D, et. al. Pediatric intracranial arachnoid cysts: comparative effectiveness of surgical treatment options. Childs Nerv Syst. 2014;30:461–9.
4. Banna M. Arachnoid cysts on computed tomography. AJR Am J Roentgenol. 1976;127:979–82.
5. Bilginer B, Onal MB, Oguz KK, Akalan N. Arachnoid cyst associated with subdural hematoma: report of three cases and review of the literature. Childs Nerv Syst. 2009;25:119–24.
6. Choi JU, Kim DS. Pathogenesis of arachnoid cyst: congenital or traumatic? Pediatr Neurosurg. 1998;29:260–6.
7. Cullis PA, Gilroy J. Arachnoid cyst with rupture into the subdural space. J Neurol Neurosurg Psychiatry. 1983;46:454–6.
8. Di Rocco C, Tamburrini G, Caldarelli M, et. al. Prolonged ICP monitoring in sylvian arachnoid cysts. Surg Neurol. 2003;60:211–8.
9. Eskandary H, Sabba M, Khajehpour F, Eskandari M. Incidental findings in brain computed tomography scans of 3000 head trauma patients. Surg Neurol. 2005;63:550–3.
10. Galassi E, Tognetti F, Gaist G, et. al. CT scan and metrizamide CT cisternography in arachnoid cysts of the middle cranial fossa: classification and pathophysiological aspects. Surg Neurol. 1982;17:363–9.
11. Gelabert-Gonzalez M, Fernandez-Villa J, Cutrin-Prieto J, Garcia AA, Martinez-Rumbo R. Arachnoid cyst rupture with subdural hygroma: report of three cases and literature review. Childs Nerv Syst. 2002;18:609–13.
12. Haino K, Serikawa T, Kikuchi A, Takakuwa K, Tanaka K. Prenatal diagnosis of fetal arachnoid cyst of the quadrigeminal cistern in ultrasonography and MRI. Prenat Diagn. 2009;29:1078–80.
13. Hall S, Smedley A, Rae S, Mathad N, Waters R, Chakraborty A, Sparrow O, Tsitouras V. Clinical and radiological outcomes following surgical treatment for intra-cranial arachnoid cysts. Clin Neurol Neurosurg. 2019;177:42–6.
14. Handa J, Nakano Y, Aii H. CT cisternography with intracranial arachnoidal cysts. Surg Neurol. 1977;8:451–4.
15. Hayashi T, Anegawa S, Honda E, et. al. Clinical analysis of arachnoid cysts in the middle fossa. Neurochirurgia (Stuttg). 1979;22:201–10.
16. Helland CA, Wester K. Intracystic pressure in patients with temporal arachnoid cysts: a prospective study of preoperative complaints and postoperative outcome. J Neurol Neurosurg Psychiatry. 2007;78:620–3.
17. Hoffman HJ, Hendrick EB, Humphreys RP, Armstrong EA. Investigation and management of suprasellar arachnoid cysts. J Neurosurg. 1982;57:597–602.
18. Johnston JC, Wester K, Sartwelle TP. Neurological fallacies leading to malpractice: a case studies approach. Neurol Clin. 2016;34(3):747–73.
19. Kang JK, Lee KS, Lee IW, Jeun SS, Son BC, Jung CK, et al. Shunt-independent surgical treatment of middle cranial fossa arachnoid cysts in children. Childs Nerv Syst. 2000;16:111–6.
20. Katzman GL, Dagher AP, Patronas NJ. Incidental findings on brain magnetic resonance imaging from 1000 asymptomatic volunteers. JAMA. 1999;282:36–9.
21. Kim BS, Illes J, Kaplan RT, Reiss A, Atlas SW. Incidental findings on pediatric MR images of the brain. AJNR Am J Neuroradiol. 2002;23:1674–7.
22. Kusaka Y, Luedemann W, Oi S, Shwardfegar R, Samii M. Fetal arachnoid cyst of the quadrigeminal cistern in MRI and ultrasound. Childs Nerv Syst. 2005;21:1065–6.
23. Lee JY, Kim JW, Phi JH, et al. Enlarging arachnoid cyst: a false alarm for infants. Childs Nerv Syst. 2012;28:1203–11.
24. Levy ML, Wang M, Aryan HE, Yoo K, Meltzer H. Microsurgical keyhole approach for middle fossa arachnoid cyst fenestration. Neurosurgery. 2003;53:1138–45.
25. Maixner VJ, Besser M, Johnston IH. Pseudotumor syndrome in treated arachnoid cysts. Childs Nerv Syst. 1992;8:207–10.
26. McDonald PJ, Rutka JT. Middle cranial fossa arachnoid cysts that come and go. Report of two cases and review of the literature. Pediatr Neurosurg. 1997;26:48–52.
27. McLone DG. The subarachnoid space: a review. Childs Brain. 1980;6:113–30.
28. Oberbauer RW, Haase J, Pucher R. Arachnoid cysts in children: a European co-operative study. Childs Nerv Syst. 1992;1992(8):281–6.

29. Okumura Y, Sakaki T, Hirabayashi H. Middle cranial fossa arachnoid cyst developing in infancy. Case report. J Neurosurg. 1995;82:1075–7.
30. Rakier A, Feinsod M. Gradual resolution of an arachnoid cyst after spontaneous rupture into the subdural space. Case report. J Neurosurg. 1995;83:1085–6.
31. Rao G, Anderson RC, Feldstein NA, Brockmeyer DL. Expansion of arachnoid cysts in children: report of two cases and review of the literature. J Neurosurg. 2005;102(3 Suppl):314–7.
32. Russo N, Domenicucci M, Beccaglia MR, et al. Spontaneous reduction of intracranial arachnoid cysts: a complete review. Br J Neurosurg. 2008;2008(22):626–9.
33. Scheel M, Bauknecht HC. Teaching neuroimages: head banging without head trauma: subdural hemorrhage in association with arachnoid cysts. Neurology. 2011;76:e60.
34. Seizeur R, Forlodou P, Coustans M, Dam-Hieu P. Spontaneous resolution of arachnoid cysts: review and features of an unusual case. Acta Neurochir. 2007;149:75–8.
35. Spacca B, Kandasamy J, Mallucci CL, Genitori L. Endoscopic treatment of middle fossa arachnoid cysts: a series of 40 patients treated endoscopically in two centres. Childs Nerv Syst. 2010;26:163–72.
36. Thomas BP, Pearson MM, Wushensky CA. Active spontaneous decompression of a suprasellar-prepontine arachnoid cyst detected with routine magnetic resonance imaging. Case report. J Neurosurg Pediatr. 2009;3:70–2.
37. Vernooij MW, Ikram MA, Tanghe HL, Vincent AJ, Hofman A, Krestin GP, et al. Incidental findings on brain MRI in the general population. N Engl J Med. 2007;357:1821–8.
38. Weber F, Knopf H. Incidental findings in magnetic resonance imaging of the brains of healthy young men. J Neurol Sci. 2006;240:81–4.
39. Weber R, Voit T, Lumenta C, Lenard HG. Spontaneous regression of a temporal arachnoid cyst. Childs Nerv Syst. 1991;7:414–5.
40. Wester K. Peculiarities of intracranial arachnoid cysts: location, sidedness, and sex distribution in 126 consecutive patients. Neurosurgery. 1999;45:775–9.

Genetics of Arachnoid Cysts

Adithi Randeni, Sydney Colvin, and Satish Krishnamurthy

1 Introduction

Arachnoid cysts (ACs) are cerebrospinal fluid-filled sacs that are enclosed by the arachnoid membrane [103, 142]. ACs have a prevalence [52] of 1.2% in the general population [138]. Men are more commonly affected than women [138, 141]. ACs are found in multiple locations of the brain and spinal cord; however, most are found in the middle cranial fossa and the retrocerebellar fossa [2]. Other frequent locations are the suprasellar and quadrigeminal cisterns, the posterior fossa, and the convexity [2, 8]. Spinal intradural ACs are rare [23]. When they do occur, anterior spinal ACs of idiopathic origins are found mostly in the cervical spine, and posterior spinal ACs are found mostly in the thoracic and thoracolumbar spine [23].

ACs are primarily asymptomatic but can present with clinical findings [141]. Intracranial abnormalities associated with ACs are more common than extracranial abnormalities [8]. Intracranial abnormalities commonly associated with ACs include ventriculomegaly, corpus callosum abnormality (agenesis or absence), microcephaly, hydrocephalus, and mass effect on adjacent structures [8, 143]. With many of these associated abnormalities such as ventriculomegaly, it is unclear whether the AC caused the abnormality or if ACs are a consequence of the abnormality [143]. Further, it is possible that the abnormality is totally unrelated to the AC and that the AC and the abnormality arose because of a third external factor. Less frequently found complications of ACs include chronic subdural hematomas (CSDH) [141]. These are common in younger patients and individuals who have had recent head trauma [141]. Neurological symptoms of ACs are more commonly found in spinal ACs and usually affect motor function [21]. These can include progressive paraparesis or quadriparesis [21]. In the pediatric population, spinal ACs usually present with motor deficits [22]. Other nonspecific clinical features of all ACs include headache, seizures, vomiting, paralysis, and spasms [52].

In addition to the clinical findings attributed to ACs, there are also syndromes associated with ACs. These include glutaric aciduria type I (GA-I) [75] and Proteus syndrome [4] among others. Whether ACs are truly an integral part of these syndromes or whether they are incidental findings will be discussed.

The development of ACs is poorly understood, but there have been genes that are proposed to

A. Randeni
Leeds School of Medicine, University of Leeds, Leeds, UK

S. Colvin
Siena College, Loudon, NY, USA

S. Krishnamurthy (✉)
Department of Neurosurgery, SUNY Upstate Medical University, Syracuse, NY, USA
e-mail: krishnsa@upstate.edu

M. Turgut et al. (eds.), *Arachnoid Cysts*, https://doi.org/10.1007/978-3-031-22701-1_8

have an impact on the formation of ACs. These include the KAL1 gene on chromosome Xp22.3 [77] and CHD7 on 8q21.1 [77]. Some of these genes such as the KAL1 gene are indirectly associated with ACs due to the role they play in a syndrome (Kallmann syndrome) that is thought to be linked to ACs [77]. This chapter will introduce and discuss some of these common genes.

2 Method

Prior to the compilation of this chapter, we conducted an extensive literature review using PubMed. We looked at papers discussing the pathogenesis of ACs, the genetics of ACs, and the syndromes associated with ACs. The results were then filtered to look at the systematic reviews and the review articles. We also specifically explored the link between ACs and hydrocephalus. The reason for this is that there is more written about the pathogenesis of hydrocephalus than that of ACs and the two seem to be related via the syndromes.

3 Pathophysiology of ACs

Multiple theories have been suggested in the past regarding the congenital formation of ACs. One theory is that the arachnoid membrane either duplicates, splits, or tears and CSF is forced through this defect by arterial pulsations [8]. The manner in which these defects arise has not been specified, and it is unclear if there are other factors, e.g., thinning of the membrane, that make ACs more likely in some individuals [8].

Another hypothesis is that defects are present in the arachnoid membrane and the cyst expands due to one of two reasons. Either choroid plexus-like tissue within the cyst produces CSF, or a ball and valve mechanism allows CSF to flow into and become trapped in the cyst [143]. Hamada et al. showed that there was choroid plexus tissue present in a 7-month-old patient whose cyst re-enlarged after resection [46]. Singleton et al. also found ectopic choroid plexus tissue in a 26-year-old patient who had an AC in her cerebellopontine angle [122]. Both of these case reports, however, concede that the presence of choroid plexus tissue within the AC is a rare finding. So, in these cases, the ACs may still be incidental findings [46, 122].

The causes of spinal intradural ACs can be idiopathic, traumatic, posthemorrhagic, or post-inflammatory [23]. However, the spinal intradural ACs may form in the same manner as other ACs (ball-valve mechanism, etc.) but remain asymptomatic. They only become symptomatic and detectable when there is trauma or inflammation and thus leads to the impression that the cyst arose because of trauma or inflammation [23].

Kouyialis et al.'s theory supports the posttraumatic and post-inflammatory causes of AC formation [65]. Leptomeningeal inflammation can cause adhesive arachnoiditis with impaired CSF dynamics and loculation that can cause the cysts to form [65]. Then a ball-valve mechanism can cause the AC to increase in size until it becomes symptomatic [65].

Dr. Evangelou, a Neurology Professor at the University of Nottingham [1], and his team's findings support the Kuhlendahl theory for the formation of ACs [23]. Kuhlendahl proposed that a vent-like CSF flow obstruction caused by arachnoid trabeculae in the spinal canal can be asymptomatic for long periods of time. A pathological process, e.g., inflammation or trauma, can increase the flow of CSF into the previously existing cyst leading to a pressure gradient development [23]. The gradient would allow CSF to flow into the cyst freely but not out and hence result in enlargement of the cyst [23, 44]. Although obstruction is discussed, it is still unclear exactly how to understand the mechanisms that draw water into the cyst in light of Dr. Grzybowski's findings [37].

Grzybowski did work on in vitro models and showed that the entire arachnoid membrane absorbs CSF. This would provide a much larger surface area for CSF absorption [37]. Further, Dr. Grzybowski found that the membrane absorbs more CSF than the granulations [61]. It was argued that the in vitro models would not be accurate as cell adhesion would not be present, but Dr. Grzybowski demonstrated that the tight junctions are preserved in the in vitro models [50].

There is insufficient evidence to prove or disprove these hypotheses. Furthermore, these theories explain how ACs expand, but do not explore how the defect in the arachnoid membrane formed. To explore this, we need to look at the syndromes and genes associated with ACs.

One hypothesis for the formation of ACs is given by Demir et al. [19]. They propose that the perimedullary mesh (endomeninx), which is a precursor to the pia and arachnoid mater, splits and duplicates anomalously during week 15 of gestation which is when CSF escapes into the layers of the mesh following rupture of the rhombic roof [19].

4 Syndromes Associated with ACs

4.1 Glutaric Aciduria Type 1 (GA-1)

This is an autosomal recessive inborn error of metabolism [75]. A deficiency in glutaryl-CoA dehydrogenase enzyme results in motor symptoms such as dystonia and psychomotor delay due to an inability to catabolize lysine, hydroxylysine, and tryptophan [75]. Macrocephaly, dystonia, and the presence of bilateral temporal ACs are considered diagnostic of GA-1 [72, 75, 115]. However, there is no clear indication of whether the ACs are directly linked to the syndrome as treating the cysts did not relieve the symptoms [75]. The severity of the symptoms has been found to be directly linked to the degree of enlargement of the fissures in the bilateral frontotemporal region around the Sylvian fissures [3, 57, 72]. There can be variation in the presentation of clinical symptoms both between and within families [26].

In a regional neurosurgical department, a total of 147 patients with ACs were found in a population of 890,000 [10, 15, 131, 134]. Of these, only two patients presented with GA-1. So, there was a 1.3% prevalence of ACs and GA-1 in the population.

There is a lot of cerebral damage associated with GA-1, and one explanation for this is that there is a direct effect of glutaric acid (or another related metabolite) on the neurons [75]. Another explanation is that the symptoms are caused by the deposition of L-carnitine in the cerebral tissue [75]. Either way, the loss of neurons, especially in the caudate and the putamen, results in reduced levels of GABA in the brain and CSF [57, 75].

Hald et al. posed an explanation as to how ACs might arise in patients with GA-1. The rapid frontotemporal atrophy would lead to changes in CSF dynamics and cause fluid accumulation [45]. If these changes took place during the folding of the neural tube, then it can result in anomalous splitting of the arachnoid layers resulting in true ACs [45]. Alabedeen et al. found that in GA-1 the location of the ACs aligns with the areas of the brain that are predisposed to atrophy (i.e., the frontotemporal region) [57]. This paper argued that the arachnoid membrane might split due to loss of brain tissue in the surrounding areas and not due to the enzyme imbalances brought about by GA-1 [57]. Other papers in the literature support this hypothesis [3, 72]. An alternative theory is that the atrophy and chronic subdural effusion might be caused by the 3-OHGA affecting endothelial structures in the brain during development and resulting in vascular dysfunction [26].

While the paper by Martinez-Lage et al. [45] discusses how ACs are a part of the GA-1 syndrome, Serarslan et al. and other papers explore how bitemporal ACs and macrocephaly can occur in the absence of GA-1 [57, 118]. GA-1 is diagnosed by the detection of a high concentration of glutaric acid in the urine and a low plasma creatinine level [118]. There were patients present with bilateral ACs and no diagnosis of GA-1 [72, 118]. Thus, ACs can occur for many reasons, but they are commonly associated with GA-1. If they are found either on scans, especially alongside macrocephaly and dystonia, doctors should consider GA-1 as a differential diagnosis [45, 72, 118]. This is extremely important because even simple surgical procedures can be dangerous in children with GA-1 [72]. Surgery would induce a catabolic state in the patient and result in worsening of the metabolic disease.

4.2 Aicardi Syndrome

The syndrome is an X-linked dominant condition characterized by infantile spasms, chorioretinal lacunae, and agenesis of the corpus callosum (either complete or partial) [16, 42, 144, 149]. Here, it is worth noting that ACs are also strongly associated with agenesis of the corpus callosum [8, 143], so it is possible that AC formation is linked to Aicardi syndrome. However, due to the rarity of the syndrome itself, it is hard to conclude this.

Aicardi syndrome has an estimated incidence of 1:105,000 live births in the United States as of 2009 [149], and the prevalence is thought to be higher than reported with an estimated survival rate of 62% at 27 years of age [149].

Yuksel et al. present the case of a female infant with Aicardi syndrome and an AC [144]. They state that these are rare additional findings of the syndrome [144] and there has been a total of nine other examples of Aicardi syndrome with ACs in the literature. Barkovich et al.'s case series describes five patients who all presented with Aicardi syndrome, but not a single one had an AC [6]. Lee et al.'s findings were also similar to those of Barkovich [68]. Thus, ACs are not always associated with Aicardi syndrome and may be a coincidental finding.

Interestingly, Mohammad et al. found a midline AC in a male patient with the 47,XXY karyotype and state that cysts in the interhemispheric fissure are a common (but less emphasized) feature of Aicardi syndrome [149]. Another paper had similar findings [16]. So, while cysts of any nature are common, it is uncommon to find ACs specifically in patients with Aicardi syndrome. This conclusion is, however, unverified as there is limited histological information about the cysts [149].

Aicardi himself re-evaluated the syndrome and stated that corpus callosum agenesis is not the sole hallmark of the disease and is not needed to diagnose the condition if other abnormalities such as cysts were present [55]. Further, the presence of intracranial cysts may indicate some other abnormalities and warrant further investigation (e.g., a fetal MRI) [16]. The findings are important to neurosurgeons consulting parents whose fetus has been diagnosed with a cyst due to the impact it would have on prognosis [16].

4.3 Sturge-Weber Syndrome

Sturge-Weber syndrome is a neurocutaneous syndrome characterized by a facial port-wine stain and hemiparesis among other symptoms [24]. Epilepsy is an essential feature for the diagnosis of this syndrome which encompasses vascular malformations of the brain, skin, and eyes [24]. Of note, GA-1, Proteus, and PHACE syndrome, which are well associated with ACs, are also accompanied by vascular dysfunction. Hence, it may be vascular dysfunction that is causing the formation of ACs.

We identified one paper that described Sturge-Weber syndrome with an AC in a 2-year-old boy [24]. Therefore, it could be that ACs are associated with the syndrome, but it is hard to tell because the syndrome itself is so rare.

4.4 Trigeminal Neuralgia

Trigeminal neuralgia usually presents with paroxysmal lancinating pain in the distributions of the trigeminal nerve and its branches [136]. It can be idiopathic, or it can be caused by compression of the nerve [136]. In the idiopathic cases, demyelination of the trigeminal nerve root has been shown, and the ignition hypothesis proposes that light touch can be interpreted as pain by the nerve due to demyelination between nerve fibers that carry pain and those that carry light touch [136]. Vascular compression is recognized as the most common cause of trigeminal neuralgia, but there have been multiple cases of ACs in various parts of the brain also causing the syndrome [5, 27].

Several papers have reported trigeminal neuralgia being caused by an AC compressing the nerve [97, 136]. Kouyialis et al. report a 55-year-old female patient who experienced pain recurrence after vascular decompression for trigeminal neuralgia [65]. They proposed that direct compression of the nerve or arterial pulsation through a cyst may have caused the pain [65]. Excision of the AC relieved the patient's symptoms, and so it was felt that the cyst was the cause of the recurrence [65]. Other papers have also reported cases in which the pain has been relieved either following the surgical excision of ACs [39, 47, 107, 126, 135, 145] or following medical therapy [38, 40]. Medical relief was most commonly employed when the AC was in Meckel's cave and eroding the greater wing of the sphenoid bone [38, 40].

One paper presented a case where the patient had trigeminal neuralgia and an AC in Meckel's cave. However, her symptoms improved despite the cyst remaining unchanged in size and location [9]. Thus, it is not only the location of the AC, but its size that impacts its ability to compress the nerve and cause trigeminal neuralgia.

There is a very strong association between ACs and trigeminal neuralgia. However, the AC was not a symptom of the syndrome but a cause.

5 Other Syndromes Associated with ACs

There are syndromes linked to ACs by one or two cases. These are listed in Table 1.

Table 1 Other syndromes associated with arachnoid cysts

Name of syndrome
Kallmann Syndrome [41, 42]
Oculo-ectodermal syndrome [43]
Empty Sella Syndrome [44, 45]
PHACE Syndrome[28]
Brown-Sequard syndrome [46–50]
Proteus Syndrome [25]
Chudley McCullough syndrome [51, 52]
Neurocutaneous melanosis [53]
Dandy-Walker Syndrome [54, 55]
Bobble-Head syndrome [56–59]
Usher Syndrome [29]
Encephalocraniocutaneous syndrome [60]
Kernohan-Woltman Notch Phenomenon [61]
Organoid Nervous syndrome [62]
Kosaki Overgrowth syndrome [62]
Septo-optic Dysplasia [63]
Sjogren syndrome [64]
Precocious puberty [65]
Kabuki Syndrome [30, 31]
Epidermal Naevus syndrome [66]
Oro-Facio-Digital syndrome Type 1[67]
Other syndromes [68–86]

We did not explore these further as we feel that they were incidental findings.

6 Genetics of ACs

There have been multiple genes that have been thought to be associated with ACs. Many papers in the literature discuss autosomal dominant polycystic kidney disease (ADPKD) and ACs. In ADPKD, cysts are found in the kidneys, pancreas, seminal vesicles, and arachnoid membrane [48]. Arachnoid membrane cysts are present in 8% of affected individuals and are mostly asymptomatic [48]. This is a large proportion given the incidence of ACs in the general population is 1.2% [138]. Table 2 lists some of the main genes involved in ADPKD.

It is unclear how the proteins are involved in the genesis or sustenance of the AC or how these defects in protein synthesis relate to CSF flow. In the case of PKD1 and PKD2, it is thought that the disruption to the protein's signaling function within the cell and in primary cilia leads to cells growing and dividing abnormally, causing cysts to develop [91, 92].

Kallmann syndrome is also linked to ACs. It is hypothesized that the syndrome is caused by a defect in the migration of GnRH-1 neurons due to abnormal development of olfactory nerves and bulbs and absence of adhesion proteins [77]. This defect in the neurodevelopmental pathway might contribute to the development of ACs. Table 3 lists some of the genes commonly found in this syndrome and hence may be linked to AC formation.

Table 2 Main genes involved in ADPKD

Name of gene [95]	Location of gene on chromosome [95]	Function of the gene [96–99]
PKD1	16p13.3	• Impact protein folding, assembly, trafficking and degradation
PKD2	4q21-23	
GANAB	11q12.3	
DNAJB11	3q27.3	

Table 3 Genes found in Kallmann syndrome

Name of gene [8]	Location of gene on chromosome [8]	Function of gene [8]
KAL1	Xp22.3	• Encodes for an extracellular glycoprotein called anosmin-1 that promotes migration of GnRH secreting neurons from the olfactory bulbs to the hypothalamus
		• X-linked transmitted and found in 10% of patients
CCDC141	2q31.2	• Similar role to KAL1 in regulation of GnRH
Fibroblast growth factor receptor-1 (FGFR1 or KAL2)	8q11.2-12	• Accounts for 10% of all cases of Kallmann syndrome
Prokinetic receptor-2 (PROKR2)	20p12.3	• Account for a further 20% - 30% of all cases of Kallmann syndrome
Prokinetin-2 (PROk2)	13p21.2	
Chromodomain helicase DNA binding protein 7 (CHD7)	8q12.2	
Fibroblast growth factor 8 (FGFS)	10q24	

Long-term epilepsy-associated tumors (LEAT) have also been associated with the formation of ACs [124]. LEAT includes gangliogliomas (GG), dysembryoplastic neuroepithelial tumors (DNT), papillary glioneuronal tumors (PGNT), and adenoid cystic carcinomas [124]. Table 4 lists some of the genes commonly associated with LEAT entities.

While mutations in any of these genes could affect the proliferation of cells, it is uncertain how these mutations ultimately lead to the development of ACs.

Oculopharyngeal dystrophy is another condition to which ACs are linked [73]. This syndrome is caused by repeat expansions in the PABP2 gene (Chr.14q11 in humans) [73] which produces a protein needed for polyadenylation [90]. It is hypothesized that the extra alanine produced by the mutation clump up within muscles leading to loss of muscle function [90]. How this relates to AC formation is still unclear, and it is likely that this gene may not be related to AC formation [90].

One paper conducted a particularly interesting study that looked at the differences in gene expression between the normal arachnoid membrane and the cyst membrane [87]. This paper found 9 (out of 33,096) genes that were different. These are listed in Table 5.

Of these genes ASGR1, SHROOM3, A2BP1, ATP10D, and TRIML1 may be the genes involved in AC formation. Other mutations could be coincidental findings.

Another paper reported on intracranial ACs that showed an X-linked dominant inheritance pattern [24]. There were four family members who all presented with large, bilateral, symmetric middle fossa ACs [24]. They were all found to have a maternally inherited 720-kb duplication of the Xp22.2 chromosome that was not present in any of the unaffected family members [24]. This chromosome region includes the genes listed in Table 6.

Loss of function of MID1 and ARHGAP6 were found due to breakpoints in the duplication [24]. Here, it seems that genes needed for appropriate disposal (or recycling) of proteins were important in the formation of ACs. The other two genes in the region may not be related to the formation of ACs.

Tuberous sclerosis complex (TCS) is a condition caused by mutations in the TSC1 (on Chr.9q34 in humans) and TSC2 (on Chr.16p13.3 in

Table 4 Genes commonly associated with LEAT entities

Name of the gene [100]	Location of the gene on chromosome [100]	Function of gene
BRAF V600E	7q34	• Linked to GGs with CD34 expression [100]
		• Involved in protein trafficking as part of the RAS/MAPK signaling pathway that controls cell proliferation, differentiation, migration and apoptosis [101]
FGFR1	8p11.23	• Linked to DNTs [100]
		• Makes a protein that is involved in proliferation and maturation of cells, wound healing and blood vessel formation [102]
		• Major role in the formation, survival and movement of nerve cells in several areas of the brain, particularly those secreting GnRH [102]
PRKCA	17q24.2	• Linked to PGNTs [100]
		• Involved in cell growth [104]
FGFR2	10q26.13	• Mutations have been recognized in common LEAT entities [100]
		• Makes a protein that is involved in proliferation and maturation of cells, wound healing and blood vessel formation [103]
		• Involved in bone growth [103]
MYB/L1	8q13.1	• Mutations have been recognized in common LEAT entities [100]
		• Associated with the formation of adenoid cyst carcinoma [105]

Table 5 Differences in gene expression between the normal arachnoid membrane and the cyst membrane

Name of the gene [109]	Location of the gene on chromosome [109]	Function of gene
ASGR1	17p13.1	• Produces a transmembrane protein involved in transport of molecules in and out of the cell [110]
DPEP2	16q22.1	• Involved in many pathways including the inflammatory pathway [111]
SOX9	17q24	• Involved in skeletal development and sex determination [112]
SHROOM3	4q21.1	• Involved in neural tube closure [113]
A2BP1	16p13.3	• Important in neuronal development and can lead to benign epilepsy with centrotemporal spikes [114]
ATP10D	4p12	• Needed for cellular transport of GlcCer from the outer to the inner leaflet of the plasma membrane [115]
TRIML1	4q35.2	• Function is as of yet unclear[116]
NMU	4q12	• Needed for muscle contraction in the GI tract [117]
BEND5	1p33	• Acts as a transcriptional repressor [118]

Table 6 Genes in the duplicated region of chromosome Xp22.2

Name of the gene [14]	Location of the gene on chromosome [14]	Function of gene
MID1	Xp22.2	• Involved in the recycling of PP2A, ITGA4 and STK36 proteins by tagging them with ubiquitin [120]
HCCS		• Needed for ATP production and the apoptosis of cells [121]
AMELX		• Needed for enamel formation on the teeth [122]
ARHGAP6		• Involved in cell motility and changes of cell morphology [123]

humans) genes that lead to over-activation of the mTOR pathway [11]. Patients with these mutations have also been found to have ACs along with other clinical manifestations, and it seems that TSC2 mutations are more commonly associated with ACs than TSC1 in these individuals [11]. Both these genes are involved in cell growth and cell size control [95].

Papers have found a correlation between skull base meningiomas and middle cranial fossa ACs [128]. The specificity of the location of the condition indicates that local factors such as alterations in intracranial pressure, vascular occlusion, and localized release of bone growth factors might explain the pathology. IGF-1 (Chr.12q23.2), IGF-2 (Chr.11p15.5), and PDGF (Chr.22q13.1) are all involved in bone formation and growth (cell proliferation) [128].

ACs have been associated with syndromes such as spastic paraplegia which is caused by a mutation in the SPG4 gene [73]. The SPG4 gene (now called the SPAST gene) found on Chr.2p21-22 in humans has a role in the functioning of microtubules that allow transport of substances in and out of cells and in cell division [94]. This gene is particularly abundant in neurons [94].

Sporadic SEDAC is thought to be caused by haplo-insufficiency of the HOXD4 gene [106]. HOXD4 is found on Chr.2q31-37 [106] and is important in determining the position of developing limb buds during embryological growth [32].

Patients with Edward's syndrome have also been found to have ACs [8]. Karyotypes include 47,XY,+18 and 47,X?,+18 [8]. The first karyotype also had severe developmental delay, and the second died neonatally [8].

Both a KAT6A de novo mutation (variant p. P528S, coding DNA c.1582 C > T—likely pathogenic variant) and an inherited USP9X X-linked mutation (variant p.E903G, coding DNA c.2708 A > G—variant of uncertain significance) presented with posterior fossa ACs (PFAC) [41]. KAT6A (Chr.8p11.21) is needed to encode proteins and is important in various parts of the body [104], and USP9X (Chr.Xp11.4) is important in chromosome alignment and segregation during centromere alignment in cell division [108].

The RERE gene (Chr.1p36.23) was found to have heterozygous missense mutations (c.2576C > T) in a 7-year-old and 6-year-old female human cousins. These patients also had intracranial ACs [137]. The RERE gene codes for a regulatory protein and is essential for the development of the brain, eyes, inner ear, heart, and kidneys [93]. The WNT1 gene on Chr.12q13.12 was also found in a patient with ACs [60]. This gene plays a role in the development of the embryonic brain and CNS [33]. Mutations in these genes may cause agenesis of brain structures, but there is not enough evidence to link this to the formation of ACs.

It has been found that lateral meningocele syndrome (LMS) is due to specific pathogenic variants in the last exon of the NOTCH3 gene (Chr.19p13.12) [12]. A paper discussed a patient who presented with this mutation and intradural and extradural ACs alongside other clinical presentations [12]. The NOTCH3 gene is important for the function and survival of vascular smooth muscle [89]. It is also thought to be necessary to maintain the blood vessels in the brain [89].

As discussed in the introduction, GA-1 is a metabolic disorder caused by a mutation in the GCDH gene at Chr.19p13 [127]. GA-1 has been commonly associated with ACs in the literature [127]. The GCDH gene is needed for the breakdown of amino acids lysine, hydroxylysine, and tryptophan [88].

The PAPB2 gene on Chr.14 was linked to genetic myopathy, oculopharyngeal muscular dystrophy (OPMD), and ACs in a family [56]. This gene might play a role in the formation of ACs, but we cannot be sure how this association occurs.

Autosomal recessive missense Rotatin (RTTN) mutations at Chr.18q22.2 have been associated with ACs [13]. In one case study, a brain MRI showed extensive dysgyria associated with nodular heterotopia, large interhemispheric ACs, and corpus callosum hypoplasia [13]. The RTTN gene is needed for left-right specification and plays a role in the maintenance of normal ciliary structure [34]. We are unsure how this relates to AC formation, and further study is needed to understand the association between mutations in this gene and ACs.

Primary ciliary dyskinesia-related MCIDAS gene mutation is associated with AC formation [116]. The reduced generation of multiple motile cilia (RGMC) and mutation in the multicilin (MCIDAS) gene on Chr.5q11.2 have been linked to a high incidence of hydrocephalus, ACs, and CPH in MCIDAS-associated RGMC [116]. The gene is also required for centriole biogenesis [35]. Thus, like a few other genes mentioned, this gene is required for cilia formation and function. However, we are unsure how this relates to AC formation or expansion.

A rare heterozygous variant in the NID1 gene on Chr.1q42.3 was associated with autosomal dominant Dandy-Walker malformation and occipital cephalocele (ADDWOC) [81]. The paper describes a three-generation family in which individuals presented with ACs in the proband and the proband's maternal grandfather, an occipital cephalocele in the proband and his brother, and a small bony defect in the proband's mother [81]. This gene is related to pathways such as MET that promote cell motility and degradation of the extracellular matrix [36]. However, there is no clear indication as to how this is associated with ACs.

A patient with a Col4A1 gene mutation (Chr.13q34) was also found to have an AC [18]. Col4A1 is needed to make one component of type IV collagen [85]. Type IV collagen is one of the main components of the basement membranes in almost all the tissue in the body including the blood vessels [85]. The basement membrane also plays a role in cell migration, proliferation, differentiation, and survival [85]. Mutations in this gene can lead to defects in the basement membrane of blood vessels and lead to impaired movement of electrolytes that may cause CSF flow to change. Igarashi et al. hypothesize that since ACs and vascular smooth muscles originate from mesenchymal cells that surround the neural tube, which also produce collagen for the extracellular matrix in cerebral vessels, both the vascular and mesenchymal structures may be forming at the same time [52]. Thus, the histogenesis of arachnoid and arterial layers may be involved at the same time [52], and defects in either or both may lead to the formation of ACs.

Microdeletions on chromosomes, specifically Chr.22q13.31q13.33 in one case report and Chr.22q13 and Chr.22q11 in another case report, were found along with ACs [43]. Both patients were human females and had other clinical features commonly associated with Phelan-McDermid syndrome (PMS) [43].

There are many other genes that are linked to ACs either through syndromes or via one or two cases in the literature. Table 7 summarizes these genes and their association with ACs.

In summary, genes associated with ACs can be grouped into four categories as shown in Fig. 1.

Given the lack of specific gene mutations associated with ACs, it is difficult to pinpoint which mutations are more impactful than others, and further research is needed to conclude if these genes are in fact related to the formation of ACs.

Some of these genes have been associated with hydrocephalus formation. For example, the primary ciliary dyskinesia-related MCIDAS gene mutation has been known to be found in patients with both ACs and hydrocephalus [35, 116].

Table 7 Other genes associated with AC formation

Gene	Location on chromosome	Function	Association with arachnoid cysts
ZIC2 [124]	13q32.2 [124]	• Produces a transcription factor essential for the development of the forebrain [125]	• A 9-month-old female patient presented with mild microcephaly, semilobar HPE and an AC alongside this mutation [124]
		• Mutations may be linked to agenesis of the corpus callosum [125]	• Agenesis of the corpus callosum is strongly linked to the presentation of ACs [125]
SOX2 [140]	3q26.33 [140]	• Critical in the formation of many different tissues and organs during embryonic development, especially the eyes [146]	• Found to be associated with an AC, microcornea, retrobulbar colobomatous orbital cyst and penoscrotal hypospadias in one paper [140]
		• It also acts as a transcription factor for other genes [146]	
Oligophrenin-1 (OPHN1) [142]	Xq12 [142]	• This gene is a Rho-GTPase activating protein [142]	• One paper discussed a family with a mild developmental delay, behavioral disturbances, facial dysmorphism, pes planus, nystagmus, strabismus, epilepsy, and occipital AC alongside a mutation in this gene [142]
		• Involved in intracellular signal transduction which affects cell migration and cell morphogenesis [147]	
Frataxin [144]	9q21.11 [144]	• Frataxin is found in the mitochondria and its role is not well understood but it is thought to be needed to assemble clusters of iron and sulfur molecules needed for the function of many proteins and for energy production within the cell [148]	• A paper discusses 2 patients with a GAA repeat expansions mutation in this gene who also have ACs [144]
			• This GAA repeat expansions mutation in this gene is also lined to Friedreich ataxia (FRDA) and cerebral lesions and demyelinating neuropathy [144]
SLC12A2 [130]	5q23 [130]	• Codes for the NKCC1 protein which is needed for the Na^+/K^+/2CL-cotransporter [130]	• This gene is significantly upregulated in ACs [130]
		• It is important for fluid transport [130]	• Upregulation may explain why CSF dynamics can be abnormal (and lead to AC expansion due to CSF accumulation) [130]
ATP1A3 [141]	19q13.2 [141]	• Needed to make one part of a protein known as Na^+/K^+ ATPase (sodium pump) [146]	• This mutation was found alongside a right temporal AC [141]

Table 7 (continued)

Gene	Location on chromosome	Function	Association with arachnoid cysts
			• Na^+/K^+ ATPase is involved in the uptake of neurotransmitters [146]. This may directly relate to CSF flow dynamics and an imbalance in this may lead to AC expansion via CSF accumulation in the cyst
FOXC2 [109]	16q24.1 [109]	• Critical for development of the lungs, eyes, kidneys and the urinary tract [109]	
		• Needed for formation of veins [109]	
GPSM2 [109]	1p13.1[109]	• Involved in cell division, particularly in the metaphase spindle orientation [119]	• A homozygous mutation of this gene was present in a pair of dizygotic twins who both presented with an interhemispheric AC [109]
PDGFRB [132]	5q32 [132]	• Important for signal transduction and signaling pathway activation [133]	
		• These signaling pathways are needed for cell proliferation, movement and survival [133]	• 19-year-old Caucasian female patient presented with a cervical spine AC along with many other CNS and cardiac abnormalities. Exome sequencing trio analysis identified a de novo previously reported pathogenic variant in this gene c.1696T>C (p.[Trp566Arg]) [132]

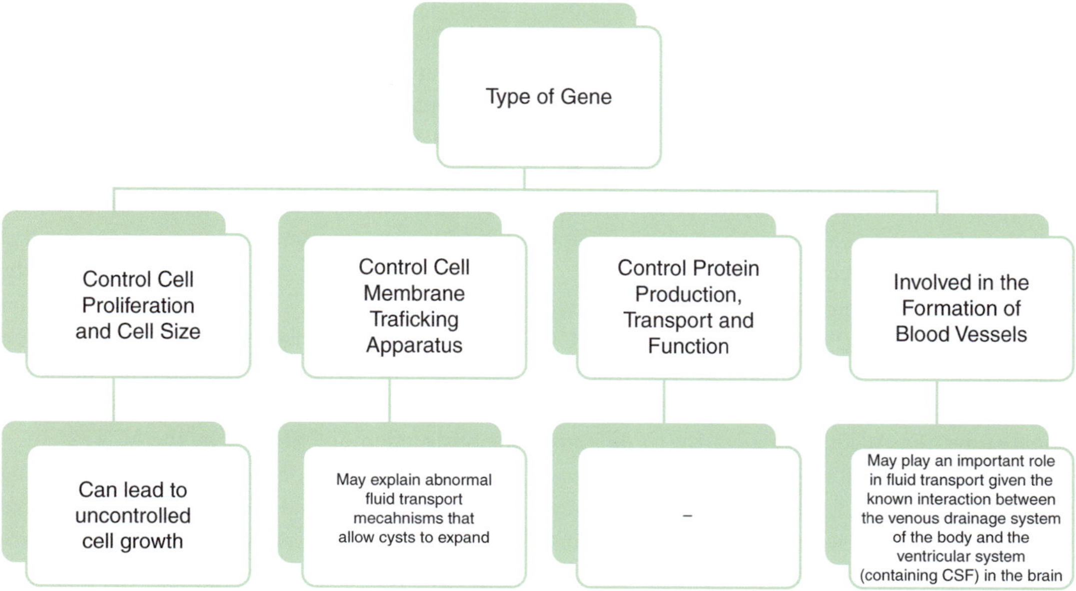

Fig. 1 Summary of types of genes associated with ACs

7 Hydrocephalus

"Hydrocephalus (HC) is classically defined as dynamic imbalance between the production and absorption of cerebrospinal fluid (CSF), leading to enlarged ventricles" [70]. Hydrocephalus is often found in midline and posterior fossa ACs [76]. It is also possible to observe ventriculomegaly in interhemispheric lesions, but it is rare to see hydrocephalus in middle fossa lesions [76]. Since ACs can be found in all areas of the brain with arachnoid mater and hydrocephalus is not found in all of these areas, it indicates that ACs may not be the sole cause of hydrocephalus.

There has been speculation that some ACs are due to disturbed CSF dynamics and that ACs may be a localized form of hydrocephalus [76]. It may be that ACs are the cause of hydrocephalus or it could be that hydrocephalus causes ACs. However, Martinez-Lage et al. state that "CSF dynamics seem to play a major role in the development of both [arachnoid] cysts and hydrocephalus" [76].

A paper by Topsakal et al. describes a 67-year-old female patient who presented with symptoms of normal pressure hydrocephalus, lower cranial nerve pareses, and pyramidal and cerebellar signs associated with respiratory disturbances [130]. She was found to have a quadrigeminal AC that was compressing the aqueduct and other brain structures [130]. Removing the cyst surgically resolved some of her symptoms including the hydrocephalus [130]. Thus, in this case, it seems that the AC was the cause of the patient's symptoms including the hydrocephalus.

Basaran et al. discuss a patient with persistent subarachnoid bleeds, hydrocephalus, and ACs [7]. Treating the hydrocephalus did not treat the patient's symptoms of headaches and diplopia, but treating the ACs did resolve the symptoms [7]. Here it is difficult to distinguish if the hydrocephalus was caused by the AC, but it does show that the AC was not caused by the hydrocephalus since treating the hydrocephalus did not treat the AC. In addition, this article illustrates once again that hydrocephalus, and ACs do occur together very frequently.

There are other papers that support the notion that ACs cause hydrocephalus in patients, most frequently by obstructing and putting pressure on the key ventricular structures of the brain [78, 109, 112, 139].

However, a paper by Pradilla et al. found that only 9% of their 20 patients that presented with ACs had hydrocephalus [111]. So, it seems that hydrocephalus is not always found with ACs and discredits the idea that ACs cause hydrocephalus. Another paper also found that out of ten patients with ACs, only three had hydrocephalus [25]. But here it can be argued that the location, size, and extent of compression caused by the AC might play a role in the development of hydrocephalus [78, 109, 112, 139].

There are also articles that focus on the presence of hydrocephalus and ACs and the role they play in the development of syringomyelia and Chiari malformation type 1 (CM-1) [20, 74, 129]. These papers do not help answer the question as to whether ACs cause hydrocephalus or vice versa, but they do indicate that the two occur together very frequently and may play a role in the formation of other secondary symptoms (such as CM-1).

Perna et al. describe 12 patients with ACs, CM-1, syringomyelia, and hydrocephalus [20]. Given the rarity of CM-1 [20], the fact that 12 cases were found with this combination of clinical symptoms provides some backing to the theory that there might be a third external factor causing the development of both hydrocephalus and ACs. Martinez-Lage et al. found a patient with this same presentation but concluded that the CM-1 and syringomyelia were caused by the hydrocephalus and AC because ventricular decompression and removal of the AC resolved the CM-1 and syringomyelia [74]. They also concur that, usually, the syringomyelia is caused by the obstruction of CSF flow by the AC [74].

ACs and hydrocephalus are closely associated with each other. Table 8 depicts some genes that are thought to be associated with both hydrocephalus and ACs. However, it is still unclear if one causes the other or if they are both the consequence of a third external factor such as a common gene mutation or syndrome.

Table 8 Genes associated with both hydrocephalus and arachnoid cysts

Name of gene [149]	Location on chromosome	Function [149]	Other mutant phenotypes [149]
TMEM67	8q22.1	• Migration of centrioles to apical membrane	Meckel Syndrome Type 3 Joubert Syndrome Type 6
		• Primary cilium formation	
FGFR2	10q26.13	• Cell growth, division, maturation, and differentiation	Apert Syndrome Pfeiffer Syndrome
		• Angiogenesis, wound healing	
GPSM2	1p13.1	• Organization	Nonsyndromic hearing loss Chudly-McCullough Syndrome
		• Development of normal hearing	
ZIC2	13q32.3	• Instructions for making forebrain development proteins	Dandy-Walker malformation Neural Tube Defects
		• Transcription factor for left-right axis formation	

8 Conclusion

From the above, we can see that there are some syndromes that have a significantly higher association with ACs than others. There are also genes that appear to be linked to AC formation. One common feature of these genes is that most of them seem to be involved in protein production, function, and (like in hydrocephalus) protein transport. Moreover, there is much coinciding between genes and syndromes of hydrocephalus and ACs, so there may be common features between hydrocephalus and ACs such as their mechanism of formation and expansion. Most ACs seem to be sporadic (nonsyndromic), but there are instances in which they occur commonly along with other clinical presentations. The presence of agenesis of the corpus callosum (which is very strongly associated with the presence of ACs) should alert clinicians to look for structural malformations that can be present. Conclusively, the mechanism of formation of ACs and pathophysiologic mechanisms involved in their expansion are poorly understood. Further research is required to understand the mechanisms presented and discussed within this chapter.

References

1. Neurology Academy 2021. Available at: https://neurologyacademy.org/profiles/dr-nikos-evangelou. Accessed 20 November 2021.
2. Al-Holou W, Terman S, Kilburg C, Garton H, Muraszko K, Maher C. Prevalence and natural history of arachnoid cysts in adults. J Neurosurg. 2013;118(2):222–31.
3. Alkan A, Baysal T, Yakinci C, Sigirci A, Kutlu R. Glutaric aciduria type I diagnosed after poliovirus immunization: magnetic resonance findings. Pediatr Neurol. 2002;26(5):405–7. https://doi.org/10.1016/s0887-8994(01)00411-8.
4. Anik Y, Anik I, Gonullu E, Inan N, Demirci A. Proteus syndrome with syringohydromyelia and arachnoid cyst. Childs Nerv Syst. 2007;23(10):1199–202.; ; discussion 1203. https://doi.org/10.1007/s00381-007-0364-z.
5. Babu R, Murali R. Arachnoid cyst of the cerebellopontine angle manifesting as contralateral trigeminal neuralgia: case report. Neurosurgery. 1991;28(6):886–7. https://doi.org/10.1097/00006123-199106000-00018.
6. Barkovich AJ, Simon EM, Walsh CA. Callosal agenesis with cyst: a better understanding and new classification. Neurology. 2001;56(2):220–7. https://doi.org/10.1212/wnl.56.2.220.
7. Basaran R, Kaksi M, Efendioglu M, Onoz M, Balkuv E, Kaner T. Spinal arachnoid cyst associated with arachnoiditis following subarachnoid haemorrhage in adult patients: A case report and literature review.

Br J Neurosurg. 2015;29(2):285–9. https://doi.org/10.3109/02688697.2014.976175. Epub 2014 Nov 3
8. Beresford C, Hall S, Smedley A, Mathad N, Waters R, Chakraborty A, Sparrow OC, Tsitouras V. Prenatal diagnosis of arachnoid cysts: a case series and systematic review. Childs Nerv Syst. 2020;36(4):729–41. https://doi.org/10.1007/s00381-019-04477-6. Epub 2020 Jan 2
9. Bigder MG, Helmi A, Kaufmann AM. Trigeminal neuropathy associated with an enlarging arachnoid cyst in Meckel's cave: case report, management strategy and review of the literature. Acta Neurochir. 2017;159(12):2309–12. https://doi.org/10.1007/s00701-017-3262-5. Epub 2017 Jul 31
10. Bijarnia S, Wiley V, Carpenter K, Christodoulou J, Ellaway CJ, Wilcken B. Glutaric aciduria type I: outcome following detection by newborn screening. J Inherit Metab Dis. 2008;31(4):503–7. https://doi.org/10.1007/s10545-008-0912-z. Epub 2008 Aug 9
11. Boronat S, Barber I. Less common manifestations in TSC. Am J Med Genet C Semin Med Genet. 2018;178(3):348–54. https://doi.org/10.1002/ajmg.c.31648. Epub 2018 Aug 29
12. Cappuccio G, Apuzzo D, Alagia M, Torella A, Pinelli M, Franco B, Corrado B, Del Giudice E, D'Amico A, Nigro V, TUDP, Brunetti-Pierri N. Expansion of the phenotype of lateral meningocele syndrome. Am J Med Genet A. 2020;182(5):1259–62. https://doi.org/10.1002/ajmg.a.61536. Epub 2020 Mar 6
13. Cavallin M, Bery A, Maillard C, Salomon LJ, Bole C, Reilly ML, Nitschké P, Boddaert N, Bahi-Buisson N. Recurrent RTTN mutation leading to severe microcephaly, polymicrogyria and growth restriction. Eur J Med Genet. 2018;61(12):755–8. https://doi.org/10.1016/j.ejmg.2018.08.001. Epub 2018 Aug 16
14. Chapman T, Mahalingam S, Ishak GE, Nixon JN, Siebert J, Dighe MK. Diagnostic imaging of posterior fossa anomalies in the fetus and neonate: part 2, posterior fossa disorders. Clin Imaging. 2015;39(2):167–75. https://doi.org/10.1016/j.clinimag.2014.10.012. Epub 2014 Oct 22
15. Christensen E, Ribes A, Merinero B, Zschocke J. Correlation of genotype and phenotype in glutaryl-CoA dehydrogenase deficiency. J Inherit Metab Dis. 2004;27(6):861–8. https://doi.org/10.1023/B:BOLI.0000045770.93429.3c.
16. Columbano L, Luedemann W, Kusaka Y, Oi S, Samii M. Prenatal diagnosed cyst of the quadrigeminal cistern in Aicardi syndrome. Childs Nerv Syst. 2009;25(5):521–2. https://doi.org/10.1007/s00381-008-0772-8. Epub 2008 Dec 24
17. Correa GG, Amaral LF, Vedolin LM. Neuroimaging of Dandy-Walker malformation: new concepts. Top Magn Reson Imaging. 2011;22(6):303–12. https://doi.org/10.1097/RMR.0b013e3182a2ca77.
18. Değerliyurt A, Ceylaner G, Koçak H, Bilginer Gürbüz B, Cihan BS, Rizzu P, Ceylaner S. A new family with autosomal dominant porencephaly with a novel Col4A1 mutation. Are arachnoid cysts related to Col4A1 mutations? Genet Couns. 2012;23(2):185–93.
19. Demir HD, Deniz FE, Yardim H. A rare brain developmental anomaly in a patient with Usher's syndrome. Int Ophthalmol. 2010;30(1):85–8. https://doi.org/10.1007/s10792-008-9277-4. Epub 2008 Nov 13
20. Di Perna G, Piatelli G, Rossi A, Consales A, Fiaschi P, Castaldo M, Pavanello M. Coexisting Retrocerebellar arachnoid cyst and Chiari type 1 malformation: 3 pediatric cases of surgical management tailored to the pathogenic mechanism and systematic review of the literature. World Neurosurg. 2021;148:44–53. https://doi.org/10.1016/j.wneu.2020.12.094. Epub 2020 Dec 29
21. Engelhardt J, Vignes J. Anterior cervical intradural arachnoid cyst, a rare cause of spinal cord compression: a case report with video systematic literature review. Eur Spine J. 2015;25(S1):19–26.
22. Evangelou P, Meixensberger J, Bernhard M, Hirsch W, Kiess W, Merkenschlager A, Nestler U, Preuss M. Operative management of idiopathic spinal intradural arachnoid cysts in children: a systematic review. Childs Nerv Syst. 2013;29(4):657–64. https://doi.org/10.1007/s00381-012-1990-7. Epub 2012 Dec 9
23. Evangelou P, Meixensberger J, Bernhard M, Hirsch W, Kiess W, Merkenschlager A, Nestler U, Preuss M. Operative management of idiopathic spinal intradural arachnoid cysts in children: a systematic review. Childs Nerv Syst. 2012;29(4):657–64.
24. Furey CG, Timberlake AT, Nelson-Williams C, Duran D, Li P, Jackson EM, Kahle KT. Xp22.2 chromosomal duplication in familial intracranial arachnoid cyst. JAMA Neurol. 2017;74(12):1503–4. https://doi.org/10.1001/jamaneurol.2017.3399.
25. Galarza M, López-Guerrero AL, Martínez-Lage JF. Posterior fossa arachnoid cysts and cerebellar tonsillar descent: short review. Neurosurg Rev. 2010;33(3):305–14.; ; discussion 314. https://doi.org/10.1007/s10143-010-0262-9.
26. Garcia P, Martins E, Diogo L, Rocha H, Marcão A, Gaspar E, Almeida M, Vaz C, Soares I, Barbot C, Vilarinho L. Outcome of three cases of untreated maternal glutaric aciduria type I. Eur J Pediatr. 2008;167(5):569–73. https://doi.org/10.1007/s00431-007-0556-2. Epub 2007 Jul 28
27. Genc E, Dogan EA, Kocaogullar Y, Emlik D. A case with prepontine (clival) arachnoid cyst manifested as trigeminal neuralgia. Headache. 2008;48(10):1525–7. https://doi.org/10.1111/j.1526-4610.2008.01147.x. Epub 2008 Jun 11
28. Genecards.org. 2021. Available at: https://www.genecards.org/cgi-bin/carddisp.pl?gene=DPEP2. Accessed 20 November 2021.
29. Genecards.org. 2021. Available at: https://www.genecards.org/cgi-bin/carddisp.pl?gene=ATP10D#:~:text=UniProtKB%2FSwiss%2DProt%20Summary%20for,leaflet%20of%20the%20

plasma%20membrane. Accessed 20 November 2021.
30. Genecards.org. 2021. Available at: https://www.genecards.org/cgi-bin/carddisp.pl?gene=NMU#:~:text=Stimulates%20muscle%20contractions%20of%20specific,the%20ileum%20and%20urinary%20bladder. Accessed 20 November 2021.
31. Genecards.org. 2021. Available at: https://www.genecards.org/cgi-bin/carddisp.pl?gene=BEND5. Accessed 20 November 2021.
32. Genecards.org. 2021. Available at: https://www.genecards.org/cgi-bin/carddisp.pl?gene=HOXD4. Accessed 20 November 2021.
33. Genecards.org. 2021. Available at: https://www.genecards.org/cgi-bin/carddisp.pl?gene=WNT1#:~:text=UniProtKB%2FSwiss%2DProt%20Summary%20for%20WNT1%20Gene&text=Plays%20an%20essential%20role%20in,23499309%2C%20PubMed%3A23656646). Accessed 20 November 2021.
34. Genecards.org. 2021. Available at: https://www.genecards.org/cgi-bin/carddisp.pl?gene=RTTN#:~:text=UniProtKB%2FSwiss%2DProt%20Summary%20for,of%20NODAL%2C%20LEFTY%20and%20PITX2. Accessed 20 November 2021.
35. Genecards.org. 2021. Available at: https://www.genecards.org/cgi-bin/carddisp.pl?gene=MCIDAS. Accessed 20 November 2021.
36. Genecards.org. 2021. Available at: https://www.genecards.org/cgi-bin/carddisp.pl?gene=NID1#:~:text=NID1%20(Nidogen%201)%20is%20a,Degradation%20of%20the%20extracellular%20matrix. Accessed 20 November 2021.
37. Glimcher SA, Holman DW, Lubow M, Grzybowski DM. Ex vivo model of cerebrospinal fluid outflow across human arachnoid granulations. Invest Ophthalmol Vis Sci. 2008;49(11):4721–8. https://doi.org/10.1167/iovs.08-2238. Epub 2008 Jul 9
38. Granata F, Alafaci C, Passalacqua M, Cacciola F, Caffo M, Salpietro FM, Vinci SL, Longo M. Non-traumatic sphenoidal intradiploic arachnoid cyst as a cause of trigeminal neuralgia. A case report. Neuroradiol J. 2011;24(6):867–71. https://doi.org/10.1177/197140091102400606. Epub 2011 Dec 23
39. Grande-Martín A, Díaz-Conejo R, Verdú-Pérez A, Hernández-Moneo JL. Trigeminal neuralgia in a child with a cerebellopontine angle arachnoid cyst. Pediatr Neurol. 2015;53(2):178–9. https://doi.org/10.1016/j.pediatrneurol.2015.03.010. Epub 2015 Mar 13
40. Grasso G, Passalacqua M, Giambartino F, Cacciola F, Caruso G, Tomasello F. Typical trigeminal neuralgia by an atypical compression: case report and review of the literature. Turk Neurosurg. 2014;24(1):82–5. https://doi.org/10.5137/1019-5149.JTN.7048-12.0.
41. Guell X, Anteraper SA, Ghosh SS, Gabrieli JDE, Schmahmann JD. Neurodevelopmental and psychiatric symptoms in patients with a cyst compressing the cerebellum: an ongoing enigma. Cerebellum. 2020;19(1):16–29. https://doi.org/10.1007/s12311-019-01050-4.
42. Guerriero S, Sciruicchio V, De Blasi R, Furino C, Smaldone G, Ciracì L, Galeone D. Chorioretinal lacunae: pathognomonic findings for Aicardi syndrome. J Pediatr Ophthalmol Strabismus. 2010;47:e1–3. https://doi.org/10.3928/01913913-20100324-03.
43. Ha JF, Ahmad A, Lesperance MM. Clinical characterization of novel chromosome 22q13 microdeletions. Int J Pediatr Otorhinolaryngol. 2017;95:121–6. https://doi.org/10.1016/j.ijporl.2016.12.008. Epub 2016 Dec 23
44. Halani SH, Safain MG, Heilman CB. Arachnoid cyst slit valves: the mechanism for arachnoid cyst enlargement. J Neurosurg Pediatr. 2013;12(1):62–6. https://doi.org/10.3171/2013.4.PEDS12609. Epub 2013 May 10
45. Hald JK, Nakstad PH, Skjeldal OH, Strømme P. Bilateral arachnoid cysts of the temporal fossa in four children with glutaric aciduria type I. AJNR Am J Neuroradiol. 1991;12(3):407–9.
46. Hamada H, Nonaka Y, Kusaka Y, Nakazaki H, Abdullah SH, Oi S. Huge arachnoid cyst incorporating choroid plexus. Childs Nerv Syst. 2006;22(4):420–3. https://doi.org/10.1007/s00381-005-1174-9. Epub 2005 Jun 3
47. Hanakita S, Oya S, Matsui T. Trigeminal neuralgia caused by an arachnoid cyst in Meckel's cave: A case report and literature review. Surg Neurol Int. 2021;10(12):45. https://doi.org/10.25259/SNI_734_2020.
48. Harris PC, Torres VE. Polycystic kidney disease, autosomal dominant. 2002 Jan 10 [updated 2018 Jul 19]. In: Adam MP, Ardinger HH, Pagon RA, Wallace SE, bean LJH, Mirzaa G, Amemiya A, editors. GeneReviews®. Seattle (WA): University of Washington, Seattle; 1993–2021.
49. Helland CA, Aarhus M, Knappskog P, Olsson LK, Lund-Johansen M, Amiry-Moghaddam M, Wester K. Increased NKCC1 expression in arachnoid cysts supports secretory basis for cyst formation. Exp Neurol. 2010;224(2):424–8. https://doi.org/10.1016/j.expneurol.2010.05.002. Epub 2010 May 21
50. Holman DW, Grzybowski DM, Mehta BC, Katz SE, Lubow M. Characterization of cytoskeletal and junctional proteins expressed by cells cultured from human arachnoid granulation tissue. Cerebrospinal Fluid Res. 2005;13(2):9. https://doi.org/10.1186/1743-8454-2-9.
51. Holmes LB, Redline RW, Brown DL, Williams AJ, Collins T. Absence/hypoplasia of tibia, polydactyly, retrocerebellar arachnoid cyst, and other anomalies: an autosomal recessive disorder. J Med Genet. 1995;32(11):896–900. https://doi.org/10.1136/jmg.32.11.896.
52. Igarashi Y, Murai Y, Yamada O, Shirokane K, Hironaka K, Sato S, Sugiyama M, Tachizawa T, Morita A. Cerebral aneurysm associated with an arachnoid cyst: 3 case reports and a systematic review

of the literature. World Neurosurg. 2018;109:e203–9. https://doi.org/10.1016/j.wneu.2017.09.139. Epub 2017 Sep 28
53. Ishizaka S, Hayashi K, Otsuka M, Fukuda S, Tsunoda K, Ushijima R, Kitagawa N, Suyama K, Nagata I. Syringomyelia and arachnoid cysts associated with spinal arachnoiditis following subarachnoid hemorrhage. Neurol Med Chir (Tokyo). 2012;52(9):686–90. https://doi.org/10.2176/nmc.52.686.
54. Islam MP. Neurocutaneous melanosis. Handb Clin Neurol. 2015;132:111–7. https://doi.org/10.1016/B978-0-444-62702-5.00007-X.
55. Iturralde D, Meyerle CB, Yannuzzi LA. Aicardi syndrome: chorioretinal lacunae without corpus callosum agenesis. Retina. 2006;26(8):977–8. https://doi.org/10.1097/01.iae.0000224937.78389.15.
56. Jadeja KJ, Grewal RP. Familial arachnoid cysts associated with oculopharyngeal muscular dystrophy. J Clin Neurosci. 2003;10(1):125–7. https://doi.org/10.1016/s0967-5868(02)00105-4.
57. Jamjoom ZA, Okamoto E, Jamjoom AH, Al-Hajery O, Abu-Melha A. Bilateral arachnoid cysts of the sylvian region in female siblings with glutaric aciduria type I. report of two cases. J Neurosurg. 1995;82(6):1078–81. https://doi.org/10.3171/jns.1995.82.6.1078.
58. Jonklaas J. Atypical presentation of a patient with both Kallmann syndrome and a craniopharyngioma: case report and literature review. Endocr Pract. 2005;11(1):30–6. https://doi.org/10.4158/EP.11.1.30.
59. Kaisho Y, Miyazaki S, Shimo-oku M, Hayashi T, Tani E. A case of suprasellar arachnoid cyst followed up for a long time. Nippon Ganka Gakkai Zasshi. 1995;99(1):109–14. Japanese
60. Kantaputra PN, Sirirungruangsarn Y, Visrutaratna P, Petcharunpaisan S, Carlson BM, Intachai W, Sudasna J, Kampuansai J, Dejkhamron P. WNT1-associated osteogenesis imperfecta with atrophic frontal lobes and arachnoid cysts. J Hum Genet. 2019;64(4):291–6. https://doi.org/10.1038/s10038-019-0565-9. Epub 2019 Jan 28
61. Kapoor KG, Katz SE, Grzybowski DM, Lubow M. Cerebrospinal fluid outflow: an evolving perspective. Brain Res Bull. 2008;77(6):327–34. https://doi.org/10.1016/j.brainresbull.2008.08.009. Epub 2008 Sep 13
62. Kara B, Kayserili H, Imer M, Calişkan M, Ozmen M. Quadrigeminal cistern arachnoid cyst in a patient with kabuki syndrome. Pediatr Neurol. 2006;34(6):478–80. https://doi.org/10.1016/j.pediatrneurol.2005.11.006.
63. Kau T, Veraguth D, Schiegl H, Scheer I, Boltshauser E. Chudley-McCullough syndrome: case report and review of the neuroimaging spectrum. Neuropediatrics. 2012;43(1):44–7. https://doi.org/10.1055/s-0032-1307451. Epub 2012 Mar 19
64. Kollias SS, Ball WS Jr, Prenger EC. Cystic malformations of the posterior fossa: differential diagnosis clarified through embryologic analysis. Radiographics. 1993;13(6):1211–31. https://doi.org/10.1148/radiographics.13.6.8031352.
65. Kouyialis AT, Stranjalis G, Boviatsis EJ, Ziaka DS, Bouras TI, Sakas DE. Recurrence of trigeminal neuralgia due to an acquired arachnoid cyst. J Clin Neurosci. 2008;15(12):1409–11. https://doi.org/10.1016/j.jocn.2006.10.027. Epub 2008 Oct 7
66. Kurt S, Cevik B, Aksoy D, Sahbaz EI, Gundogdu Eken A, Basak AN. Atypical features in a large turkish family affected with friedreich ataxia. Case Rep Neurol Med. 2016;2016:4515938. https://doi.org/10.1155/2016/4515938. Epub 2016 Sep 7
67. Lee HJ, Cho DY. Symptomatic spinal intradural arachnoid cysts in the pediatric age group: description of three new cases and review of the literature. Pediatr Neurosurg. 2001;35(4):181–7. https://doi.org/10.1159/000050419.
68. Lee SW, Kim KS, Cho SM, Lee SJ. An atypical case of Aicardi syndrome with favorable outcome. Korean J Ophthalmol. 2004;18(1):79–83. https://doi.org/10.3341/kjo.2004.18.1.79.
69. Leibovitz Z, Guibaud L, Garel C, Massoud M, Karl K, Malinger G, Haratz KK, Gindes L, Tamarkin M, Ben-Sira L, Lev D, Shalev J, Brasseur-Daudruy M, Gutierrez C, de Piñeres CA, Lerman-Sagie T. The cerebellar "tilted telephone receiver sign" enables prenatal diagnosis of PHACES syndrome. Eur J Paediatr Neurol. 2018;22(6):900–9. https://doi.org/10.1016/j.ejpn.2018.08.006. Epub 2018 Sep 1
70. Leinonen V, Vanninen R, Rauramaa T. Cerebrospinal fluid circulation and hydrocephalus. Handb Clin Neurol. 2018;145:39–50.
71. Lerman-Sagie T, Prayer D, Stöcklein S, Malinger G. Fetal cerebellar disorders. Handb Clin Neurol. 2018;155:3–23. https://doi.org/10.1016/B978-0-444-64189-2.00001-9.
72. Lütcherath V, Waaler PE, Jellum E, Wester K. Children with bilateral temporal arachnoid cysts may have glutaric aciduria type 1 (GAT1); operation without knowing that may be harmful. Acta Neurochir. 2000;142(9):1025–30. https://doi.org/10.1007/s007010070058.
73. Martin MM, Lockspieler T, Slavotinek AM. Oculo-ectodermal syndrome: is arachnoid cyst a common finding? Clin Dysmorphol. 2007;16(1):35–8. https://doi.org/10.1097/MCD.0b013e328010b7f9.
74. Martínez-Lage JF, Almagro MJ, de San R, Pedro J, Ruiz-Espejo A, Felipe-Murcia M. Regression of syringomyelia and tonsillar herniation after posterior fossa arachnoid cyst excision. Case report and literature review. Neurocirugia (Astur). 2007;18(3):227–31.
75. Martínez-Lage JF, Casas C, Fernández MA, Puche A, Rodriguez Costa T, Poza M. Macrocephaly, dystonia, and bilateral temporal arachnoid cysts: glutaric aciduria type 1. Childs Nerv Syst. 1994;10(3):198–203. https://doi.org/10.1007/BF00301092.
76. Martínez-Lage JF, Pérez-Espejo MA, Almagro MJ, López-Guerrero AL. Hydrocephalus and arachnoid cysts. Childs Nerv Syst. 2011;27(10):1643–52.

https://doi.org/10.1007/s00381-011-1481-2. Epub 2011 Sep 17
77. Massimi L, Izzo A, Paternoster G, Frassanito P, Di Rocco C. Arachnoid cyst: a further anomaly associated with Kallmann syndrome? Childs Nerv Syst. 2016;32(9):1607–14. https://doi.org/10.1007/s00381-016-3154-7. Epub 2016 Jul 5
78. Mattox A, Choi JD, Leith-Gray L, Grant GA, Adamson DC. Guidelines for the management of obstructive hydrocephalus from suprasellar-prepontine arachnoid cysts using endoscopic third ventriculocystocisternostomy. Surg Innov. 2010;17(3):206–16. https://doi.org/10.1177/1553350610377212. Epub 2010 Aug 5
79. Mayo Clinic. 2021. Hydrocephalus—symptoms and causes. Available at: https://www.mayoclinic.org/diseases-conditions/hydrocephalus/symptoms-causes/syc-20373604. Accessed 20 November 2021.
80. McKnight I, Hart C, Park IH, Shim JW. Genes causing congenital hydrocephalus: their chromosomal characteristics of telomere proximity and DNA compositions. Exp Neurol. 2021;335:113523. https://doi.org/10.1016/j.expneurol.2020.113523. Epub 2020 Nov 4
81. McNiven V, Ito YA, Hartley T, Kernohan K, Miller E, Care4Rare Canada, Armour CM. NID1 variant associated with occipital cephaloceles in a family expressing a spectrum of phenotypes. Am J Med Genet A. 2019;179(5):837–41. https://doi.org/10.1002/ajmg.a.61095. Epub 2019 Feb 17
82. Medlineplus.gov. 2021. AMELX gene: MedlinePlus Genetics. Available at: https://medlineplus.gov/genetics/gene/amelx/. Accessed 20 November 2021.
83. Medlineplus.gov. 2021. ATP1A3 gene: MedlinePlus Genetics. Available at: https://medlineplus.gov/genetics/gene/atp1a3/. Accessed 20 November 2021.
84. Medlineplus.gov. 2021. BRAF gene: MedlinePlus Genetics. Available at: https://medlineplus.gov/genetics/gene/braf/#conditions. Accessed 20 November 2021.
85. Medlineplus.gov. 2021. COL4A1 gene: MedlinePlus Genetics. Available at: https://medlineplus.gov/genetics/gene/col4a1/. Accessed 20 November 2021.
86. Medlineplus.gov. 2021. FGFR1 gene: MedlinePlus Genetics. Available at: https://medlineplus.gov/genetics/gene/fgfr1/. Accessed 20 November 2021.
87. Medlineplus.gov. 2021. FOXC2 gene: MedlinePlus Genetics. Available at: https://medlineplus.gov/genetics/gene/foxc2/#conditions. Accessed 20 November 2021.
88. Medlineplus.gov. 2021. GCDH gene: MedlinePlus Genetics. Available at: https://medlineplus.gov/genetics/gene/gcdh/#:~:text=The%20GCDH%20gene%20provides%20instructions,are%20building%20blocks%20of%20proteins. Accessed 20 November 2021.
89. Medlineplus.gov. 2021. NOTCH3 gene: MedlinePlus Genetics. Available at: https://medlineplus.gov/genetics/gene/notch3/#:~:text=The%20NOTCH3%20protein%20plays%20a,supply%20blood%20to%20the%20brain. Accessed 20 November 2021.
90. Medlineplus.gov. 2021. PABPN1 gene: MedlinePlus Genetics. Available at: https://medlineplus.gov/genetics/gene/pabpn1/#conditions. Accessed 20 November 2021.
91. Medlineplus.gov. 2021. PKD1 gene: MedlinePlus Genetics. Available at: https://medlineplus.gov/genetics/gene/pkd1/#:~:text=Normal%20Function&text=The%20PKD1%20gene%20provides%20instructions,made%20in%20normal%20adult%20kidneys. Accessed 20 November 2021.
92. Medlineplus.gov. 2021. PKD2 gene: MedlinePlus Genetics. Available at: https://medlineplus.gov/genetics/gene/pkd2/#:~:text=Normal%20Function&text=The%20PKD2%20gene%20provides%20instructions,and%20in%20many%20adult%20tissues. Accessed 20 November 2021.
93. Medlineplus.gov. 2021. RERE gene: MedlinePlus Genetics. Available at: https://medlineplus.gov/genetics/gene/rere/. Accessed 20 November 2021.
94. Medlineplus.gov. 2021. SPAST gene: MedlinePlus Genetics. Available at: https://medlineplus.gov/genetics/gene/spast/. Accessed 20 November 2021.
95. Medlineplus.gov. 2021. TSC1 gene: MedlinePlus Genetics. Available at: https://medlineplus.gov/genetics/gene/tsc1/. Accessed 20 November 2021.
96. Medlineplus.gov. 2021. ZIC2 gene: MedlinePlus Genetics. [online] Available at: https://medlineplus.gov/genetics/gene/zic2/#:~:text=The%20ZIC2%20gene%20provides%20instructions,the%20activity%20of%20certain%20genes. Accessed 20 November 2021.
97. Mitsos AP, Samelis AI, Panteleakou-Sameli HM, Kottas GD. Arachnoid cyst of quadrigeminal cistern presenting as trigeminal neuralgia. Acta Neurochir. 2006;148(1):93–4.; ; discussion 94. https://doi.org/10.1007/s00701-005-0640-1.
98. Miyake S, Tamaki N, Nagashima T, Kurata H, Eguchi T, Kimura H. Idiopathic spinal cord herniation. Report of two cases and review of the literature. J Neurosurg. 1998;88(2):331–5. https://doi.org/10.3171/jns.1998.88.2.0331.
99. Miyamoto T, Ebisudani D, Kitamura K, Ohshima T, Horiguchi H, Nagahiro S. Surgical management of symptomatic intrasellar arachnoid cysts--two case reports. Neurol Med Chir (Tokyo). 1999;39(13):941–5. https://doi.org/10.2176/nmc.39.941.
100. Mussell HG, Dure LS, Percy AK, Grabb PS. Bobble-head doll syndrome: report of a case and review of the literature. Mov Disord. 1997;12(5):810–4. https://doi.org/10.1002/mds.870120534.
101. Nadkarni TD, Menon RK, Shah AH, Goel A. Chudley McCullough syndrome. Childs Nerv Syst. 2008;24(5):541–4. https://doi.org/10.1007/s00381-007-0518-z. Epub 2007 Oct 26
102. Najjar MW, Baeesa SS, Lingawi SS. Idiopathic spinal cord herniation: a new theory of pathogenesis. Surg Neurol. 2004;62(2):161–70; discussion 170–1. https://doi.org/10.1016/j.surneu.2003.10.030.

103. Ninds.nih.gov. 2021. Arachnoid Cysts Information Page|National Institute of Neurological Disorders and Stroke. Available at: https://www.ninds.nih.gov/Disorders/All-Disorders/Arachnoid-Cysts-Information-Page. Accessed 20 November 2021.
104. NORD (National Organization for Rare Disorders). 2021. KAT6A Syndrome—NORD (National Organization for Rare Disorders). Available at: https://rarediseases.org/rare-diseases/kat6a-syndrome/#:~:text=The%20KAT6A%20gene%20contains%20instructions,a%20type%20of%20histone%20acetyltransferase. Accessed 20 November 2021.
105. Odent S, Le Marec B, Toutain A, David A, Vigneron J, Tréguier C, Jouan H, Milon J, Fryns JP, Verloes A. Central nervous system malformations and early end-stage renal disease in oro-facio-digital syndrome type I: a review. Am J Med Genet. 1998;75(4):389–94.
106. Ogura Y, Miyake N, Kou I, Iida A, Nakajima M, Takeda K, Fujibayashi S, Shiina M, Okada E, Toyama Y, Iwanami A, Ishii K, Ogata K, Asahara H, Matsumoto N, Nakamura M, Matsumoto M, Ikegawa S. Identification of HOXD4 mutations in spinal extradural arachnoid cyst. PLoS One. 2015;10(11):e0142126. https://doi.org/10.1371/journal.pone.0142126.
107. Ohnishi YI, Fujimoto Y, Taniguchi M, Tsuzuki T, Taki T. Neuroendoscopically assisted cyst-cisternal shunting for a quadrigeminal arachnoid cyst causing typical trigeminal neuralgia. Minim Invasive Neurosurg. 2007;50(2):124–7. https://doi.org/10.1055/s-2007-982507.
108. Omim.org. 2021. OMIM Entry—* 300072—UBIQUITIN-SPECIFIC PROTEASE 9, X-LINKED; USP9X. Available at: https://www.omim.org/entry/300072. Accessed 20 November 2021.
109. Park SW, Cho KH, Shin YS, Kim SH, Ahn YH, Cho KG, Huh JS, Yoon SH. Helmetlike skull deformity with a large arachnoid cyst. Surg Neurol. 2006;65(1):95–8; discussion 98. https://doi.org/10.1016/j.surneu.2005.03.039.
110. Peter JC, Fieggen G. Congenital malformations of the brain--a neurosurgical perspective at the close of the twentieth century. Childs Nerv Syst. 1999;15(11–12):635–45. https://doi.org/10.1007/s003810050452.
111. Pradilla G, Jallo G. Arachnoid cysts: case series and review of the literature. Neurosurg Focus. 2007;22(2):E7. https://doi.org/10.3171/foc.2007.22.2.7.
112. Price SJ, David KM, O'Donovan DG, Aspoas AR. Arachnoid cyst of the craniocervical junction: case report. Neurosurgery. 2001;49(1):212–5. https://doi.org/10.1097/00006123-200107000-00034.
113. Qin X, Wang Y, Xu S, Hong X. Familial arachnoid cysts: a review of 35 families. Childs Nerv Syst. 2019;35(4):607–12. https://doi.org/10.1007/s00381-019-04060-z. Epub 2019 Jan 23
114. Quillo-Olvera J, Quillo-Reséndiz J, Gutiérrez-Partida CF, Rodríguez-García M. Quiste aracnoideo extradural espinal: reporte de un caso y revisión de la literatura [Spinal extradural arachnoid cyst: A case report and review of literature]. Cir Cir. 2017;85(6):544–8. https://doi.org/10.1016/j.circir.2016.09.003. Epub 2016 Oct 14
115. Renner C, Razeghi S, Uberall MA, Hartmann P, Lehnert W. Clinically asymptomatic glutaric aciduria type I in a 4 5/12-year-old girl with bilateral temporal arachnoid cysts. J Inherit Metab Dis. 1997;20(6):840–1. https://doi.org/10.1023/a:1005348624375.
116. Robson EA, Dixon L, Causon L, Dawes W, Benenati M, Fassad M, Hirst RA, Kenia P, Moya EF, Patel M, Peckham D, Rutman A, Mitchison HM, Mankad K, O'Callaghan C. Hydrocephalus and diffuse choroid plexus hyperplasia in primary ciliary dyskinesia-related MCIDAS mutation. Neurol Genet. 2020;6(4):e482. https://doi.org/10.1212/NXG.0000000000000482.
117. Sakellaridis N, Panagopoulos D, Mahera H. Sacral epidural noncommunicating arachnoid cyst. Case report and review of the literature. J Neurosurg Spine. 2007;6(5):473–8. https://doi.org/10.3171/spi.2007.6.5.473.
118. Serarslan Y, Melek IM, Sangün O, Akçora B, Akdemir G. Macrocephaly and bitemporal arachnoid cysts not associated with glutaric aciduria type I in a child. Turk Neurosurg. 2008;18(2):172–6.
119. Shekdar K. Posterior fossa malformations. Semin Ultrasound CT MR. 2011;32(3):228–41. https://doi.org/10.1053/j.sult.2011.02.003.
120. Shields JA, Shields CL, Eagle RC Jr, Arevalo F, De Potter P. Ophthalmic features of the organoid nevus syndrome. Trans Am Ophthalmol Soc. 1996;94:65–86; discussion 86–7. https://doi.org/10.1016/s0002-9394(14)70161-8.
121. Siddiqui S, Naaz S, Ahmad M, Khan ZA, Wahab S, Rashid BA. Encephalocraniocutaneous lipomatosis: A case report with review of literature. Neuroradiol J. 2017;30(6):578–82. https://doi.org/10.1177/1971400917693638. Epub 2017 Jul 14
122. Singleton WG, Lawrence T, Green AL, Jeans A, Kerr RS. Cerebellopontine angle arachnoid cyst containing ectopic choroid plexus--case report. Acta Neurochir. 2010;152(5):881–3. https://doi.org/10.1007/s00701-009-0516-x. Epub 2009 Oct 6
123. Sioutos P, Arbit E, Tsairis P, Gargan R. Spontaneous thoracic spinal cord herniation. A case report. Spine. 1996;21(14):1710–3. https://doi.org/10.1097/00007632-199607150-00019.
124. Slegers RJ, Blumcke I. Low-grade developmental and epilepsy associated brain tumors: a critical update 2020. Acta Neuropathol Commun. 2020;8(1):27. https://doi.org/10.1186/s40478-020-00904-x.
125. Society for Maternal-Fetal Medicine (SMFM), Yeaton-Massey A, Monteagudo A. Intracranial

cysts. Am J Obstet Gynecol. 2020;223(6):B42–6. https://doi.org/10.1016/j.ajog.2020.08.185. Epub 2020 Nov 7
126. Sugita K, Niizuma H, Suzuki J, Tsuburaya K. A case of arachnoid cyst in the middle cranial fossa presenting with trigeminal neuralgia. No Shinkei Geka. 1986;14(12):1481–5.
127. Suzuki H, Takanashi J, Sugita K, Barkovich AJ, Kohno Y. Retrocerebellar arachnoid cysts in siblings with mental retardation and undescended testis. Brain and Development. 2002;24(5):310–3. https://doi.org/10.1016/s0387-7604(02)00061-x.
128. Sweatman J, Beltechi R. Pneumosinus Dilatans: an exploration into the association between arachnoid cyst, meningioma and the pathogenesis of Pneumosinus Dilatans. Clin Neurol Neurosurg. 2019;185:105462. https://doi.org/10.1016/j.clineuro.2019.105462. Epub 2019 Aug 14
129. Thotakura AK, Marabathina NR. Acquired Chiari I malformation with syringomyelia secondary to colloid cyst with hydrocephalus-case report and review of literature. World Neurosurg. 2017;108:995.e1–4. https://doi.org/10.1016/j.wneu.2017.09.012. Epub 2017 Sep 9
130. Topsakal C, Kaplan M, Erol F, Cetin H, Ozercan I. Unusual arachnoid cyst of the quadrigeminal cistern in an adult presenting with apneic spells and normal pressure hydrocephalus--case report. Neurol Med Chir (Tokyo). 2002;42(1):44–50. https://doi.org/10.2176/nmc.42.44.
131. Tsai FC, Lee HJ, Wang AG, Hsieh SC, Lu YH, Lee MC, Pai JS, Chu TH, Yang CF, Hsu TR, Lai CJ, Tsai MT, Ho PH, Lin MC, Cheng LY, Chuang YC, Niu DM. Experiences during newborn screening for glutaric aciduria type 1: diagnosis, treatment, genotype, phenotype, and outcomes. J Chin Med Assoc. 2017;80(4):253–61. https://doi.org/10.1016/j.jcma.2016.07.006. Epub 2017 Mar 13
132. Utsunomiya H, Yamashita S, Takano K, Ueda Y, Fujii A. Midline cystic malformations of the brain: imaging diagnosis and classification based on embryologic analysis. Radiat Med. 2006;24(6):471–81. https://doi.org/10.1007/s11604-006-0049-7.
133. Vallée B, Mercier P, Menei P, Bouhour F, Fischer C, Fournier D, Bougeard R, Diabira S, Mahla K. Ventral transdural herniation of the thoracic spinal cord: surgical treatment in four cases and review of literature. Acta Neurochir. 1999;141(9):907–13. https://doi.org/10.1007/s007010050396.
134. van der Watt G, Owen EP, Berman P, Meldau S, Watermeyer N, Olpin SE, Manning NJ, Baumgarten I, Leisegang F, Henderson H. Glutaric aciduria type 1 in South Africa-high incidence of glutaryl-CoA dehydrogenase deficiency in black south Africans. Mol Genet Metab. 2010;101(2-3):178–82. https://doi.org/10.1016/j.ymgme.2010.07.018. Epub 2010 Aug 3
135. Verghese J, Mahore A, Goel A. Arachnoid cyst associated with painful tic convulsif. J Clin Neurosci. 2012;19(5):763–4. https://doi.org/10.1016/j.jocn.2011.07.039. Epub 2012 Feb 8
136. Visagan R, Wright D, Jayamohan J. Trigeminal neuralgia in a paediatric patient caused by arachnoid cyst. Br J Neurosurg. 2015;29(1):103–4. https://doi.org/10.3109/02688697.2014.957161. Epub 2014 Sep 15
137. Wang Y, Cui J, Qin X, Hong X. Familial intracranial arachnoid cysts with a missense mutation (c.2576C>T) in RERE: A case report. Medicine (Baltimore). 2018;97(50):e13665. https://doi.org/10.1097/MD.0000000000013665.
138. Database G. 2022. RTTN Gene - GeneCards | RTTN Protein|RTTN Antibody. Genecards.org. Available at: https://www.genecards.org/cgi-bin/carddisp.pl?gene=RTTN#:~:text=UniProtKB%2FSwiss%2DProt%20Summary%20for,of%20NODAL%2C%20LEFTY%20and%20PITX2. Accessed 1 September 2022.
139. Westermaier T, Vince GH, Meinhardt M, Monoranu C, Roosen K, Matthies C. Arachnoid cysts of the fourth ventricle - short illustrated review. Acta Neurochir. 2010;152(1):119–24. https://doi.org/10.1007/s00701-009-0309-2. Epub 2009 Apr 23
140. Wiese JA, Gentry LR, Menezes AH. Bobble-head doll syndrome: review of the pathophysiology and CSF dynamics. Pediatr Neurol. 1985;1(6):361–6. https://doi.org/10.1016/0887-8994(85)90073-6.
141. Wu X, Li G, Zhao J, Zhu X, Zhang Y, Hou K. Arachnoid cyst–associated chronic subdural hematoma: report of 14 cases and a systematic literature review. World Neurosurg. 2018;109:e118–30.
142. Yeaton-Massey A, Monteagudo A. Intracranial cysts. Am J Obstet Gynecol. 2020;223(6):B42–6.
143. Youssef A, D'Antonio F, Khalil A, Papageorghiou A, Ciardulli A, Lanzone A, Rizzo G, Thilaganathan B, Pilu G. Outcome of fetuses with supratentorial extra-axial intracranial cysts: A systematic review. Fetal Diagn Ther. 2016;40(1):1–12.
144. Yüksel D, Yilmaz D, Usak E, Senbil N, Gürer Y. Arachnoid cyst and costovertebral defects in Aicardi syndrome. J Paediatr Child Health. 2009;45(6):391–2. https://doi.org/10.1111/j.1440-1754.2009.01520.x.
145. Zakaria J, Wemhoff M, Anderson D. Microvascular decompression and arachnoid cyst fenestration for treatment of medulla oblongata compression caused by arachnoid cyst-vascular loop complex. World Neurosurg. 2018;113:293–5. https://doi.org/10.1016/j.wneu.2018.02.104. Epub 2018 Feb 25
146. Zarate YA, Boccuto L, Srikanth S, Pauly R, Ocal E, Balmakund T, Hinkle K, Stefans V, Schaefer GB, Collins RT 2nd. Constitutive activation of the PI3K-AKT pathway and cardiovascular abnormalities in an individual with Kosaki overgrowth syndrome. Am J Med Genet A. 2019;179(6):1047–52. https://doi.org/10.1002/ajmg.a.61145. Epub 2019 Apr 2
147. Zhang N, Qi Z, Zhang X, Zhong F, Yao H, Xu X, Liu J, Huang Y. Dandy-Walker syndrome associated

with syringomyelia in an adult: a case report and literature review. J Int Med Res. 2019;47(4):1771–7. https://doi.org/10.1177/0300060518808961. Epub 2019 Feb 24
148. Zieliński G, Podgórski JK, Koziarski A, Potakiewicz Z. Sródsiodłowa torbiel pajeczynówki. Opis przypadku i przeglad piśmiennictwa [Intrasellar arachnoid cyst. A case report and review of the literature]. Neurol Neurochir Pol. 2006;40(4):347–52; discussion 353
149. Zubairi MS, Carter RF, Ronen GM. A male phenotype with Aicardi syndrome. J Child Neurol. 2009;24(2):204–7. https://doi.org/10.1177/0883073808322337.

Natural History of Arachnoid Cysts

Alexander E. Braley and Walter A. Hall

1 Introduction

Arachnoid cysts (ACs) are localized collections of cerebrospinal fluid (CSF)-like fluid that may be present intracranially or within the spinal canal. They were first described by Richard Bright in 1831 [8]. These lesions have an incidence of around 3% in children and 1.4% in adults [6]. These cysts are lined by a membranous capsule and generally are asymptomatic and found incidentally on imaging studies. There is a small subset of patients who will experience AC growth through mechanisms which vary and are often disputed. Patients who develop symptoms may do so after cyst enlargement or even without a cyst size change. These symptoms vary from headaches and nausea to focal neurological deficits or endocrinologic aberrations depending on the size and location of the cyst. Asymptomatic lesions are typically monitored unless radiologic studies demonstrate progressive growth or until clinical symptoms develop. Around 5% of patients with intracranial ACs develop symptoms [6]. The symptomatology of these lesions is often difficult to characterize because patients often attribute a variety of symptoms to these lesions, especially after they are discovered incidentally, which may not demonstrate clear physiologic ties to causality [1]. These symptoms may or may not improve with surgery. A variety of surgical techniques are utilized to treat these lesions which include resection, fenestration, and shunting. However, less clear is the natural history of ACs.

A. E. Braley (✉) · W. A. Hall
Department of Neurosurgery, SUNY Upstate Medical University, Syracuse, NY, USA
e-mail: Braleya@upstate.edu; Hallw@upstate.edu

2 Natural History

The natural history of ACs is poorly understood in part because of the benign nature of these lesions. Given that the lesions are often found incidentally, it is also not surprising that the incidence of these lesions is higher in autopsy studies, and as routine imaging becomes more available and more commonplace, it is expected that these numbers will continue to increase [2, 6]. What is known about the natural history of ACs is that the vast majority are asymptomatic and will not enlarge enough to cause symptoms in the patient's lifetime (Fig. 1). The questions that are difficult to answer regarding ACs are when the cyst formed, how long it has been present, whether it will continue to increase in size, the rate at which the lesion may enlarge or shrink, and how to predict which lesions may become symptomatic in the future, in addition to whether pharmacologic or surgical intervention may prevent or delay this occurrence.

Al-Houlou et al. authored two large case series addressing the natural history of ACs in adults and children. For children, they showed that the lesions tended to be approximately 0.5 cm larger

M. Turgut et al. (eds.), *Arachnoid Cysts*, https://doi.org/10.1007/978-3-031-22701-1_9

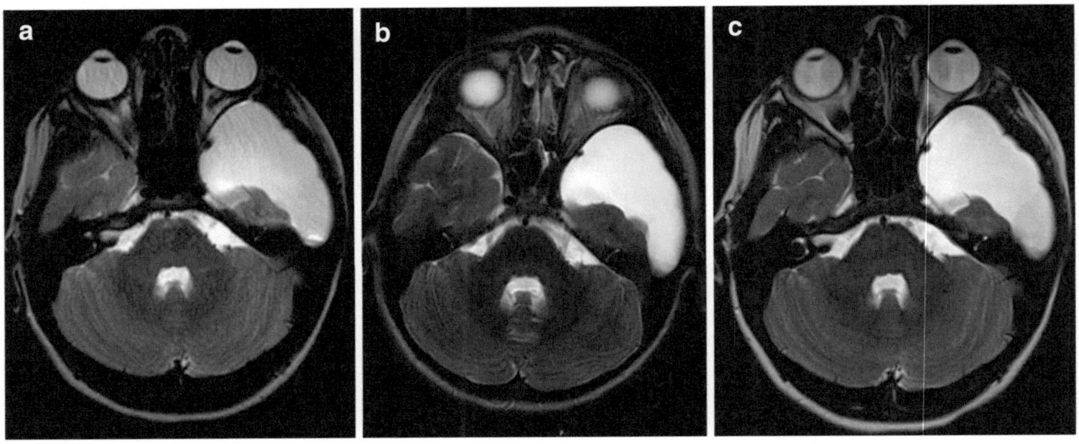

Fig. 1 Axial magnetic resonance imaging demonstrating a left middle fossa AC that was diagnosed in a 6-year-old female who presented with vomiting, fever, and headaches (**a**). The patient was diagnosed with rotavirus, and her symptoms were resolved with the passage of the viral infection. Conservative management was chosen for the AC. The cyst did enlarge on her 8-year-old follow-up MRI (**b**), but she remained asymptomatic. Another follow-up MRI at 11 years old (**c**) demonstrates stability of the lesion

in males (~3 cm^3 vs. 2.5 cm^3). They reported that the middle fossa was the most common location for development in 47% of patients. The posterior fossa was the next most common location in 38%. The remaining locations such as over the cerebral convexity, within the ventricles, the parasellar region, the interhemispheric fissure, or over the quadrigeminal plate were much less common. Most lesions are on the left side of the brain compared to the midline or on the right side (47% vs. 28% and 27%, respectively) [6]. Not surprisingly, larger cysts were highly correlated with symptom presence and eventual intervention. Anterior fossa and quadrigeminal plate cysts were more likely than posterior fossa lesions to require surgical treatment. Younger age at presentation correlated with cyst enlargement and the need for future intervention. Only 1 patient out of 309 suffered a posttraumatic hemorrhage into the AC [2].

In their adult series, Al-Houlou et al. demonstrated an incidence of 1.4% and that males had a higher incidence. The most common location was in the middle fossa (34%) in children. The next most common location for ACs was retrocerebellar, followed by convexity ACs which occur in 33% of patients and 14%, respectively [1]. The mean cyst size was approximately 2.5 cm^3. Middle fossa cysts tended to be on the left side of the brain, and cerebellopontine angle cysts tended to be on the right. Symptoms described in decreasing order of frequency ranged from headache, ataxia, seizures, dizziness, visual changes, nausea, vomiting, hearing loss, vertigo, and speech issues. Hydrocephalus and cervical myelopathy with syrinx have also been reported. Of the 203 patients with ACs followed on average for 3.8 years, 5 cysts showed to be enlarged and 2 cysts decreased in size with only 2 of the cysts that had enlarged causing the development of new symptoms [1].

Although symptomatic lesions usually undergo surgical intervention, asymptomatic lesions often do not change in size or character, and most neurosurgeons do not recommend serial imaging unless the lesions are large or are in a location at a higher risk for causing hydrocephalus in the future [6]. With this philosophy, these lesions often go for long intervals of time without being reimaged. Additionally, given that the cyst is mostly empty space, it is possible for the dimensions of the lesion to increase with growth of the skull, but this should not be regarded as actual growth of the lesion because the enlargement is proportional to the size of the skull. Studies show low rates of growth and symptomatic conversion for both adults and children; however, children tend to have a slightly higher risk of enlargement and the development of symptoms. Rates of lesion growth in children is around 10%, and symptoms develop in around 1% [2, 6, 7]. The growth rates for adults are often lower at around 2–3% increase in size where less than 1% become symptomatic [1, 6]. Huang et al. noted that 99% of their 412 ACs that received conservative management did not enlarge on follow-up imaging [7].

3 Growth and Resolution

The exact statistics on the proportion of patients who undergo cyst enlargement and the rate of growth, stagnation, and resolution are difficult to estimate because many patients who do not develop symptoms later in life never go on to receive further imaging. Although it may be safe to assume that patients who did not develop symptoms did not likely experience significant growth of their AC, there remains the possibility that the lesion may have enlarged. Rarely these lesions can decrease in size or even resolve spontaneously. Hall et al. reported a patient in their series who experienced headaches that were attributed to their AC and was scheduled for surgery; however, preoperative imaging showed complete resolution of the lesion [6]. These outcomes indicate that at least some of the lesions are blamed for symptoms that they are not causing, artificially increasing the number of "symptomatic" lesions [6].

The formation and growth of the lesions are not well understood. The creation is often described as an abnormal formation, splitting, or duplication of the arachnoid mater during development [3, 6]. Congenital ACs are thought to develop in the embryo during defective development of mesenchymal cells, or they are related to aberrant CSF flow [5, 7]. Previous concerns that ACs were caused by ischemic, traumatic, or infectious insults have been largely abandoned [8]. Pathologic evaluation of AC walls demonstrates duplicated layers of normal arachnoid that may have an increased collagen content, hyperplastic arachnoid cells, and will lack trabeculations seen in normal arachnoid [8]. Enlargement of ACs are hypothesized to occur by a one-way slit valve mechanism, osmotic gradient, or direct fluid secretion by the cyst lining cells [8, 10]. The spontaneous resolution of ACs has occurred albeit rarely. There have been associations with trauma leading to spontaneous resolution of an AC; however, cysts have resolved similarly without injury [3]. The mechanism of cyst resolution is not known; however, its association with trauma suggests a traumatic rupture of a membrane or the obliteration of a slit valve mechanism triggering the involution of the cyst.

4 Management

The management of ACs continues to be controversial for several reasons. First, there is difficulty in ascribing clinical symptoms definitively to the AC in question which will lead some surgeons to recommend surgery, whereas other surgeons might determine that the same lesion is not responsible for the symptoms that are present. There are many instances in patients who have had symptoms attributed to a cyst where they had surgical intervention without resolution of their symptoms. Alternatively, a patient who has a "symptomatic" cyst may have resolution of their symptoms without a change in the size of the lesion, calling into question the symptomatic nature of the lesion. There is a small risk of posttraumatic hemorrhage into an AC which leads some surgeons to consider this as a reason to offer surgery for an asymptomatic lesion; however, this risk is small, and patients who have hemorrhage into their AC tend to do well either with or without surgical evacuation of the hemorrhage [4, 8, 9]. As noted earlier, Al-Holou et al. noted that only 1 pediatric patient out of 309 patients with an AC had evidence of a posttraumatic intra-cystic hemorrhage [2]. Cress M et al. observed in a small case-control study that cysts with a cross-sectional diameter of over 5 cm were at an increased risk of rupture compared to those below 5 cm [4].

5 Conclusion

Intracranial ACs are relatively common intracranial lesions that are often discovered incidentally. These lesions may develop congenitally or may be acquired later in life. Their clinical course is usually benign in the vast majority of cases. Symptoms attributed to these cysts depend on their size and location but commonly include headaches and focal neurological deficits. Symptomatic lesions are likely overestimated in their incidence, and the vast majority are asymptomatic. We do not advocate for prophylactic surgery based on size or location. Conservative management should be the mainstay of treatment for ACs unless they are obviously symptomatic.

References

1. Al-Holou WN, Terman S, Kilburg C, Garton HJL, Muraszko KM, Maher CO. Prevalence and natural history of arachnoid cysts in adults. J Neurosurg. 2013;118:222–31.
2. Al-Holou WN, Yew AY, Boomsaad ZE, Garton HJL, Muraszko KM, Maher CO. Prevalence and natural history of arachnoid cysts in children. J Neurosurg Pediatr. 2010;5:578–85. https://doi.org/10.3171/2010.2.PEDS09464.
3. Cincu R, Agrawal A, Eiras J. Intracranial arachnoid cysts: current concepts and treatment alternatives. Clin Neurol Neurosurg. 2007;109:837–43. https://doi.org/10.1016/J.CLINEURO.2007.07.013.
4. Cress M, Kestle JRW, Holubkov R, Riva-Cambrin J. Risk factors for pediatric arachnoid cyst rupture/hemorrhage: a case-control study. Neurosurgery. 2013;72:716–22. https://doi.org/10.1227/NEU.0b013e318285b3a4.
5. Grossman TB, Uribe-Cardenas R, Radwanski RE, Souweidane MM, Hoffman CE. Arachnoid cysts: using prenatal imaging and need for pediatric neurosurgical intervention to better understand their natural history and prognosis. J Matern Fetal Neonatal Med. 2022;35(24):4728–33. https://doi.org/10.1080/14767058.2020.1863361.
6. Hall S, Smedley A, Sparrow O, Mathad N, Waters R, Chakraborty A, Tsitouras V. Natural history of intracranial arachnoid cysts. World Neurosurg. 2019;126:e1315–20. https://doi.org/10.1016/j.wneu.2019.03.087.
7. Huang JH, Mei WZ, Chen Y, Chen JW, Lin ZX. Analysis on clinical characteristics of intracranial arachnoid cysts in 488 pediatric cases. Int J Clin Exp Med. 2015;8(10):18343–50. http://www.ncbi.nlm.nih.gov/pubmed/26770437
8. Jafrani R, Raskin JS, Kaufman A, Lam S. Intracranial arachnoid cysts: pediatric neurosurgery update. Surg Neurol Int. 2019;10(1):15. https://doi.org/10.4103/sni.sni_320_18.
9. Parsch CS, Krauss J, Hofmann E, Meixensberger J, Roosen K. Arachnoid cysts associated with subdural hematomas and hygromas: analysis of 16 cases, long-term follow-up, and review of the literature. Neurosurgery. 1997;40:483–90. https://doi.org/10.1097/00006123-199703000-00010.
10. Santamarta D, Aguas J, Ferrer E. The natural history of arachnoid cysts: endoscopic and cine-mode MRI evidence of a slit-valve mechanism. Minim Invasive Neurosurg. 1995;38:133–7. https://doi.org/10.1055/s-2008-1053473.

Anatomic Locations of Arachnoid Cysts

Ali Akhaddar

1 Introduction

Arachnoid cysts (ACs), also known as "leptomeningeal cysts," are vesicles of cerebrospinal fluid (CSF) or CSF-like fluid found adjacent to normal CSF spaces. These cysts are extra axial and are limited by arachnoid membranes (a single layer of flattened mature and normal arachnoid cells) that may or may not communicate with the subarachnoid space [4, 19, 45]. These structures are benign, and most are congenital in origin (developmental lesions), although a small group may develop following inflammation, infection, bleeding, trauma, or even surgery [18, 34, 60]. ACs have various localizations in the central nervous system and are oriented by the anatomical location involved. Most cysts are located supratentorially with respect to an arachnoid cistern [7]. However, other locations are also reported, particularly in the posterior fossa and even in the spinal canal [2, 17, 45]. The incidence of spinal AC is much lower than those found in the intracranial space. Some congenital cysts may be associated with other neural anomalies [4, 22, 23, 41]. Clinical symptoms are highly variable and depend primarily on their anatomic location, cyst volume, and the patient's age.

With the widespread use of neuroimaging techniques, many incidental asymptomatic cysts are being discovered on computed tomography (CT) scans (Fig. 1) and magnetic resonance imaging (MRI) (Fig. 2) within all age groups. However, symptomatic cases occur mainly in early childhood. Although many authors recommend no treatment for small or asymptomatic cysts, there is still some debate regarding the best treatment strategy for symptomatic cysts requiring surgical decompression, excision, ligation of the communication site, fenestration, marsupialization, or shunting [7, 48, 58].

A summary of the intracranial and intraspinal distributions of AC is provided in this chapter realizing that the different classifications of AC will be discussed in Chap. 11 of the same book.

A. Akhaddar (✉)
Department of Neurosurgery, Mohammed V University in Rabat, Rabat, Morocco

Department of Neurosurgery, Avicenne Military Hospital of Marrakech, Mohammed V University in Rabat, Rabat, Morocco

M. Turgut et al. (eds.), *Arachnoid Cysts*, https://doi.org/10.1007/978-3-031-22701-1_10

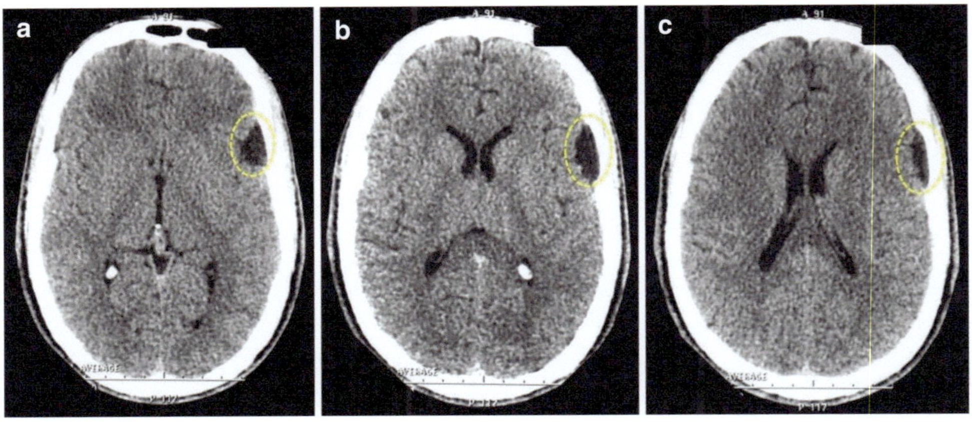

Fig. 1 Axial CT scan (**a–c**) demonstrating a small "asymptomatic" Sylvian fissure AC on the left side (dotted oval circle)

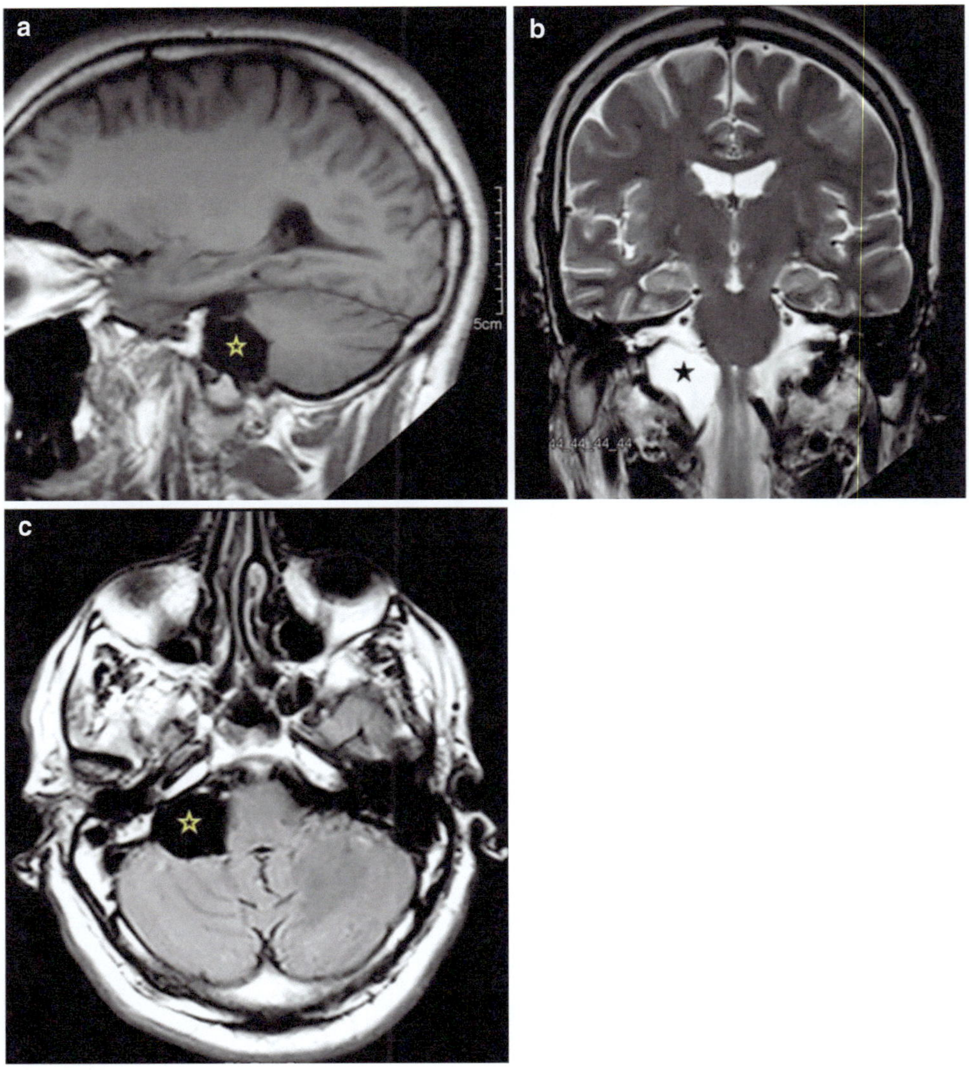

Fig. 2 "Asymptomatic" AC of the right cerebellopontine angle (stars). Sagittal T1-weighted MRI (**a**), coronal T2-weighted image (**b**), and axial FLAIR image (**c**)

2 Intracranial Locations of Arachnoid Cysts

Most intracranial ACs are in the supratentorial compartment [7, 25, 45]. About two-thirds occur in the Sylvian fissure and middle cranial fossa, anteromedial to the temporal lobe (Fig. 3). The second most common localization is in the posterior fossa (about 15%), which includes the cerebellopontine angle cistern (Fig. 2) and the retrocerebellar area (Figs. 4, 5, 6, 7 and 8). The next most frequent locations are the quadrigeminal (supracollicular) cistern (Fig. 9) and the sellar/suprasellar areas (Fig. 10) (10% each). Other supratentorial ACs are uncommon, such as over the brain convexities (principally the frontal lobes) (Fig. 11 and 12) and those in the interhemispheric fissure [4, 7, 19, 25, 53].

Some locations are rarely reported such as in the prepontine cistern (also known as retroclival),

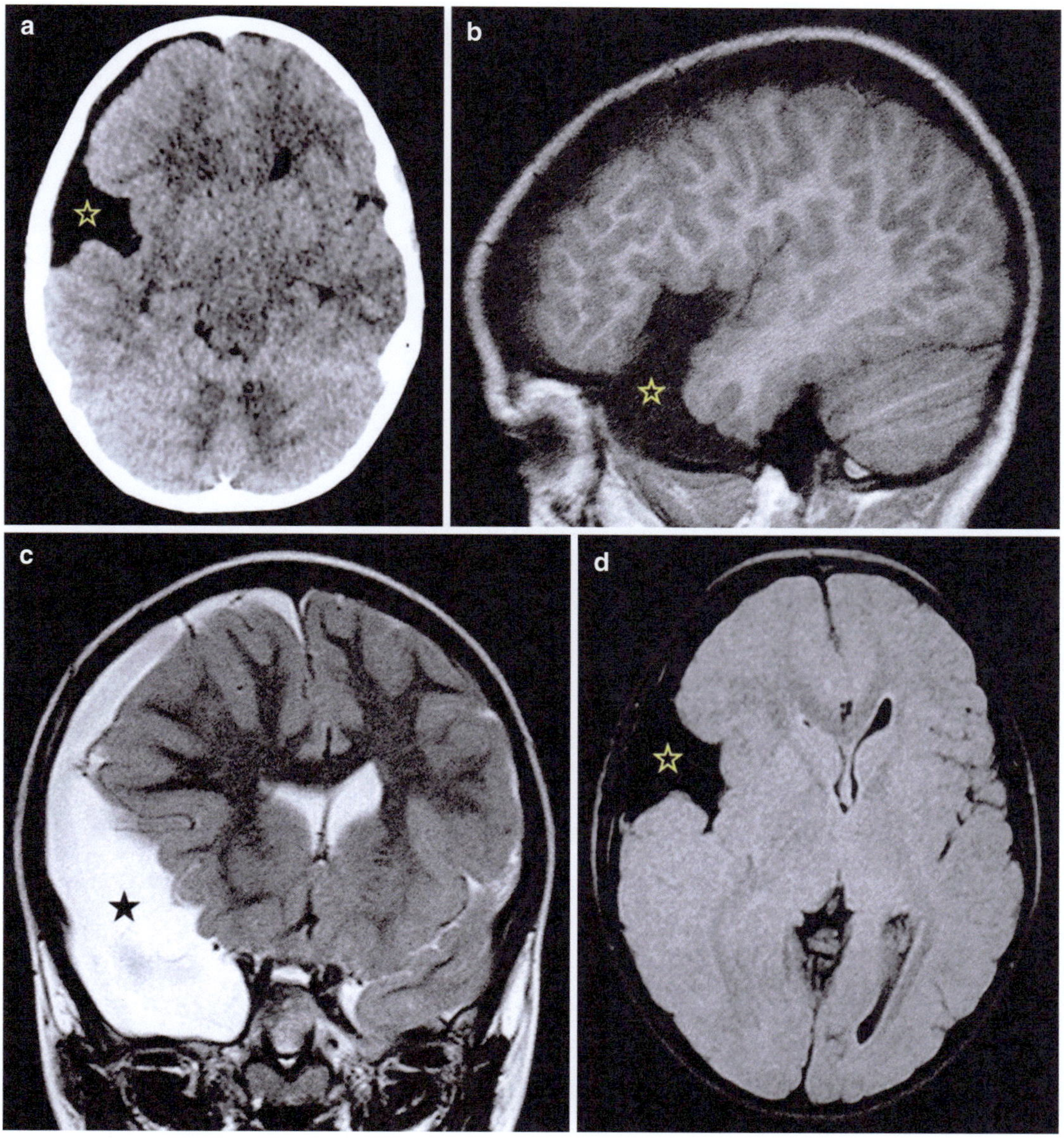

Fig. 3 Axial CT scan (**a**), sagittal T1-weighted MRI (**b**), coronal T2-weighted image (**c**), and axial fluid-attenuated inversion recovery (FLAIR) image (**d**) showing a middle cranial fossa AC on the right side (stars)

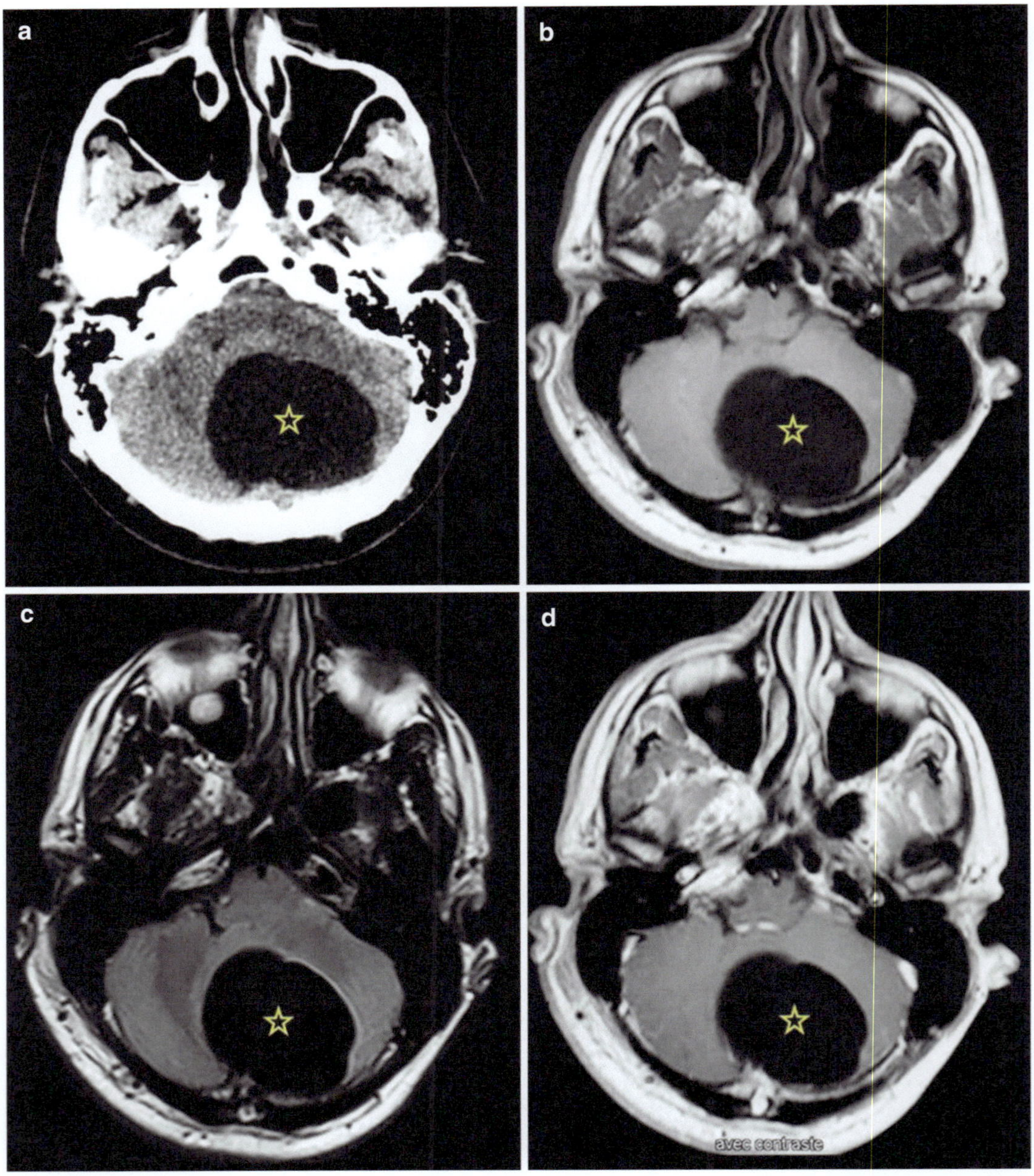

Fig. 4 Cerebellar AC. Axial CT scan (**a**), axial T1-weighted MRI (**b**), axial FLAIR image (**c**), and axial T1-weighted image following gadolinium administration (**d**)

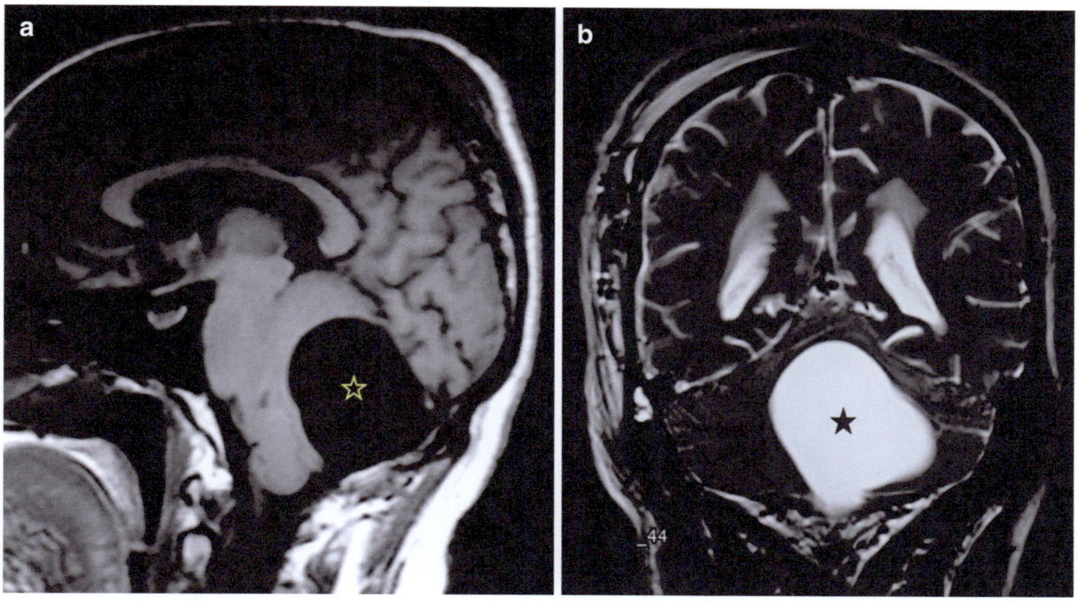

Fig. 5 Same case as Fig. 4. Cerebellar AC on MRI (stars). Sagittal T1-weighted MRI (**a**) and coronal T2-weighted image (**b**)

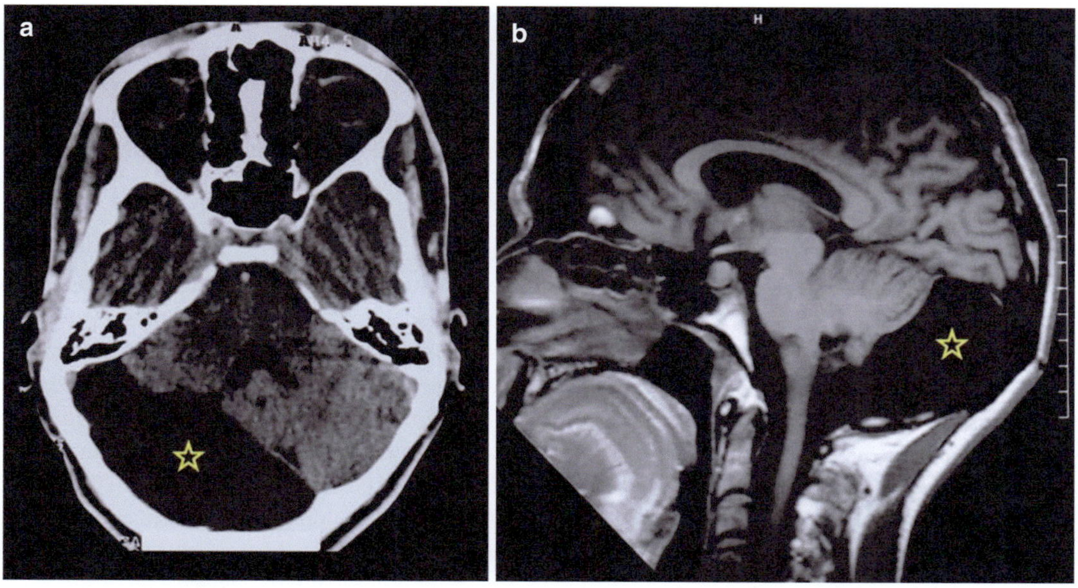

Fig. 6 Retrocerebellar AC (stars). Axial CT scan (**a**), sagittal T1-weighted MRI (**b**), axial T2-weighted image (**c**), and axial proton density-weighted image (**d**)

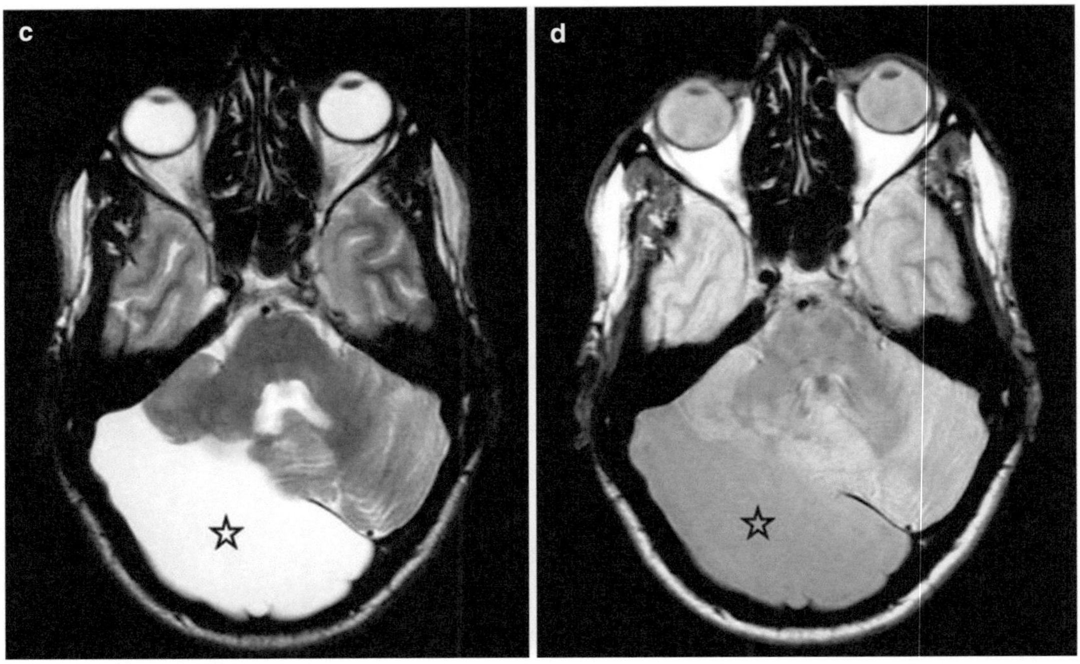

Fig. 6 (continued)

in the cervico-medullary junction area, and within the ventricular system [33, 40, 44, 49, 59]. A few other anecdotal cases have been described in the cavernous sinus [12, 31], within the internal auditory canal, in the perigeniculate region [32], in the foramen of Magendie [14], and also there are those that are extradural and intradiploic over the convexity [21, 27, 51].

ACs are usually unilateral and unilocular, but some multiple, multilocular, and bilateral cases have been reported principally in the middle cranial fossa and in the cerebellopontine angle [1, 42, 50, 55]. Regarding gender distribution and sidedness predominance, some studies have suggested that there is a left-sided and male preponderance for middle cranial fossa cysts as well as right sidedness and female preponderance for cerebellopontine angle ACs [4, 25].

ACs are present in different sizes, with some being small "incidental" asymptomatic cysts and others being large space-occupying lesions. Headaches are by far the most common symptom seen among patients with symptomatic intracranial AC [7]. Sometimes, the origin of large ACs is difficult to determine because these voluminous lesions are not restricted to a single anatomic location. In the presence of such a difficult determination, further neuroimaging studies should be requested whenever necessary. This may help in specifying the exact topography of the cysts and their internal structures, defining the precise margins of the collections, and determining their relationship to adjacent anatomic formations. Assessment of any communication between the cyst and the surrounding subarachnoid space is also very important in the pretreatment evaluation.

Large temporal cysts often have suprasellar extension, and suprasellar cysts may have prepontine components. Also, large cysts in the lateral cerebellomedullary cistern can often have both cranial and cervical expansions [33, 40, 44, 59]. On the other hand, some suprasellar AC may elevate the floor of the third ventricle causing obstructive hydrocephalus, and these cysts appear to originate within the ventricle on MR imaging. In addition, some large suprasellar AC may extend downward into the sella. True intrasellar ACs without suprasellar extension are unusual

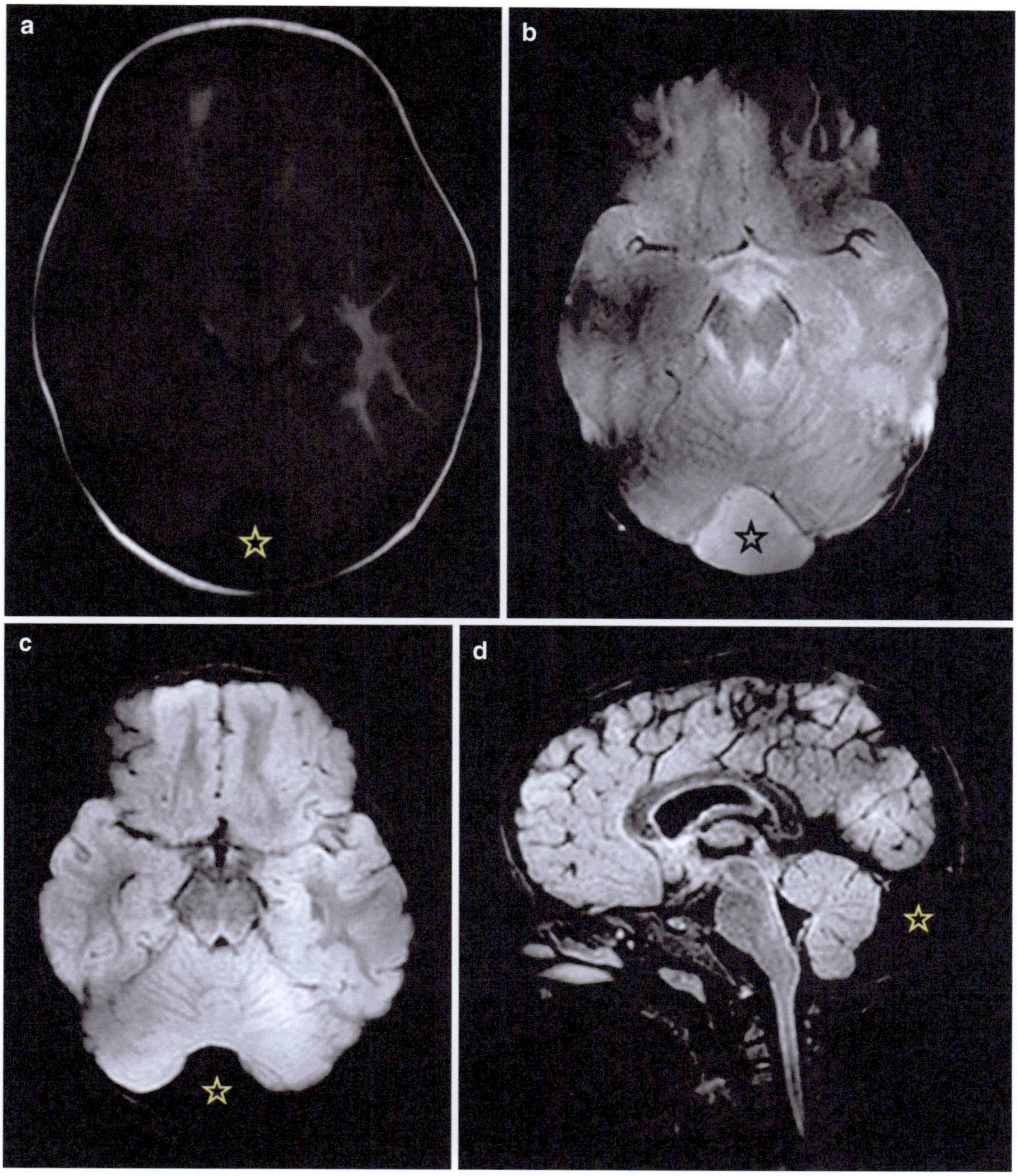

Fig. 7 Retrocerebellar AC (stars). Axial T1- (**a**) and T2-weighted MRI (**b**). Axial (**c**) and sagittal FLAIR images (**d**)

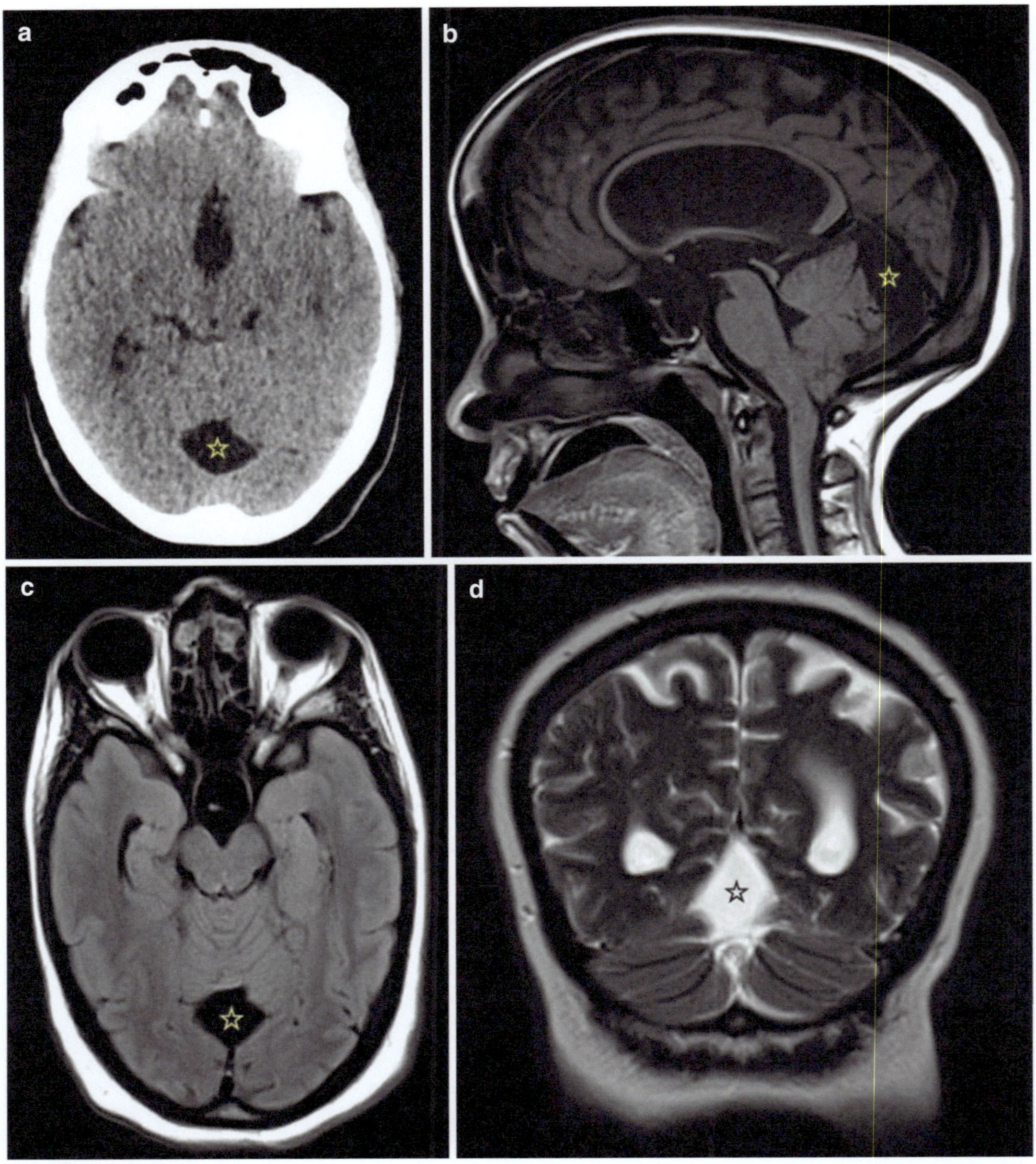

Fig. 8 Retrocerebellar and supracerebellar AC (stars). Axial CT scan (**a**), sagittal T1-weighted MRI (**b**), axial FLAIR image (**c**), and coronal T2-weighted image (**d**)

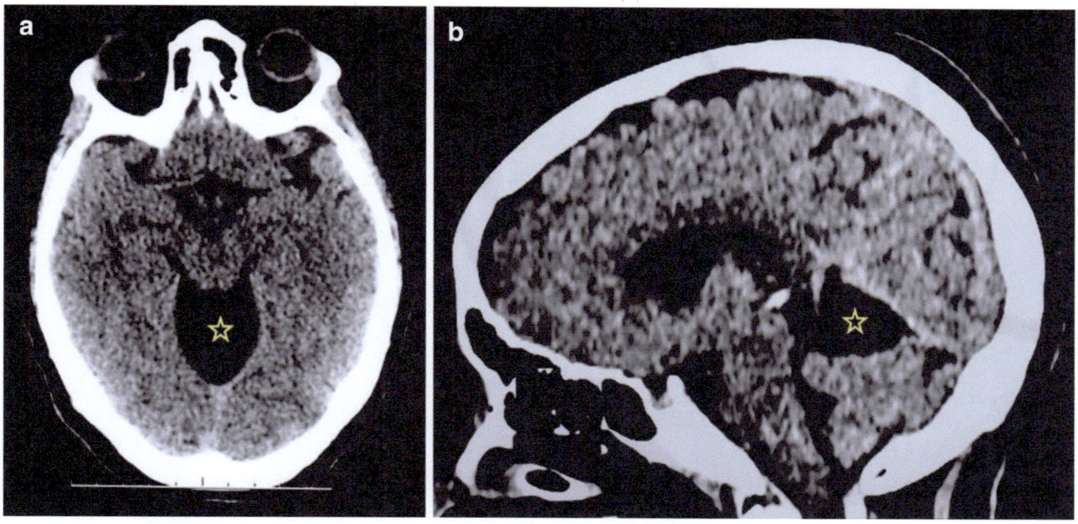

Fig. 9 Supracerebellar and quadrigeminal AC (stars). Axial (**a**) and sagittal CT scans (**b**)

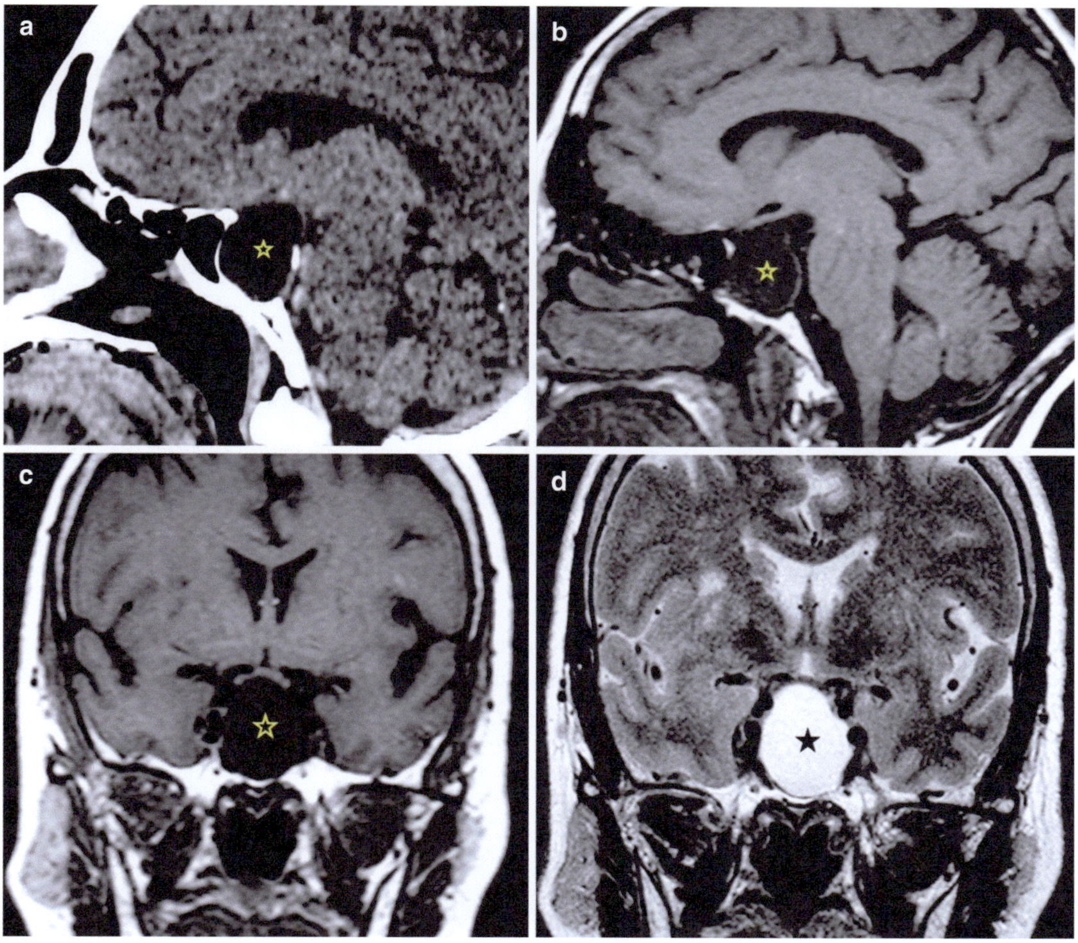

Fig. 10 Intrasellar and suprasellar AC (stars). Sagittal CT scan (**a**), sagittal T1-weighted MRI (**b**), and coronal T1- (**c**) and T2-weighted images (**d**)

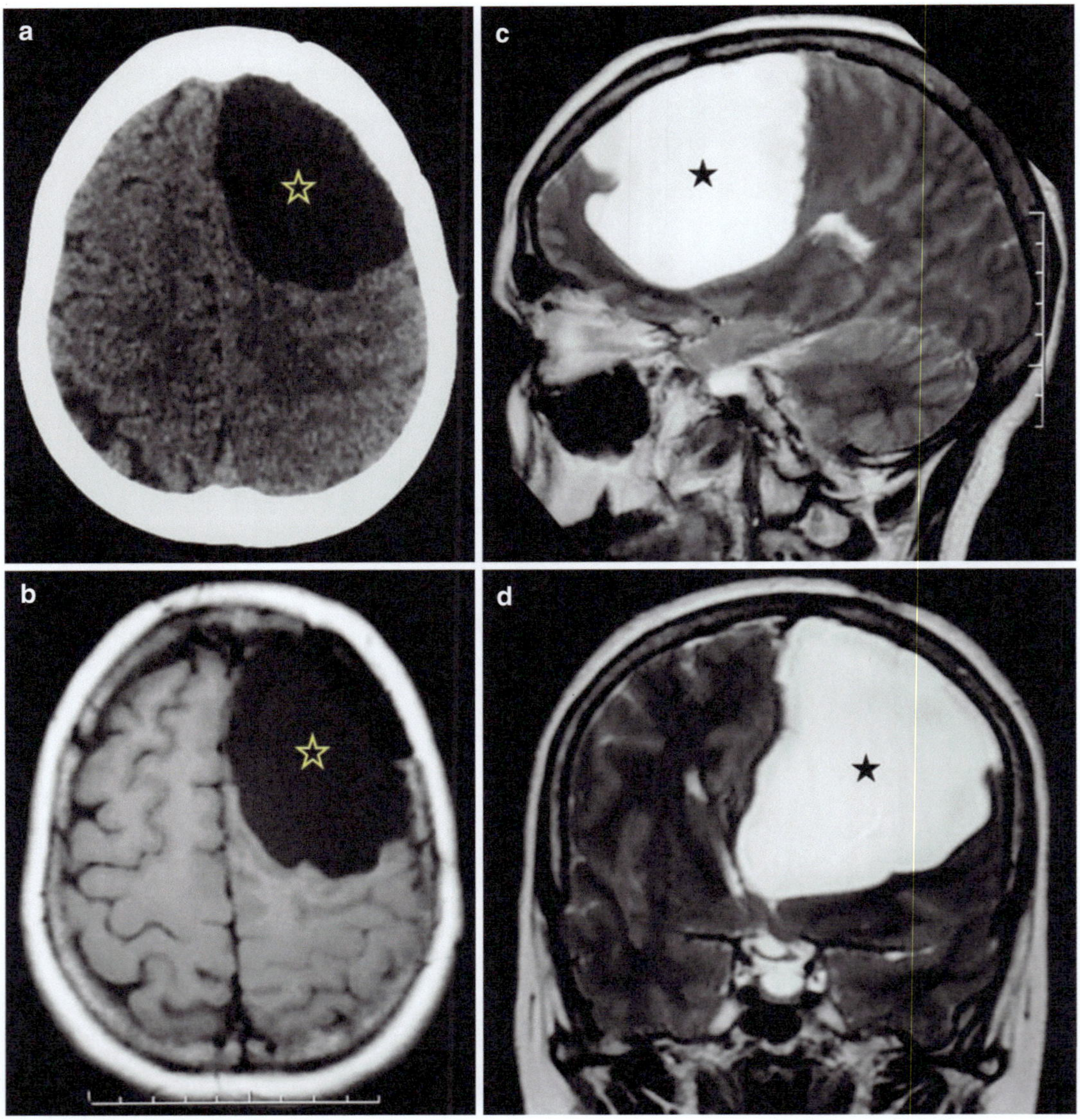

Fig. 11 Axial CT scan (**a**), axial T1-weighted MRI (**b**), and sagittal (**c**) and coronal T2-weighted image (**d**) revealing a frontal cerebral convexity AC on the left side (stars)

conditions that are sometimes confused or associated with cases of empty sella syndrome [23]. Over time, cranial bone and neural and vascular structures contiguous with the cystic lesion may be compressed and/or displaced. Also, some ACs may have an extracranial extension with or without spontaneous CSF fistula formation [24, 32, 47]. Intraneural ACs are rare, but some optic nerve cysts have been described within the orbit [3, 9, 11, 13].

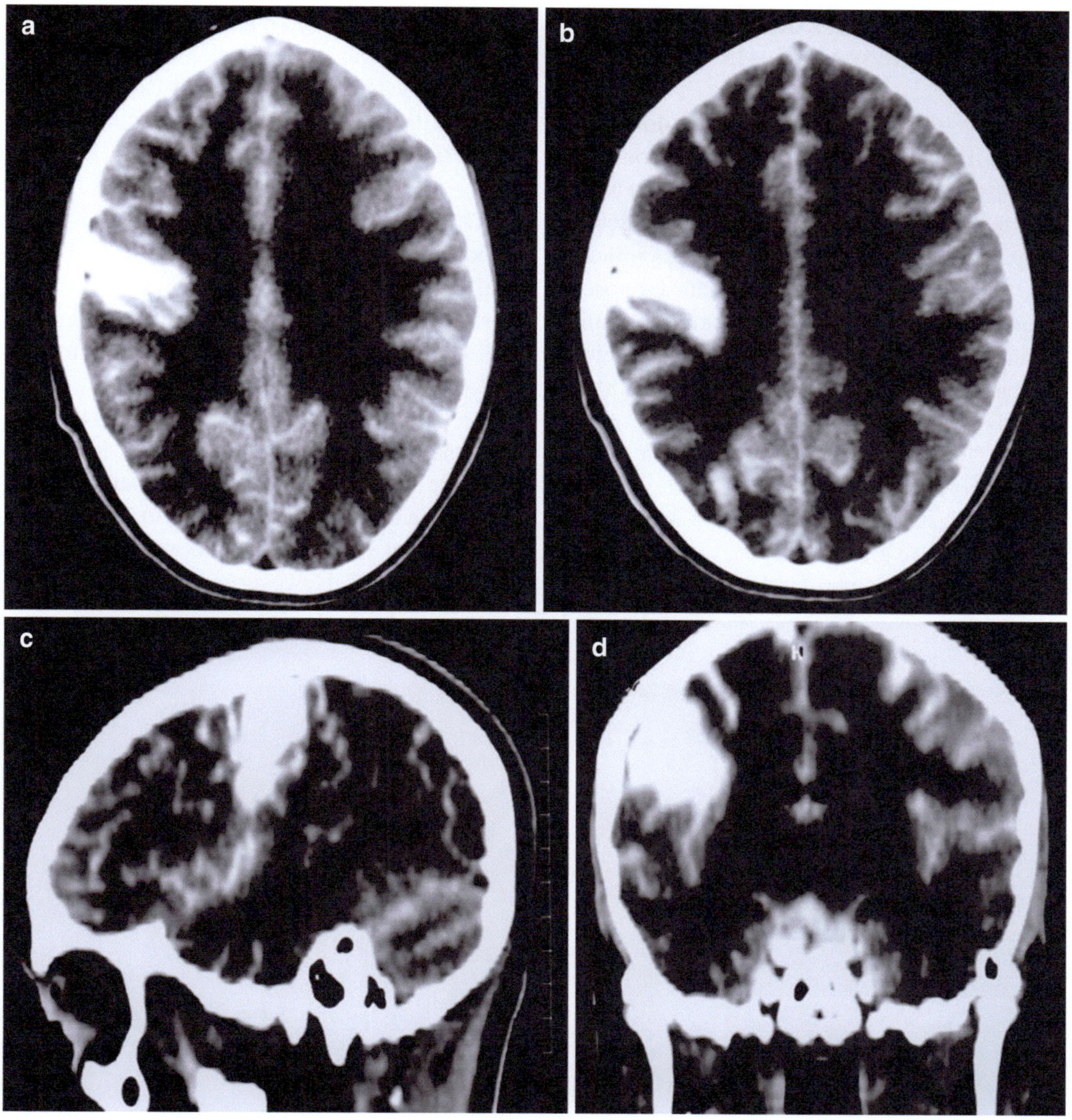

Fig. 12 Communicating AC with the subdural space in the right frontoparietal area. CT cisternography image showing filling of the cyst 2 h after metrizamide intrathecal injection. Axial (**a**, **b**), sagittal (**c**), and coronal (**d**) images

3 Intraspinal Locations of Arachnoid Cysts

The incidence of spinal AC is much lower than that of the intracranial cysts. The literature on spinal AC is sparse and generally limited to case reports and small case series [8, 17, 20, 26, 30]. They can be intradural, extradural, or perineural [20, 50, 52]. In 1988, Nabors' team proposed a simplified well-known classification of spinal meningeal cysts, containing three main categories based on their topographic location [38]:

Type I: Cysts are extradural without spinal nerve root fibers.
Type II: Cysts are extradural with spinal nerve root fibers (e.g., Tarlov cyst).
Type III: Cysts are intradural.

Type I was subdivided into extradural cysts (type *IA*) and sacral meningoceles (type *IB*).
Type III cysts can be intradural extramedullary (type *IIIA*) or intradural intramedullary (type *IIIB*).

The most common site of spinal AC is in the middle or lower thoracic spine with several vertebral segments being involved (Figs. 13 and 14). Less common locations are, in decreasing order of frequency, as follows: lumbar and lumbosacral, thoracolumbar, and sacral. The cervical spine is rarely involved with AC [46, 48]. The vast majority of cysts are typically limited to three or four vertebral body segments craniocaudally and therefore restricted to a single spinal segment or a junction between two spinal segments [6, 20]. However, extensive ACs involv-

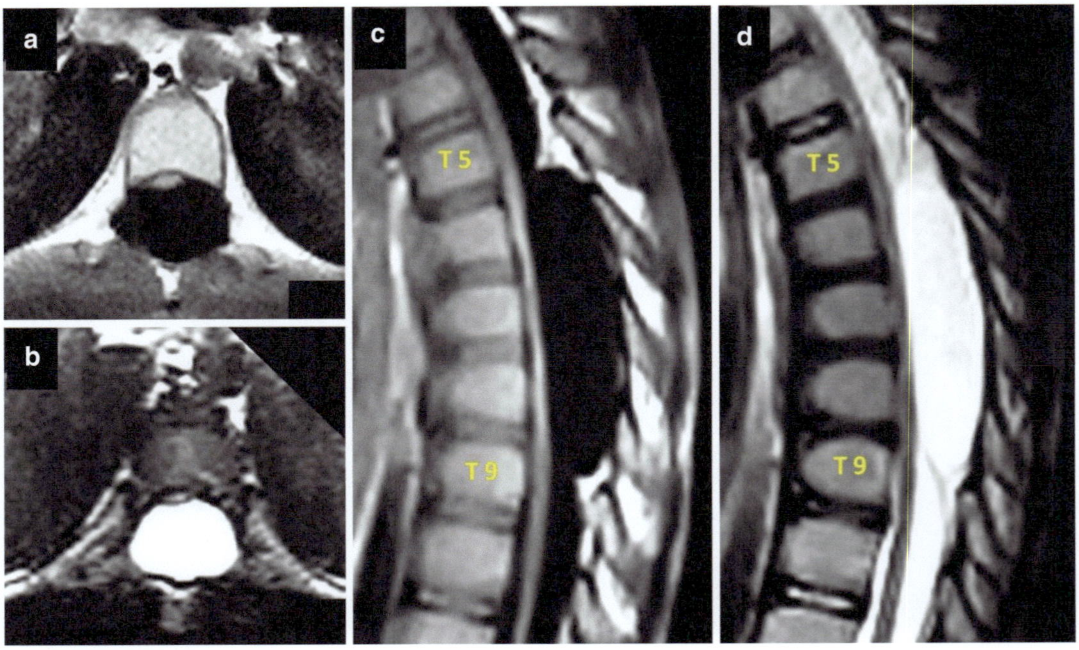

Fig. 13 T5–T9 spinal extradural AC located posterior to the spinal cord in an 11-year-old girl. Axial T1- (**a**) and T2-weighted (**b**) MRI, sagittal T1- (**c**) and T2-weighted images (**d**)

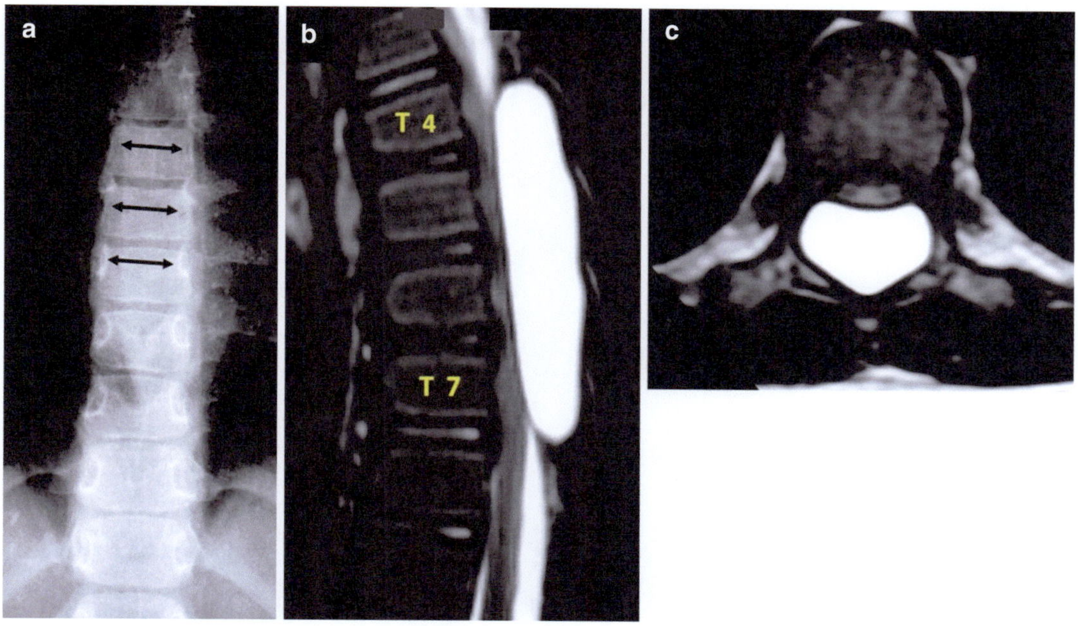

Fig. 14 T4–T7 spinal extradural AC with posterior spinal cord compression in an 8-year-old boy. Enlarged spinal canal (double arrows) on anteroposterior spinal thoracic radiogram (**a**). Sagittal (**b**) and axial T2-weighted MRI (**c**)

ing multiple segments of the spinal axis *have been* already *described* [18, 28, 37, 48]. *Furthermore, large s*pinal extradural cysts may have significant paraspinal extension or intra-abdominal organ compression [54].

The predominance of the disease in the thoracic spine may be because it is the longest part of the spine and also has a narrow diameter, allowing for faster neurologic symptoms to develop when the spinal cord is compressed [57]. Furthermore, for many authors, intradural ACs arise from the septum posticum (the fibrous membrane joining the arachnoid and pia along the posterior line of the spinal cord) which is principally sited in the posterior thoracic spine [43, 46]. The majority of ACs are most likely related to an idiopathic condition (more than 90%), whereas less than 10% may result from secondary conditions such as intraspinal inflammation, infection (Fig. 15), hemorrhage, and injury, following a spinal anesthetic procedure or even secondary to spinal surgery [18, 34, 36, 39, 56, 58, 60].

Associated congenital anomalies such as syringomyelia, spina bifida, tethered cord, diastematomyelia, meningocele, or Chiari malformations [22, 35, 41] are more common in the pediatric population principally among patients with intradural AC. Most spinal ACs are single, but multiloculated and multiple epidural cysts have been previously described [10, 15, 28, 35, 37, 48]. ACs with multiple septations are more often related to secondary etiologies, especially those resulting from delayed postinfectious meningitis (Fig. 15).

Extradural spinal ACs are commonly located posterior to the spinal cord at the thecal sac nerve root sleeve junction, in the dorsal midline, or in the nerve root sleeve itself (Figs. 13 and 14). A

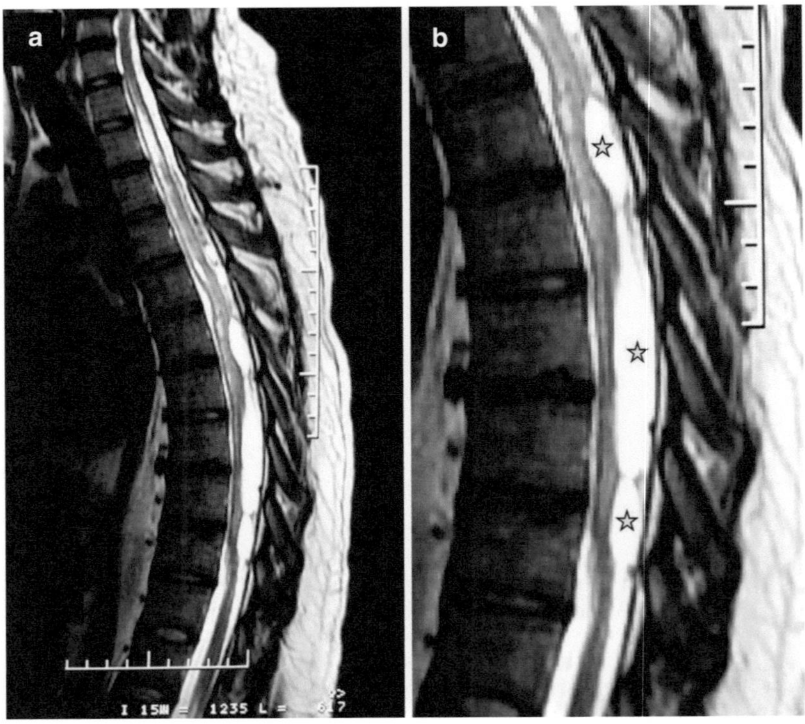

Fig. 15 Intradural multiloculated AC (stars): complications of tuberculous meningitis (stars). Sagittal (**a**, **b**) T2-weighted MRI

few have been reported to extend into or through the neural foramen. There is usually a dural defect that allows the cyst to communicate with the intradural arachnoid space through a narrow channel [20, 45]. Spinal ACs generally develop among adolescents; however, all age groups can be affected. Thoracic cysts typically occur among young adolescents, whereas lumbar and sacral cysts are more often found among adults in the fourth decade of life. About twice as many cases occur in males compared to female patients. Most perineural cysts are known as Tarlov cysts located in the sacrum (Figs. 16 and 17).

Intradural cysts are generally located retromedullary (posterior) in more than 75%; however, a few cases have been found pre-medullary (anterior) [29, 57] and even intramedullary (within the spinal cord) [16, 26, 30, 46]. Indeed, fewer than 20 cases of intramedullary ACs have been reported in the literature [26]. In addition, intradural ACs may be associated with an intramedullary syrinx (Fig. 15) in more than 66% of cases [46]. Some authors have suggested that this association is related to a delayed complication of spinal surgery or spinal cord injury [5].

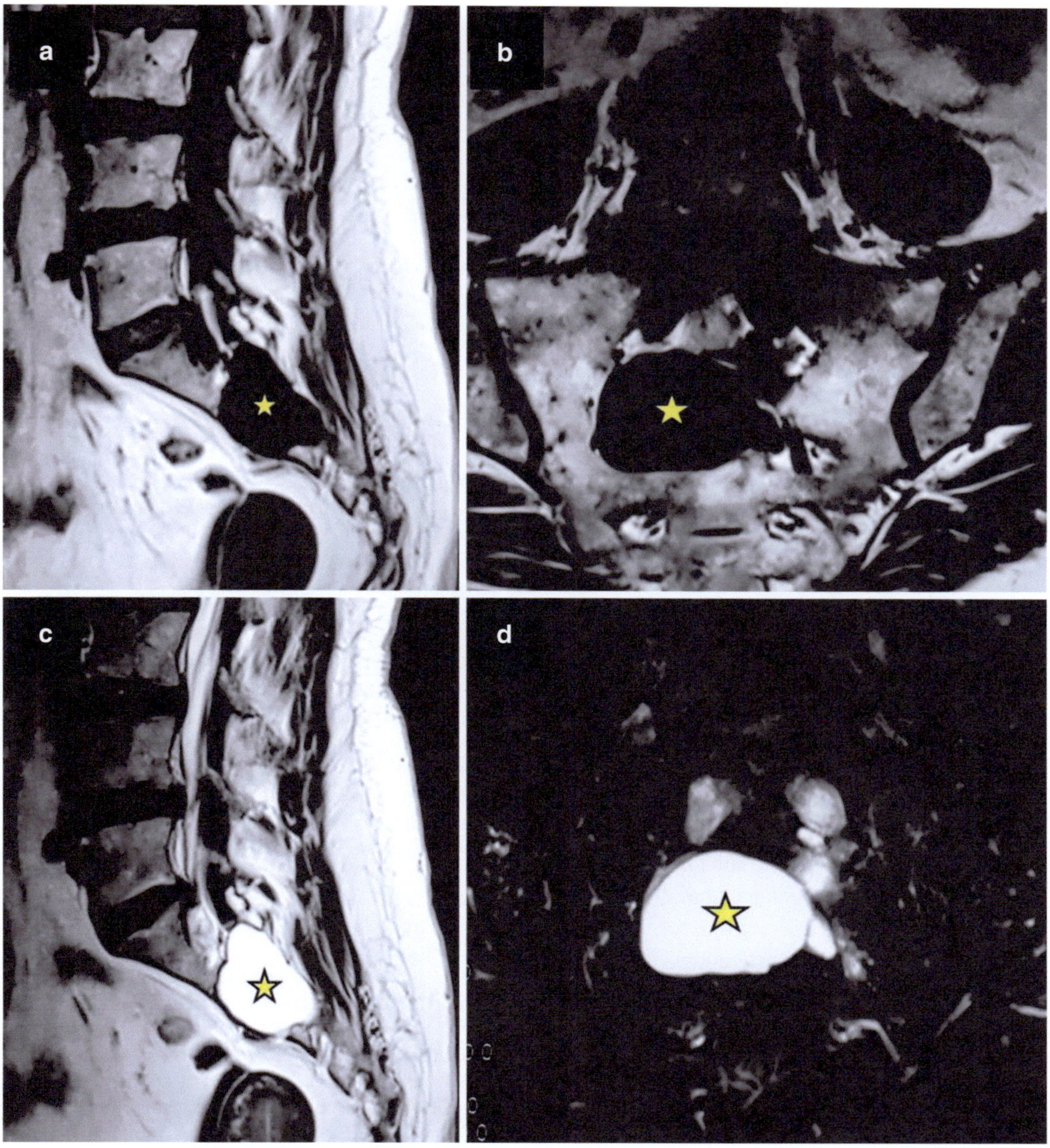

Fig. 16 S2 Tarlov cyst in an adult (stars). Sagittal (**a**) and coronal (**b**) T1-weighted MRI. Sagittal T2-weighted image (**c**), and coronal MR image on STIR sequence (**d**)

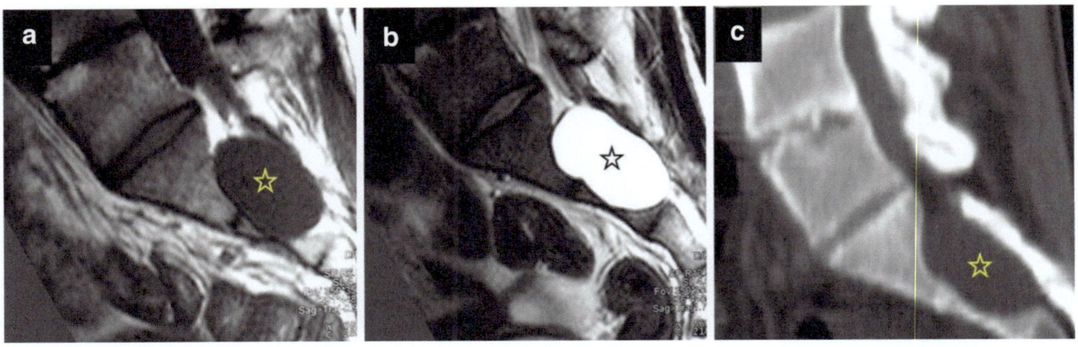

Fig. 17 S1–S2 Tarlov cyst in an adult (stars). Sagittal T1- (**a**) and T2-weighted MRI (**b**). Sagittal spinal CT scan on bone window (**c**)

4 Conclusion

AC is an uncommon heterogeneous pathologic entity that is more complex than was previously thought. These cystic lesions appear in various shapes, sizes, and anatomic localizations. These locations include cranial, spinal, intradural, extradural, perineural, intraventricular, intraparenchymatous, primitive, or secondary forms that are seen in all age groups. Topographic considerations and the relationship between the cysts and the meninges as well as other adjacent neurologic structures are necessary to better assess the clinical and neuroimaging findings and enhance our ability to discuss the best therapeutic option for each case. Future supplementary investigations focusing on etiology and pathogenesis and pathophysiology should be conducted for a better understanding of the development of AC and a more accurate diagnosis associated with better therapeutic results.

References

1. Abbas M, Khairy S, AlWohaibi M, Aloraidi A, AlQurashi WW. Bilateral temporal extradural hematoma on top of bilateral temporal arachnoid cyst: first case report and extensive literature review. World Neurosurg. 2018;115:134–7. https://doi.org/10.1016/j.wneu.2018.04.040.
2. Aithala GR, Sztriha L, Amirlak I, Devadas K, Ohlsson I. Spinal arachnoid cyst with weakness in the limbs and abdominal pain. Pediatr Neurol. 1999;20:155–6. https://doi.org/10.1016/s0887-8994(98)00131-3.
3. Akor C, Wojno TH, Newman NJ, Grossniklaus HE. Arachnoid cyst of the optic nerve: report of two cases and review of the literature. Ophthalmic Plast Reconstr Surg. 2003;19:466–9. https://doi.org/10.1097/01.IOP.0000092798.36098.9C.
4. Al-Holou WN, Terman S, Kilburg C, Garton HJ, Muraszko KM, Maher CO. Prevalence and natural history of arachnoid cysts in adults. J Neurosurg. 2013;118:222–31. https://doi.org/10.3171/2012.10.JNS12548.
5. Andrews BT, Weinstein PR, Rosenblum ML, Barbaro NM. Intradural arachnoid cysts of the spinal canal associated with intramedullary cysts. J Neurosurg. 1988;68:544–9. https://doi.org/10.3171/jns.1988.68.4.0544.
6. Bond AE, Zada G, Bowen I, McComb JG, Krieger MD. Spinal arachnoid cysts in the pediatric population: report of 31 cases and a review of the literature. J Neurosurg Pediatr. 2012;9:432–41. https://doi.org/10.3171/2012.1.PEDS11391.
7. Boutarbouch M, El Ouahabi A, Rifi L, Arkha Y, Derraz S, El Khamlichi A. Management of intracranial arachnoid cysts: institutional experience with initial 32 cases and review of the literature. Clin Neurol Neurosurg. 2008;110:1–7. https://doi.org/10.1016/j.clineuro.2007.08.009.
8. Bowman JJ, Edwards CC 2nd. Extradural arachnoid cyst with bony erosion: a rare case report. J Spine Surg. 2020;6:736–42. https://doi.org/10.21037/jss-20-590.
9. Brewington D, Petrov D, Whitmore R, Liu G, Wolf R, Zager EL. De novo intraneural arachnoid cyst presenting with complete third nerve palsy: case report and literature review. World Neurosurg. 2017;98:873.e27–31. https://doi.org/10.1016/j.wneu.2016.11.124.
10. Cavalcante-Neto JF, e Silva-Neto LS, PRL L, CHS M, EML R, Cristino-Filho G, et al. Multiple extradural spinal arachnoid cysts: a case report. Surg Neurol Int. 2021;12:101. https://doi.org/10.25259/SNI_105_2021.
11. Celli P, Palma L, Palatisky E. Congenital extradural cyst of the orbital optic nerve: case report. Neurosurgery. 1983;13:208–10. https://doi.org/10.1227/00006123-198308000-00020.

12. Cheng CH, Lin HL, Cho DY, Chen CC, Liu YF, Chiou SM. Intracavernous sinus arachnoid cyst with optic neuropathy. J Clin Neurosci. 2010;17:267–9. https://doi.org/10.1016/j.jocn.2009.05.027.
13. Das D, Deka P, Deka AC, Bhattacharjee K, Bhattacharjee H, Das JK, Kuri GC. An unusual case of retrobulbar arachnoid cyst and its management. Orbit. 2009;28:169–71. https://doi.org/10.1080/01676830902765933.
14. de Oliveira Filho ÍT, Romero PC, Fontoura EAF, de Oliveira SD, Botelho RV. Symptomatic foramen of Magendie arachnoid cyst in an elderly patient: the second case report in the literature. Surg Neurol Int. 2019;10:189. https://doi.org/10.25259/SNI_380_2019.
15. Fam MD, Woodroffe RW, Helland L, Noeller J, Dahdaleh NS, Menezes AH, et al. Spinal arachnoid cysts in adults: diagnosis and management. A single-center experience. J Neurosurg Spine. 2018;29:711–9. https://doi.org/10.3171/2018.5.SPINE1820.
16. Fortuna A, Mercuri S. Intradural spinal cysts. Acta Neurochir. 1983;68:289–314. https://doi.org/10.1007/BF01401186.
17. French H, Somasundaram A, Biggs M, Parkinson J, Allan R, Ball J, et al. Idiopathic intradural dorsal thoracic arachnoid cysts: a case series and review of the literature. J Clin Neurosci. 2017;40:147–52. https://doi.org/10.1016/j.jocn.2017.02.051.
18. Fukumoto H, Samura K, Katsuta T, Miki K, Fukuda K, Inoue T. Extensive multilocular spinal extradural meningeal cyst that developed 16 years after traumatic brachial plexus injury: a case report. World Neurosurg. 2016;86(510):e5–10. https://doi.org/10.1016/j.wneu.2015.10.027.
19. Galassi E, Tognetti F, Gaist G, Fagioli L, Frank F, Frank G. CT scan and metrizamide CT cisternography in arachnoid cysts of the middle cranial fossa: classification and pathophysiological aspects. Surg Neurol. 1982;17:363–9. https://doi.org/10.1016/0090-3019(82)90315-9.
20. Garg K, Borkar SA, Kale SS, Sharma BS. Spinal arachnoid cysts—our experience and review of literature. Br J Neurosurg. 2017;31:172–8. https://doi.org/10.1080/02688697.2016.1229747.
21. Gorgulu A, Albayrak BS. Giant intradiploic leptomeningeal cyst of the posterior fossa. Acta Neurochir. 2006;148:923–4. https://doi.org/10.1007/s00701-006-0791-8.
22. Habibi Z, Hanaei S, Nejat F. Sacral extradural arachnoid cyst in association with split cord malformation. Spine J. 2016;16:1109–15. https://doi.org/10.1016/j.spinee.2016.05.016.
23. Hatipoğlu HG, Cetin MA, Gürses MA, Dağlioğlu E, Sakman B, Yüksel E. Petrous apex cephalocele and empty Sella/arachnoid cyst coexistence: a clue for cerebrospinal fluid pressure imbalance? Diagn Interv Radiol. 2010;16:7–9. https://doi.org/10.4261/1305-3825.DIR.2650-09.2.
24. Hayashi Y, Futami K, Munemoto S, Hamada Y, Soma M, Yamashita J, et al. Congenital arachnoid cyst mimicking meningocele. Pediatr Neurosurg. 2002;36:324–8. https://doi.org/10.1159/000063537.
25. Helland CA, Lund-Johansen M, Wester K. Location, sidedness, and sex distribution of intracranial arachnoid cysts in a population-based sample. J Neurosurg. 2010;113:934–9. https://doi.org/10.3171/2009.11.JNS081663.
26. Ichinose T, Miyashita K, Tanaka S, Oikawa N, Oishi M, Nambu I, et al. Recurrent spinal intramedullary arachnoid cyst: case report and literature review. World Neurosurg. 2020;138:68–72. https://doi.org/10.1016/j.wneu.2020.02.106.
27. Iplikcioglu AC, Dinc C, Bikmaz K, Bek S, Gokduman CA, Cosar M. Non-traumatic intradiploic arachnoid cyst. Acta Neurochir. 2006;148:659–62. https://doi.org/10.1007/s00701-006-0746-0.
28. Kahraman S, Anik I, Gocmen S, Sirin S. Extradural giant multiloculated arachnoid cyst causing spinal cord compression in a child. J Spinal Cord Med. 2008;31:306–8. https://doi.org/10.1080/10790268.2008.11760728.
29. Kazan S, Ozdemir O, Akyüz M, Tuncer R. Spinal intradural arachnoid cysts located anterior to the cervical spinal cord. Report of two cases and review of the literature. J Neurosurg. 1999;91(2 Suppl):211–5. https://doi.org/10.3171/spi.1999.91.2.0211.
30. Kendall BE, Valentine AR, Keis B. Spinal arachnoid cysts: clinical and radiological correlation with prognosis. Neuroradiology. 1982;22:225–34. https://doi.org/10.1007/BF00342069.
31. Kidani N, Onishi M, Kurozumi K, Date I. The supposed intracavernous sinus arachnoid cyst with abducens neuropathy: a case report. Neurol Med Chir (Tokyo). 2014;54:582–6. https://doi.org/10.2176/nmc.cr.2013-0092.
32. Lee EE, Andresen NS, McKenzie B, Sharon JD, Francis HW, Sun DQ. Perigeniculate arachnoid cysts and CSF fistulae of the fallopian canal: histopathologic correlates of a rare clinical entity. World J Otorhinolaryngol Head Neck Surg. 2021;7:71–81. https://doi.org/10.1016/j.wjorl.2020.12.005.
33. Manzo M, D'Urso PI. Craniocervical junction arachnoid cyst. Surg Neurol Int. 2020;11:34. https://doi.org/10.25259/SNI_609_2019.
34. Mao HQ, Yang HL, Geng DC, Bao ZH, Tang TS. Spinal extradural arachnoid cyst following percutaneous vertebroplasty. Eur Spine J. 2011;20(2(Suppl 2)):S206–10. https://doi.org/10.1007/s00586-010-1569-5.
35. Moses ZB, Friedman GN, Penn DL, Solomon IH, Chi JH. Intradural spinal arachnoid cyst resection: implications of duraplasty in a large case series. J Neurosurg Spine. 2018;28:548–54. https://doi.org/10.3171/2017.8.SPINE17605.
36. Muthukumar N. Anterior cervical arachnoid cyst presenting with traumatic quadriplegia. Childs Nerv Syst. 2004;20:757–60. https://doi.org/10.1007/s00381-003-0903-1.
37. Myles LM, Gupta N, Armstrong D, Rutka JT. Multiple extradural arachnoid cysts as a cause of spinal cord compression in a child. Case report. J Neurosurg.

1999;91(1 Suppl):116–20. https://doi.org/10.3171/spi.1999.91.1.0116.
38. Nabors MW, Pait TG, Byrd EB, Karim NO, Davis DO, Kobrine AI, et al. Updated assessment and current classification of spinal meningeal cysts. J Neurosurg. 1988;68:366–77. https://doi.org/10.3171/jns.1988.68.3.0366.
39. Nath PC, Mishra SS, Deo RC, Satapathy MC. Intradural spinal arachnoid cyst: a long-term Postlaminectomy complication: a case report and review of the literature. World Neurosurg. 2016;85(367):e1–4. https://doi.org/10.1016/j.wneu.2015.09.058.
40. Panigrahi S, Mishra SS, Das S, Patra SK, Satpathy PC. Large intradural craniospinal arachnoid cyst: a case report and review of literature. J Craniovertebr Junction Spine. 2012;3:16–8. https://doi.org/10.4103/0974-8237.110119.
41. Patankar AP. Spinal intradural arachnoid cyst associated with diastematomyelia in an adult: a case report and review of literature. Br J Neurosurg. 2019;17:1–3. https://doi.org/10.1080/02688697.2019.1666087.
42. Patel RA, Levy ML, Crawford JR. Spontaneous subdural haemorrhage in a child with bilateral middle cranial fossa arachnoid cysts. BMJ Case Rep. 2013;2013:bcr2013200802. https://doi.org/10.1136/bcr-2013-200802.
43. Perret G, Green D, Keller J. Diagnosis and treatment of intradural arachnoid cysts of the thoracic spine. Radiology. 1962;79:425–9. https://doi.org/10.1148/79.3.425.
44. Price SJ, David KM, O'Donovan DG, Aspoas AR. Arachnoid cyst of the craniocervical junction: case report. Neurosurgery. 2001;49:212–5. https://doi.org/10.1097/00006123-200107000-00034.
45. Rengachary SS, Watanabe I. Ultrastructure and pathogenesis of intracranial arachnoid cysts. J Neuropathol Exp Neurol. 1981;40:61–83.
46. Sadek AR, Nader-Sepahi A. Spinal arachnoid cysts: presentation, management and pathophysiology. Clin Neurol Neurosurg. 2019;180:87–96. https://doi.org/10.1016/j.clineuro.2019.03.014.
47. Sagardoy T, de Mones E, Bonnard D, Darrouzet V, Franco-Vidal V. Arachnoid cyst of the fallopian canal and geniculate ganglion area: our experience of 9 cases. Clin Otolaryngol. 2017;42:461–6. https://doi.org/10.1111/coa.12629.
48. Samura K, Morioka T, Miyagi Y, Nagata S, Mizoguchi M, Mihara F, et al. Surgical strategy for multiple huge spinal extradural meningeal cysts. Case report. J Neurosurg. 2007;107(4 Suppl):297–302. https://doi.org/10.3171/PED-07/10/297.
49. Sarica C, Ziyal MI. Retroclival arachnoid cysts: case series, literature review, and new classification proposal. World Neurosurg. 2019;121:e898–907. https://doi.org/10.1016/j.wneu.2018.10.006.
50. Sharma A, Sharma A, Mittal RS, Gandhi A. Bilateral cerebellopontine arachnoid cyst: a rare entity. Br J Neurosurg. 2015;29:576–8. https://doi.org/10.3109/02688697.2015.1015100.
51. Sharma R, Gupta P, Mahajan M, Sharma P, Gupta A, Khurana A. Giant nontraumatic intradiploic arachnoid cyst in a young male. Radiol Bras. 2016;49:337–9. https://doi.org/10.1590/0100-3984.2013.0022.
52. Singh S, Bhaisora KS, Sardhara J, Das KK, Attri G, Mehrotra A, et al. Symptomatic extradural spinal arachnoid cyst: more than a simple herniated sac. J Craniovertebr Junction Spine. 2019;10:64–71. https://doi.org/10.4103/jcvjs.JCVJS_12_19.
53. Spennato P, Ruggiero C, Aliberti F, Buonocore MC, Trischitta V, Cinalli G. Interhemispheric and quadrigeminal cysts. World Neurosurg. 2013;79((2 Suppl)):S20.e1-7. https://doi.org/10.1016/j.wneu.2012.02.010.
54. Srinivas B, Joseph V, Chacko G, Rajshekhar V. Extradural developmental dural root sleeve cyst presenting as a lumbar paraspinal mass with renal compression in an infant. J Neurosurg Pediatr. 2010;5:586–90. https://doi.org/10.3171/2010.2.PEDS09324.
55. Tatli M, Guzel A. Bilateral temporal arachnoid cysts associated with tuberous sclerosis complex. J Child Neurol. 2007;22:775–9. https://doi.org/10.1177/0883073807304014.
56. Velz J, Fierstra J, Regli L, Germans MR. Spontaneous spinal subarachnoid hemorrhage with development of an arachnoid cyst-a case report and review of the literature. World Neurosurg. 2018;119:374–80. https://doi.org/10.1016/j.wneu.2018.08.108.
57. Wang MY, Levi AD, Green BA. Intradural spinal arachnoid cysts in adults. Surg Neurol. 2003;60:49–55. https://doi.org/10.1016/s0090-3019(03)00149-6.
58. Werner C, Mathkour M, Scullen T, Dallapiazza RF, Dumont AS, Maulucci CM. Recurrent arachnoid cysts secondary to spinal adhesive arachnoiditis successfully treated with a ventriculoperitoneal shunt. Clin Neurol Neurosurg. 2020;194:105835. https://doi.org/10.1016/j.clineuro.2020.105835.
59. Yanaka K, Hyodo A, Fujimori H, Yoshii Y, Nose T. Foramen magnum meningioma and arachnoid cyst coinciding in the lateral cerebellomedullary cistern--case report. Neurol Med Chir (Tokyo). 1992;32:581–4. https://doi.org/10.2176/nmc.32.581.
60. Yuen J, McGavin L, Adams W, Haden N. Intradural symptomatic arachnoid cyst formation following noninstrumented lumbar decompression. Br J Neurosurg. 2021;35:352–7. https://doi.org/10.1080/02688697.2020.1817313.

Classification of Arachnoid Cysts

Mehmet Saim Kazan and Ahmet Özak

1 Introduction

Arachnoid cysts (ACs) are non-tumorous pathological entities in which a cavity is filled with a cerebrospinal fluid (CSF)-like fluid, frequently communicating with the subarachnoid space, containing collagen and cells within the arachnoid membrane [7, 47]. Bright described the ACs more than 170 years ago (1831) and noted correctly in his monograph that such cysts were found "... in connection with the arachnoid, and apparently lying between the layers ..." and that they were "... formed by the splitting of the arachnoid membrane..." [50].

ACs often arise within and expand the margins of CSF cisterns rich in arachnoid membrane (i.e., Sylvian fissures, suprasellar, quadrigeminal, cerebellopontine angle, and posterior infratentorial midline cisterns) [1, 3, 9, 18] (Fig. 1). It may be difficult to distinguish between porencephalic cysts and ACs, since the structures they originate from are cisternal compartments (Fig. 2). ACs comprise 1% of all intracranial space-occupying lesions. The prevalence in adults is approximately 1.4% with a female preponderance, while the prevalence in children is 2.6% [2, 3, 32, 40]. Based on 208 reported cases in the literature in 1981, Watanabe and Rengachary found the following distribution in their comprehensive study: Sylvian fissure 103 (49%), cerebellopontine angle 22 (11%), supracollicular area 21 (10%), vermian area 19 (9%), sellar and suprasellar area 18 (9%), interhemispheric fissure 10 (5%), cerebral convexity 9 (4%) (Fig. 3), and clival area 6 (3%) [43] (Fig. 4). Rarely, ACs are also seen in intraventricular location (Fig. 5).

The increasing widespread use of imaging modalities has undoubtedly lowered the threshold for radiological examinations of patients with headache, which is the dominating symptom in patients with intracranial ACs. As a consequence, the diagnosis of ACs is now made more often than before. In a population-based study, the intracranial distribution among 299 patients with 305 cysts (6 patients with bitemporal cysts) was as follows: the vast majority "198 patients (66.2%)" had cysts located in the middle cranial fossa (included the 6 patients with bitemporal cysts), 42 (14%) had frontal cysts, 36 (12%) had cysts in the posterior fossa, and 23 (7.7%) had cysts located in various other places of the neurocranium [21, 49]. ACs very rarely occur within the ventricular system, where no arachnoid tissue exists. However, intraventricular AC might be originated from the arachnoid layer drawn into the choroidal fissure with choroidal vascular mesenchyme [36].

ACs can be congenital (primer, developmental, splitting, or duplication of the primitive arachnoid membrane) cysts (also called "true" ACs and occur to be the most common type) often or secondary ACs. This should be differen-

M. S. Kazan (✉) · A. Özak
Department of Neurosurgery, Akdeniz University School of Medicine, Antalya, Turkey

M. Turgut et al. (eds.), *Arachnoid Cysts*, https://doi.org/10.1007/978-3-031-22701-1_11

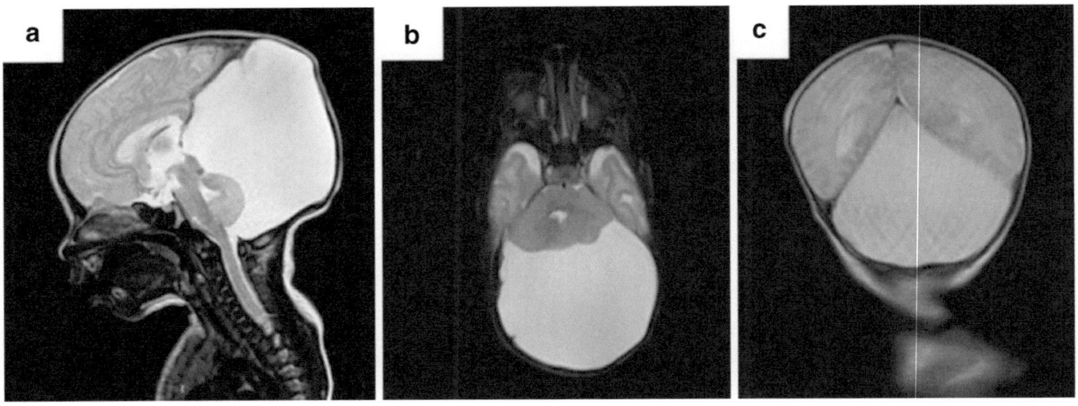

Fig. 1 Giant posterior fossa AC. T2-weighted sequence sagittal, axial, and coronal view

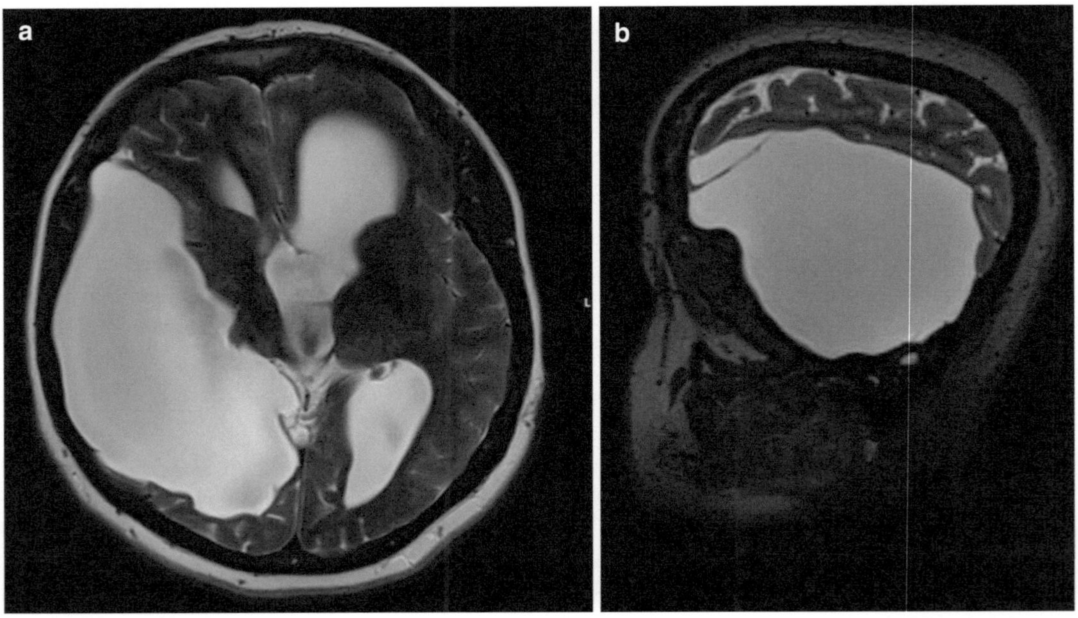

Fig. 2 A 42-year-old female case. Asymptomatic, incidentally detected right temporal cystic lesion. Axial and sagittal views of T2-weighted sequence MRI. Differentiation between arachnoid and porencephalic cysts can be difficult

tiated from other types of cysts that result from CSF sequestration due to inflammation, brain trauma, surgery, hemorrhage, chemical irritation, and tumors; these are called secondary ACs. They differ from secondary (acquired) cysts by the structure of their cyst walls, which contains arachnoid cells connected with unaltered arachnoid matter. In secondary cysts, which usually occur after inflammatory or traumatic process, the loculations of CSF are surrounded by arachnoid adhesions. The intracranial ACs (both congenital and acquired forms) are invariably intradural, while the spinal cyst may be either intradural or extradural [6, 8–10, 43, 48].

A variety of classification systems exist for ACs. Huang et al. used CT cisternography (CTC) to divide the ACs into (1) noncommunicating ACs (NCIACs), where the cyst and subarachnoid space are not connected, and (2) communicating ACs (CIACs), where the cysts and subarachnoid space are interlinked and CSF can flow freely between the two parts. CTC has

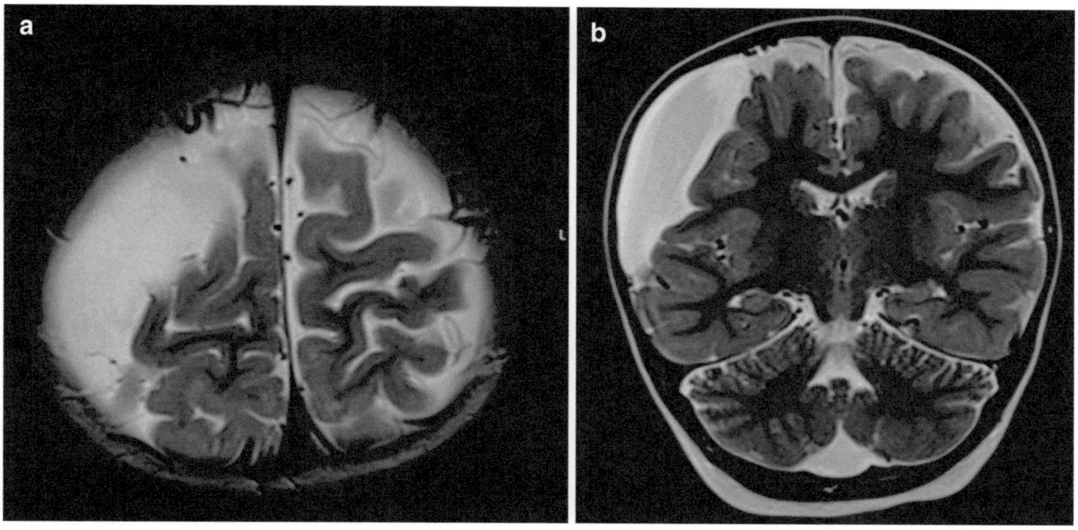

Fig. 3 Right parietal convexity AC T2-weighted sequence MRI axial and coronal views

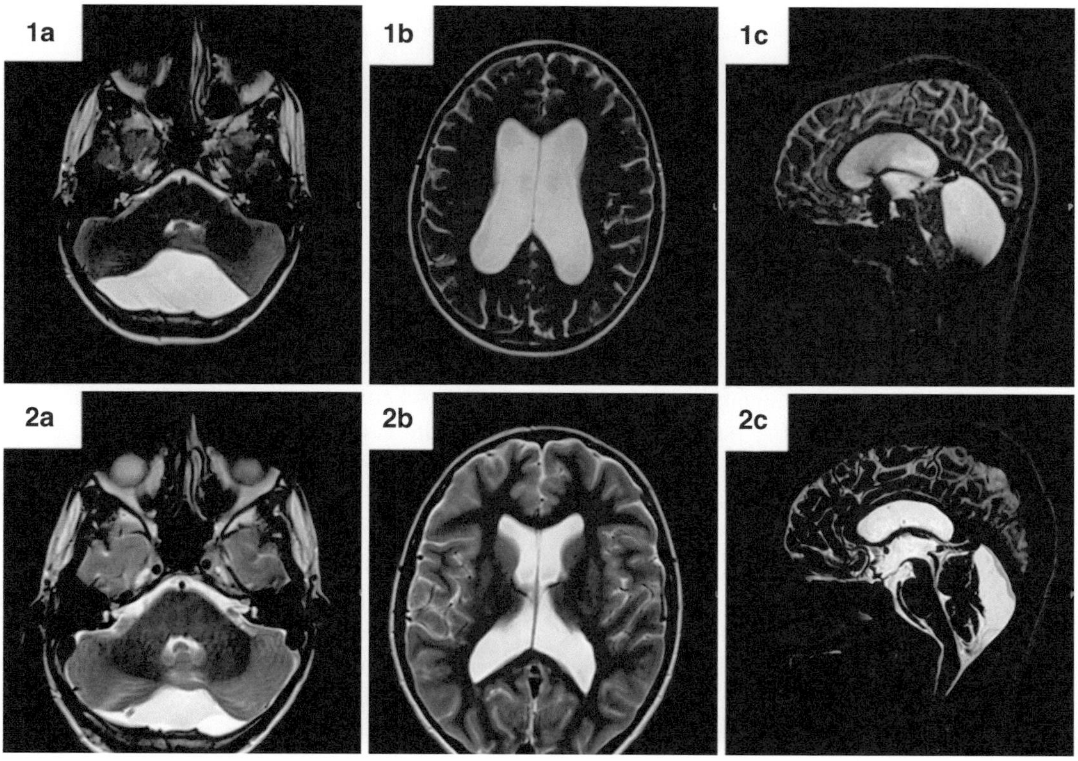

Fig. 4 Retrocerebellar AC that also caused hydrocephalus by compression of the IV ventricle and aqueductus sylvii. Preoperative T2-weighted sagittal and axial MR images (1**a**, **b**, **c**). T2-weighted axial and sagittal MR images of the same patient in the early period after cystoperitoneal shunt application (2**a**, **b**, **c**). Axial and sagittal reconstruction cranial CT images in the late postoperative term. Cerebellar compression disappeared and hydrocephalus improved (3**a**, **b**, **c**)

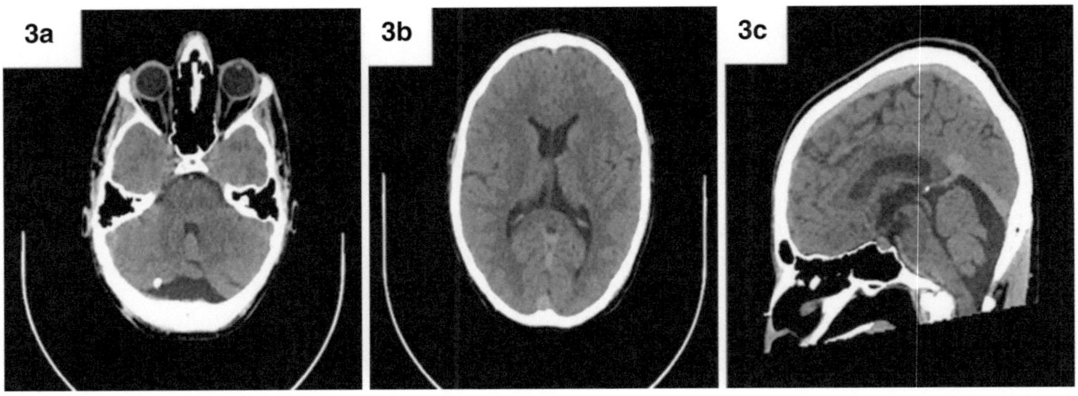

Fig. 4 (continued)

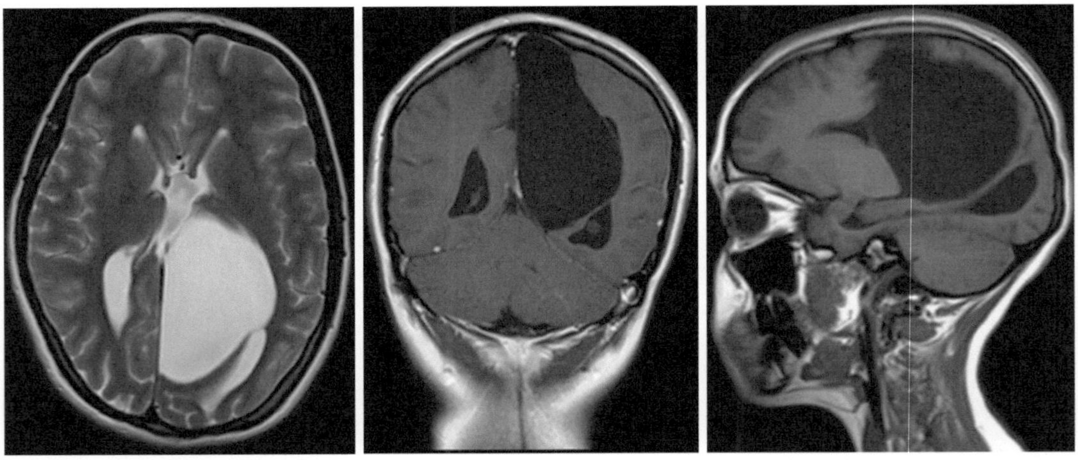

Fig. 5 Intraventricular AC. T2-weighted sequence axial view, T1-weighted sequence coronal and sagittal view

been an effective way to diagnose communicating/noncommunicating ACs, but it is an invasive, radioactive, and relatively time-consuming examination that is not used in standard clinical practice [22, 27, 35].

2 Classification of Middle Fossa Temporal Cysts

2.1 Galassi Classification

Approximately 50–65% of intracranial ACs occur in the middle cranial fossa [20, 32]. The widely used Galassi classification (1982) provides a schematic radiological classification of the middle fossa temporal cysts [17, 23]. Based on CT (computerized tomography) scan and (metrizamide) CT cisternography (CTC), Galassi et al. provided a useful classification of middle fossa temporal ACs based on their size, the segment of the Sylvian fissure involved, the evidence of a mass effect, and the presence/absence of what they referred to as communication with the subarachnoid space [17].

There are three types of temporal fossa ACs based on their size and degree of mass effect [16, 17, 23, 51]:

Type I cysts (Galassi named it as "mildest" form) are characterized by the following: lens-

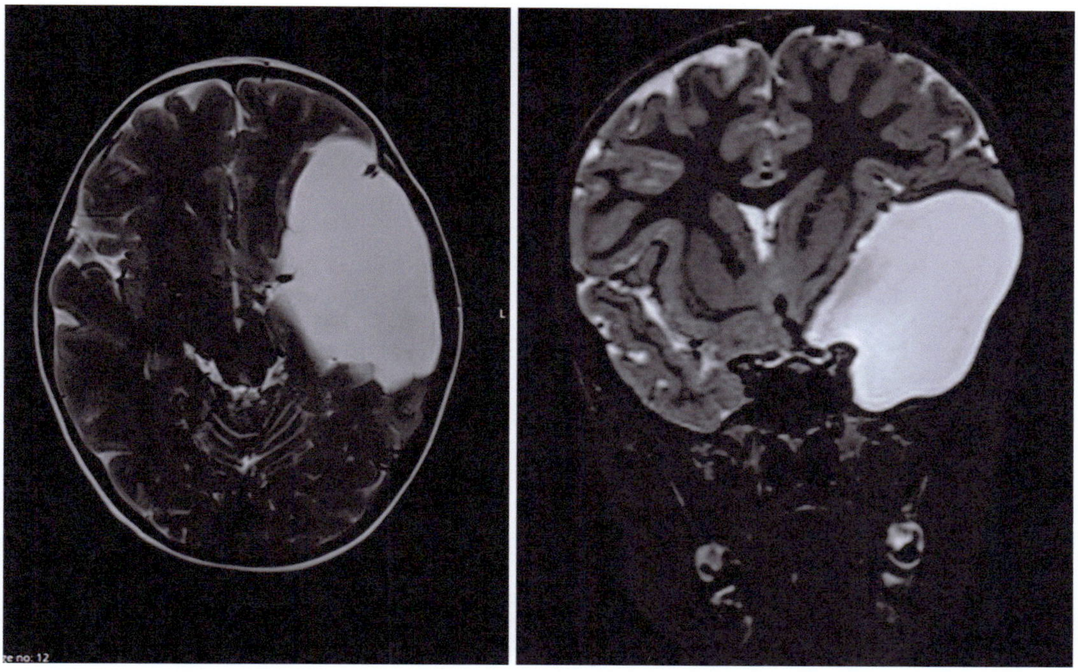

Fig. 6 Left Sylvian Galassi type II AC. Axial and coronal views of T2-weighted sequence MRI

shaped, located at the anterior tip of the middle temporal fossa, and freely communicate with CSF/surrounding subarachnoid space on MR/CT ventriculography. They rarely require surgery.

Type II cysts (Galassi named it as "classic" form) are characterized by intermediate size and more rectangular morphology than type I, extend into the Sylvian fissure (anterior and middle part of temporal fossa), have variable communication with CSF pathways, and exert local mass effect on the temporal lobe. They sometimes require surgery (Fig. 6).

Type III cysts (Galassi named it "most severe" form) constitute the largest size group, generally extend the full length of the Sylvian fissure, exert significant mass effect (often with midline shift), and do not communicate with the subarachnoid space. They usually require surgery [16, 17, 23, 51].

Based on the communication studies, Galassi et al. assumed the presence of communication in type I and II cysts, whereas type III lesions did not communicate with the rest of the subarachnoid space [17].

3 Suprasellar Arachnoid Cyst Classification

Several subtypes of suprasellar AC (SAC) have been described based on anatomic findings. All these observations are very relevant, but none of these studies has made a correlation between the clinical presentation and anatomic findings. Furthermore, surgical strategies remain unclear. Arthur Andre et al. distinguished three main subtypes of SAC, according to the clinical and radiological presentations [4, 28, 30, 37]:

SAC-1 subtype is characterized by the pure suprasellar cysts with early blockage of the foramen of Monro and ventriculomegaly that seem to come from an expansion of the chiasmatic cistern or the diencephalic leaf of the Liliequist membrane. For SAC-1 subtype, hydrocephalus with intracranial hypertension is the primary symptom. Surgical intervention is necessary, and the outcome is usually favorable when the hydrocephalus is resolved [4, 28, 37] (Fig. 7).

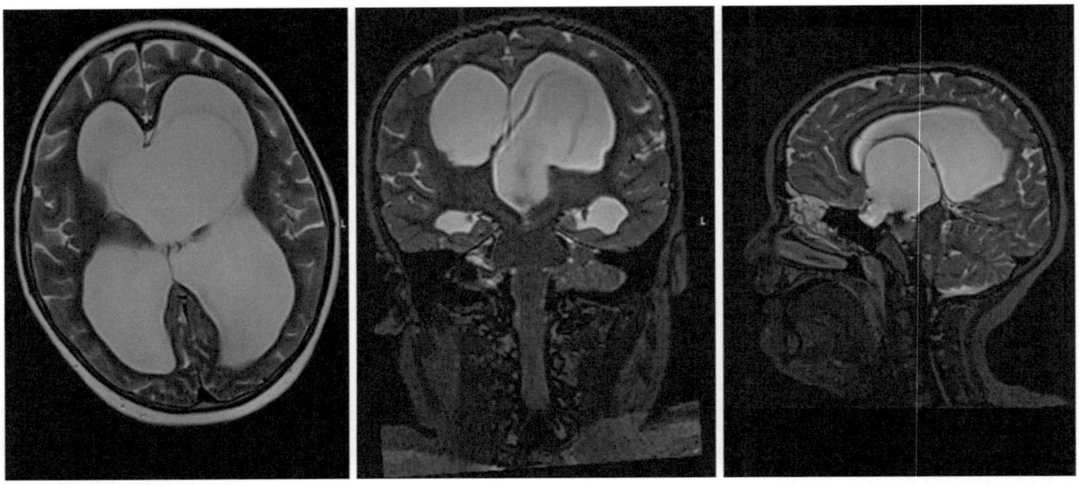

Fig. 7 Suprasellar intraventricular AC (SAC-1 subtype). Axial, coronal, and sagittal views of T2-weighted MRI sequence

SAC-2 subtype represents a dilatation of the interpeduncular cistern with elevated Liliequist membrane but free third ventricle. The defect of the mesencephalic leaf of the Liliequist membrane may be the pathological mechanism of SAC-2 subtype. SAC-2 subtype is usually diagnosed antenatally and might remain stable in time without requiring any surgical intervention. Both SAC-1 and SAC-2 subtypes may result in a mass effect on the pituitary stalk and cause endocrine disorders. Patients with endocrinological disturbances showed no or little improvement after surgical treatment, whereas developmental delay improved significantly [4, 28, 30, 37].

SAC-3 subtype is characterized by the asymmetrical forms with an involvement of other subarachnoid space, mainly presenting with macrocrania with mild/no hydrocephalus. SAC-3 subtypes are radiologically similar to SAC type 2 with lateral extension. They have good prognostic outcomes when surgically treated. These ACs may have a mass effect on the pituitary stalk with less CSF flow coming from the infratentorial to the supratentorial space [4, 37].

4 Retroclival Arachnoid Cyst Classification

Understanding the suprasellar region and clivus anatomy, in particular the arachnoid membrane anatomical architecture, is essential for understanding the pathogenesis of ACs and planning effective surgical strategies. The basal region arachnoid membrane originates from the superior wall of the cavernous sinus and optic canals and continuing as the Liliequist membrane (LM) over the posterior clinoids. The LM often splits into two leaves, the diencephalic leaf (DL) of the LM and the mesencephalic leaf (ML) of the LM. The diencephalic and mesencephalic leaves separate the chiasmatic-interpeduncular cisterns and the interpeduncular-prepontine cisterns, respectively [5, 15, 19, 28, 45]. On the basis of anatomical knowledge, the origins of the ACs of the ventral midline cisterns can be grouped into the following five categories:

1. Intra-arachnoid ACs that originate between two leaves of the diencephalic membrane [30].
2. True ACs that arise from the interpeduncular cistern arachnoid membranes [28].
3. Cystic dilatation of the interpeduncular cistern [14, 46].
4. True ACs that arise from the prepontine cistern arachnoid membranes [28].
5. True ACs that arise from the premedullary cistern arachnoid membranes [4, 45].

Clinically, the first three groups can be categorized as "suprasellar ACs" which have already been categorized by Andre et al. [4] Interpeduncular cistern arachnoid formations (categories 1 and 2) are classified as suprasellar SAC-1. The cystic enlargement of the interpeduncular cistern (category 3), which has been explained using a slit-valve mechanism by Schroeder and Gaab, is classified as SAC-2 subtype. SAC-3 subtype is radiologically similar to SAC type 2 with lateral extension [4, 28, 30, 45, 46].

Sarica and Ziyal classified the prepontine and premedullary ACs (categories 4 and 5) into three subtypes, which can have different clinical presentations and treatment approaches [45]:

Retroclival AC (RAC) type 1 (RAC-1), the "suprasellar type," is characterized by the cysts located in the prepontine and/or premedullary cisterns that extend beyond the borders of the DL of the LM, further compressing the third ventricle floor and causing hydrocephalus. RAC-1 should be treated using a similar approach as that for SAC-1. Currently, transfrontal endoscopic procedures are the reference standard for the treatment of these cysts in hydrocephalic patients [4, 11, 29, 37].

RAC type 2 (RAC- 2), the "retroclival type," is characterized by the cysts located in the prepontine and/or premedullary cisterns that do not cross the border of the DL of the LM or only mildly deflect the third ventricle floor, unlike the classical suprasellar cysts; these cysts mostly present with cranial nerve deficits. RAC-2 can be managed using either endoscopic or open surgery. To reach the clival region surgically, various trajectories with limitations and advantages have been formulated, such as anteromedial (endonasal route), anterolateral (orbitozygomatic approach and anterior petrosectomy), lateral (transpetrous presigmoideposterior petrosectomy), and posterior (retromastoid retrosigmoid approach) [31, 45].

RAC type 3 (RAC-3), the "retroclival type with spinal extension," is characterized by the RAC-2 cysts that extend to the anterior spinal cistern. RAC-3 might require a more extended surgical approach or additional surgical approaches than those required for RAC-2, in particular if total cyst wall excision has been planned. RAC-3 can be approached in a manner similar to that used for RAC-2 type. However, for total excision or dual fenestration, an extended approach should frequently be used [4, 11, 31, 37, 45].

5 Spinal Arachnoid Cysts

Spinal ACs are rare pathological entities that usually present with back pain or myelopathy [12]. Theories on the physiopathology of spinal ACs, suggesting that they arise from diverticula in the septum posticum or ectopic arachnoid granulations, have not been substantiated [13, 26, 38, 39, 42]. In most cases, no underlying cause for the spinal ACs can be identified and is considered as an idiopathic. In some cases, spinal ACs can develop from arachnoid adhesions following spine trauma or inflammatory or infectious causes (Fig. 8). Surgical etiologies of ACs (iatrogenic ACs) have also been described after conducting various procedures, such as a lumbar myelography, vertebroplasty, and laminectomy [25, 34].

Spinal meningeal/ACs in humans have been categorized by Nabors et al. in 1988, in which

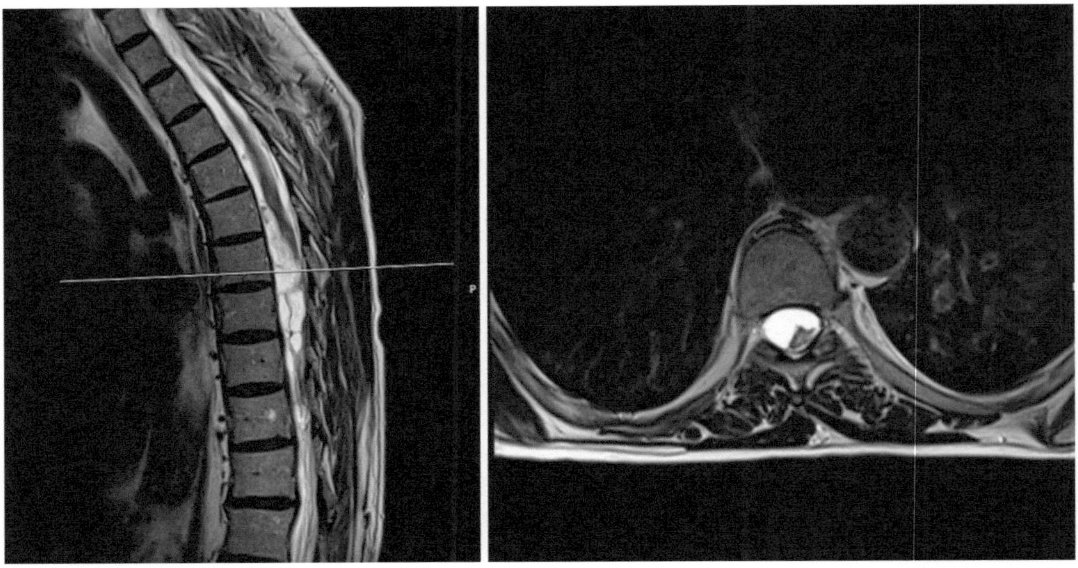

Fig. 8 Sagittal and axial T2-weighted sequence MR views of a postmeningitic, anteriorly located AC in the thoracic spinal cord

three types are identified by operative and light microscopic examination. In this classification, *type I* cysts are extradural without involvement of spinal nerve root fiber, *type II* cysts are extradural cysts with spinal nerve root fiber involvement, and *type III* cysts are classified as intradural cysts [24, 33]. However, Qi J et al. advocated another classification system. In this classification system, spinal ACs are divided into five types: (1) intramedullary cysts/syrinxes, (2) subdural extramedullary, (3) subdural/epidural, (4) intraspinal epidural, and (5) intraspinal/extraspinal. Intraspinal epidural spinal ACs (subgroup 4) are more common than other cyst types, followed by subdural extramedullary (subgroup 2) and intramedullary cysts/syrinxes (subgroup 1) [41].

Adhesion of arachnoid membrane especially after spine surgery (postoperative ACs) can also form a one-way valve entrapping circulating CSF, ultimately resulting in the formation of spinal ACs [38, 44]. Surgical management of the spinal ACs consists of surgical exploration of the cyst and decompression via total cyst excision, marsupialization, fenestration, ligation of the communication site if possible or shunting, or a combination of these techniques [12].

6 Conclusion

ACs are non-tumorous lesions and considered as benign developmental/acquired anomalies. ACs are not exact neurodegenerative disorders; rather, the underlying defect of the architecture of the arachnoid layer is probably congenital in nature. They can occur sporadically or can be associated with other congenital malformations or disorders. There are multiple classifications for ACs, most depending on their location. The classification systems are made difficult by the anatomical variability of the arachnoid membranes and cisterns and the possible occupation of several cisterns or regions depending on the size of the cysts. An agreement between the different professionals is necessary in order to establish a consensus classification.

References

1. Aicardi J, Bauman F. Supratentorial extracerebral cysts in infants and children. J Neurol Neurosurg Psychiatry. 1975;38(1):57–68.
2. Al-Holou WN, Terman S, Kilburg C, Garton HJ, Muraszko KM, Maher CO. Prevalence and natural history of arachnoid cysts in adults. J Neurosurg. 2013;118(2):222–31.
3. Al-Holou WN, Yew AY, Boomsaad ZE, Garton HJ, Muraszko KM, Maher CO. Prevalence and natural history of arachnoid cysts in children. J Neurosurg Pediatr. 2010;5(6):578–85.
4. Andre A, Zerah M, Roujeau T, Brunelle F, Blauwblomme T, Puget S, et al. Suprasellar arachnoid cysts: toward a new simple classification based on prognosis and treatment modality. Neurosurgery. 2016;78(3):370–9; discussion 9–80
5. Anik I, Ceylan S, Koc K, Tugasaygi M, Sirin G, Gazioglu N, et al. Microsurgical and endoscopic anatomy of Liliequist's membrane and the prepontine membranes: cadaveric study and clinical implications. Acta Neurochir. 2011;153(8):1701–11.
6. Catala M, Poirier J. Arachnoid cysts: histologic, embryologic and physiopathologic review. Rev Neurol (Paris). 1998;154(6–7):489–501.
7. Choi JU, Kim DS. Pathogenesis of arachnoid cyst: congenital or traumatic? Pediatr Neurosurg. 1998;29(5):260–6.
8. Choux M, Raybaud C, Pinsard N, Hassoun J, Gambarelli D. Intracranial supratentorial cysts in children excluding tumor and parasitic cysts. Childs Brain. 1978;4(1):15–32.
9. Cincu R, Agrawal A, Eiras J. Intracranial arachnoid cysts: current concepts and treatment alternatives. Clin Neurol Neurosurg. 2007;109(10):837–43.
10. Clemenceau S, Carpentier A. Intracranial arachnoid cysts. A review. Rev Neurol (Paris). 1999;155(8):604–8.
11. Ersahin Y, Kesikci H, Ruksen M, Aydin C, Mutluer S. Endoscopic treatment of suprasellar arachnoid cysts. Childs Nerv Syst. 2008;24(9):1013–20.
12. Fam MD, Woodroffe RW, Helland L, Noeller J, Dahdaleh NS, Menezes AH, et al. Spinal arachnoid cysts in adults: diagnosis and management. A single-center experience. J Neurosurg Spine. 2018;29(6):711–9.
13. Fortuna A, Mercuri S. Intradural spinal cysts. Acta Neurochir. 1983;68(3–4):289–314.
14. Fox JL, Al-Mefty O. Suprasellar arachnoid cysts: an extension of the membrane of Liliequist. Neurosurgery. 1980;7(6):615–8.
15. Froelich SC, Abdel Aziz KM, Cohen PD, van Loveren HR, Keller JT. Microsurgical and endoscopic anatomy of Liliequist's membrane: a complex and variable structure of the basal cisterns. Neurosurgery. 2008;63(1 Suppl 1):ONS1-8; discussion ONS-9
16. Fulkerson DH, Vogel TD, Baker AA, Patel NB, Ackerman LL, Smith JL, et al. Cyst-ventricle stent as primary or salvage treatment for posterior fossa arachnoid cysts. J Neurosurg Pediatr. 2011;7(5):549–56.
17. Galassi E, Tognetti F, Gaist G, Fagioli L, Frank F, Frank G. CT scan and metrizamide CT cisternography in arachnoid cysts of the middle cranial fossa: classification and pathophysiological aspects. Surg Neurol. 1982;17(5):363–9.
18. Gandy SE, Heier LA. Clinical and magnetic resonance features of primary intracranial arachnoid cysts. Ann Neurol. 1987;21(4):342–8.
19. Goksu E, Kazan S. Spontaneous shrinkage of a suprasellar arachnoid cyst diagnosed with prenatal sonography and fetal magnetic resonance imaging: case report and review of the literature. Turk Neurosurg. 2015;25(4):670–3.
20. Goswami P, Medhi N, Sarma PK, Sarmah BJ. Case report: middle cranial fossa arachnoid cyst in association with subdural hygroma. Indian J Radiol Imaging. 2008;18(3):222–3.
21. Helland CA, Lund-Johansen M, Wester K. Location, sidedness, and sex distribution of intracranial arachnoid cysts in a population-based sample. J Neurosurg. 2010;113(5):934–9.
22. Huang Q, Wang D, Guo Y, Zhou X, Wang X, Li X. The diagnosis and neuroendoscopic treatment of noncommunicating intracranial arachnoid cysts. Surg Neurol. 2007;68(2):149–54; discussion 54
23. Jafrani R, Raskin JS, Kaufman A, Lam S. Intracranial arachnoid cysts: pediatric neurosurgery update. Surg Neurol Int. 2019;10:15.
24. Kazan S, Ozdemir O, Akyuz M, Tuncer R. Spinal intradural arachnoid cysts located anterior to the cervical spinal cord. Report of two cases and review of the literature. J Neurosurg. 1999;91(2 Suppl):211–5.
25. Kriss TC, Kriss VM. Symptomatic spinal intradural arachnoid cyst development after lumbar myelography. Case report and review of the literature. Spine. 1997;22(5):568–72.
26. Lake PA, Minckler J, Scanlan RL. Spinal epidural cyst: theories of pathogenesis. Case report. J Neurosurg. 1974;40(6):774–8.
27. Li L, Zhang Y, Li Y, Zhai X, Zhou Y, Liang P. The clinical classification and treatment of middle cranial fossa arachnoid cysts in children. Clin Neurol Neurosurg. 2013;115(4):411–8.
28. Lyu J. Possible origins of suprasellar arachnoid cysts based on anatomical considerations. World Neurosurg. 2014;82(3–4):e570–3.
29. Mattox A, Choi JD, Leith-Gray L, Grant GA, Adamson DC. Guidelines for the management of obstructive hydrocephalus from suprasellar-prepontine arachnoid cysts using endoscopic third ventriculocystocisternostomy. Surg Innov. 2010;17(3):206–16.
30. Miyajima M, Arai H, Okuda O, Hishii M, Nakanishi H, Sato K. Possible origin of suprasellar arachnoid

cysts: neuroimaging and neurosurgical observations in nine cases. J Neurosurg. 2000;93(1):62–7.
31. Mohyeldin A, Prevedello DM, Jamshidi AO, Ditzel Filho LF, Carrau RL. Nuances in the treatment of malignant tumors of the clival and petroclival region. Int Arch Otorhinolaryngol. 2014;18(Suppl 2):S157–72.
32. Mustansir F, Bashir S, Darbar A. Management of Arachnoid Cysts: a comprehensive review. Cureus. 2018;10(4):e2458.
33. Nabors MW, Pait TG, Byrd EB, Karim NO, Davis DO, Kobrine AI, et al. Updated assessment and current classification of spinal meningeal cysts. J Neurosurg. 1988;68(3):366–77.
34. Nath PC, Mishra SS, Deo RC, Satapathy MC. Intradural spinal arachnoid cyst: a long-term Postlaminectomy complication: a case report and review of the literature. World Neurosurg. 2016;85(367):e1–4.
35. Nijm GM, Sahakian AV, Swiryn S, Carr JC, Sheehan JJ, Larson AC. Comparison of self-gated cine MRI retrospective cardiac synchronization algorithms. J Magn Reson Imaging. 2008;28(3):767–72.
36. Okamura K, Watanabe M, Inoue N, Kanoh M, Ohno T, Mitsui Y, et al. Intraventricular arachnoid cyst--on the origin of intraventricular arachnoid cysts. No To Shinkei. 1996;48(11):1015–21.
37. Ozek MM, Urgun K. Neuroendoscopic management of suprasellar arachnoid cysts. World Neurosurg. 2013;79(2 Suppl):S19. e3–8
38. Paramore CG. Dorsal arachnoid web with spinal cord compression: variant of an arachnoid cyst? Report of two cases. J Neurosurg. 2000;93(2 Suppl):287–90.
39. Perret G, Green D, Keller J. Diagnosis and treatment of intradural arachnoid cysts of the thoracic spine. Radiology. 1962;79:425–9.
40. Pradilla G, Jallo G. Arachnoid cysts: case series and review of the literature. Neurosurg Focus. 2007;22(2):E7.
41. Qi J, Yang J, Wang G. A novel five-category multimodal T1-weighted and T2-weighted magnetic resonance imaging-based stratification system for the selection of spinal arachnoid cyst treatment: a 15-year experience of 81 cases. Neuropsychiatr Dis Treat. 2014;10:499–506.
42. Rabb CH, McComb JG, Raffel C, Kennedy JG. Spinal arachnoid cysts in the pediatric age group: an association with neural tube defects. J Neurosurg. 1992;77(3):369–72.
43. Rengachary SS, Watanabe I. Ultrastructure and pathogenesis of intracranial arachnoid cysts. J Neuropathol Exp Neurol. 1981;40(1):61–83.
44. Rohrer DC, Burchiel KJ, Gruber DP. Intraspinal extradural meningeal cyst demonstrating ball-valve mechanism of formation. Case report. J Neurosurg. 1993;78(1):122–5.
45. Sarica C, Ziyal MI. Retroclival arachnoid cysts: case series, literature review, and new classification proposal. World Neurosurg. 2019;121:e898–907.
46. Schroeder HW, Gaab MR. Endoscopic observation of a slit-valve mechanism in a suprasellar prepontine arachnoid cyst: case report. Neurosurgery. 1997;40(1):198–200.
47. Starkman SP, Brown TC, Linell EA. Cerebral arachnoid cysts. J Neuropathol Exp Neurol. 1958;17(3):484–500.
48. Ucar T, Akyuz M, Kazan S, Tuncer R. Bilateral cerebellopontine angle arachnoid cysts: case report. Neurosurgery. 2000;47(4):966–8.
49. Wester K. Gender distribution and sidedness of middle fossa arachnoid cysts: a review of cases diagnosed with computed imaging. Neurosurgery. 1992;31(5):940–4.
50. Wester K. Peculiarities of intracranial arachnoid cysts: location, sidedness, and sex distribution in 126 consecutive patients. Neurosurgery. 1999;45(4):775–9.
51. Yildiz H, Erdogan C, Yalcin R, Yazici Z, Hakyemez B, Parlak M, et al. Evaluation of communication between intracranial arachnoid cysts and cisterns with phase-contrast cine MR imaging. AJNR Am J Neuroradiol. 2005;26(1):145–51.

Intracranial Hemorrhage Associated with Arachnoid Cysts

Haydn Hoffman and Grahame C. Gould

1 Introduction

Arachnoid cysts (ACs) are congenital anomalies of the arachnoid membrane that are usually diagnosed in children. They are believed to be due to abnormal splitting of the arachnoid layer during folding of the neural tube [11]. Diagnosis of ACs is increasing due to greater utilization of neuroimaging, and their prevalence is estimated to be 2.3% [10].

While ACs are frequently incidental findings, they may cause symptoms due to local mass effect, increased intracranial pressure (ICP), and obstruction of cerebrospinal fluid (CSF) flow. Asymptomatic ACs are often associated with benign natural histories [1], while symptomatic ACs may be considered for surgical treatments including fenestration, marsupialization, and shunting. ACs may also become symptomatic due to hemorrhage. This is rare, and the annual risk of hemorrhage for patients with middle fossa ACs is estimated to be <0.1% [4]. AC-associated hemorrhage (ACH) may be related to cyst rupture, trauma, chronic subdural hematoma (cSDH) formation, or surgery. Frequently, patients who present with ACH had never experienced symptoms due to their AC. Here, we describe the etiology, risk factors, treatment, and outcome of ACH.

H. Hoffman (✉) · G. C. Gould
Department of Neurosurgery, State University of New York Upstate Medical University, Syracuse, NY, USA
e-mail: hoffmanh@upstate.edu; gouldg@upstate.edu

2 Etiology and Classification

ACH may be classified according to its etiology (spontaneous or traumatic) and intracranial compartment (subdural, epidural, or intracystic). Figure 1 provides an overview of these categories.

Trauma is implicated in most cases of ACH. Multiple theories regarding the pathophysiology of traumatic ACH have been proposed. Intraoperatively, ACs have been observed to be associated with fragile bridging veins that connect between the outer layer of the AC and the dura. The bridging veins may traverse the cyst wall, and their rupture may lead to SDH. Another potential mechanism is direct injury to the cyst wall itself, which may create a communication with the cyst cavity and the subdural space. Tears in the cyst wall could also lead to inflow of CSF, increase in intracystic pressure, and rupture of vessels within or around the AC. Finally, ACs may be less compliant than normal brain tissue, leading to greater transfer of force to the brain during trauma [12].

ACHs may also occur spontaneously and have been reported to involve intracystic and subdural compartments. Prior reports have attributed these bleeds to cyst "rupture," but do not describe why this could have occurred. As with traumatic ACH, bridging veins have been implicated, which could be stretched by cyst growth causing spontaneous hemorrhage similar to cSDH in elderly patients [15]. The AC membrane itself, which has been observed intraoperatively to be highly vascular,

M. Turgut et al. (eds.), *Arachnoid Cysts*, https://doi.org/10.1007/978-3-031-22701-1_12

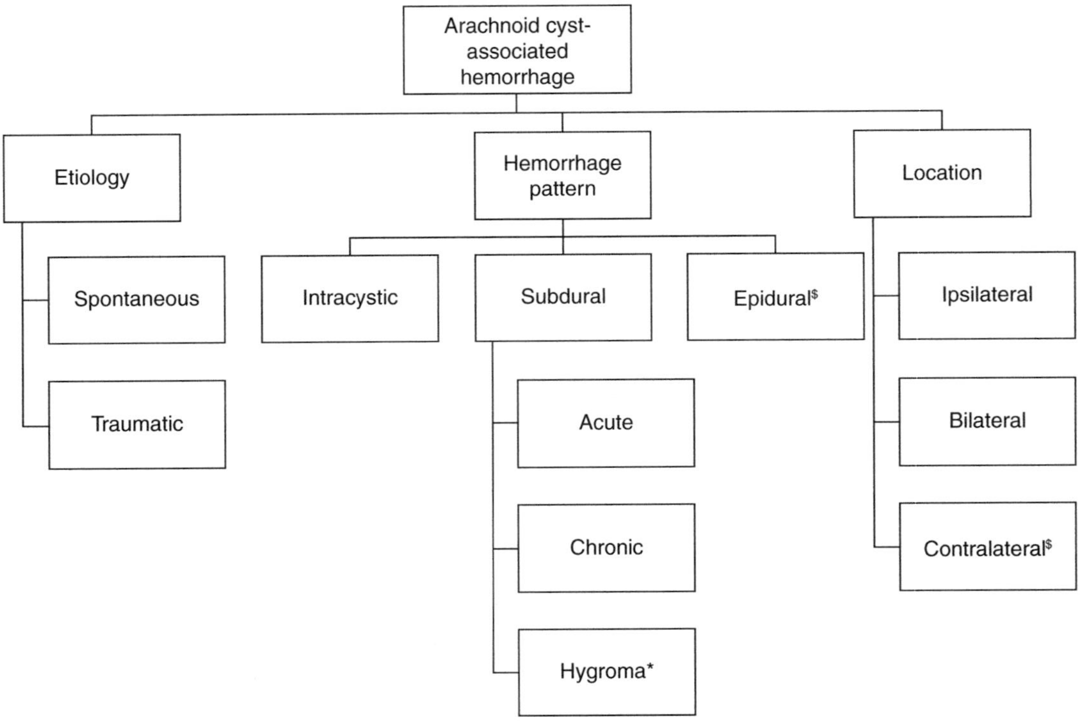

Fig. 1 Categorization of AC-associated hemorrhage by etiology and hematoma location. (*Although hygromas do not include blood products, they are included due to their relationship with chronic subdural hematomas. $Rare)

could theoretically be prone to hemorrhage in a similar fashion. The inflammation and angiogenesis commonly implicated in cSDH of the elderly are less frequently described for SDH associated with ACs.

Subdural hematoma is the most frequent pattern of ACH reported in the literature. These may be acute or chronic. The latter in a pediatric patient should raise suspicion for an underlying AC. Intracystic hemorrhage is typically associated with SDH but has been reported to occur independently after trauma [5].

3 Risk Factors

Characterization of risk factors for ACH is limited by the rarity of the event, which makes obtaining large enough samples for statistical analysis challenging. In their literature review, Wu et al. reported a mean age of 24 years among 182 patients with ACH and proposed that patients 10–20 years old are at greatest risk for ACH [14]. The majority of reported ACH cases involve males, although this may just reflect the greater incidence of AC in males [14]. The only case-control study comparing patients with and without hemorrhage of their ACs found a history of head trauma and greater cyst diameter to be associated with hemorrhage [2]. Another study found that middle fossa location was more common in patients whose ACs bled [13]. The authors related this to their intraoperative finding that the AC membrane is only loosely attached to the middle fossa dura and detachment leads to dural venous oozing. Parsch et al. identified a preponderance of Galassi type II ACs in their series of ACH and in the literature, but no difference in Galassi type was noted in another series [9, 13].

4 Diagnosis and Presentation

Patients with ACH often present in their second or third decade of life. This is contrary to non-AC-associated cSDH, which is primarily found in the elderly. Trauma is commonly implicated in ACH, so many patients present after a head injury. The trauma may be distant, with a mean duration of 8 weeks before presentation in one ACH series [8]. Patients with spontaneous ACH may present with symptoms of elevated ICP such as headache and vomiting. Lethargy is less frequently observed due to the often chronic nature of ACH, but acute uncal herniation requiring emergency surgery has been reported [6]. Symptoms of elevated ICP are more common from cSDH associated with AC than cSDH in the elderly, likely due to the presence of cerebral atrophy in the latter [8]. Patients may also develop seizures or a focal neurologic deficit such as hemiparesis.

cSDH is the most common pattern of ACH (93.4%) followed by intracystic (55.1%) and epidural hematoma [14]. ACH is typically ipsilateral to the AC; however, bilateral and contralateral cSDH have been reported. In a large systematic review of ACH, bilateral hematomas were observed in 6.5% of patients who presented with cSDH [14].

5 Treatment

Given the rarity of ACH, surgery for otherwise asymptomatic ACs to prevent bleeding events is not justified. Most patients who develop ACH present with cSDH, and acute management follows the typical principles of non-AC-associated cSDH. Patients with absent or minimal symptoms and without mass effect on CT may be managed expectantly with serial imaging. Resolution is often observed for these smaller collections. Hygromas may have a particularly favorable prognosis, with seven of eight patients in one series not requiring surgery [7]. In those who are symptomatic, initial treatment is aimed at evacuating the hematoma through a burr hole or craniotomy. There is no clear preference for burr hole or craniotomy in the AC literature.

It is unclear whether concurrent treatment of the AC with fenestration into the basal cisterns or membrane removal is warranted. Although ACs typically have a benign natural history, those that have bled may represent a higher risk subset. Parsch et al. proposed that ACH can usually be managed without treatment of the cyst itself and reported excellent outcomes in 16 patients with this approach [9]. They reserved treatment of the AC for those with persistent symptoms after hematoma evacuation. Domenicucci et al. advocated for the same approach based on their experience with eight patients [3]. ACs associated with hygromas have been reported to spontaneously resolve, possibly because the hygroma is formed by a tear in the cyst lining that functions similar to a surgical fenestration [7]. A proposed treatment algorithm is shown in Fig. 2.

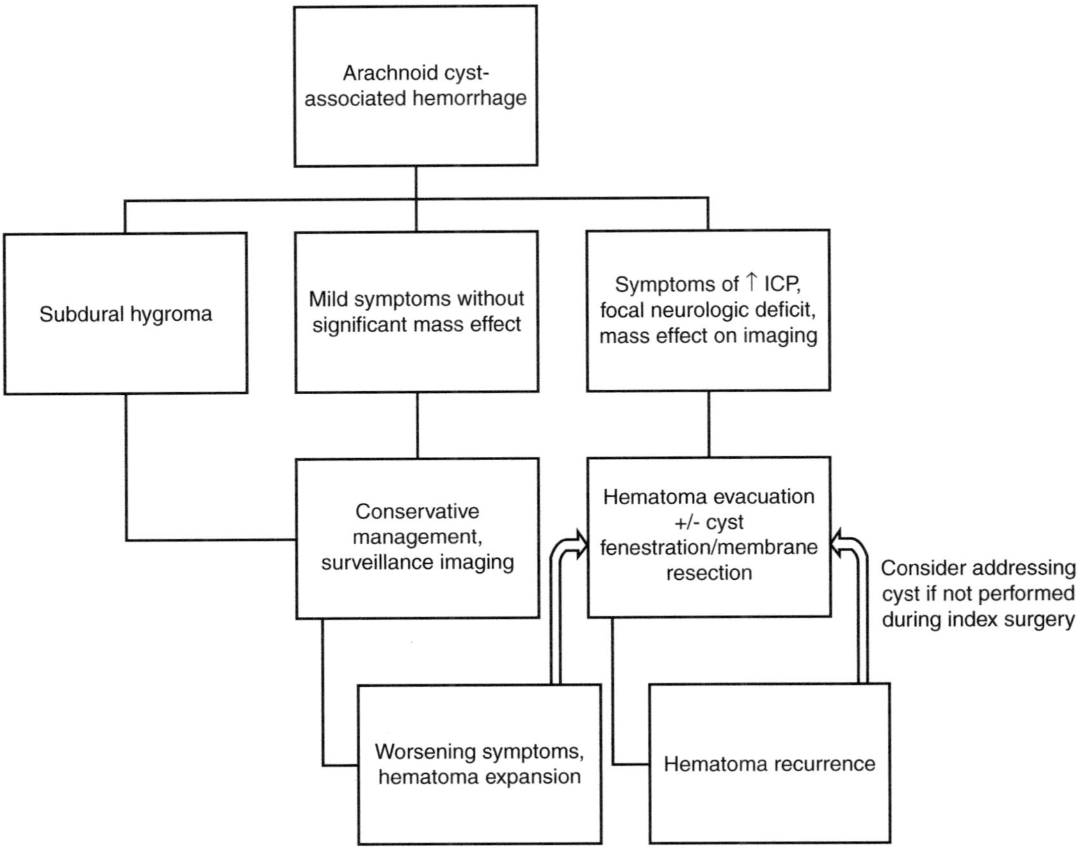

Fig. 2 Proposed treatment algorithm for AC-associated hemorrhage

6 Outcome

Published outcomes following ACH are favorable with low rates of morbidity and high rates of symptom resolution. These should be interpreted with caution, however, given the high potential for publication bias with case reports and small series. Wu et al. reported a 98.8% rate of favorable outcomes (defined as a Glasgow Outcome Scale of 5) among 161 cases in the literature [14]. The excellent outcomes may be explained by the higher rate of brain expansion after evacuation of AC-associated cSDH compared to non-AC-associated cSDH [8].

The primary complication following surgery for ACH is cSDH recurrence. In the elderly population, this is a major cause of morbidity; however, it appears to be less problematic in younger patients with ACs. A systematic review of 182 patients with ACH reported an 8.2% recurrence rate [14]. Those with recurrence underwent burr hole drainage, craniotomy, or burr hole drainage with middle meningeal artery embolization. None of the patients with recurrence experienced a negative outcome related to the bleed [14]. Treatment of the AC may be considered if it was not addressed in the index surgery. Additional complications include CSF leak.

7 Case Presentation

A 16-year-old male with no significant past medical history presented to the Emergency Department (ED) with subacute lower back pain that radiated down the left leg. There was no history of trauma, and his neurologic exam was unremarkable. MRI of the lumbar spine demonstrated a dorsal SDH at L5-S1. Further imaging of the neuroaxis was performed, which revealed a left type III middle fossa AC with bilateral subacute SDHs (Fig. 3). Subacute intracystic hemorrhage was also present. Given the patient was neurologically intact without symptoms attributable to the cyst or intracranial SDH, he was initially managed expectantly with the plan for close outpatient follow-up. He returned to the ED 5 days later with worsening headache and nuchal rigidity. Head CT showed stable subacute cSDH and intracystic hemorrhage. Given his worsening symptoms, surgical treatment was pursued with plan for simultaneous AC fenestration and bilat-

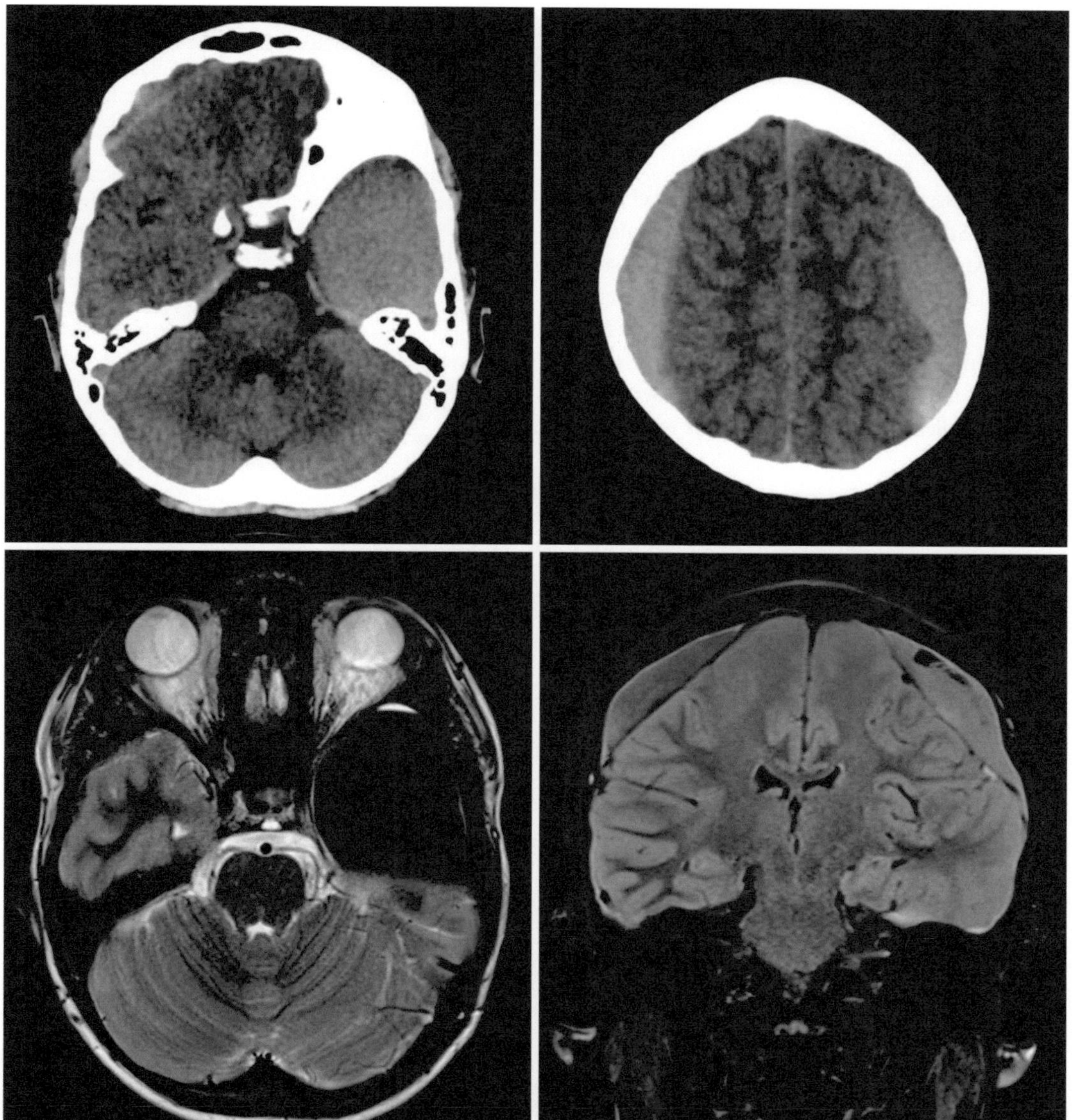

Fig. 3 Preoperative axial CT demonstrates a left type III middle fossa AC containing subacute blood (top left) as well as bilateral subacute convexity subdural hematomas (top right). Preoperative T2-weighted axial MRI demonstrates subacute blood within the cyst as well as a small rim of hyperintensity anteriorly, which likely corresponds to the cyst's normal cerebrospinal fluid content (bottom left). The coronal T2-FLAIR sequence shows both subdural hematomas (bottom right). The hematoma ipsilateral to the cyst is slightly larger and contains a fluid level

eral cSDH evacuation. The AC was fenestrated medially into the opticocarotid cistern through a left mini-pterional approach. Small craniotomies were created over each cSDH to evacuate the blood and resect the hematoma membrane. Subdural drains were left in place and removed on postoperative day (POD) #2. The patient remained neurologically intact and was discharged home on POD #5. At 1 month follow-up, the patient's headaches were resolved.

8 Conclusion

ACH is a rare phenomenon that is usually characterized by cSDH ipsilateral to the cyst. Potential risk factors for ACH include trauma, larger cyst size, and middle fossa location. Conservative management may be pursued for smaller hematomas without significant symptoms or mass effect. Excellent outcomes are reported after surgical evacuation of ACH regardless of whether the cyst is fenestrated.

References

1. Al-Holou WN, Terman S, Kilburg C, et al. Prevalence and natural history of arachnoid cysts in adults. J Neurosurg. 2013;118:222–31.
2. Cress M, Kestle JR, Holubkov R, et al. Risk factors for pediatric arachnoid cyst rupture/hemorrhage: a case-control study. Neurosurgery. 2013;72:716–22.
3. Domenicucci M, Russo N, Giugni E, et al. Relationship between supratentorial arachnoid cyst and chronic subdural hematoma: neuroradiological evidence and surgical treatment. J Neurosurg. 2009;110:1250–5.
4. Iaconetta G, Esposito M, Maiuri F, et al. Arachnoid cyst with intracystic haemorrhage and subdural haematoma: case report and literature review. Neurol Sci. 2006;26:451–5.
5. Ildan F, Cetinalp E, Bağdatoğlu H, et al. Arachnoid cyst with traumatic intracystic hemorrhage unassociated with subdural hematoma. Neurosurg Rev. 1994;17:229–32.
6. Kode S, Hegde A, Menon G. Chronic subdural hematoma associated with congenital arachnoid cysts: management dilemmas. Cureus. 2018;10:e2550.
7. Maher CO, Garton HJ, Al-Holou WN, et al. Management of subdural hygromas associated with arachnoid cysts. J Neurosurg Pediatr. 2013;12:434–43.
8. Mori K, Yamamoto T, Horinaka N, et al. Arachnoid cyst is a risk factor for chronic subdural hematoma in juveniles: twelve cases of chronic subdural hematoma associated with arachnoid cyst. J Neurotrauma. 2002;19:1017–27.
9. Parsch CS, Krauss J, Hofmann E, et al. Arachnoid cysts associated with subdural hematomas and hygromas: analysis of 16 cases, long-term follow-up, and review of the literature. Neurosurgery. 1997;40:483–90.
10. Rabiei K, Jaraj D, Marlow T, et al. Prevalence and symptoms of intracranial arachnoid cysts: a population-based study. J Neurol. 2016;263:689–94.
11. Rengachary SS, Watanabe I. Ultrastructure and pathogenesis of intracranial arachnoid cysts. J Neuropathol Exp Neurol. 1981;40:61–83.
12. Takizawa K, Sorimach T, Honda Y, et al. Chronic subdural hematomas associated with arachnoid cysts: significance in young patients with chronic subdural hematomas. Neurol Med Chir (Tokyo). 2015;55:727–34.
13. Wester K, Helland CA. How often do chronic extracerebral haematomas occur in patients with intracranial arachnoid cysts? J Neurol Neurosurg Psychiatry. 2008;79:72–5.
14. Wu X, Li G, Zhao J, et al. Arachnoid cyst-associated chronic subdural hematoma: report of 14 cases and a systematic literature review. World Neurosurg. 2018;109:e118–30.
15. Yüksel MO, Gürbüz MS, Senol M, et al. Spontaneous subdural haematoma developing secondary to arachnoid cyst rupture. J Clin Diagn Res. 2016;10:PD05–6.

Spontaneous Resolution of Arachnoid Cysts

Ved Prakash Maurya, Priyadarshi Dikshit, Mayank Singh, Maruti Nandan, Guramritpal Singh, Vikas Dwivedi, and Sanjay Behari

1 Introduction

Arachnoid cysts (ACs) are rare intracranial space occupying lesions and represent less than 1% of all the intracranial lesions [32]. Despite the extensive research and clinical studies being performed on them, several facts regarding the origin, presentation, and natural course of the disease still remain an enigma [34]. A high incidence of ACs is now being diagnosed with the advent of newer diagnostic modalities.

To date, the natural history of ACs has not been completely elucidated. The phenomena of spontaneous resolution are sparsely described, either in the form of case reports or review articles. There is a relative lack of literature regarding the natural history of an asymptomatic AC. There exists no correlation between an individual's age and the size of the AC. The rate of spontaneous resolution of ACs at various positions is also undetermined.

2 Historical Background

In 1830, Bright brought the attention of the world towards this innocuous lesion of the intracranial cavity. The lesion, with its usual extra-axial location, is mostly avascular and usually does not cause a significant mass effect. Some reports also indicate a rare, malignant transformation of these lesions [25]. Another tendency of these benign lesions is to undergo reduction in their size. This very uncommon event has been noticed in less than three percent of the patient population, who are diagnosed to be harboring an AC [11].

It took almost six decades to report the first case of an AC that had undergone spontaneous reduction or total resolution. In 1987, Beltramello reported the first case of spontaneous resolution of an AC without the need for any surgical intervention. It was hypothesized that this rare event of spontaneous resolution usually occurs in the first or second decades of life [6].

3 Impact of the Disease

Middle cranial fossa contributes to more than 50% of intracranial ACs. The other less common locations where ACs may be found are the cerebral convexity, the parasellar region, the quadrigeminal as well as cerebellopontine angle cisterns, and the subarachnoid spaces of the posterior cranial fossa, in a decreasing order of frequency. The actual prevalence of an AC in the society may be higher as it may have been present, and yet, may not have produced any clinical manifestations [23, 24]. The incidence of hematoma formation following a craniotomy or a burr-hole drainage of ACs has been well documented in literature [26]. The incidence

V. P. Maurya · P. Dikshit · M. Singh · M. Nandan · G. Singh · V. Dwivedi · S. Behari (✉)
Department of Neurosurgery, Sanjay Gandhi Postgraduate Institute of Medical Sciences, Lucknow, India

M. Turgut et al. (eds.), *Arachnoid Cysts*, https://doi.org/10.1007/978-3-031-22701-1_13

of spontaneous resolution has been reported following the sustenance of a head injury; however, this phenomenon may also occur without any history of injury. The event of spontaneous resolution is most commonly encountered in the middle cranial fossa lesions, followed by anterior fossa lesions, and least commonly in the posterior cranial fossa lesions [27]. Most of these cysts are congenital in origin. Many of them enlarge during the early years of life and become symptomatic at the time of adolescence. The male population is affected twice as often when compared to the female one [28].

4 Radiological Evaluation of Arachnoid Cysts

Most of the ACs are noticed incidentally during the workup performed for other ailments, or during the conduction of a routine antenatal ultrasonography. ACs in the intrauterine life are observed as hypoechoic cystic lesions, and most of these become obscure by the time of the child's first birthday. The CT scan appearance is characteristic and is similar to the appearance of cerebrospinal fluid (CSF) in the ventricles. A hypodense appearance on a CT scan image, without adjoining cerebral edema, with the lesion having no contrast uptake, is a characteristic radiological feature of an AC. On MRI, ACs appear as hypointense lesions on T-weighted image (WI) and as hyperintense lesions on T2WI. The diffusion-weighted image (DWI) and fluid-attenuated inversion recovery (FLAIR) sequences are highly useful in diagnosing these lesions and in differentiating ACs from other cystic lesions of the brain [39]. Upon diagnostic intrathecal contrast CT cisternography, there appears to be avid filling of the contrast in type I ACs, while type II ACs fill after a small latency period. On the other hand, type III ACs do not fill upon contrast administration. On the basis of contrast filling and communication with the cerebral cisterns, type I and II ACs are considered as arachnoid diverticula. On the contrary, type III ACs are regarded as true and non-communicating ACs [15].

5 Clinical Manifestations of ACs

Primary ACs arise as a result of splitting of two layers of the arachnoidal membrane while secondary ACs appear following head trauma, surgery, infection as well as intracranial bleed. The prevalence of ACs is around 1.4%, with the predominant involvement of female patients, while it is 2.6% in the pediatric age group. The clinical presentation depends upon the location of the cysts, which in turn is the result of neurovascular compression. On the basis of clinical symptomatology, Choi et al. advocated the occurrence of three categories of ACs [8].

Sommer and Smit conducted a review of 19 patients with ACs in various locations of the cranial cavity (both supratentorial and infratentorial). There was a significant variation in clinical symptoms in accordance with their location, but most of these cysts were detected incidentally and remain asymptomatic throughout their life. Robust evidence is lacking regarding the influence of size of ACs on the severity of clinical symptoms [36].

6 Management of AC

Galassi and colleagues classified ACs of the middle cranial fossa into three types, depending upon their size as well as the severity of clinical symptoms.

Type I: Mildest form of ACs, which are small lesions having spindle-shaped appearance and are not associated with any mass effect in the form of compression of brain matter or midline shift. Type II: These cysts are larger than the type I variety and are associated with mass effect in the form of compression on the ventricular system in more than half of the cases. Type III: These are ACs with the severest forms of manifestations. These cysts are large in size and are often associated with a significant mass effect on the cerebral cortex as well as the ventricular system [13]. According to Smith and Smith, the surgical interventions that are most prevalent in the man-

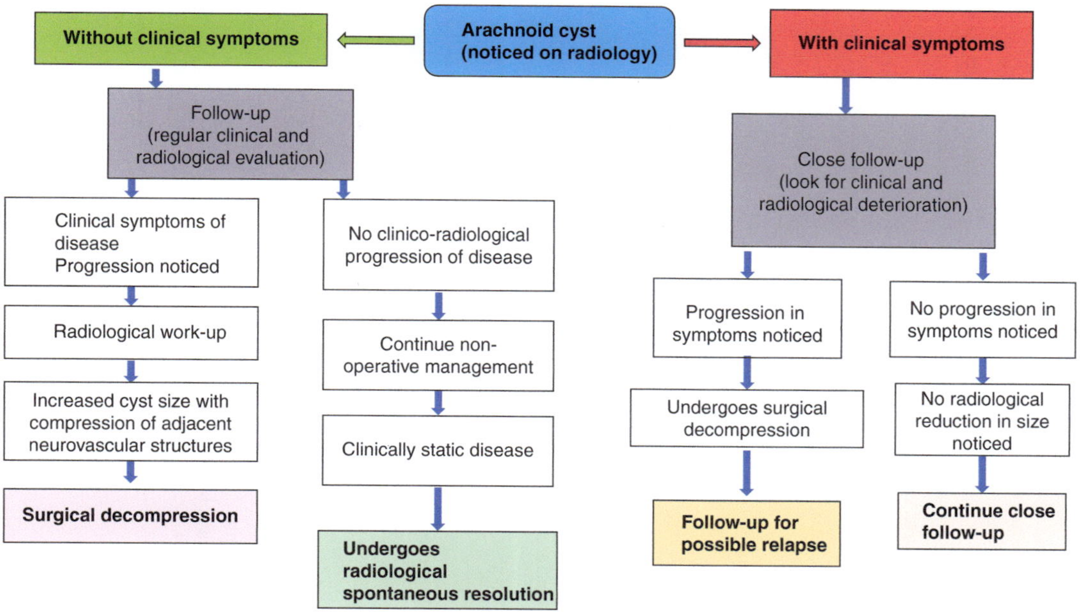

Fig. 1 The proposed algorithm for management of ACs

agement of ACs are craniotomy with arachnoid membrane removal, and cystic fenestration into potential cisternal spaces [1].

The management of symptomatic and asymptomatic ACs may be according to the proposed algorithm (Fig. 1).

7 Pathophysiology of Spontaneous Resolution of AC

The phenomenon of spontaneous resolution (also called spontaneous regression) of ACs is a gradual and time-taking process, and hence, left unnoticed in most of the cases. ACs undergoing spontaneous resolution constitute a very small proportion of cases, which are reported and published in the form of case reports or case series (Table 1).

The microanatomical location of ACs revealed that these cysts appear due to the splitting of arachnoidal layers and the creation of a potential space between the two thin layers of arachnoid. The split between these two layers is localized and the size depends upon the capaciousness of the cistern of cerebral lobes involved. Sometimes, the phenomena that are responsible for the origin and expansion of ACs exceed the threshold limits and result in the release of contents into the surrounding spaces. The ball-valve mechanism (ingress of fluid into the cyst that cannot escape back into the extracyst tissues), the osmotic gradient theory (the attraction of fluid into the cyst due to the osmotic gradient existing between the cyst and the extracyst environment), the malformation theory (considering cyst as the trapped fluid associated with cerebral lobe agenesis), and the hypersecretion of fluid by the cyst lining are among the proposed mechanisms responsible for the origin of ACs [4]. No time limit dictates the duration after which spontaneous resolution of an AC is noticed. Thus, the time interval after diagnosis of these intracranial ACs to their spontaneous resolution varies from weeks to years.

Table 1 Tabular demonstration of AC undergoing spontaneous resolution mentioned in literature

Author, (year), [ref.#]	Gender	Side	Location	Underlying event	Presenting complaints	Time required for spontaneous resolution	Outcome (extent of resolution)
Bamber and Prabhu, (2016) [3]	F	Left	Posterior fossa	Fall from height	Headache and vomiting	4 weeks	Good
Beltramello and Mazza, (1985) [5]	M	Left	Middle fossa	None	GTCS	2 yrs	Complete
Yamanouchi et al., (1986) [43]	M	Left	Middle fossa	Head injury	Headache	6 mos	Complete
Inoue et al., (1987) [17]	M	Right	Middle fossa	SDH following trauma	Headache	18 mos	Almost complete
Takagi et al., (1987) [37]	M	Left	CP angle	None	Meningitis	2 yrs	Complete
Wester et al., (1991) [42]	M	Left	Middle fossa	None	Headache	3 yrs	Complete
Weber et al., (1991) [41]	M	Right	Middle fossa	None	Headache	10 yrs	Complete
Takizawa et al., (1991) [38]	M	Left	Middle fossa	Head injury	Headache	10 mos	Complete
Mokri et al., (1994) [21]	F	Right	Frontal lobe	None	Left focal seizures	13 yrs	Good
Rakier and Feinsod, (1995) [30]	F	Right	Middle fossa	None		6 yrs	Almost complete
Mori et al., (1995) [24]	M	Middle—2 Anterior—2	Temporal lobe—2, Frontal—2	Head injury	Chronic subdural effusion/ hematoma	5 mos	Good
Przybylo et al., (1997) [29]	M	Right	Temporal fossa	None	Ataxia, somnolence (hepatic encephalopathy)	1.5 yrs	Complete

McDonald and Rutka, (1997) [20]	M	Left	Middle fossa	None	None	1 yr	Complete
Yoshioka et al., (1998) [45]	M	Left	Middle fossa	Suppurative meningitis	Headache	2 mos	Complete
Yamauchi et al., (1999) [44]	M	Right	Middle fossa	None	Increasing head circumference	7 yrs	Complete
Dodd et al., (2002) [12]	F	Midline	Prepontine	None	Routine screening	2 yrs	Nearly complete
Liu et al., (2016) [19]	M	Left	Middle cranial fossa/ temporal lobe	Nothing obvious	Increasing head circumference	2 yrs	Good
Pandey et al., (2001) [25]	M	Midline	Posterior fossa	None	Increasing head circumference	6 mos	Good
Seizeur et al., (2006) [34]	M	Left	Middle cranial fossa	Head injury	Right frontal EDH	16 mos	Good
Bristol et al., (2007) [6]	M	Midline	Prepontine cistern	Head injury	Post-traumatic headache	1 month	Good
Turgut M, (2002) [40]	M	Right	Cerebellum	None	Complex febrile seizure	3 yrs	Good
Moorthy et al., (2017) [22]	M	C5-C7	Intradural extramedullary	None	Tingling paresthesia	3 weeks	Good

F female, *M* male, *mos* months, *yrs* years

8 Preferential Resolution of AC According to Its Site

The lesions located at the base of skull are more prone to spontaneous rupture due to the presence of basal rugosities. These rugosities may cause a spontaneous rupture of the ACs with even a minimal mechanical impact. The possible reason for the maximum resolution of the cyst in the middle cranial fossa may be because of their high frequency in this region, which in turn is the result of the presence of several arachnoidal reflections. During development, the bones of skull follow the lobes of brain. This often leads to a focal thinning of the inner table of skull at the site of occurrence of the convexity AC. The surfacing cysts are more prone to rupture even after mild impact over the head due to their proximity to the overlying bone of the skull.

9 Proposed Mechanism for the Spontaneous Resolution of ACs

The possible mechanisms responsible for the spontaneous resolution of ACs are as follows:

1. The ball-valve mechanism (ingress of cerebrospinal fluid that is unable to find an outlet through the cyst membrane) leads to a progression in the cyst size. At a point, the intracystic pressure exceeds the threshold pressure within the cyst, leading to its rupture. The ball-valve mechanism of fluid ingress into the AC may also get spontaneously reversed leading to resolution of the cyst or a decrease in the cyst size. This phenomenon is more common in the middle cranial fossa ACs.
2. The osmotic gradient reversal may lead to a resolution of the cyst. The osmolality of the microenvironment surrounding the AC may usually be higher than the AC itself leading to fluid inflow into the cyst. Occasionally, the oncotic pressure of the extra-cystic fluid may be higher resulting in the diffusion of the fluid across the AC membrane, leading to a spontaneous resolution of the AC. This may especially occur due to the use of hypertonic fluid to combat raised intracranial pressure. The hypertonicity induced into the intravascular compartment dehydrates the brain parenchyma, and this change in oncotic pressure results in efflux of fluid from the cyst into the surrounding extracellular and the neurovascular compartment.
3. The decompression or excision of a concomitantly existing space occupying lesion (SOL) may lead to the reduction of intracranial pressure (ICP) and the compensatory expansion of the brain tissue compressed by the SOL. Pascal's law may determine the physiological changes in the AC. According to Pascal's law, the pressure applied anywhere in a confined incompressible fluid (in this situation, the CSF is considered as a non-compressible liquid) is transmitted equally in all directions throughout that fluid. The tumor excision leads to a fall of the pericystic pressure, which consequently may lead to the sudden stretching of the cyst wall. This sudden expansion in the cyst wall leads to the cyst rupture, and hence, to the resolution of the cyst.
4. Kato et al. proposed that the disappearance of ACs following surgical intervention could be as a result of the establishment of an aberrant communication of the cyst with the subarachnoid space [18].
5. The phenomenon of subarachnoid hemorrhage (SAH) or chronic meningitis initiates a cascade of events which include scarring of variable degree in the subarachnoid space, leading to considerable tethering of the cyst walls to each other and to the surrounding tissue. This may lead to the obliteration of the cyst cavity. The bleed in the brain tissue or the increase in the protein content in CSF causes deposition of significant amount of ferritin as well as other osmotically active materials. This leads to subtle but constant inflammation of the cerebral tissue along with the osmotic gradient across the cyst wall. The presence of subarachnoid hemor-

rhage or chronic meningitis may occasionally result in a gradual resolution in the size of the AC.

6. The expanding cyst wall may cause a breach of the pia mater and may lead to white matter edema. The semipermeable membrane of the AC is vulnerable to the synchronous and pulsatile cardiorespiratory excursions, leading to gradual egress of fluid into the brain parenchyma. An impact on the AC wall during maneuvers such as coughing, rigorous breathing, and sports-related activity may produce adequate amount of stress to cause the breakthrough release of the AC cavity pressure. This may be the reason for the spontaneous resolutions of ACs to be more noticeable in the younger population [38].
7. The increasing size of the cyst that are located adjacent to the ventricles and rarely within the ventricles may lead to the simultaneous breach of the cyst and ependymal wall of the ventricle. This may cause a sudden decompression of the cyst cavity.
8. The fragile nature of the vessel wall is noticed due to an underlying connective/collagen tissue disorder in conditions such as microscopic polyangiitis, Wegener's granulomatosis, scleroderma, etc. The traversing/peri cystic arterioles are under continuous stretch/tension and often rupture due to the mass affect. The lack of a tamponade effect leads to continuous bleeding in and around the cyst. This sudden bleeding leads to cyst volume augmentation, causing the cyst wall rupture and release of contents to the subdural space or the subarachnoid space.
9. The CSF diversion performed to manage obstructive hydrocephalus leads to a significant reduction in intracranial pressure. The significant pressure gradient across the cyst wall and the sudden change in fluid dynamics lead to shrinkage of cyst size or the rupture of the cyst wall.
10. The walls of the convexity ACs are in close proximity to the dura mater. Even a trivial blow to the head, such as minor blow on the head or a trivial fall from height that may often go unnoticed, may lead to cyst decompression towards the less pliable side, that is, towards dural side (Fig. 2).
11. The cysts located at the lateral aspect are prone to undergo compression due to weight of the lobes. These mechanical compressions sometimes lead to gradual resolution of the cyst due to a spontaneous rupture of the cyst wall or the gradual egress of its contents due to the differential hydrostatic pressure across the cyst wall. The larger ACs of the temporal lobe (as suggested by Robinson) may decompress but occasionally fail to resolve completely, even after surgical intervention, due to the residual mass effect of the lobes that cause the cyst outlet to close after a partial ejection of its contents [18, 31].

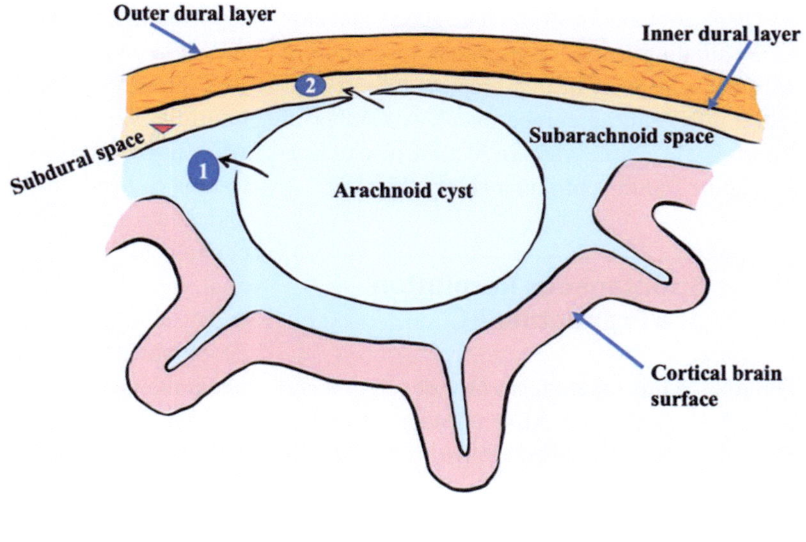

Fig. 2 Schematic diagram showing the proposed pathway for the spontaneous resolution of ACs. Number 1 (in blue circle): subarachnoid space; Number 2 (in blue circle)/Red triangle: subdural space (Thanks Dr. Indubala Maurya, medical illustrator for this drawing)

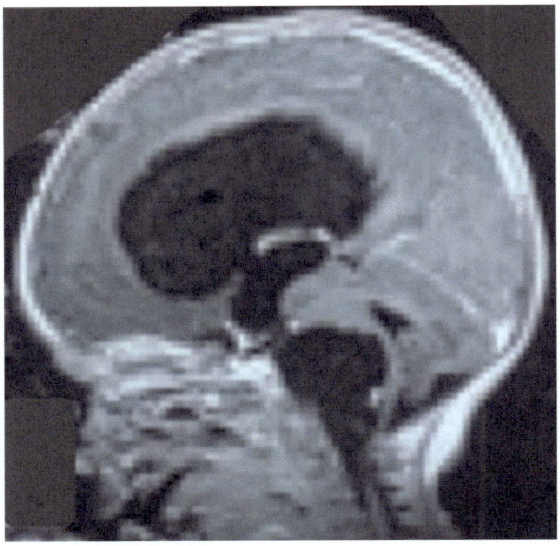

Fig. 3 The sagittal section of a T1WI MRI scan of a child showing a hypointense lesion (AC) entrapped in the cavity of fourth ventricle

12. Resolution of a spinal AC is an extremely uncommon phenomenon and only a single case report has been mentioned in literature (Table 1). The space constraint in the spinal cord as well as the robust musculoskeletal anatomy prevents mechanical impact over these ACs. Drainage of CSF following a lumbar puncture as well as following several spinal epidural anesthetic procedures generates significant pressure gradient across the thin wall of spinal ACs. This phenomenon may lead to a gradual and relatively asymptomatic resolution of the spinal AC.

There exist a number of case reports and case series alluding to the spontaneous resolution of ACs, but a majority of these reports refer to ACs in the infratentorial compartment. A number of reports are available wherein ACs are also noticeable in the fourth ventricular cavity (Fig. 3).

10 Spontaneous Resolution of a Prepontine AC

The ACs in this location are also developmental anomalies similar to ACs at other locations. These lesions are noticed almost exclusively in the pediatric age group. These patients present with features of raised intracranial pressure in the form of visual disturbances, headache, vomiting, endocrine dysfunction, and/or cranial neuropathies. Some of these cysts are diagnosed incidentally when routine prenatal or postnatal imaging is formed. The presence of vital structures in the vicinity of the prepontine AC warrants a lower threshold for surgical intervention. Dodd et al. reported a case of a prepontine AC that underwent a spontaneous resolution following close observation for a period of 5 years [12]. The prepontine location of an AC is among the rarest location and this AC often extends upward into the suprasellar region. On the basis of neuroimaging (cine-mode MRI) and neuroendoscopy, Fitzpatrick and Barlow suggested that the cysts in the suprasellar region originates in the prepontine arachnoid space and expands in the upward direction. The basic pathophysiology behind the origin of these cysts is the presence of a slit-valve mechanism, which appears due to the piercing of arachnoid membrane in the prepontine cistern by the basilar artery. Hence, a few authors refer to these lesions as the suprasellar-prepontine ACs [14]. In order to relieve the symptoms of raised intracranial pressure, these cysts are occasionally subjected to stereotactic aspiration, in addition to the standard surgical modalities employed for diversion of the cyst contents or for excision of the cyst wall [33].

A series by Beltramello and Mazza, in 1985, reported the first spontaneous resolution of an AC, in a patient having a middle cranial fossa AC, presenting with seizures. In literature, multiple reports of spontaneous resolution of ACs have been described following minor trauma to head, the development of meningitis and among patients with asymmetric macrocephaly in the pediatric population. Yoshioka et al. reported a case of spontaneous resolution of an AC in a 2-month-old child following the development of meningitis. In this case, the phenomenon of spontaneous resolution was noticed 10 days later, following the process of initial expansion of the cyst. The possible mechanism underlying this resolution may have been rupture of the cyst wall into the subdural space [45].

Inoue et al. reported a case where the AC resolved spontaneously once the associated thin subdural hematoma underwent resolution on its own. The mean duration taken for the cysts to undergo spontaneous regression was 9 months for the traumatic cases, while it was 50 months for the nontraumatic cases. There was no significant difference in the age group of the individuals undergoing spontaneous resolution of the ACs [17].

There are reports where ACs have been noticed in the intrauterine life during the performance of antenatal ultrasonography and these have undergone spontaneous resolution following childbirth.

The choice of intervention depends upon the location of the AC. The latest literature supports the usage of endoscopic fenestration as the preferred mode of treatment over microsurgical decompression.

11 Spontaneous Resolution of a Middle Cranial Fossa AC

More than half (50–65%) of the ACs occur in the middle cranial fossa (Fig. 4). The possible reason for this high incidence in this location is the presence of maximal arachnoidal reflections in the Sylvian fissure as well as in the base of the skull. The popular classification proposed by Galassi is applicable for middle cranial fossa ACs.

Type I: They remain asymptomatic and majority of the cases are located in the anterior part of middle fossa.

Type II: They extend upwards along the Sylvian fissure and occasionally displace the temporal lobe. Features of compression of the brain matter are obvious.

Type III: These lesions are significantly larger in size and occupy almost the entire middle cranial fossa cavity. These lesions not only displace the temporal lobe by virtue of their size but also cause compression over the frontal and parietal lobe [2].

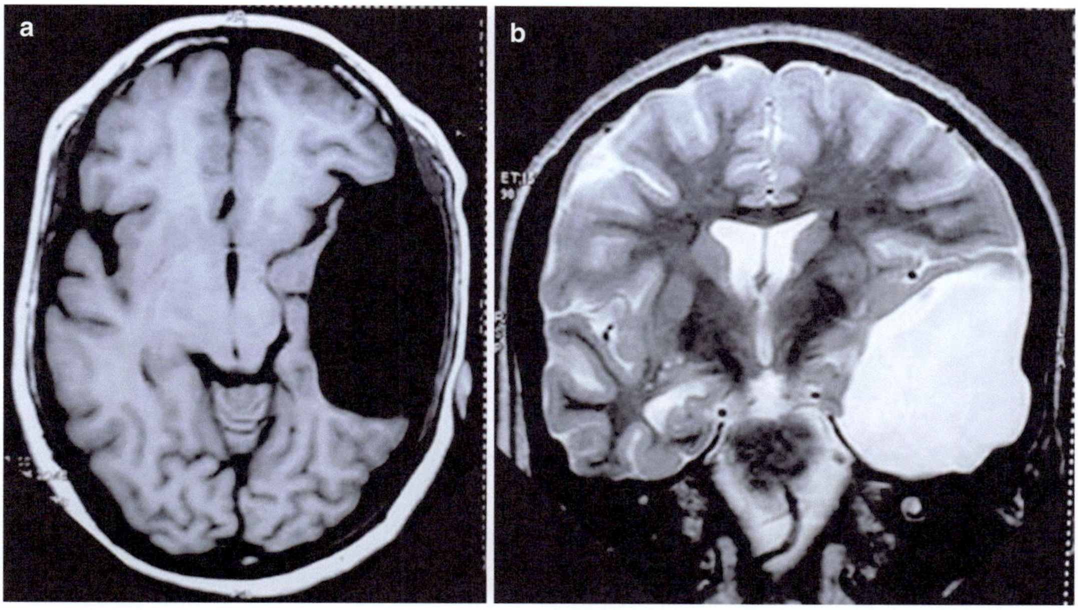

Fig. 4 (**a**) The axial view of T1WI MRI scan shows a hypointense well-defined cystic lesion in the region of left Sylvian fissure. There is significant crowding of the gyri on the posterior aspect of the lesion. (**b**) The T2WI scan shows a hyperintense lesion with edema extending to the adjoining white matter

11.1 Surgical Nuances

The available treatment options for managing ACs of middle cranial fossa are endoscopic or microsurgical fenestration of the cyst, craniotomy and removal of the cyst wall, as well as the diversion of the cyst fluid with the help of a CSF diversion procedure (Fig. 5). The selection of the treatment modality depends on the structure of the AC and its relation to the adjacent neurovascular structure. The radiological appearance of the chiasmatic and interpeduncular cisterns acts as an indicator in deciding the modality of treatment [9].

1. When there is adequate space in the opticocarotid cistern, as well as between the tentorial notch and the oculomotor nerve, with the cyst having a thin-walled membrane, an endoscopic cyst fenestration in the cisternal space is preferred.
2. In the case when the cyst wall is thicker and the cyst is in close proximity to adjacent vital structures, the preferred modality is microsurgical fenestration of the cyst.

A recent meta-analysis advocated that despite availability of several treatment options, the endoscopic modality should be favored as it is less invasive and causes lesser postoperative complications [7].

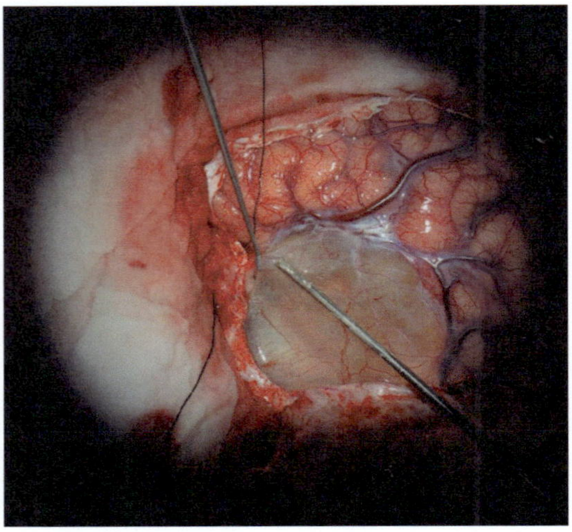

Fig. 5 Intraoperative photograph showing a large Sylvian AC of the left side. The cyst is causing significant compression of the frontal and temporal lobes

12 Spontaneous Resolution of an Interhemispheric AC

Mori at al. categorized the cysts in this area into the midline and parasagittal ACs. The presence of midline cysts indicates agenesis of the corpus callosum, as well as significant compression on the roof of the ventricles. Such cysts are noticeable at the time of birth, are often multi-loculated on screening sonography, and usually lead to hydrocephalus. The treatment consists of fenestrating the cyst into the roof of third ventricle as well removal of the septations. On the other hand, a parasagittal location of the cysts is often found in toddlers, and corpus callosum agenesis is infrequent. Being located in the paramedian plane, there are less chances of developing hydrocephalus. Therefore, cyst wall excision remains the treatment of choice [24].

13 Spontaneous Resolution of a Suprasellar AC

The anatomical proximity of these cysts to the third ventricle results in hydrocephalus being one of the chief presenting complaints. Endoscopic fenestration of the cysts is considered as the preferred treatment modality. Gui et al. suggested that among the endoscopic procedures, the ventriculocystocisternostomy is associated with much higher success rate than solely a ventriculocystostomy or cystocisternostomy [16]. The spontaneous fenestration of the cyst through the third ventricular floor may also be a possible mechanism for its spontaneous resolution.

14 Spontaneous Resolution of a Quadrigeminal AC

ACs of this region are extremely rare with less than 100 cases reported to date.

The cysts of the quadrilateral cistern are categorized into three types. Type I cysts are those having supratentorial as well as infratentorial extension; those with only infratentorial extension are labeled as Type II cysts (these include the supracerebellar or the supra-retrocerebellar cysts);

and those cysts having a lateral extension towards the temporal lobe are grouped as the Type III ACs. ACs of the quadrigeminal cistern, due to an early compression of the cerebral aqueduct, lead to ventricular dilatation as an early manifestation. These lesions manifest with an increasing head size, headache, vomiting, failure to thrive, and disorders of the ocular movement. In view of the significant mass effect and obvious symptoms, these lesions require urgent attention. A study conducted by Cinalli et al. proposed endoscopic decompression as the preferred modality of treatment with a 90% success rate. The higher success rate was associated with the combined endoscopic third ventriculostomy and ventriculocystostomy as the treatment modality [10].

A literature review conducted by Bristol et al., from 1985 to 2007, revealed a higher incidence of spontaneous resolution of middle cranial fossa ACs when compared to cysts at other sites. The possible explanation underlying the higher rate of resolution of ACs in this location was an increased surface area of the AC, which was exposed to the dorsolateral surface of the middle cranial fossa cavity. The lesion being more exposed to the bony surface is more at risk to undergo tear or injury to the arachnoidal wall following even minor trauma. These events are noticed more in the pediatric or the adolescent age group. The events which precipitate spontaneous resolution include sports-related activity, prolonged coughing, hyperventilation, or minor head trauma [6].

15 Spontaneous Resolution of Cerebellar AC

The incidence of cerebellar AC is extremely rare and spontaneous resolution of AC at this location is of utmost rarity. Turgut M. (2002) described an intra-axial AC in the right cerebellar hemisphere of a 1-year-old boy. He made an uneventful recovery over the period of 3 years. The subsequent imaging of brain revealed complete spontaneous resolution of AC [40].

16 Spontaneous Resolution of a Spinal AC

Limited literature is available regarding the spontaneous resolution of a spinal AC (Fig. 6). A single case report of spontaneous resolution

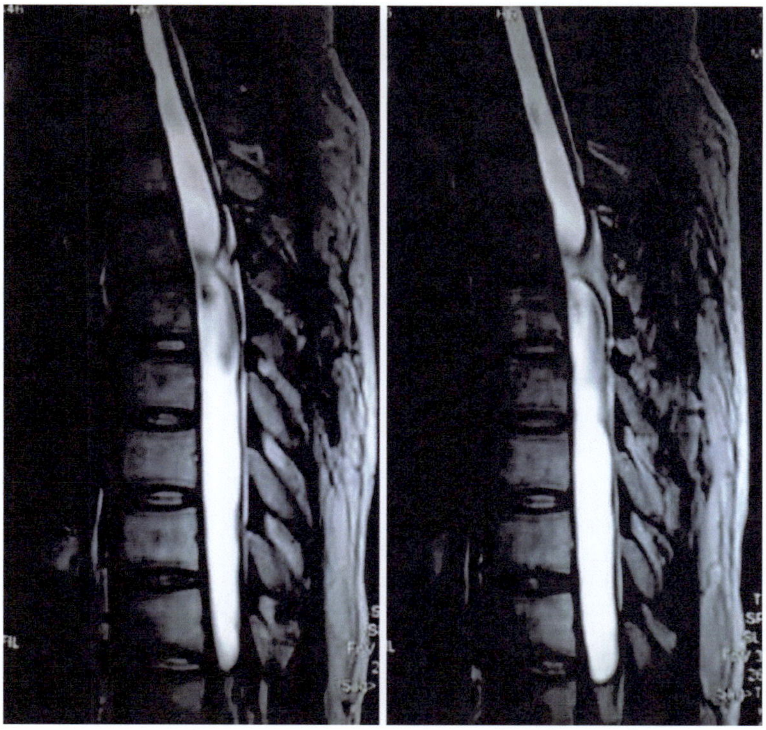

Fig. 6 The sagittal view of T2WI of MRI spine shows an intradural extramedullary AC (from T3 to T11) with two loculations

of spinal AC in the cervical segment was reported by Moorthy et al. in 2017. In this report, the C5 to C7 intradural extramedullary AC resolved completely over a period of 3 weeks following the establishment of its diagnosis on MRI [22].

17 Lesions Mimicking an AC, with Varied Presentation

There are lesions which often mimic an AC on radiological evaluation but have an entirely different origin and a natural course of the disease. These include suprasellar cystic lesions, such as Rathke's cleft cysts, epidermoids, cystic craniopharyngiomas, parasitic infestation (inactive form of neurocysticercotic cyst) as well as developmental anomaly such as porencephalic cysts. Most of the time, rupture of these infective as well as neoplastic lesions leads to vasospasm and meningitis. On the contrary, the rupture of ACs is associated with subdural hygroma, hematoma formation, or spontaneous resolution [35].

18 Conclusion

ACs are benign lesions and their natural progression takes a variable course. The treatment options of ACs depend upon the clinico-radiological correlation rather than its radiological appearance. A case-wise decision making is desirable. The patient should be educated about the clinical signs of deterioration and the risks associated with observation versus surgical intervention. The need for surgical intervention must be reserved for patients who either show disease progression or clinical deterioration.

References

1. Auer LM, Gallhofer B, Ladurner G, Sager WD, Heppner F, Lechner H. Diagnosis and treatment of middle fossa arachnoid cysts and subdural hematomas. J Neurosurg. 1981;54:366–9.
2. Azab WA, Almanabri M, Yosef W. Endoscopic treatment of middle fossa arachnoid cysts. Acta Neurochir (Wien). 2017;159:2313–31.
3. Bamber NI, Prabhu VC. Spontaneous resolution of a posterior fossa arachnoid cyst following a closed head injury: a case report. J Neurosurg Imaging Techniques. 2016;1:84–8.
4. Basaldella L, Orvieto E, Tos AP, Barbera MD, Valente M, Longatti P. Causes of arachnoid cyst development and expansion. Neurosurg Focus. 2007;2:E4.
5. Beltramello A, Mazza C. Spontaneous disappearance of a large middle fossa arachnoid cyst. Surg Neurol. 1985;24:181–3.
6. Bristol RE, Albuquerque FC, McDougall C, Spetzler RF. Arachnoid cysts: spontaneous resolution distinct from traumatic rupture. Neurosurg Focus. 2007;22:E2.
7. Chen Y, Fang HJ, Li ZF. Treatment of middle cranial fossa arachnoid cysts: a systematic review and meta-analysis. World Neurosurg. 2016;92:480–90.
8. Choi JW, Lee JY, Phi JH, Kim SK, Wang KC. Stricter indications are recommended for fenestration surgery in intracranial arachnoid cysts of children. Childs Nerv Sys. 2015;31:77–86.
9. Cinalli G, Cappabianca P, de Falco R. Current state and future development of intracranial neuroendoscopic surgery. Expert Rev Med Devices. 2005;2:351–73.
10. Cinalli G, Spennato P, Columbano L. Neuroendoscopic treatment of arachnoid cysts of the quadrigeminal cistern: a series of 14 cases. J Neurosurg Pediatr. 2010;6:489–97.
11. Cokluk C, Senel A, Celik F, Ergur H. Spontaneous disappearance of two asymptomatic arachnoid cysts in two different locations. Minim Invasive Neurosurg. 2003;46:110–2.
12. Dodd RL, Barnes PD, Huhn SL. Spontaneous resolution of a prepontine arachnoid cyst. Case report and review of the literature. Pediatr Neurosurg. 2002;37:152–7.
13. Dyck P, Gruskin P. Supratentorial arachnoid cysts in adults. Arch Neurol. 1977;34:276–9.
14. Fitzpatrick MO, Barlow P. Endoscopic treatment of prepontine arachnoid cysts. Br J Neurosurg. 2001;15:234–8.
15. Galassi E, Tognetti F, Gaist G, Fagioli L, Frank F, Frank G. CT scan and metrizamide CT cisternography in arachnoid cysts of the middle cranial fossa: classification and pathophysiological aspects. Surg Neurol. 1982;17:363–9.
16. Gui SB, Wang XS, Zong XY, Zhang YZ, Li CZ. Suprasellar cysts: clinical presentation, surgical indications, and optimal surgical treatment. BMC Neurol. 2011;11:5.
17. Inoue T, Matsushima T, Tashima S, Fukui M, Hasuo K. Spontaneous disappearance of a middle fossa arachnoid cyst associated with subdural hematoma. Surg Neurol. 1987;28:447–50.
18. Kato M, Nakada Y, Ariga N, Kokubo Y, Makino H. Prognosis of four cases of primary middle fossa arachnoid cyst in children. Childs Brain. 1980;7:195–204.
19. Liu Z, Li J, Xu J. Teaching neuroimages: spontaneous resolution of a giant intracranial arachnoid cyst. Neurology. 2016;86:199–200.

20. McDonald PJ, Rutka JT. Middle cranial fossa arachnoid cysts that come and go. Report of two cases and review of the literature. Pediatr Neurosurg. 1997;26:48–52.
21. Mokri B, Houser OW, Dinapoli RP. Spontaneous resolution of arachnoid cysts. J Neuroimaging. 1994;4:165–8.
22. Moorthy S, Garg K, Aggarwal A, Kale SS, Sharma BS, Mahapatra AK. Spontaneous resolution of a spinal arachnoid cyst. Neurology India. 2017;65:1416–7.
23. Mori K, Yamamoto T, Horinaka N, Maeda M. Arachnoid cyst is a risk factor for chronic subdural hematoma in juveniles: twelve cases of chronic subdural hematoma associated with arachnoid cyst. J Neurotrauma. 2002;19:1017–27.
24. Mori T, Fujimoto M, Sakae K, Sakakibara T, Shin H, Yamaki T, et al. Disappearance of arachnoid cysts after head injury. Neurosurgery. 1995;36:938–42.
25. Pandey P, Tripathi M, Chandra PS, Sigh VP, Mehta VS. Spontaneous decompression of a posterior fossa arachnoid cyst: a case report. Pediatr Neurosurg. 2001;35:162–3.
26. Parsch CS, Krauss J, Hofmann E, Meixensberger J, Roosen K. Arachnoid cysts associated with subdural hematomas and hygromas: analysis of 16 cases, long-term follow up, and review of the literature. Neurosurgery. 1997;40:483–90.
27. Prabhu VC, Bailes JE. Chronic subdural hematoma complicating arachnoid cyst secondary to soccer-related head injury: case report. Neurosurgery. 2002;50:195–7.
28. Pradilla G, Jallo G. Arachnoid cysts. Case series and review of the literature. Neurosurg Focus. 2007;22:E7.
29. Przybylo HJ, Radkowski MA, Przybylo J, McLone D. Spontaneous resolution of an asymptomatic arachnoid cyst. Pediatr Neurosurg. 1997;26:312–4.
30. Rakier A, Feinsod M. Gradual resolution of an arachnoid cyst after spontaneous rupture into the subdural space. Case Rep. 1995;83:1085–6.
31. Robinson RG. The temporal lobe agenesis syndrome. Brain. 1964;87:87–106.
32. Russo N, Domenicucci M, Rojas Beccaglla M, Santoro A. Spontaneous reduction of intracranial arachnoid cysts: a complete review. Br J Neurosurg. 2008;22:626–9.
33. Schroeder HW, Gaab MR. Endoscopic observation of a slit-valve mechanism in a suprasellar prepontine arachnoid cyst: case report. Neurosurgery. 1997;40:198–200.
34. Seizeur R, Forlodou P, Coustans M, Dam-Hein P. Spontaneous resolution of arachnoid cyst: review and features of an unusual case. Acta Neurochir (Wein). 2007;19:361–4.
35. Shida N, Nakasato N, Mizoi K, Kanaki M, Yoshimoto T. Symptomatic vessel narrowing caused by spontaneous rupture of craniopharyngioma cyst-case report. Neurol Med Chir (Tokyo). 1998;38:666–8.
36. Sommer IE, Smit LM. Congenital supratentorial arachnoidal and giant cysts in children: a clinical study with arguments for a conservative approach. Childs Nerv Syst. 1997;13:8–12.
37. Takagi K, Sasaki T, Basugi N. Spontaneous disappearance of cerebellopontine angle arachnoid cyst: report of a case (in Japanese). No Shinkei Geka. 1987;15:295–9.
38. Takizawa H, Sugiura K, Kudo C, Kadoyama S. Spontaneous disappearance of a middle fossa arachnoid cyst—a case report. No To Shinkei. 1991;43:987–9.
39. Tsuruda JS, Chew WM, Moseley ME, Norman D. Diffusion-weighted MR imaging of the brain: value of differentiating between extraaxial cysts and epidermoid tumors. AJNR Am J Neuroradiol. 1990;11:925–34.
40. Turgut M. Complete spontaneous resolution of an intra-axial cystic lesion in the cerebellum: a case report. Curr Pediatr Res. 2002;6:33–4.
41. Weber R, Voit T, Lumenta C, Lenard HG. Spontaneous regression of a temporal arachnoid cyst. Childs Nerv Syst. 1991;7:414–5.
42. Wester K, Gilhus NE, Hugdahl K, Larsen JL. Spontaneous disappearance of an arachnoid cyst in the middle intracranial fossa. Neurology. 1991;41:1524–6.
43. Yamanouchi Y, Someda K, Oka N. Spontaneous disappearance of middle fossa arachnoid cyst after head injury. Childs Nerv Syst. 1986;2:40–3.
44. Yamauchi T, Saeki N, Yamaura A. Spontaneous disappearance of temporo-frontal arachnoid cyst in a child. Acta Neurochir (Wien). 1999;141:537–40.
45. Yoshioka H, Kurisu K, Arita K, Eguchi K, Tominaga A, Mizoguchi N, et al. Spontaneous disappearance of a middle cranial fossa arachnoid cyst after suppurative meningitis. Surg Neurol. 1998;50:487–91.

Part III

Neuroimaging of Arachnoid Cysts

Editor's Summary

In this "Part III: Neuroimaging of Arachnoid Cysts," there are a total of four chapters describing the various forms of neuroimaging that is employed to evaluate these fluid-filled collections. Even today, the diagnosis of arachnoid cysts (ACs) can at times be difficult for clinicians to determine. This part begins with the routine radiological evaluation of ACs which is primarily performed using computed tomography (CT) and magnetic resonance imaging, in addition to x-ray and myelography. Now, these basic imaging techniques are usually sufficient for obtaining an accurate diagnosis of the presence of an AC. Occasionally, the intrauterine diagnosis of ACs can be made during routine obstetrical monitoring during pregnancy via ultrasonography as is described in 15. Although not usually necessary for the evaluation of patients with ACs, metrizamide CT cisternography can be occasionally useful as is discussed in the next chapter. This part concludes with the nuclear medicine tomographic imaging technique known as SPECT imaging for providing additional information for diagnosing ACs.

Radiological Evaluation of Arachnoid Cysts

Pinar İlhan Demir, Almila Coşkun Bilge, and Ahmet T. Turgut

1 Introduction

In 1831, English physician Bright first described arachnoid cysts (ACs) as serous cysts surrounded by a wall related to the arachnoid membrane [68]. ACs are the most common benign, non-neoplastic, intra-arachnoid abnormalities of the brain. ACs are encapsulated by the arachnoid membrane which is filled with a fluid like cerebrospinal fluid (CSF). They are usually asymptomatic. When they are symptomatic, symptoms are usually related to the mass effect on adjacent structures and locations. Prenatal ultrasound (US) screening and the widespread use of magnetic resonance imaging (MRI) and computed tomography (CT) for other head pathologies lead to incidentally diagnosed ACs [11, 41, 81].

The incidence of ACs is controversial because the asymptomatic course of ACs obscures the true incidence. In the literature, the incidence of ACs is reported as approximately 0.5–1.5% of the population [41, 82, 85]. Al-Holou et al. studied 11,738 patients aged 18 years or younger who had undergone brain MRI and found that the prevalence in childhood was about 2.6%. In another study in adults by Al-Holou et al., 661 of 48,417 patients had ACs, with a 1.4% prevalence [4, 5].

ACs can be seen throughout life, but nearly 75% of ACs are diagnosed in childhood. Males are twice more likely to be affected, and the left hemisphere is predominantly affected although the etiology is unknown [4, 5, 25, 30]. ACs are usually sporadic and present as a single malformation. Multiple ACs may occur in syndromes and metabolic disorders such as glutaric aciduria type 1, polycystic kidney disease, Down syndrome, neurofibromatosis, etc. in which the incidence of ACs increases [30, 48].

The location of the ACs in the cranial cavity varies; in adults, 60–70% of ACs are found in the middle cranial fossa and Sylvian fissure (Figs. 1 and 2). Infratentorial ACs are 10% of ACs and are located in the cerebellopontine angle or retrocerebellar area (Fig. 3). Infratentorial ACs are more common in children than in adults. ACs are also rarely found in the suprasellar, interhemispheric, intraventricular, and cerebellopontine angles and in the spinal region [4, 19]. Most ACs remain stable, but rarely progression or regression can be seen [5, 66, 73].

P. İ. Demir (✉)
Department of Radiology, Ankara Bilkent City Hospital, Çankaya, Ankara, Turkey

A. C. Bilge
Department of Radiology, Dr. Abdurrahman Yurtaslan Ankara Oncology Training and Research Hospital, Yenimahalle, Ankara, Turkey

A. T. Turgut
Department of Radiology, Ankara Medipol University School of Medicine, Çankaya, Ankara, Turkey

M. Turgut et al. (eds.), *Arachnoid Cysts*, https://doi.org/10.1007/978-3-031-22701-1_14

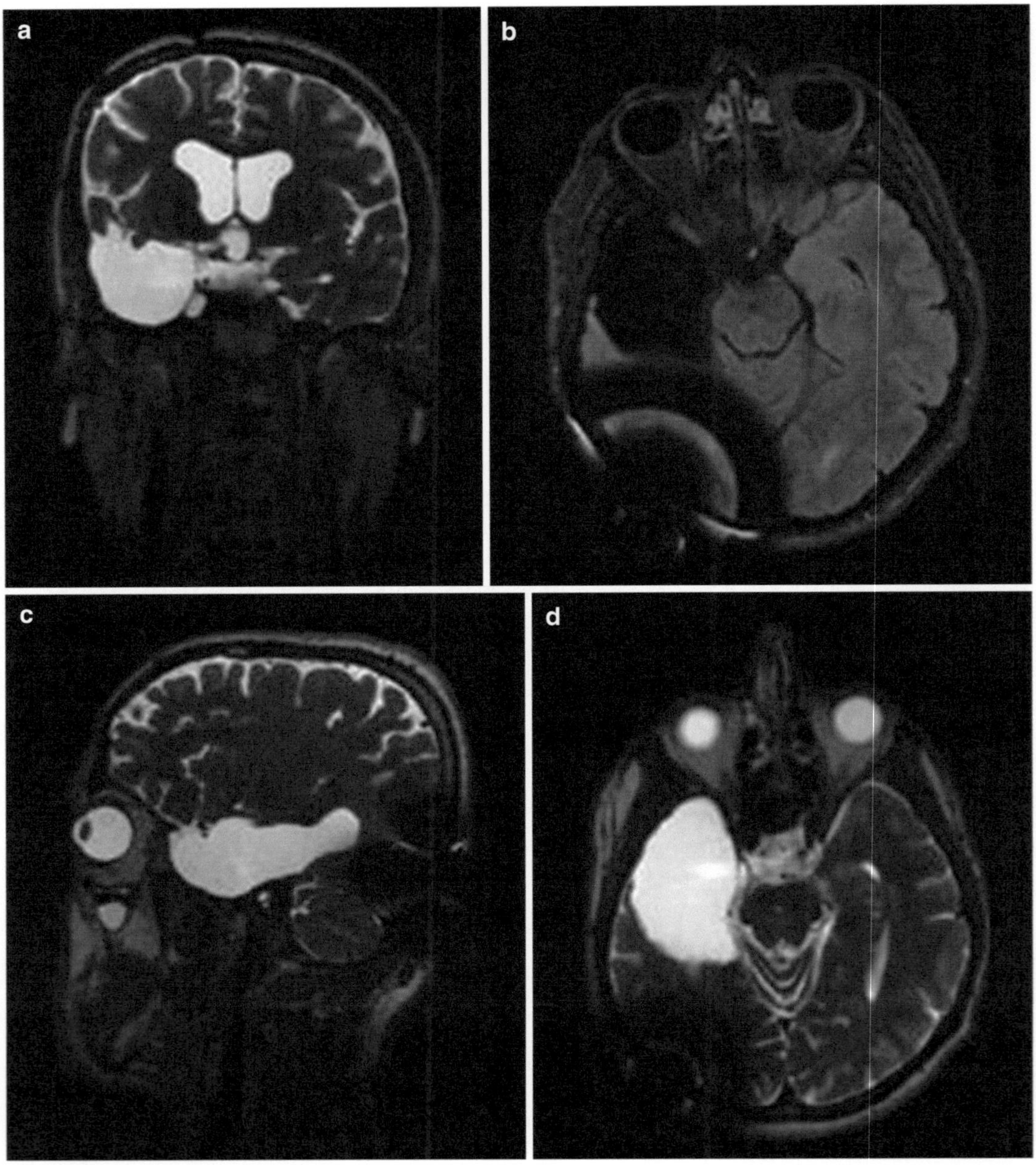

Fig. 1 (**a–d**) MRI of the brain of a 55-year-old patient; AC is anterior to the right temporal lobe. A V-P shunt catheter used to treat AC is depicted. Temporal remodeling and mass effect of the AC are clearly seen

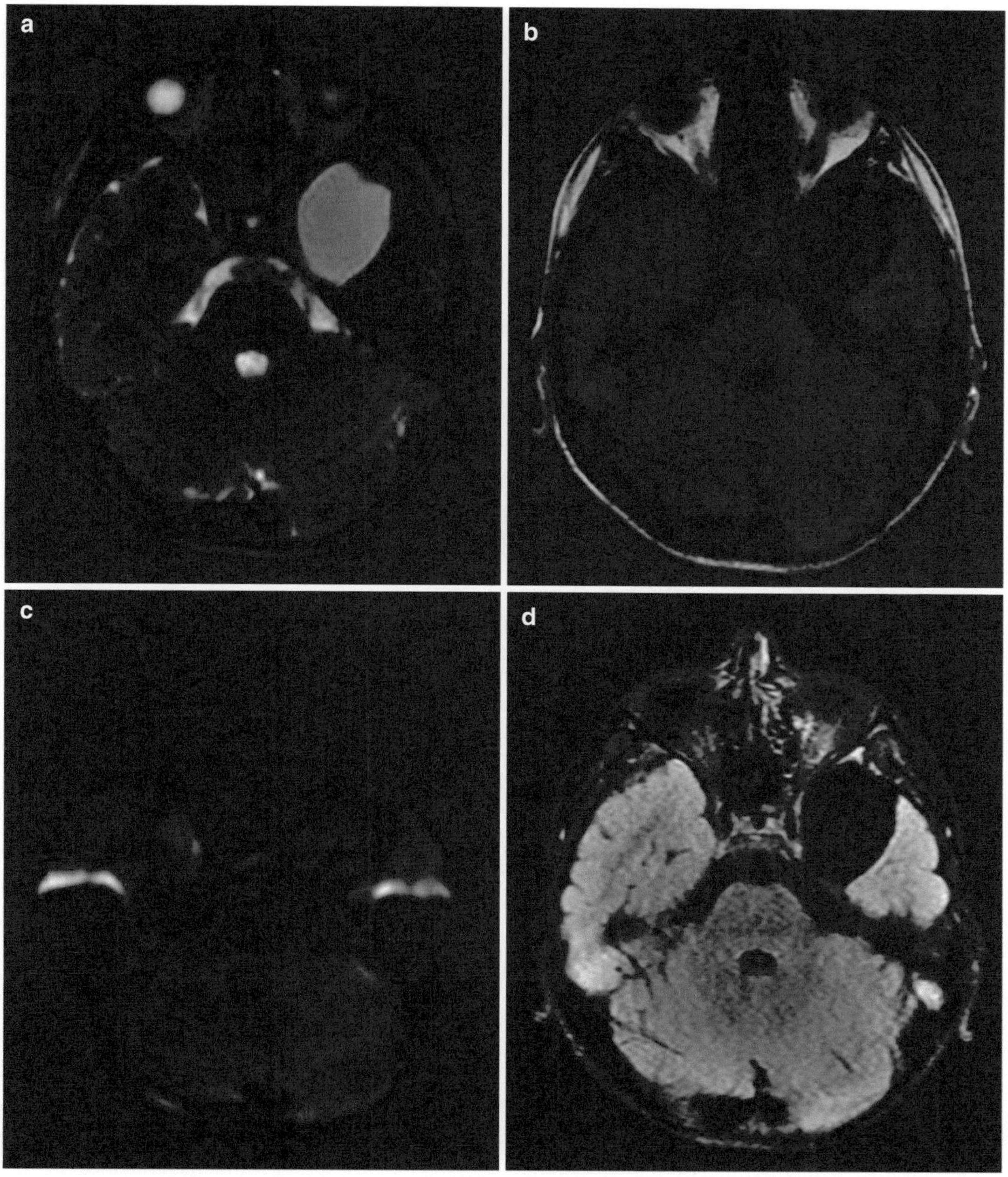

Fig. 2 (**a**–**d**) MRI of the brain of a 6-year-old child. There is an AC at the left temporal pole that was diagnosed incidentally during fetal ultrasonography. After several years of follow-up, the AC was stable in volume and shape. There is remodeling of the skull near the sphenoid bone and orbital walls

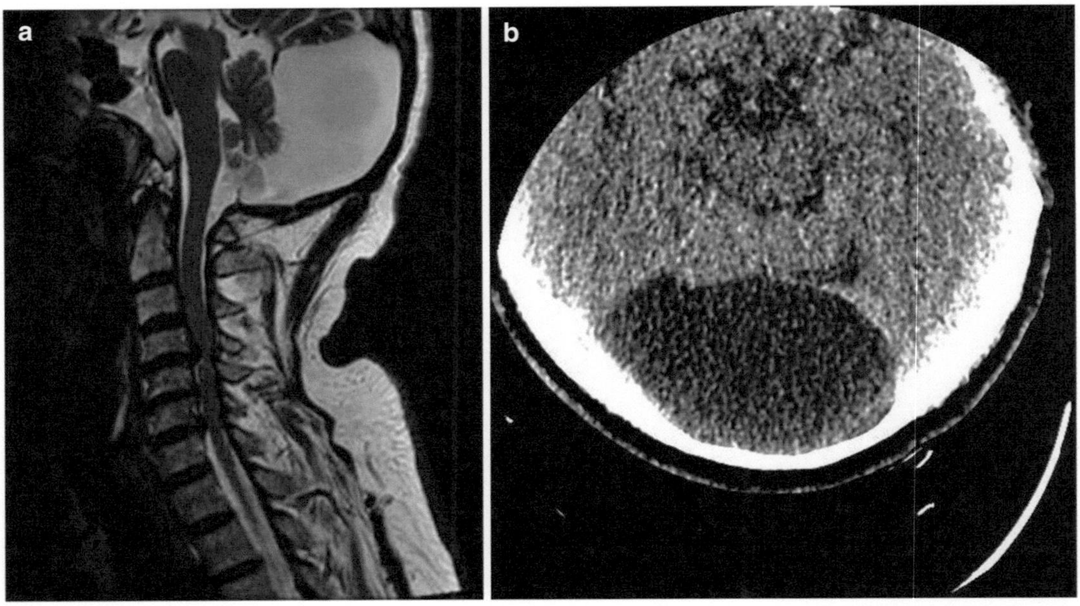

Fig. 3 (**a**, **b**) Infratentorial AC was diagnosed incidentally while evaluating for neck pain. T2-weighted MRI images show hyperintense cystic collection. (**b**) CT shows hypodense cystic collection that compresses the cerebellum

2 Pathology, Etiology, and Clinical Symptoms

ACs are fluid-filled arachnoid layers formed by cleavage of the arachnoid membrane due to congenital malformation or as a result of intracranial pathology. Primary ACs are a congenital developmental anomaly of the arachnoid mater due to cleavage of the arachnoid membrane at the edge of the cyst, which fills with CSF-like fluid, also called true ACs [8, 67]. Primary ACs are located in the arachnoid space and are surrounded by a vascularized collagen wall lined with multilayered hyperplastic arachnoid cells. ACs are distinguished from arachnoid granulations and membranes by a thick collagen wall lined with hyperplastic arachnoid cells and by the absence of trabecular processes. The inner and outer layers of the ACs are fused at the border, and they continue as normal arachnoid membrane. Choroid plexus and neuroglial cells can be seen in some cases of suprasellar or posterior fossa ACs. Primary ACs are the most common type [59, 67].

Secondary ACs are required ACs as a result of head trauma, infection, inflammation, etc., in which CSF-like fluid accumulates in the arachnoid space. Pericystic gliosis and hemosiderosis may accompany the cyst. The contents may be proteinaceous or xanthochromic, and an arachnoid cell layer is not present [59, 78].

ACs can be also classified as communicating and noncommunicating cysts depending on their relationship to the subarachnoid CSF space. In communicating ACs, there is a connection between the AC and the surrounding subarachnoid space, allowing CSF to enter the cyst space (Fig. 4). As for noncommunicating ACs, the AC has no communication, and CSF cannot enter the cyst. If surgical intervention is required for treatment of ACs, the difference between communicating and noncommunicating cysts should be established for treatment management [67].

ACs filled with CSF-like fluid are clear and contain no cellular debris, proteinaceous material, hemosiderin, or inflammatory cells with the same osmolarity and concentration of sodium, potassium, chloride, calcium, magnesium, and glucose. But some proteins and enzymes are minimal or absent, such as hemoglobin, carbonic anhydrate, lactate dehydrogenase, and alpha-1-antitrypsin, which distinguish CSF from ACs [9, 72].

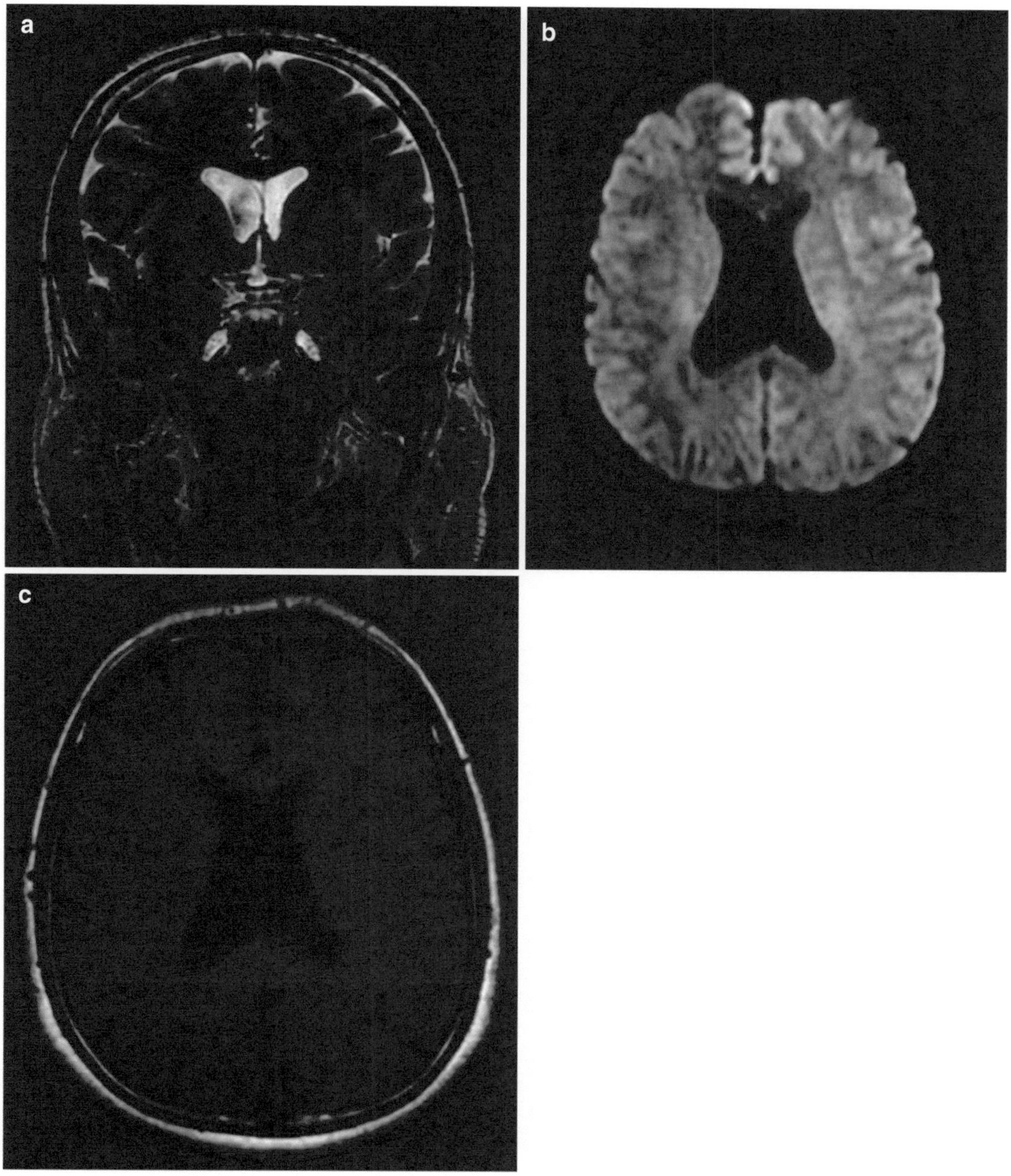

Fig. 4 (**a**–**c**) A 55-year-old male patient with recurrent syncope. An intraventricular AC is seen on coronal T2-weighted, DWI-weighted, and T1-weighted MR images, and CSF flow is seen as a signal void in the cyst on T2-weighted images. Communicated cyst

ACs are often stable in size and behavior. Occasionally, they regress and disappear entirely [19, 69, 73, 80]. ACs rarely enlarge resulting in remodeling of the calvarium, mass effects on surrounding tissue, and other symptoms [19]. There are several theories that explain the enlargement of ACs. In the one-way valve mechanism theory, CSF enters the cyst space but cannot escape. The osmotic gradient theory explains the expansion by the hyperosmolar intracystic space and the influx of fluid into the cyst from the iso-osmolar environment. The other theory explains the expansion of the ACs by secretory arachnoid cells lining the inner wall of the ACs and secreting CSF-like fluid [14, 71]. It is believed that the combination of these three mechanisms contribute to the development of ACs, but this is still controversial [23].

Most ACs (80–90%) are located in the supratentorial space. The vast majority of ACs in the supratentorial space arise from the Sylvian fissure (50–60% of all intracranial ACs) and are located in the temporal fossa (Figs. 1 and 2). The quadrigeminal plate region and the chiasmatic cistern are other common sites for supratentorial ACs (Fig. 5). The interhemispheric fissure and convexity are less frequent sites of origin [4, 19] (Fig. 6). The lateral cerebellopontine (CP) angles (Fig. 7) and the midline retrocerebellar cisterns are fairly equivalent, whereas the interpeduncular and prepontine cisterns are a rare site of origin of the infratentorial ACs. Unlike in children, the retrocerebellar location of ACs in adults is as common as that of ACs in the middle

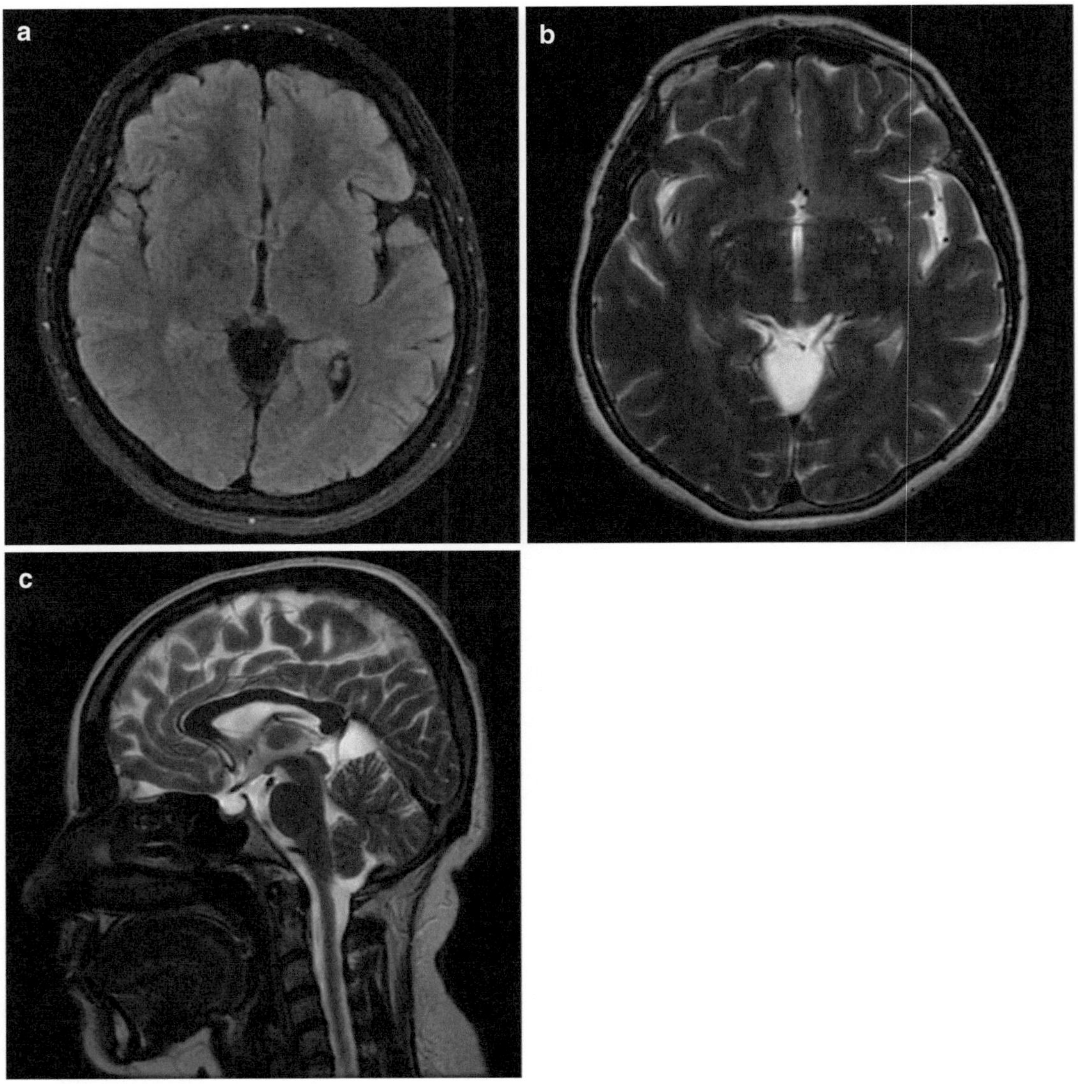

Fig. 5 (**a–c**) This is a quadrigeminal plate AC in a 25-year-old male patient complaining of headache and compressing the medial temporal lobes and cerebellum

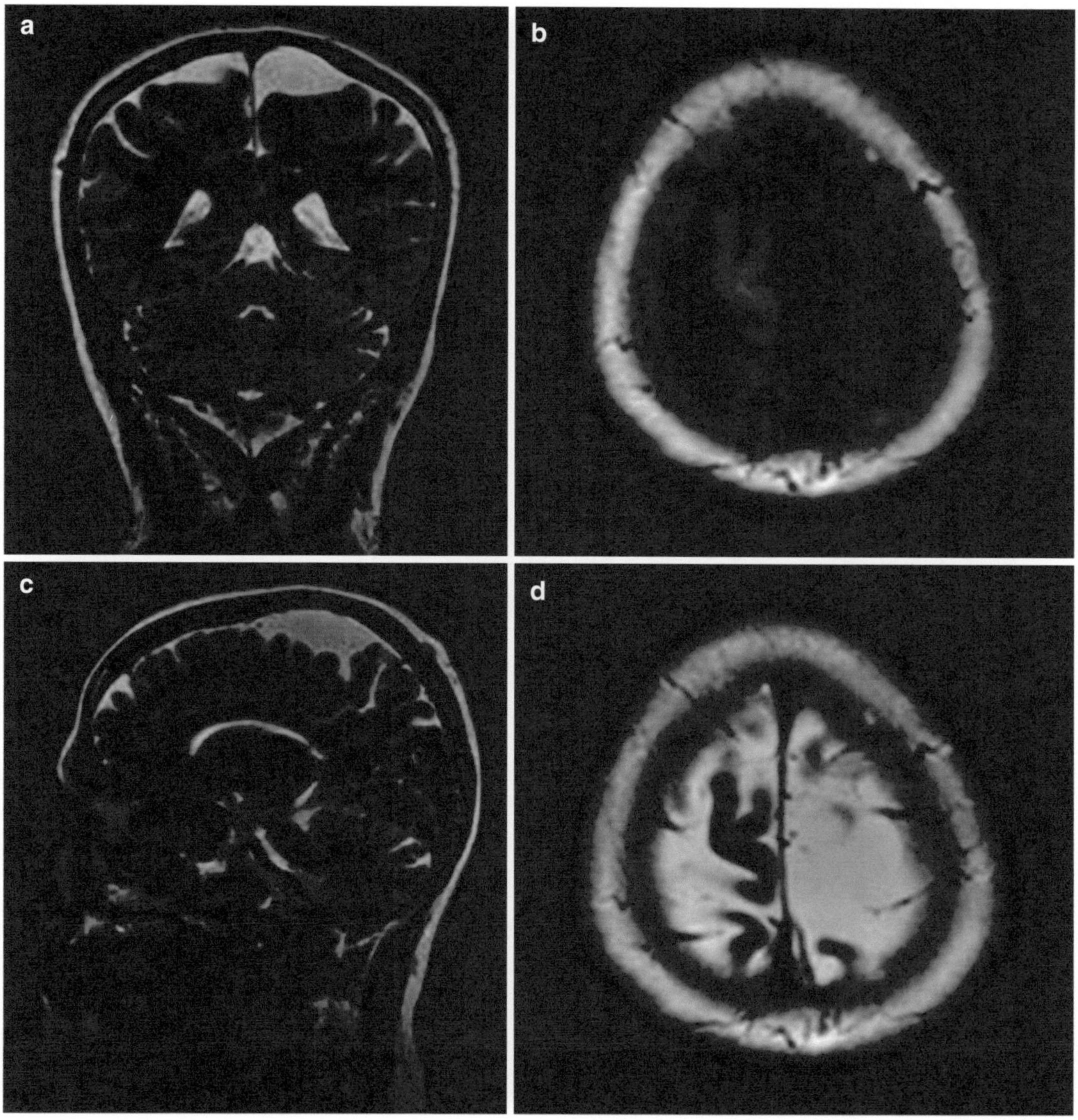

Fig. 6 (**a**–**d**) A 43-year-old female patient complains of headache. MRI shows no contrast enhancement and no diffusion-restricted extraaxial lesion that can be diagnosed as AC

cranial fossa [4, 5]. Some ACs located in the suprasellar and quadrigeminal plate may grow toward and into the cerebral ventricles (Fig. 5). Paraventricular cysts are usually primary ACs. The purely intraventricular cysts generally develop secondary to tumoral, inflammatory, posthemorrhagic, or postinfectious processes or are secondary to malformative lesions (cavum septi) or arise from the choroid plexus or ependyma [50, 63] (Fig. 4).

Symptoms of ACs usually depend on the location and size. Headache, seizures, hydrocephalus, macrocrania, hormonal deficits, visual loss, hearing loss, and facial sensory loss can be observed. After head trauma, cyst rupture, hemorrhage, intracystic hemorrhage, or hygroma development leads the asymptomatic cysts to become symptomatic. Patients with ACs are prone to develop subdural hematomas after minor head trauma [4, 33, 34, 37, 53, 55].

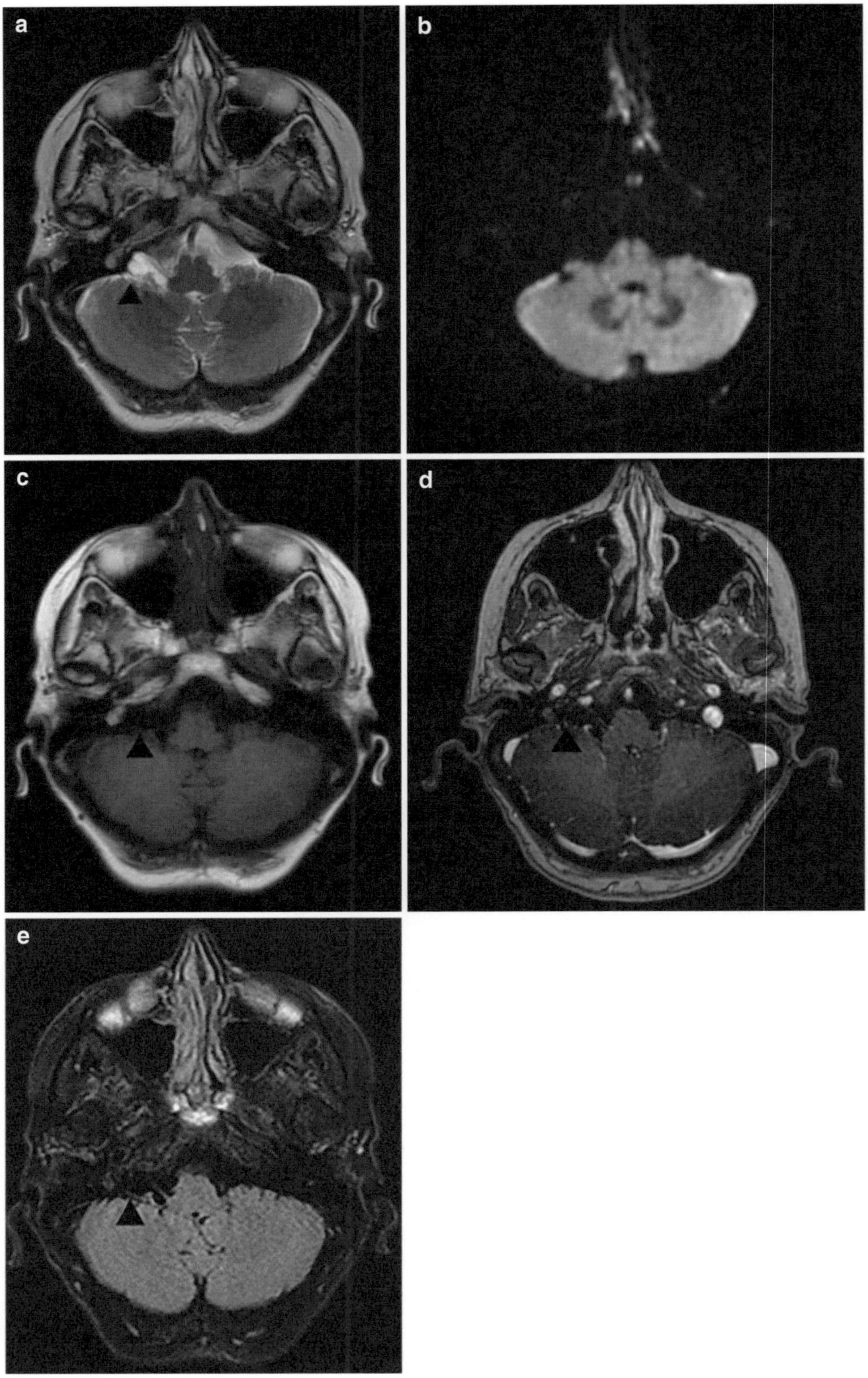

Fig. 7 (**a**–**e**) A 63-year-old woman complains of dizziness and tinnitus. There is a cystic lesion in the right pontocerebellar cistern leading to these symptoms. The diagnosis is AC

3 Radiological Diagnosis of Arachnoid Cysts

3.1 Antenatal Ultrasonography

US has a role in diagnosing ACs, predominantly in prenatal, infantile, and early childhood periods. As the cranial bones thicken in the advanced ages, sonographic resolution decreases considerably and does not allow intracranial evaluation [83]. US is useful as a noninvasive, widely available, cost-effective, and radiation-free imaging technique with a high yield for detecting and characterizing cystic masses [10]. These features of US also allow serial examination in the follow-up of the AC and its complications [90].

The standard prenatal approach for evaluating the central nervous system (CNS) is US imaging [33]. Although rare, ACs of developmental origin (primary) can be detected in prenatal screening (0.2%) [31]. Prenatal US can reveal an AC as early as 20 weeks of gestation. However, there is a case in the literature diagnosed as a posterior fossa AC by transvaginal US at 13 weeks of gestation [15, 29, 90]. Most children with a prenatal diagnosis have a normal neurodevelopmental course. Large size (>2 cm), syndromic/genetic diagnosis, and/or presence of other intracranial abnormalities are reported as the predictors of pathological outcomes [17, 31]. Maternal obesity, oligohydramnios, fetal head engagement during late pregnancy, or acoustic shadowing by surrounding bony structures may impair sonographic imaging [10, 13]. In such restrictive situations, transvaginal neurosonography can be used. Convex probe (1–6 MHz), sector probe (3–5 MHz), and transvaginal probes (5–10 MHz) are used in the prenatal US [13, 90]. Fetal brain images are examined predominantly in the transverse axial plane, additionally in the coronal and parasagittal planes [13]. ACs are imaged as avascular extraaxial anechoic-hypoechoic lesions of variable dimensions with a thin regular outline, with or without septa on antenatal US [10, 16, 60, 90]. They do not communicate with the lateral ventricles and are not associated with loss of brain tissue. Larger cysts may cause compression in the adjacent cerebral parenchyma. The cysts are usually located in supratentorial (50–65% middle cranial fossa) and rarely infratentorial areas [15, 57, 89]. If the cyst blocks the foramen of Monro or the aqueduct, secondary hydrocephalus develops, and ventriculomegaly is observed on US [29, 90]. In addition, ACs and chromosomal abnormalities may co-exist, and accompanying structural abnormalities of the CNS such as frontal polymicrogyria, an abnormal corpus callosum, cerebellar dysplasia, and gray matter heterotopia can be visualized on the prenatal US [15, 17]. In the differential diagnosis of ACs in prenatal US, porencephalic cysts, choroid plexus cysts, aneurysms of the vein of Galen, schizencephaly, cystic neoplasms, and intracranial hemorrhage should be considered US [15, 17, 90].

AC consists of 1% of neonatal intracranial masses [15, 17, 29]. Transcranial US is a crucial diagnostic tool to evaluate the ACs during the first year of life. It is limited by the closure of the anterior fontanelle, which generally occurs in full-term infants 9–18 months of age. A sector probe (1–4 MHz) was used for the transcranial US. A high-frequency linear probe (5–10 MHz) is used for detailed visualization of superficial structures. Anterior-posterior-sphenoidal fontanelle, temporal area, high parietal convexity, supraorbital areas, and foramen magnum can be used as an acoustic window while performing US. Infratentorial structures are evaluated using acoustic windows, including posterior-lateral fontanelle, temporal approach, and foramen magnum. The sellar region is a challenging area for the transcranial US to evaluate small space-occupying lesions. Images should be symmetrical in the coronal and sagittal planes. ACs are imaged as extraaxial well-circumscribed smooth thin-walled anechoic-hypoechoic lesions. Color Doppler interrogation helps to assess the vascularization of lesions [32, 83]. ACs are avascular, which can be demonstrated by color Doppler imaging. Hydrocephalus and brain herniation, which may develop due to the mass effect caused by large cysts, can be determined in the US. The differential diagnosis of an AC is a subdural hygroma, dilatation of normal subarachnoid space secondary to underlying atrophy or encephalomalacia, and epidermoid cyst [58].

US can be used in the diagnosis of ACs as well as throughout surgical treatment. During the operation, intraoperative US can clearly define ACs, and treatment of these cysts, including drainage and fenestration of septations, is easily facilitated by intraoperative US guidance. Direct intraoperative real-time US of the brain and spinal cord is made with scan heads small enough for use after craniotomy/laminectomy or even through a burr hole. The sector probe (3–10 MHz) is generally used as the intraoperative probe [7, 40]. The cysts' location and extent are evaluated before the neurosurgical approach for drainage or excision [40]. Thus, a safer and much more effective surgery becomes possible.

3.2 Computed Tomography

ACs are usually discovered incidentally during imaging studies (Fig. 3). On CT, ACs are sharply demarcated, unilocular, homogeneous, extraaxial lesions that have identical density with CSF. Hounsfield attenuation values range from 10 to 20 (hypodense). In the case of intracystic hemorrhage, they may be hyperintense. ACs do not usually enhance after intravenous injection of iodinated contrast medium, but ACs may enhance with delayed imaging. Bone remodeling such as calvarial bone thinning, bulging of the skull, and sphenoid wing displacements can be best distinguished on CT. ACs usually obliterate the subarachnoid space and compress surrounding tissue. ACs vary in size and may be unilocular or septated [30, 62, 87].

When CT is compared with MRI, soft tissue contrast is lower, and scanning CT requires an ionizing dose of radiation, which is a disadvantage in the pediatric population. But CT is a faster, cheaper, and more available neuroimaging test than MRI. CT is also helpful in detecting intracystic hemorrhage. CT imaging is often sufficient to establish the diagnosis of an AC. Thin-walled cysts that have CSF-like density at the usual locations generally help to determine the presence of ACs [30, 87, 88].

3.3 Magnetic Resonance Imaging

MRI is the gold standard imaging tool for ACs and distinguishes them from other intracranial cystic lesions. MRI is the most useful diagnostic tool for evaluating ACs to confirm their extraaxial location. On T2-weighted images, ACs exhibit hyperintense signal that attenuates on fluid-attenuated inversion recovery (FLAIR) images similar to that of CSF [24, 30, 87]. On T1-weighted images, the ACs have hypointense signal to the brain. Diffusion-weighted imaging is essential for distinguishing ACs from epidermoid cysts. Both ACs and epidermoid cysts generally have the same appearance on T1- and T2- weighted images (Figs. 1, 2, 3, 4, 5, 6, 7, 8, 9, 10, 11, 12, and 13). If ACs rupture or bleed into the cystic space, blooming can be seen on gradient echo (GRE) sequences. Uncomplicated ACs show no blooming on GRE [24, 75]. ACs do not enhance after gadolinium administration and do not have diffusion restriction, whereas epidermoid cysts usually restrict the diffusion on DWI [15] (Figs. 2, 6, 7, and 8).

For radiological evolution, the radiologist must first be informed with an accurate history of the patient by the clinician. During the radiological process, the radiologist must assess the mass effect on the adjacent tissues of the brain structures, such as nerves, vessels, and affected tissues. In addition, the radiologist must inform the physician about the cysts that may cause hydrocephalus or large cysts that may lead to cerebral herniation. CT imaging is often sufficient to establish the diagnosis of an AC. When additional information is needed about the anatomic location, size, and structural involvement of an AC or for follow-up, MRI is the best choice [88].

3.4 Cisternography

CT cisternography (CTC) and MR cisternography (MRC) can be performed to make a decision for surgery and to further evaluate an AC with adjacent tissue (small vessels, cranial nerves,

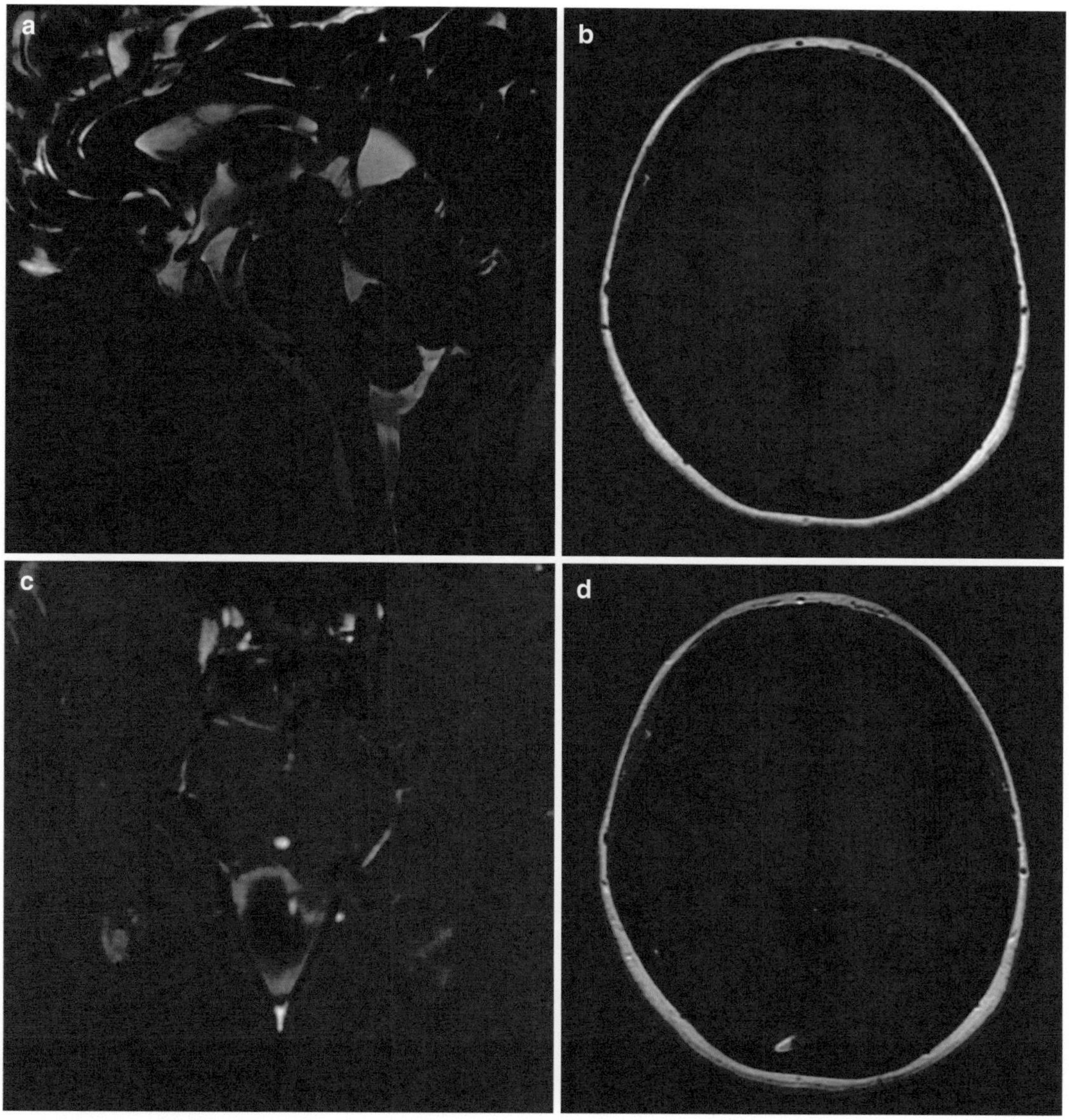

Fig. 8 (**a–d**) Quadrigeminal plate AC. (**c**) Cine images show a signal void due to flow. Since no contrast agent is administered intrathecally, MRI cine cisternography is one of the noninvasive tools for diagnosing flow in the cyst

etc.). Communication of ACs with the subarachnoid CSF space can be demonstrated by cisternography [26, 88]. In CTC, a safe, nonionic iodinated contrast agent is injected intrathecally, and the amount of filling and the time it takes to fill the cyst (dynamic images) can be obtained from CT imaging of the ACs. When cysts fill quickly and completely, they are considered as freely communicating ACs and treatment management changes [26, 84]. Communicating cysts are considered as subarachnoid space diverticulas. But slow-filling noncommunicating ACs are usually regarded as true ACs [88]. When ACs expand, it is because of an osmotic gradient, ball valve mechanism, or fluid-secreting arachnoid cells lining the cyst wall [14, 71].

MRC is another method to assess the connections of the ACs with the CSF space. MRC can be performed in two ways. Intrathecal injection of gadolinium and dynamic imaging of cyst filling

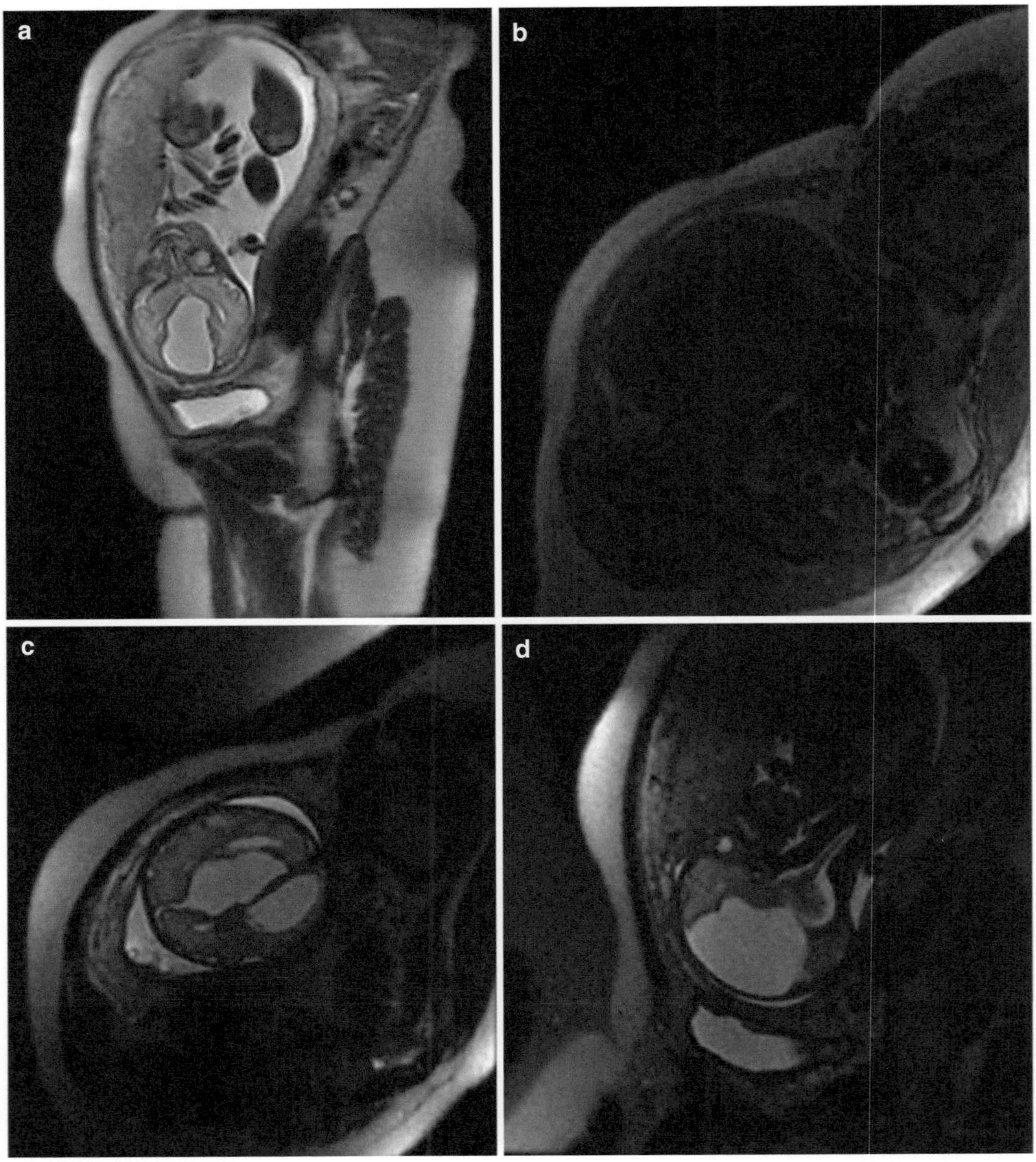

Fig. 9 (**a–d**) A 26-year-old female patient was found to have a cystic lesion after prenatal ultrasonography at 25 months of gestation, and MRI was performed for differential diagnosis. A giant AC was found in the interhemispheric region accompanied by callosal agnesia

can be demonstrated. 0.5–1-mL gadopentetate dimeglumine (Gd-DPTA) is injected intrathecally into the subarachnoid space, and serial fat-saturated T1-weighted images are acquired in three orthogonal planes. As the cyst fluid enhances, the connection between the cyst and the subarachnoid space becomes visible [1–3, 89]. In the other technique, lumbar puncture is not required, and it is more invasive than classical MRC (Fig. 8). High-resolution sequences will allow delineation of the cyst wall and neighboring structures. Constructive interference in steady state (CISS),

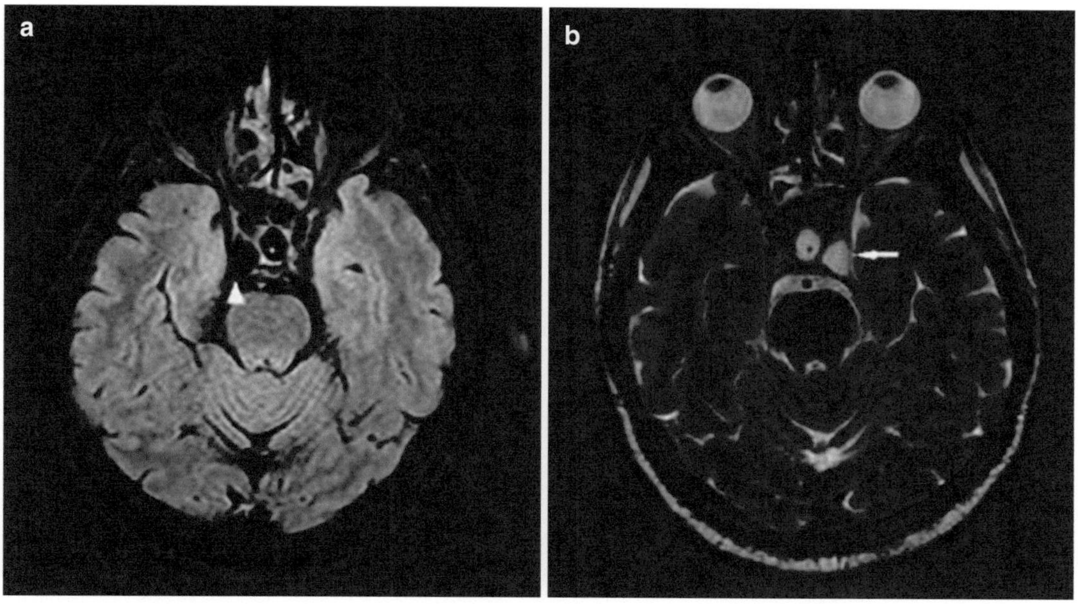

Fig. 10 (**a**, **b**) A 63-year-old man with headache and tremor. Axial noncontrast MRI of the brain showing a left extraaxial cyst in the parasellar cistern with CSF intensity on T2-weighted and FLAIR sequences (*arrows*). This was an asymptomatic AC in the left sellar region, so no further imaging was required

fast imaging employing steady-state acquisition (FIESTA), and 3D T2-weighted sampling perfection with application-optimized contrast with different flip-angle evolutions (3D SPACE) can demonstrate the possible communications of the AC wall and CSF space and also the relationship between ACs and surrounding structures such as cranial nerves and vessels. Phase-contrast cine MRI combination with cardiac gating can be performed to detect CSF connection to an AC. It is usually preferred over CT cisternography because of its minimally invasive nature. If minimally invasive techniques demonstrate the connection, contrast-enhanced MRC should be performed to avoid false-positive results. MRC also provides the ability to distinguish ACs from enlarged subarachnoid spaces [35, 89].

An accurate history of the patient must be obtained from the clinician for radiological evolution. The radiologist must assess the mass effect on the adjacent tissues of the brain structures (nerves, vessels, affected tissues) and inform the clinician about the urgent situations such as hydrocephalus or large cysts that may lead to cerebral herniation.

3.5 Fetal Magnetic Resonance Imaging

Fetal MRI is an advanced diagnostic and evaluation modality. Approximately 80% of all fetal MRI examinations are performed to evaluate fetal CNS pathologies. Fetal MRI is a complementary tool for evaluating the various fetal pathologies diagnosed by ultrasound (US). Indications for fetal MRI include evaluation of an abnormality identified by US; even if the US examination is normal, there is a high risk of pathology due to familial, environmental, or laboratory findings. In cases such as maternal obesity, oligohydramnios, and fetal malposition, where US examination is suboptimal, fetal MRI is critical for diagnosis and management. In CNS pathologies, fetal MRI is usually used to check for ventriculomegaly, underlying pathologies such as hydrocephalus, dysgenesis of the corpus callosum, and posterior fossa anomalies, and to identify brain anomalies such as cortical dysgenesis that cannot be detected on US. MRI is more sensitive than US in fetuses with CNS anomalies [36, 51] (Fig. 9).

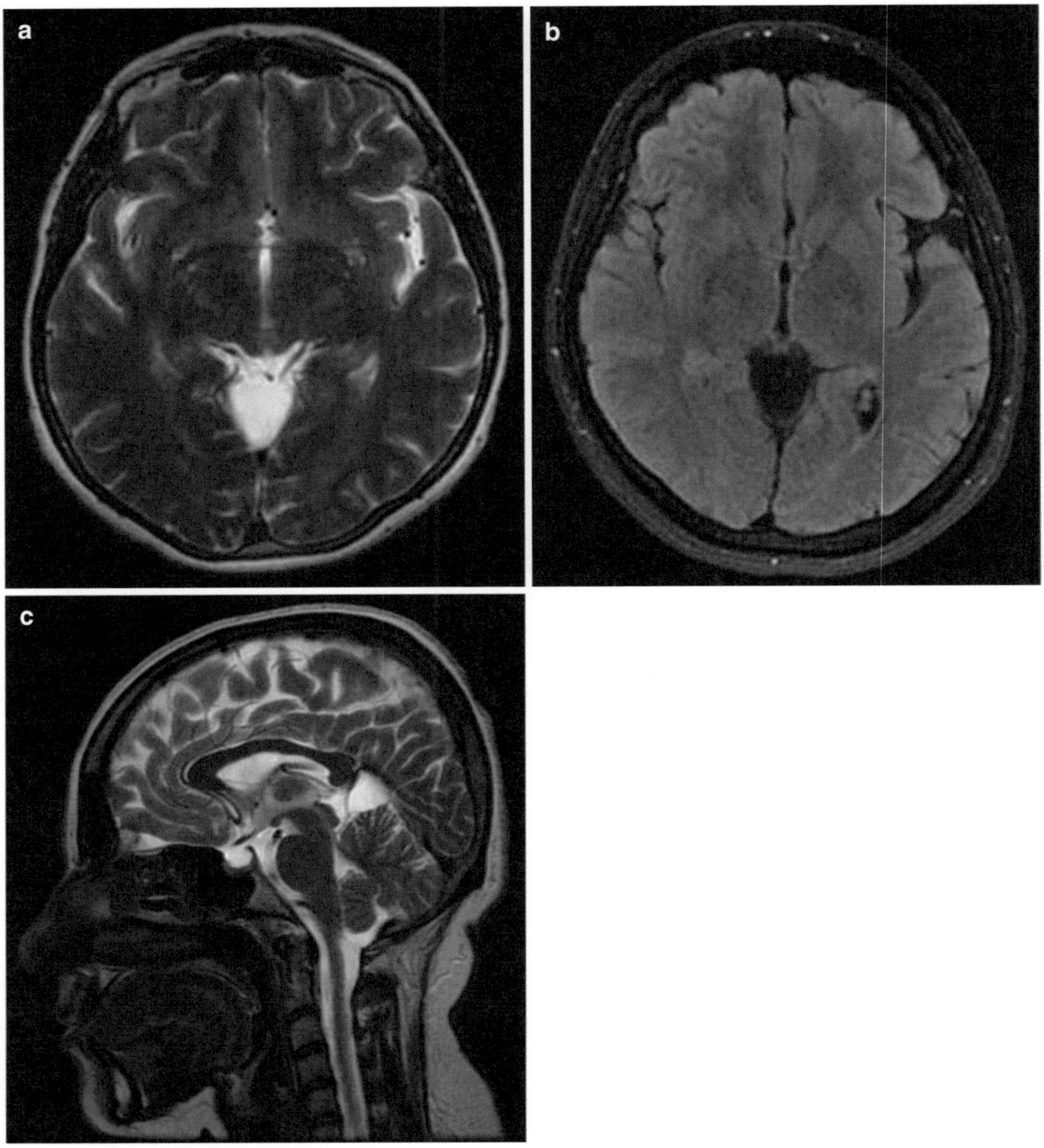

Fig. 11 (**a–c**) A 32-year-old female patient with numbness in the left arm and left leg. Cystic lesion in the lateral ventricle without diffusion restriction and hyperintense on T2-weighted images. The diagnosis is AC

Currently, the effects of MRI exposure on the fetus are not known with certainty, regardless of the fetal week of gestation. However, due to the progressive development of the fetal brain, MRI of the CNS cannot be performed before 19 weeks of gestation. Fetal MRI is often performed with a phased array torso surface coil on 1.5-T MR devices, which has been shown to be sufficient to solve a standard clinical problem. In some centers, 3T fetal MRI is also used [21, 51]. Intravenous gadolinium-based contrast agents are not FDA-approved for use during pregnancy and are not recommended for fetal MRI. The development of fast MRI sequences has significantly reduced fetal motion artifacts and eliminates the need for fetal sedation. Single-shot fast spin-echo (SSFSE) T2-weighted sequences are used as the standard [70]. Ultrafast T2-weighted

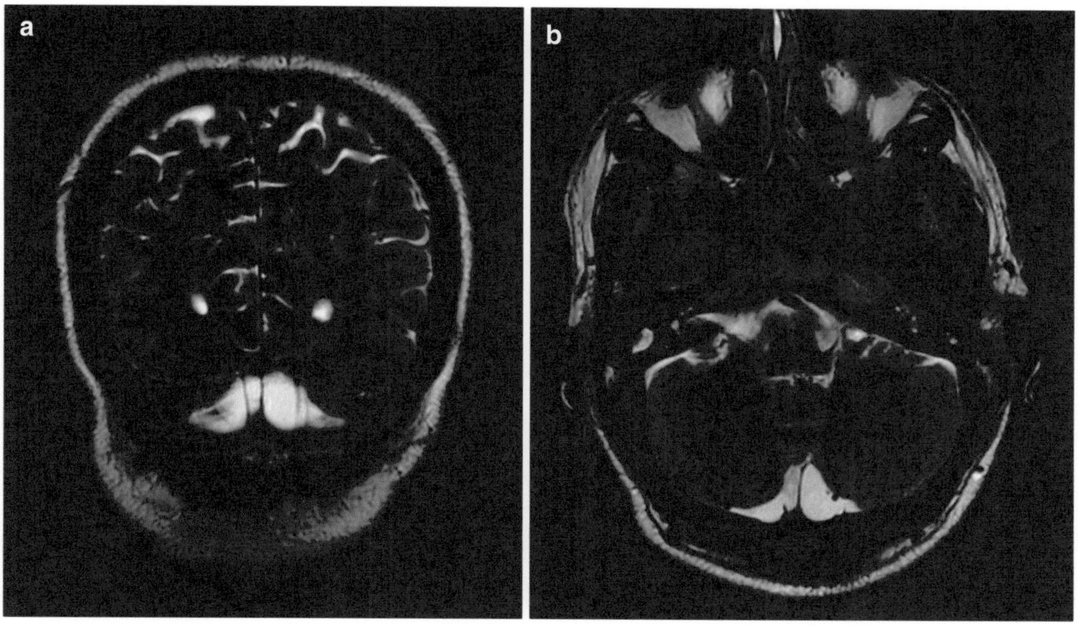

Fig. 12 (**a**, **b**) A 19-year-old male complains of seizure. An AC adjacent to the right frontal lobe is seen and bone remodeling accompanies the cyst

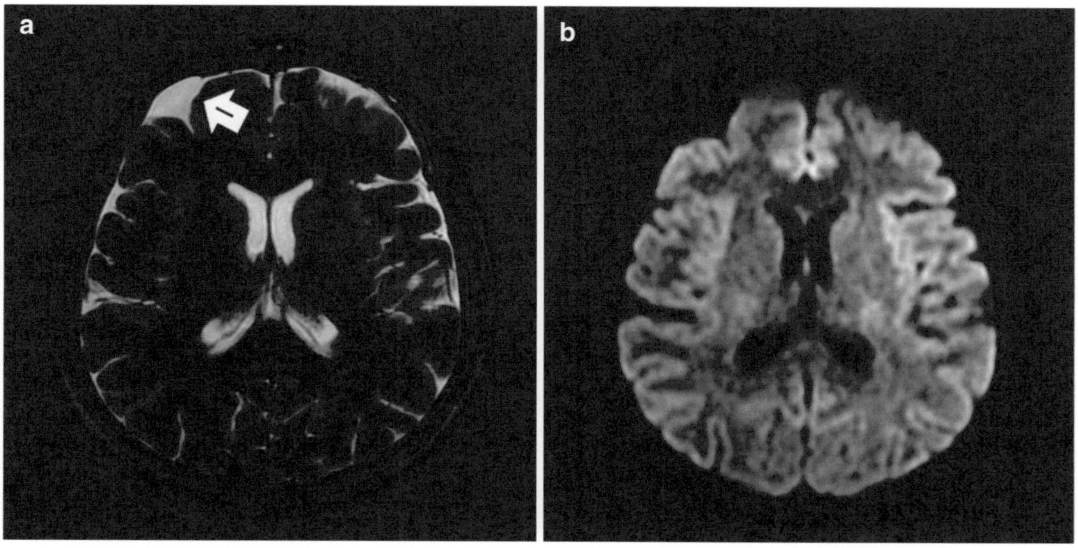

Fig. 13 (**a**–**d**) A 36-year-old man incidentally diagnosed with a homogeneous cystic lesion on examination for multiple sclerosis. An extraaxial lesion with T1 and FLAIR hypointense, T2 hyperintense signals without diffusion restriction. The diagnosis is AC

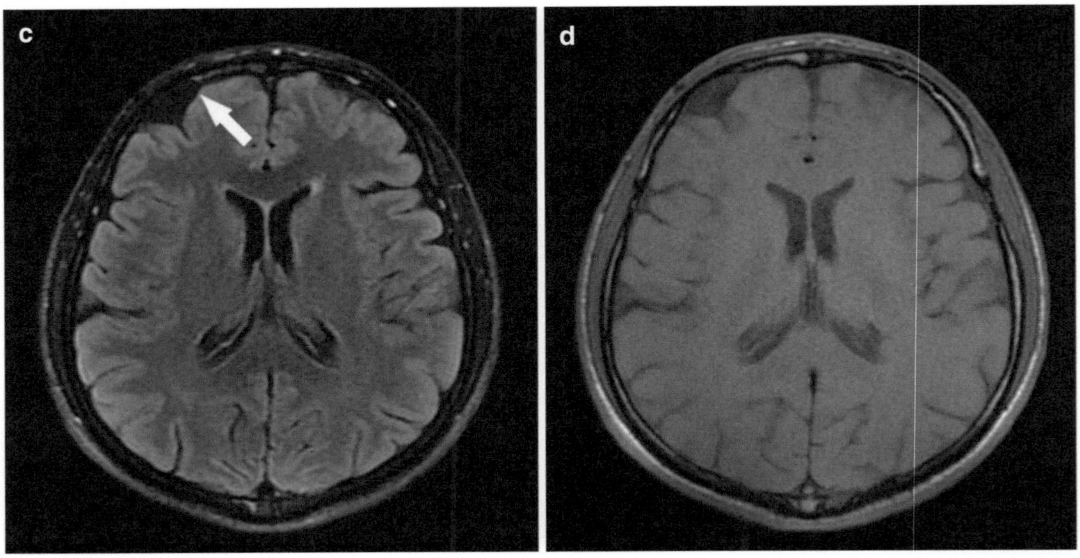

Fig. 13 (continued)

(W) sequences provide excellent visualization of fetal intracranial anatomy by optimizing the high tissue contrast between amniotic fluid and fetal tissue. T1W sequences are primarily used to visualize hemorrhage, fat, and calcium deposits. Balanced steady-state free precession (SSFP) sequences are useful for imaging fetal structures, particularly the vasculature. Diffusion-weighted imaging (DWI) plays an important role in assessing developmental and destructive processes in the brain [51, 70]. On fetal MRI, the AC is observed as a sharply demarcated and homogeneous mass with the same signal as the CSF in all sequences, resulting in displacement of the adjacent parenchyma. The location, size, and compression findings of the cyst are assessed on MRI images [20]. Prenatal MRI can detect CNS abnormalities (compression of the aqueduct, aberrant communication with the ventricles, dysgenesis of the corpus callosum, ventriculomegaly, other brain abnormalities) that often accompany ACs [20, 51].

4 Symptoms and Management of ACs

Clinical symptoms of ACs are often nonspecific and variable. Incidentally diagnosed ACs do not show any clinical symptoms [4]. When they become symptomatic, this is due to progressive enlargement or bleeding into the cyst. Clinical findings depend on the cyst's size, its anatomic location, and its effect on CSF flow. Cysts may be small and clinically symptomatic because of their location, or they may enlarge and cause mass effect on the surrounding neuronal tissue, cranial nerves, and vessels, and then symptoms occur [4, 5, 30, 37, 41, 55, 58, 66, 87, 88].

There is a general consensus for treating patients with clear symptoms. Headache, epilepsy, psychomotor retardation, attention deficit, hyperactivity, maniac depression, schizophrenia-like symptoms, paranoia, psychoses, anosmia, Menière's disease, and hearing loss are commonly encountered symptoms, but these clinical findings can rarely be entirely attributed to the cyst. Detailed history and examination must be performed for appropriate treatment. If the symptoms are attributable to the cyst, ACs need treatment [34, 57, 64].

Cyst fenestration or endoscopic fenestration (formation of a communication between the cyst and the subarachnoid space) may be suitable for small, nonobstructive, nonseptated cysts in the first instance. Ventriculocystostomy or ventriculocisternostomy is also a good choice for long-term treatment [20, 38, 44]. Placement of a cystoperitoneal shunt is also one of the surgical treatments for ACs [18, 39]. However, the rate of long-term complications is higher than with other surgical management. Appropriate surgery is almost always curative, but recurrences have been reported. Re-accumulation of the cyst requires shunt placement [65, 87]. In this manner, there is a higher risk of complications such as shunt blockage, infection, overdrainage, craniocerebral disproportion, and shunt dependency [6, 47, 79]. Craniotomy must be performed for complete resection of intracranial ACs, and temporal cysts are more often treated [57].

There is still controversy about treatment protocols for ACs. If the AC is asymptomatic and harmless, treatments with a high risk of unnecessary complications must be avoided. However, the results of the mentioned surgical methods are satisfactory for cysts that are demonstrably symptomatic.

ACs may require emergency treatment with the acute onset of symptoms such as obstructive hydrocephalus, acute myelopathy due to expansion or hemorrhage of a spinal AC, hemorrhage into a cyst, sudden onset of headache, and neurologic deficit. If symptoms are acute, appropriate surgical treatment must be performed immediately [37, 39, 57].

A symptomatic patient should be considered as asymptomatic if they are without symptoms related to the cyst. Most of the cases need no treatment. Most ACs in children are discovered incidentally, but in the case of expansion tendency, rupture, and subdural effusion, ACs can be treated conservatively [76]. Most pediatric neurosurgeons advise a "wait-and-see" approach when ACs are diagnosed incidentally and do not recommend further diagnostic examinations in asymptomatic patients. However, close clinical and radiological follow-up is recommended [57, 79]. MRI is the best choice for radiological follow-up. The timing of follow-up must be determined according to the size and location of the cyst and the age of the patient. Larger cysts in patients of younger age must be closely followed [52].

5 Intracranial Location of Arachnoid Cysts

5.1 Sylvian Fissure/Middle Cranial Fossa

In children, when ACs increase in volume, they may open the fissure and expose the middle cerebral artery. This exposure can lead to compression and underdevelopment of the anterior superior surface of the temporal lobe. In adults and children, nearly 50–60% of ACs are located in the middle cranial fossa—most commonly temporal lobe—or Sylvian fissure. The left hemisphere is predominantly affected, and headache is the most common presenting symptom [4, 30, 86] (Figs. 1 and 2).

The origin of middle cranial fossa ACs is controversial since either they may originate directly from the meninges adjacent to the temporal pole or partial agenesis of the temporal lobe may lead to a potential space for cyst formation [27]. ACs of the middle cranial fossa were classified into types 1–3 by Galassi in 1989 on CT [26]. Type 1 cysts are small and usually spindle-shaped. They are located below the sphenoid ridge and limited to the anterior portion of the middle cranial fossa. Type 2 cysts lie along the Sylvian fissure and displace the temporal lobe. Type 3 types of ACs fill the middle cranial fossa, are very large, and compress adjacent lobes such as the temporal, anterior, and parietal lobes. In type 3 ACs, proptosis, contralateral motor weakness and seizures, and mental impairment with developmental delay are more common in these patients. Asymmetric bulging of the skull and macrocrania may occur in infants [6, 25, 30, 34, 87]. Symptomatic patients are usually treated with surgery, but children with bitemporal ACs may have glutaric aciduria type 1 (GAT1), so even simple surgical procedures may be harmful for them. All pediatric patients with bitemporal ACs should be evaluated for GAT1 before surgical treatment, especially if there is also macrocephaly, acute encephalitis-like disease, or a dystonic cerebral palsy-like condition [48]. Bitemporal ACs are rare but may occur in other diseases such as neurofibromatosis [50]. Middle cranial fossa ACs most commonly present with headache, seizures, and motor deficits [6, 30, 87]. Symptoms are usually related to the size of the cyst and the mass effect on adjacent neuronal structures. However, the relationship between ACs and epilepsy, cognitive impairment, nausea, and dizziness is unclear [42].

5.2 Sellar Region

ACs in the sellar region are located in the suprasellar or intrasellar part of the sella turcica. They usually occur in pediatric patients and account for 10% of ACs [26]. Suprasellar cysts are located between the diaphragma sella and the optic chiasm. Because of their mass affect, they may cause obstruction of the third ventricle at the level of the foramen of Monro. Hydrocephalus and enlargement of the head may occur. If they compress the optic chiasm or intracerebral portions of the optic nerve, visual impairment such as unilateral or bilateral decrease in visual acuity and/or bitemporal hemianopsia may occur. Compression of the infundibulum, hypothalamus, or pituitary gland may lead to endocrine dysfunction. Growth retardation and developmental delay may occur [23, 55, 56, 91]. Due to compression of the third ventricle and dorsal thalamic nuclei by large suprasellar ACs, a rare condition called bobble-head doll syndrome may occur, with anteroposterior involuntary movements of the head, gait ataxia, and opisthotonus [38]. On MRI, suprasellar ACs are usually smooth, oval, or round masses that may push the pituitary gland down and the chiasm up, occasionally with erosion of the sella turcica [56, 91]. The differential diagnosis of ACs in the sellar region includes sellar diverticulum of the suprasellar cistern, also known as empty sella, Rathke's cleft cyst and cystic craniopharyngioma, and epidermoid cysts [74]. Bypass shunt and resection are surgical options for ACs in the sella region [56] (Fig. 10).

5.3 Interhemispheric Region

ACs arise from the cistern of the corpus callosum. Although their formation is associated with compression of the corpus callosum and disruption of its development by the mechanical mass effect of the cyst, agenesis of the corpus callosum can be observed even in the presence of a small AC. When a normally formed corpus callosum is observed, these are referred to as "parasagittal" ACs [22]. These ACs have a relatively higher frequency of signs and symptoms of increased intracranial pressure (ICP) and are found in up to two-thirds of cases, more often than other sites of the ACs [46].

Asymmetric macrocrania is the most common clinical sign usually seen in infants. When the sutures are closed, headache and vomiting may be observed in older children and are more likely to be associated with hydrocephalus. Epilepsy, developmental delay, hemiparesis, hypotonia, and ocular changes are other symptoms observed [12]. MRI is usually the first choice for imaging when there is a large, giant parafalcine cyst compressing the adjacent brain or partial or complete agenesis of the corpus callosum and the absence of a normal falx cerebri [45] (Fig. 8).

5.4 Convexity

ACs of the convexity have no relationship to a subarachnoid cistern and are therefore distinct from other ACs. As mentioned earlier, clinical symptoms depend on the age of the patient and the size of the cyst. Thus, focal thinning and scalloping of the bone, asymmetric macrocrania, and sutural diastasis may occur in infants. Sometimes, giant convexity ACs can be asymptomatic in the first years of life and then show symptoms such as headache, neurologic deficits, and seizures, and these symptoms can also be observed in adults [46]. Subdural hygroma may be among the differential diagnoses, which is usually symptomatic and has a history of head injury.

Radiological studies may reveal local thinning/bulging of the overlying bone. On MRI, an extraaxial, CSF-like, fluid-filled mass can be seen that is hypointense on T1-weighted sequences and hyperintense on T2-weighted sequences, with varying degrees of compression of the underlying brain (Fig. 6).

5.5 Quadrigeminal Plate

The quadrigeminal plate is located between supratentorial and infratentorial spaces. Quadrigeminal cistern ACs present with different symptoms because adjacent structures such as the cisterna ambiens, superior cerebellum, interhemispheric fissure, posterior part of the third ventricle, mesencephalon, and the vein of Galen can be affected. Therefore, the clinical presentation may vary. Possible obstruction of the Sylvius aqueduct and resulting hydrocephalus may cause symptoms of increased ICP. Compression of the colliculus can lead to parinaud syndrome, with upward gaze paralysis and pupillary dysfunction, nystagmus, and hearing impairment. Compression of the brain stem can lead to paralysis of the trochlear nerve, respiratory failure, and limb weakness. Pineal gland suppression leads to premature puberty. Gait ataxia due to cerebellar compression and seizures due to temporal lobe compression are other symptoms. Like suprasellar ACs, quadrigeminal plate ACs are found mainly in children and rarely in adolescents and adults, probably because of the occurrence of hydrocephalus during their early natural development [28] (Fig. 9).

5.6 Intraventricular Region

Intraventricular ACs are very rare and appear to arise from ectopic remnants of the arachnoid or invagination of the arachnoid into the choroid or from the arachnoid layer in the choroidal fissure [49]. With the aid of high-resolution MRI, which provides a reliable differential diagnosis, intraventricular ACs are being identified with increasing frequency, especially in infants. Indeed, most intraventricular cystic lesions such as choroid plexus, ependymal tumor, or inflammatory cysts resemble ACs. Distortion and enlargement of the ventricles can be observed, and these ACs become symptomatic as soon as hydrocephalus occurs (Figs. 4 and 11).

5.7 Infratentorial Region

Infratentorial ACs account for 10% of all ACs. In the pediatric population, infratentorial ACs are more common than in adults. The retrocerebellar region or the CPA are affected. Retrocerebellar ACs must be distinguished from other cystic malformations of the posterior fossa, such as Dandy-Walker malformation or mega cisterna magna. The foramen of Magendie is present in ACs, but in Dandy-Walker malformation, the foramen of Magendie is not seen, and concomitant vermin hypoplasia or aplasia may be observed. Obstruction of the foramen of Magendie and enlargement of the fourth ventricle and rotation or upward displacement of the cerebellar vermis may be observed in Dandy-Walker malformation. In mega cisterna magna, cystic enlargement of the subarachnoid space, connected to the fourth ventricle by the foramen of Magendie, is observed [30, 63, 87] (Figs. 3, 7 and 12).

6 Differential Diagnosis

The cisterna magna is the largest subarachnoid cistern, located posteroinferior to the cerebellum, dorsal to the brain stem, and superior to the foramen magnum [77]. On sagittal plane imaging, the distance between the dorsal surface of the vermis and the internal table of the occipital bone in the posterior fossa is greater than 10 mm, called the mega cisterna magna (MCM). It is accepted as an asymptomatic normal variant in which the posterior fossa is slightly enlarged on imaging [54]. Because the foramen of Luschka and Magendie are open, they are in direct contact with the subarachnoid space. Therefore, CSF obstruction or hydrocephalus does not occur. Typically, the development of the cerebellar hemispheres and cerebellar vermis is normal, and atrophy is not expected in these locations. However, in large MCM, it may be difficult to distinguish from a retrocerebellar AC if there is a mild compressive effect on the cerebellar hemispheres and vermis. Free falx cerebelli and posterior dural folds are present in about half of MCM cases, and this finding is helpful in distinguishing them from retrocerebellar ACs.

In retrocerebellar ACs, the posterior fossa is usually normal in size, but scalloping may be seen in the internal table of the adjacent occipital bone. Although scalloping is a finding classically suggestive of a retrocerebellar AC, it can sometimes be seen in MCM cases. Hydrocephalus does not occur in the vast majority of retrocerebellar ACs and may cause a very mild, asymptomatic mass effect on the cerebellar hemispheres. However, when they become large, they can cause a mass effect on the cerebellum, resulting in compression of the fourth ventricle and obstruction of CSF flow [43] (Figs. 3 and 12).

This finding plays an important role in distinguishing it from MCM. Retrocerebellar ACs are separated from the subarachnoid space by a membrane, and this membrane can occasionally be visualized by thin section, gradient echo T2WI technique, or by cisternography. Because it is associated with the subarachnoid space in MCM, bright and black signals reflecting normal CSF flow are seen in the phase images of the CSF flow study, depending on the systole and diastole of the cardiac cycle. However, retrocerebellar ACs, which are separated from the subarachnoid space by a thin membrane, are often not expected to show a signal change reflecting CSF flow in the phase images. However, some retrocerebellar ACs are associated with CSF, and in such cases, cisternography is not helpful in distinguishing them from MCM. Therefore, the mass effect on the cerebellum and hydrocephalus seen in retrocerebellar ACs may be considered more useful findings in distinguishing MCM from retrocerebellar ACs.

Both ACs and epidermoid cysts can have the same appearance on T1- and T2-weighted images, but epidermoid cysts have a heterogeneous signal, and the ACs do not [16, 58]. After head trauma, subdural hygromas may occur as a result of chronic leakage of CSF from the damaged meninges. They usually contain blood products that alter the fluid signal on T1-weighted and FLAIR sequences, so they typically do not follow CSF signal intensity on MRI. In contrast-enhanced sequences, they may have a peripherally enhanced membrane. Leptomeningeal cysts are also usually posttraumatic, and they are found near posttraumatic encephalomalacia and skull fractures. Cystic tumors include pilocytic astrocytomas and hemangioblastomas. They have brightly enhancing mural nodules and may have calcifications. Hemangioblastomas are associated with von Hippel Lindau disease. On CT, neurenteric cysts are slightly denser than CSF and do not show contrast enhancement. On MRI, they are isointense to hyperintense compared with CSF on T1-weighted images and hyperintense compared with CSF on T2-weighted images. On FLAIR sequences, the fluid content does not suppress. Neuroenteric cysts show facilitated diffusion on DWI/ADC imaging. Neuroglial cysts are located along the neuroaxis and are intraaxial cysts, whereas ACs are usually extraaxial. Porencephalic cysts communicate with the lateral ventricles, and gliosis is seen in the surrounding tissue. Ependymal cysts are located in the periventricular area. Choroidal fissure cysts are located in the choroidal fissure in the medial temporal lobe, where they are particularly common. Cerebral hydatid cysts are usually spherical and cannot be distinguished from ACs. Neurocysticercosis are usually small and may enhance peripherally [30, 58, 59, 61, 87].

For more information on differential diagnosis of intracranial ACs, please refer to chapter "Differential Diagnosis of Intracranial Arachnoid Cysts".

7 Conclusion

ACs are benign intracranial cystic lesions, usually extraaxial, that are usually diagnosed incidentally during imaging procedures because they are usually asymptomatic [11, 41, 81]. They comprise 1% of all intracranial masses. With the widespread use of prenatal and cross-sectional imaging modalities, many ACs are discovered at a young age. Males are twice more likely to be affected compared to females. Symptoms of an AC depend on its size and/or location. When adjacent neuronal structures are affected, symptoms become more prominent. ACs are prone to rupture and hemorrhage after mild intracranial trauma, and complications such as rupture or hemorrhage require immediate treatment. ACs are usually stable in size, but they rarely regress or enlarge during follow-up. As a result of CSF flow obstruction or cyst enlargement, there may be an increase in intracranial pressure, resulting in headache, dizziness, and tinnitus [4, 85]. MRI is the gold standard and further imaging tool for ACs and distinguishes them from other intracranial cystic lesions [24, 30, 87]. Cisternography is performed for determining surgical indications [26, 88]. If there is a doubt about complication presence, CT is the best faster, cheaper tool for evoluation [30, 87].

References

1. Albayram S, Kilic F, Ozer H, Baghaki S, Kocer N, Islak C. Gadolinium-enhanced MR cisternography to evaluate dural leaks in intracranial hypotension syndrome. AJNR Am J Neuroradiol. 2008;29(1):116–21.
2. Algin O, Turkbey B. Intrathecal gadolinium-enhanced MR cisternography: a comprehensive review. AJNR Am J Neuroradiol. 2013;34(1):14–22.
3. Algin O, Hakyemez B, Parlak M. Phase-contrast MRI and 3D-CISS versus contrast-enhanced MR cisternography on the evaluation of the aqueductal stenosis. Neuroradiology. 2010;52(2):99–108.
4. Al-Holou WN, Yew AY, Boomsaad ZE, Garton HJ, Muraszko KM, Maher CO. Prevalence and natural history of arachnoid cysts in children. J Neurosurg Pediatr. 2010;5(6):578–85.
5. Al-Holou WN, Terman S, Kilburg C, Garton HJ, Muraszko KM, Maher CO. Prevalence and natural history of arachnoid cysts in adults. J Neurosurg. 2013;118(2):222–31.
6. Arai H, Sato K, Wachi A, Okuda O, Takeda N. Arachnoid cysts of the middle cranial fossa: experience with 77 patients who were treated with cystoperitoneal shunting. Neurosurgery. 1996;39(6):1108–12; discussion 12–3.
7. Auer LM, van Velthoven V. Intraoperative ultrasound (US) imaging. Comparison of pathomorphological findings in US and CT. Acta Neurochir (Wien). 1990;104(3–4):84–95.
8. Bannister CM, Russell SA, Rimmer S, Mowle DH. Fetal arachnoid cysts: their site, progress, prognosis and differential diagnosis. Eur J Pediatr Surg. 1999;9(Suppl 1):27–8.
9. Berle M, Wester KG, Ulvik RJ, Kroksveen AC, Haaland OA, Amiry-Moghaddam M, Berven FS, Helland CA. Arachnoid cysts do not contain cerebrospinal fluid: a comparative chemical analysis of arachnoid cyst fluid and cerebrospinal fluid in adults. Cerebrospinal Fluid Res. 2010;7:8.
10. Blaicher W, Prayer D, Bernaschek G. Magnetic resonance imaging and ultrasound in the assessment of the fetal central nervous system. J Perinat Med. 2003;31(6):459–68.
11. Bretelle F, Senat MV, Bernard JP, Hillion Y, Ville Y. First-trimester diagnosis of fetal arachnoid cyst: prenatal implication. Ultrasound Obstet Gynecol. 2002;20(4):400–2.
12. Caldarelli M, Di Rocco C. Surgical options in the treatment of interhemispheric arachnoid cysts. Surg Neurol. 1996;46(3):212–21.
13. Callen PW. The obstetric ultrasound examination. In: Callen PW, editor. Ultrasonography in obstetrics and gynecology. 5th ed. Philadelphia, PA: Saunders-Elseiver; 2008.
14. Catala M, Poirier J. [Arachnoid cysts: histologic, embryologic and physiopathologic review]. Rev Neurol (Paris). 1998;154(6–7):489–501.
15. Chen CP. Prenatal diagnosis of arachnoid cysts. Taiwan J Obstet Gynecol. 2007;46(3):187–98.
16. Chen CP, Chang TY, Wang W. Third-trimester ultrasound evaluation of arachnoid cysts. Taiwan J Obstet Gynecol. 2007;46(4):427–8.
17. Chen CY, Wong JS, Hsieh SC, Chu JS, Chan WP. Intracranial epidermoid cyst with hemorrhage: MR imaging findings. AJNR Am J Neuroradiol. 2006;27(2):427–9.
18. Cinalli G, Peretta P, Spennato P, Savarese L, Varone A, Vedova P, Grimaldi G, Ragazzi P, Ruggiero C, Cianciulli E, Maggi G. Neuroendoscopic management of interhemispheric cysts in children. J Neurosurg. 2006;105(3 Suppl):194–202.
19. Cincu R, Agrawal A, Eiras J. Intracranial arachnoid cysts: current concepts and treatment alternatives. Clin Neurol Neurosurg. 2007;109(10):837–43.
20. Cooper S, Bar-Yosef O, Berkenstadt M, Hoffmann C, Achiron R, Katorza E. Prenatal evaluation, imaging features, and neurodevelopmental outcome of prenatally diagnosed periventricular pseudocysts. AJNR Am J Neuroradiol. 2016;37(12):2382–8.

21. da Silva N, Adolfo JV, Sarian LO, Cognard C, Sévely A. Magnetic resonance imaging of the fetal brain at 3 Tesla. Medicine. 2018;97(40):e12602.
22. di Rocco C, Caldarelli M, di Trapani G. Infratentorial arachnoid cysts in children. Childs Brain. 1981;8(2):119–33.
23. Dubuisson AS, Stevenaert A, Martin DH, Flandroy PP. Intrasellar arachnoid cysts. Neurosurgery. 2007;61(3):505–13; discussion 13.
24. Dutt SN, Mirza S, Chavda SV, Irving RM. Radiologic differentiation of intracranial epidermoids from arachnoid cysts. Otol Neurotol. 2002;23(1):84–92.
25. Fewel ME, Levy ML, McComb JG. Surgical treatment of 95 children with 102 intracranial arachnoid cysts. Pediatr Neurosurg. 1996;25(4):165–73.
26. Galassi E, Tognetti F, Gaist G, Fagioli L, Frank F, Frank G. CT scan and metrizamide CT cisternography in arachnoid cysts of the middle cranial fossa: classification and pathophysiological aspects. Surg Neurol. 1982;17(5):363–9.
27. García Santos JM, Martínez-Lage J, Gilabert Ubeda A, Capel Alemán A, Climent Oltrá V. Arachnoid cysts of the middle cranial fossa: a consideration of their origins based on imaging. Neuroradiology. 1993;35(5):355–8.
28. Garg K, Tandon V, Sharma S, Suri A, Chandra PS, Kumar R, Mahapatra AK, Sharma BS. Quadrigeminal cistern arachnoid cyst: a series of 18 patients and a review of literature. Br J Neurosurg. 2015;29(1):70–6.
29. Gedikbasi A, Palabiyik F, Oztarhan A, Yildirim G, Eren C, Ozyurt SS, Ceylan Y. Prenatal diagnosis of a suprasellar arachnoid cyst with 2- and 3-dimensional sonography and fetal magnetic resonance imaging: difficulties in management and review of the literature. J Ultrasound Med. 2010;29(10):1487–93.
30. Gosalakkal JA. Intracranial arachnoid cysts in children: a review of pathogenesis, clinical features, and management. Pediatr Neurol. 2002;26(2):93–8.
31. Grossman TB, Uribe-Cardenas R, Radwanski RE, Souweidane MM, Hoffman CE. Arachnoid cysts: using prenatal imaging and need for pediatric neurosurgical intervention to better understand their natural history and prognosis. J Matern Fetal Neonatal Med. 2022;35(24):4728–33.
32. Gupta N, Grover H, Bansal I, Hooda K, Sapire JM, Anand R, Kumar Y. Neonatal cranial sonography: ultrasound findings in neonatal meningitis—a pictorial review. Quant Imaging Med Surg. 2017;7(1):123–31.
33. Hanieh A, Simpson DA, North JB. Arachnoid cysts: a critical review of 41 cases. Childs Nerv Syst. 1988;4(2):92–6.
34. Helland CA, Wester K. A population-based study of intracranial arachnoid cysts: clinical and neuroimaging outcomes following surgical cyst decompression in children. J Neurosurg. 2006;105(5 Suppl):385–90.
35. Hoffmann KT, Hosten N, Meyer BU, Röricht S, Sprung C, Oellinger J, Gutberlet M, Felix R. Csf flow studies of intracranial cysts and cyst-like lesions achieved using reversed fast imaging with steady-state precession MR sequences. AJNR Am J Neuroradiol. 2000;21(3):493–502.
36. Hosny IA, Elghawabi HS. Ultrafast MRI of the fetus: an increasingly important tool in prenatal diagnosis of congenital anomalies. Magn Reson Imaging. 2010;28(10):1431–9.
37. Ildan F, Cetinalp E, Bağdatoğlu H, Boyar B, Uzuneyüoglu Z. Arachnoid cyst with traumatic intracystic hemorrhage unassociated with subdural hematoma. Neurosurg Rev. 1994;17(3):229–32.
38. Ishihara M, Nonaka M, Oshida N, Hamada Y, Nakajima S, Yamasaki M. "No-no" type bobble-head doll syndrome in an infant with an arachnoid cyst of the posterior fossa: a case report. Pediatr Neurol. 2013;49(6):474–6.
39. Jafrani R, Raskin JS, Kaufman A, Lam S. Intracranial arachnoid cysts: pediatric neurosurgery update. Surg Neurol Int. 2019;10:15.
40. Kane RA, Kruskal JB. Intraoperative ultrasonography of the brain and spine. Ultrasound Q. 2007;23(1):23–39.
41. Katzman GL, Dagher AP, Patronas NJ. Incidental findings on brain magnetic resonance imaging from 1000 asymptomatic volunteers. JAMA. 1999;282(1):36–9.
42. Koch CA, Voth D, Kraemer G, Schwarz M. Arachnoid cysts: does surgery improve epileptic seizures and headaches? Neurosurg Rev. 1995;18(3):173–81.
43. Kornienko VN, Pronin IN. Arachnoid cysts. In: Pronin IN, Kornienko VN, editors. Springer; 2008.
44. Kumar A, Sakia R, Singh K, Sharma V. Spinal arachnoid cyst. J Clin Neurosci. 2011;18(9):1189–92.
45. Lena G, van Calenberg F, Genitori L, Choux M. Supratentorial interhemispheric cysts associated with callosal agenesis: surgical treatment and outcome in 16 children. Childs Nerv Syst. 1995;11(10):568–73.
46. Li C, Yin L, Jiang T, Ma Z, Jia G. Shunt dependency syndrome after cystoperitoneal shunting of arachnoid cysts. Childs Nerv Syst. 2014;30(3):471–6.
47. Li L, Zhang Y, Li Y, Zhai X, Zhou Y, Liang P. The clinical classification and treatment of middle cranial fossa arachnoid cysts in children. Clin Neurol Neurosurg. 2013;115(4):411–8.
48. Lütcherath V, Waaler PE, Jellum E, Wester K. Children with bilateral temporal arachnoid cysts may have glutaric aciduria type 1 (GAT1); operation without knowing that may be harmful. Acta Neurochir (Wien). 2000;142(9):1025–30.
49. Maiuri F, Iaconetta G, Gangemi M. Arachnoid cyst of the lateral ventricle. Surg Neurol. 1997;48(4):401–4.
50. Martínez-Lage JF, Poza M, Sola J, Puche A. Congenital arachnoid cyst of the lateral ventricles in children. Childs Nerv Syst. 1992;8(4):203–6.
51. Masselli G, Vaccaro Notte MR, Zacharzewska-Gondek A, Laghi F, Manganaro L, Brunelli R. Fetal MRI of CNS abnormalities. Clin Radiol. 2020;75(8):640.e1–11.
52. Massimi L, Caldarelli M, Di Rocco C. Intracranial congenital arachnoid cysts. In: Di Rocco C, Pang D, Rutka JT, editors. Textbook of pediatric neurosurgery. Cham: Springer; 2020. p. 789–829.

53. Mastronardi L, Nardi M, Puzzilli F. Pupillary enlargement caused by an acute extradural haematoma associated with a non-symptomatic arachnoid cyst, from compression of the optic rather than the oculomotor nerve. Br J Neurosurg. 1999;13(3):341–2.
54. McKinney AM. Mega cisterna magna and retrocerebellar arachnoid cysts. In: Atlas of normal imaging variations of the brain, skull, and craniocervical vasculature. Springer; 2017.
55. Meyer FB, Carpenter SM, Laws ER Jr. Intrasellar arachnoid cysts. Surg Neurol. 1987;28(2):105–10.
56. Murakami M, Okumura H, Kakita K. Recurrent intrasellar arachnoid cyst. Neurol Med Chir (Tokyo). 2003;43(6):312–5.
57. Mustansir F, Bashir S, Darbar A. Management of arachnoid cysts: a comprehensive review. Cureus. 2018;10(4):e2458.
58. Nadgir R, Yousem D. Congenital anomalies of the central nervous system. In: Yousem D, Nadgir R, editors. Neuroradiology: the requisites the core requisites. 4th ed. Philadelphia, PA: Elseiver; 2016.
59. Oberbauer RW, Haase J, Pucher R. Arachnoid cysts in children: a European co-operative study. Childs Nerv Syst. 1992;8(5):281–6.
60. Paladini D, Volpe P. Central and peripheral nervous system anomalies. In: Paladini D, editor. Ultrasound of congenital fetal anomalies. 2nd ed. CRC Press; 2014.
61. Pascual-Castroviejo I, Roche MC, Martínez Bermejo A, Arcas J, García Blázquez M. Primary intracranial arachnoidal cysts. A study of 67 childhood cases. Childs Nerv Syst. 1991;7(5):257–63.
62. Patel AP, Oliverio PJ, Kurtom KH, Roberti F. Spontaneous subdural hematoma and intracystic hemorrhage in an arachnoid cyst. Radiol Case Rep. 2009;4(3):298.
63. Pierre-Kahn A, Hanlo P, Sonigo P, Parisot D, McConnell RS. The contribution of prenatal diagnosis to the understanding of malformative intracranial cysts: state of the art. Childs Nerv Syst. 2000;16(10–11):619–26.
64. Rabiei K, Jaraj D, Marlow T, Jensen C, Skoog I, Wikkelsø C. Prevalence and symptoms of intracranial arachnoid cysts: a population-based study. J Neurol. 2016;263(4):689–94.
65. Raffel C, McComb JG. To shunt or to fenestrate: which is the best surgical treatment for arachnoid cysts in pediatric patients? Neurosurgery. 1988;23(3):338–42.
66. Rao G, Anderson RC, Feldstein NA, Brockmeyer DL. Expansion of arachnoid cysts in children: report of two cases and review of the literature. J Neurosurg. 2005;102(3 Suppl):314–7.
67. Rengachary SS, Watanabe I, Brackett CE. Pathogenesis of intracranial arachnoid cysts. Surg Neurol. 1978;9(2):139–44.
68. Reports of medical cases, selected with a view of illustrating the symptoms and cure of diseases, by a reference to morbid anatomy. Med Chir Rev. 1831;15(30):289–330.
69. Russo N, Domenicucci M, Beccaglia MR, Santoro A. Spontaneous reduction of intracranial arachnoid cysts: a complete review. Br J Neurosurg. 2008;22(5):626–9.
70. Saleem SN. Fetal MRI: an approach to practice: a review. J Adv Res. 2014;5(5):507–23.
71. Santamarta D, Aguas J, Ferrer E. The natural history of arachnoid cysts: endoscopic and cine-mode MRI evidence of a slit-valve mechanism. Minim Invasive Neurosurg. 1995;38(4):133–7.
72. Schachenmayr W, Friede RL. Fine structure of arachnoid cysts. J Neuropathol Exp Neurol. 1979;38(4):434–46.
73. Seizeur R, Forlodou P, Coustans M, Dam-Hieu P. Spontaneous resolution of arachnoid cysts: review and features of an unusual case. Acta Neurochir (Wien). 2007;149(1):75–8; discussion 78.
74. Shin JL, Asa SL, Woodhouse LJ, Smyth HS, Ezzat S. Cystic lesions of the pituitary: clinicopathological features distinguishing craniopharyngioma, Rathke's cleft cyst, and arachnoid cyst. J Clin Endocrinol Metab. 1999;84(11):3972–82.
75. Silbergleit R, Brunberg JA, Patel SC, Mehta BA, Aravapalli SR. Imaging of spinal intradural arachnoid cysts: MRI, myelography and CT. Neuroradiology. 1998;40(10):664–8.
76. Sprung C, Armbruster B, Koeppen D, Cabraja M. Arachnoid cysts of the middle cranial fossa accompanied by subdural effusions—experience with 60 consecutive cases. Acta Neurochir (Wien). 2011;153(1):75–84; discussion 84.
77. Standring S. Gray's anatomy. 39th ed. Elsevier under the Churchill Livingstone imprint; 2011.
78. Talamonti G, D'Aliberti G, Picano M, Debernardi A, Collice M. Intracranial cysts containing cerebrospinal fluid-like fluid: results of endoscopic neurosurgery in a series of 64 consecutive cases. Neurosurgery. 2011;68(3):788–803; discussion 03.
79. Tamburrini G, Dal Fabbro M, Di Rocco C. Sylvian fissure arachnoid cysts: a survey on their diagnostic workout and practical management. Childs Nerv Syst. 2008;24(5):593–604.
80. Thomas BP, Pearson MM, Wushensky CA. Active spontaneous decompression of a suprasellar-prepontine arachnoid cyst detected with routine magnetic resonance imaging. Case report. J Neurosurg Pediatr. 2009;3(1):70–2.
81. Timor-Tritsch IE, Monteagudo AR, Cohen HL. Ultrasonography of the prenatal and neonatal brain. Appleton & Lange; 1996.
82. Vernooij MW, Ikram MA, Tanghe HL, Vincent AJ, Hofman A, Krestin GP, Niessen WJ, Breteler MM, van der Lugt A. Incidental findings on brain MRI in the general population. N Engl J Med. 2007;357(18):1821–8.
83. Wang HS, Kuo MF, Huang SC, Chou ML, Hung PC, Lin KL. Transcranial ultrasound diagnosis of intracranial lesions in children with headaches. Pediatr Neurol. 2002;26(1):43–6.

84. Wang X, Chen JX, You C, Jiang S. CT cisternography in intracranial symptomatic arachnoid cysts: classification and treatment. J Neurol Sci. 2012;318(1–2):125–30.
85. Weber F, Knopf H. Incidental findings in magnetic resonance imaging of the brains of healthy young men. J Neurol Sci. 2006;240(1-2):81–4.
86. Wester K. Peculiarities of intracranial arachnoid cysts: location, sidedness, and sex distribution in 126 consecutive patients. Neurosurgery. 1999;45(4):775–9.
87. Westermaier T, Schweitzer T, Ernestus RI. Arachnoid cysts. Adv Exp Med Biol. 2012;724:37–50.
88. White ML, Das JM. Arachnoid cysts. In: StatPearls. Treasure Island (FL): StatPearls Publishing. Copyright © 2022, StatPearls Publishing LLC; 2022.
89. Yildiz H, Erdogan C, Yalcin R, Yazici Z, Hakyemez B, Parlak M, Tuncel E. Evaluation of communication between intracranial arachnoid cysts and cisterns with phase-contrast cine MR imaging. AJNR Am J Neuroradiol. 2005;26(1):145–51.
90. Yin L, Yang Z, Pan Q, Zhang J, Li X, Wang F, Ye Y, Deng X, Hu C. Sonographic diagnosis and prognosis of fetal arachnoid cysts. J Clin Ultrasound. 2018;46(2):96–102.
91. Zada G, Lopes MBS, Mukundan S, Laws E. Sellar region arachnoid cysts. In: Lopes M, Zada G, Mukundan Jr S, Laws Jr E, editors. Atlas of sellar and parasellar lesions. Springer; 2016.

Intrauterine Detection of Arachnoid Cysts

Farideh Nejat

1 Introduction

The literature describes numerous physicians around the world who were managing the medical problems of human beings with the available diagnostic and surgical tools related to that specific time period. At least some documents concerning medical and surgical management of early humans date back to more than 12,000 years ago [11]. Parallel to the advancement in engineering and technology, the medications and medical tools improved, and with good cooperation between knowledgeable engineers and physicians, more development in the diagnostic and medical armamentarium were achieved.

The first report of the ultrasound application in obstetrics and gynecology was documented in 1958 in a manuscript from Glasgow which demonstrated a gynecological mass associated with the first ultrasonic image of a fetus [9]. Technological advances such as solid-state circuitry, real-time imaging, and Doppler, transvaginal, and three- and four-dimensional ultrasound have developed the investigation and management of patients, especially the evaluation of the fetus for fetal anomalies[6]. The first report of prenatal diagnosis of a central nervous system (CNS) anomaly known as anencephaly was published in the late second or third trimester of pregnancy in 1964 [6]. The second CNS anomaly was reported after diagnosis of spina bifida by ultrasound in 1975 [5].

Major advancements in the expertise of sonographers and also the technology of fetal neurosonography specifically transvaginal and 3D ultrasound have increased the detection rate of CNS malformations in up to 90–95% of cases [19]. With a standardized anatomical protocol, severe structural anomalies could be detected even in the first trimester [16]. Intrauterine MRI as an excellent supplementary method to ultrasound found a fundamental role to reconfirm the anomalies discovered by ultrasound [19]. Furthermore, third trimester MRI can detect additional CNS anomalies in 15% of cases [18].

Arachnoid cysts (ACs) are rare intracranial masses which are located within the cerebrospinal fluid cisterns and the major cerebral fissures. The etiology of congenital ACs is not well understood. The natural course of ACs after prenatal detection is unknown. Some pregnancies are ended as termination or stillbirth, but in surviving neonates, the course is relatively diverse. In most cases, the malformation remains stable or progresses [4] in size but rarely regresses [12].

The outcome is dependent to the patient's age at the time of diagnosis, the size and location of lesion, the rate of cyst growth, the brain integrity [20] and more importantly the associated abnormalities that are present, and the severity of the ventriculomegaly [2, 7].

F. Nejat (✉)
Department of Pediatric Neurosurgery, Children's Medical Center, Tehran University of Medical Sciences, Tehran, Iran
e-mail: nejat@sina.tums.ac.ir; nejat@tums.ac.ir

M. Turgut et al. (eds.), *Arachnoid Cysts*, https://doi.org/10.1007/978-3-031-22701-1_15

2 Case Presentation of Prenatal Detection of the Arachnoid Cyst

A 30-year-old primigravid lady was scanned routinely at 32 weeks of gestation of her twin fetus pregnancy. During the brain study of one male fetus, a noncommunicating anechoic 50 × 45 mm mass in the left parietal paramidline with compression on the lateral ventricle was found. There was also agenesis of the corpus callosum. The lesion was absent on the previous ultrasound scan at 20 weeks of pregnancy. The scan was repeated after 4 weeks which demonstrated mild increase in the size of the cyst (Fig. 1a). The twin neonates were born through uneventful caesarian section.

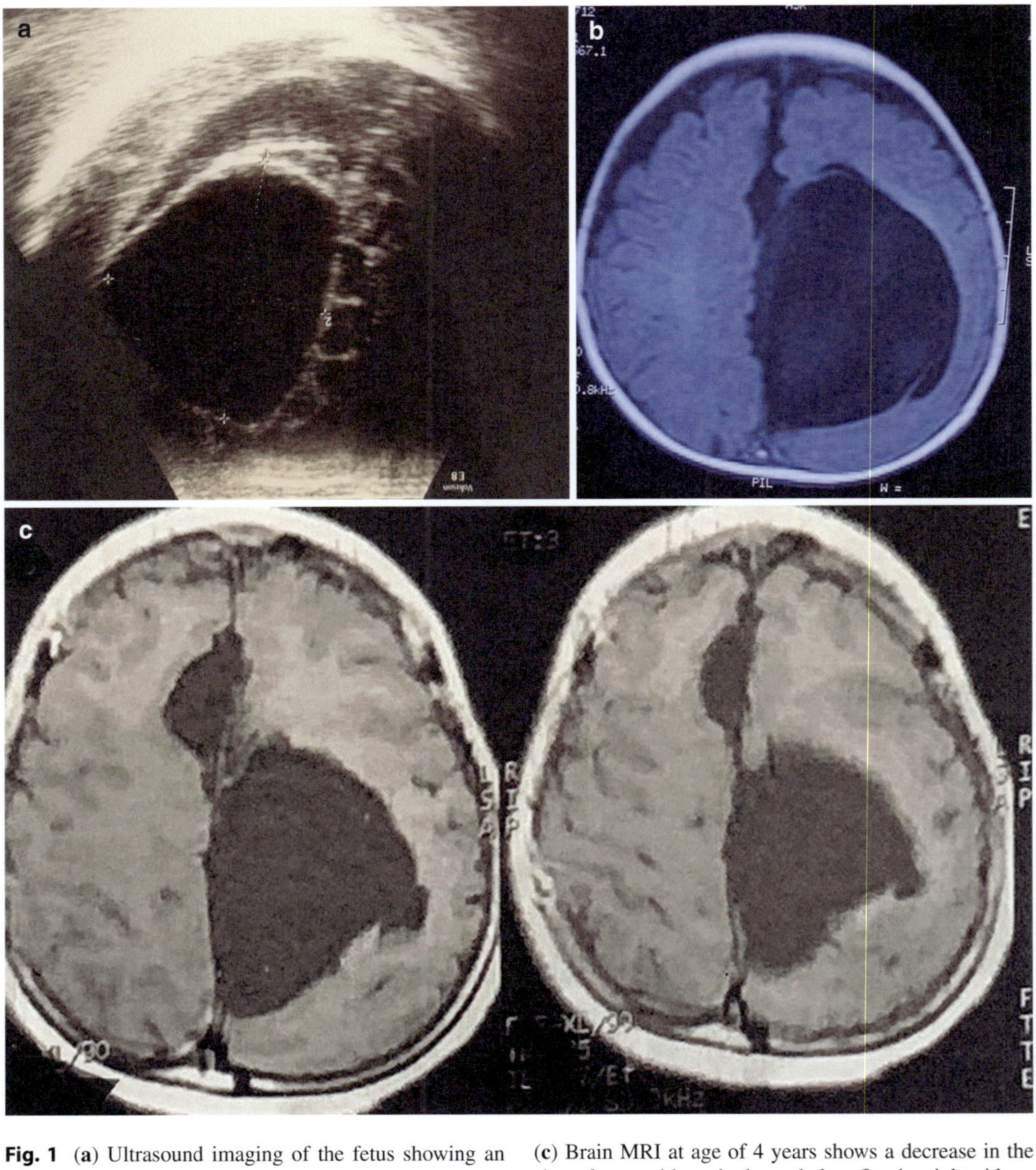

Fig. 1 (**a**) Ultrasound imaging of the fetus showing an interhemispheric cyst. (**b**) Brain postnatal MRI confirms the prenatal diagnosis of an interhemispheric cyst and corpus callosum agenesis. The cyst found increased in size. (**c**) Brain MRI at age of 4 years shows a decrease in the size of cyst without hydrocephalus. On the right side, a small interhemispheric AC is obvious

The child with the AC had head growth and fontanel position like his brother. Postnatal MRI at age of 2 months revealed a huge interhemispheric AC with compression on the adjacent ventricular system (Fig. 1b). Considering normal development and normal increase of head circumstance similar to that of his sibling, the parents' request for conservative treatment was considered. His follow-up was performed with repeat brain MRI which confirmed gradual regression of the cyst size and a new small size AC in the right interhemispheric fissure which was not obvious on prenatal and first postnatal imaging possibly because of the huge size of the lesion and its mass effect (Fig. 1c). Now at the age of 9 years old, the child is totally normal according to neurodevelopment, visual field, and ophthalmological examination.

3 Discussion

Primary ACs are congenital malformations caused by abnormal embryogenesis of the arachnoid and irregular splitting of arachnoid membrane. AC can occur anywhere in the neuraxis but are most commonly in the middle fossa and are not in communication with the surrounding subarachnoid space [4, 7]. Most ACs are diagnosed postnatally during evaluation of a head injury, abnormal development, or progressive increase of head size and most commonly are an incidental finding [7]:

3.1 Prenatal Diagnosis

Prenatal detection of CNS malformations in fetuses is possible subsequent to the routine use of a new generation of ultrasound and appropriate use of magnetic resonance imaging (MRI) [1]. Therefore, prenatal imaging has increased the detection rate and accurate diagnosis of some CNS anomalies like ACs. However, the clinical importance of prenatal detection of ACs is not well known [20]. The prevalence of ACs on imaging is about 2% [1]. These cysts are illustrated as hypoechoic masses which can be diagnosed by ultrasound as early as 13 weeks of pregnancy [1, 7]. Most ACs are found in a supratentorial location with middle fossa cysts being the most frequent [7].

3.2 Natural Course

ACs may be unchanged, enlarged, or even regress during development after prenatal diagnosis [7, 8]. Most cases of ACs with prenatal diagnosis remain asymptomatic and don't need any surgical intervention. Some cases become symptomatic with progressive increase in size or high intracranial pressure and sometimes after head trauma and bleeding inside the cyst or with cyst rupture which need surgical intervention [10, 13].

3.3 Size Change

After prenatal diagnosis, the dimensions of ACs might demonstrate any kind of changes. These cysts may increase in size, remain stable, or reduce in size [3, 4]. The course of size change of prenatally detected ACs is not well known. There is no evidence to further delineate high-risk periods for cyst growth, and thus more clinical studies will still be needed on how to best monitor these children. It has even been stated that [15] there is no cyst growth after age of 4 years, suggesting that close monitoring of cyst size with neuroimaging is only necessary in early years [4].

3.4 Pregnancy Situation After Prenatal Diagnosis

Prenatal counseling about ACs leads to the parents' decision for termination or continuing the pregnancy. The rate of pregnancy termination is unknown, and it is not the same in different countries according to the severity of malformations and cultural or religious issues. Pregnancies were terminated in 4–50% of cases in different studies [8, 21].

3.5 Associated Anatomical Abnormalities

Additional anatomical abnormalities could be found when an AC has been detected or later during follow-up of ACs. The correct rate of discovery is not obvious, but nearly 50% of fetuses have been reported to have another intracranial or extracranial anomaly [4]. Intracranial abnormalities are more common than extracranial anomalies with ventriculomegaly and corpus callosum dysgenesis being the most frequent accompanying findings. A genetic disorder is not very common but has been reported in less than 10% in some series [4, 22].

3.6 Neurodevelopment

Neurodevelopmental status of infants with AC has been reported to be normal, especially in cases with isolated ACs [6]. Most studies suggested that the cyst size or location is not on such importance, but the associated anomalies, chromosomal abnormalities, and a brain compromised by AC or associated problems are more concerning for the future developmental state [7, 14, 20].

3.7 Fetal Outcome

The outcome is nearly related to the presence or absence of other congenital malformations, chromosomal abnormalities, progression of associated ventriculomegaly, integrity of the cerebral parenchyma, and progressive increase in cyst size. Currently, postnatal less invasive surgical intervention such as the endoscopic approach has also improved the final outcome [7, 17, 18]. Overall, the outcome of a prenatal detected AC remains unclear, but favorable outcomes occur with isolated cysts without associated anatomical and chromosomal abnormalities [4].

4 Conclusion

Prenatal detection of ACs is possible with new generations of ultrasound. The natural course and outcome of ACs are not well investigated. Nevertheless, according to current literature, most ACs remain stable in size and if isolated are commonly associated with normal neurodevelopmental status. If the size of cyst changes, it is usually documented to occur in the first years of life. Therefore, close monitoring of patients with neuroimaging of these children during the first few years is advised.

References

1. Asimakopoulos G, Antsaklis P, Theodora M, Sindos M, Rodolakis A, Loutradis D, Daskalakis G. Prenatal diagnosis of a large suprasellar arachnoid cyst. HJOG. 2020;19(1):51–8.
2. Barjot P, Theobald PV, Refahi N, Delautre V, Herlicoviez M. Diagnosis of arachnoid cysts on prenatal ultrasound. Fetal Diagn Ther. 1999;14(5):306–9.
3. Basaldella L, Orvieto E, Dei Tos AP, Barbera MD, Valente M, Longatti P. Causes of arachnoid cyst development and expansion. Neurosurg Focus. 2007;22(2):E4, 1–4.
4. Beresford C, Hall S, Smedley A, Mathad N, Waters R, Chakraborty A, Sparrow OC, Tsitouras V. Prenatal diagnosis of arachnoid cysts: a case series and systematic review. Childs Nerv Syst. 2020;36:729–41.
5. Campbell S. Early prenatal diagnosis of neural tube defects by ultrasound. Clin Obstet Gynecol. 1977;20:351–9.
6. Campbell S. A short history of sonography in obstetrics and gynaecology. Facts Views Vis Obgyn. 2013;5(3):213–29.
7. Chen CP. Prenatal diagnosis of arachnoid cysts. Taiwan J Obstet Gynecol. 2007;46(3):187–98.
8. De Keersmaecker B, Ramaekers P, Claus F, Witters I, Ortibus I, Naulaers G, Van Calenbergh F, De Catte L. Outcome of 12 antenatally diagnosed fetal arachnoid cysts: case series and review of the literature. Eur J Paediatr Neurol. 2015;19(2):114–21.
9. Donald I, MacVicar J, Brown TG. Investigation of abdominal masses by pulsed ultrasound. Lancet. 1958;1:1188–95.
10. Elbers S, Furness M. Resolution of presumed arachnoid cyst in utero. Ultrasound Obstet Gynecol. 1999;14(5):353–5.

11. Garrison FH. An introduction to the history of medicine, revised and enlarged. 4th ed. Philadelphia: W.B. Saunders; 1929.
12. Goksu E, Kazan S. Spontaneous shrinkage of a suprasellar arachnoid cyst diagnosed with prenatal sonography and fetal magnetic resonance imaging: case report and review of the literature. Turk Neurosurg. 2015;25(4):670–3.
13. Hayward R. Prenatal diagnosis of neural tube defects. Prenat Diagn. 2009;29:396–401.
14. Langer B, Haddad J, Favre R, Frigue V, Schlaeder G. Fetal arachnoid cyst: report of two cases. Ultrasound Obstet Gynecol. 1994;4:68–72.
15. Lee JY, Kim JW, Phi JH, Kim SK, Cho BK, Wang KC. Enlarging arachnoid cyst: a false alarm for infants. Childs Nerv Syst. 2012;28:1203–11.
16. Liao Y, Wen H, Ouyang S, Yuan Y, Bi J, Guan Y, Fu Q, Yang X, Guo W, Huang Y, Zeng Q, Qin Y, Xiang H, Li S. Routine first-trimester ultrasound screening using a standardized anatomical protocol. Am J Obstet Gynecol. 2021;224(4):396.e1–15.
17. Nakamura Y, Mizukawa K, Yamamoto K, Nagashima T. Endoscopic treatment for a huge neonatal prepontine-suprasellar arachnoid cyst: a case report. Pediatr Neurosurg. 2001;35:220–4.
18. Santirocco M, Rodó C, Illescas T, Vázquez E, Garrido M, Higueras T, Arévalo S, Maiz N, Carreras E. Accuracy of prenatal ultrasound in the diagnosis of corpus callosum anomalies. J Matern Fetal Neonatal Med. 2021;34(3):439–44.
19. Tercanli S, Prüfer F. Fetal neurosonogaphy: ultrasound and magnetic resonance imaging in competition. Ultraschall Med. 2016;37(6):555–7.
20. Yahala O, Katorzac E, Zvic E, Berkenstadte M, Hoffmand C, Achirond R, Bar-Yosefa O. Prenatal diagnosis of arachnoid cysts: MRI features and neurodevelopmental outcome. Eur J Radiol. 2019;113:232–7.
21. Yin L, Yang Z, Pan Q, Zhang J, Li X, Wang F, Ye Y, Deng X, Hu C. Sonographic diagnosis and prognosis of fetal arachnoid cysts. J Clin Ultrasound. 2018;46(2):96–102.
22. Youssef A, D'Antonio F, Khalil A, Papageorghiou AT, Ciardulli A, Lanzone A, Rizzo G, Thilaganathan B, Pilu G. Outcome of fetuses with supratentorial extra-axial intracranial cysts: a systematic review. Fetal Diagn Ther. 2016;40:1–12.

Cisternography of Arachnoid Cysts

Yasin Celal Güneş and Oktay Algın

1 Introduction

In the literature, the first imaging clues for arachnoid cysts (ACs) were made by Robinson in the mid-1960s [50]. Thinning and bulging of the temporal bones adjacent to the ACs on the head radiographs and elevation in the middle cranial fossa and the sphenoid wing were noted [50]. Unfortunately, these findings were misnamed by the author as indirect findings of temporal lobe agenesis [50]. The term AC has been widely used in the nomenclature since the 1960s [39].

Surgical treatment options for ACs are open surgery, endoscopic fenestration, cysto-peritoneal shunt, and a combination of these techniques [40, 41]. Among these treatments, endoscopic fenestration is an important option [59]. In making the surgical treatment decision, the relationship between AC and adjacent CSF spaces should be revealed [60].

Y. C. Güneş
Department of Radiology, Kecioren Training and Research Hospital, Ankara, Turkey

Department of Radiology, City Hospital, Bilkent, Ankara, Turkey

O. Algın (✉)
Department of Radiology, City Hospital, Bilkent, Ankara, Turkey

Department of Radiology, Yıldırım Beyazıt University School of Medicine, Ankara, Turkey

National MR Research Center (UMRAM), Bilkent University, Ankara, Turkey
e-mail: oktay.algin@umram.bilkent.edu.tr

With the introduction of computed tomography (CT) into routine use, the diagnosis of ACs has increased [38]. Although conventional CT methods are a successful technique in terms of providing morphological information, they are insufficient to evaluate the kinetics and physiology of the cerebrospinal fluid (CSF). For this purpose, historical neuroradiological methods such as invasive pneumoencephalography, ventriculography, and angiography have been used [22, 37, 61].

Cisternography is defined as the imaging procedure performed after intrathecal administration of contrast material to the subarachnoid space for the evaluation of the CSF and related structures. For the last 60 years, cisternography studies have been used to evaluate intracranial CSF-filled spaces, skull base, and vertebral column. If images are obtained only for the spinal canal, the process is also called myelography [2, 19] (Fig. 1). After intrathecal contrast agent injection, patients do not stand up until cisternography images are taken. Also, waiting in the prone or Trendelenburg position facilitates the distribution or diffusion of the contrast agent to the CSF-containing spaces. Approximately 4 h later, contrast material enhancement was observed from the basal cisterns to the Sylvian fissure. Contrast media reaches the convexity at the 20th hour. In some cases, it has been reported that this procedure is extended to the late period of up to the 48th hour.

M. Turgut et al. (eds.), *Arachnoid Cysts*, https://doi.org/10.1007/978-3-031-22701-1_16

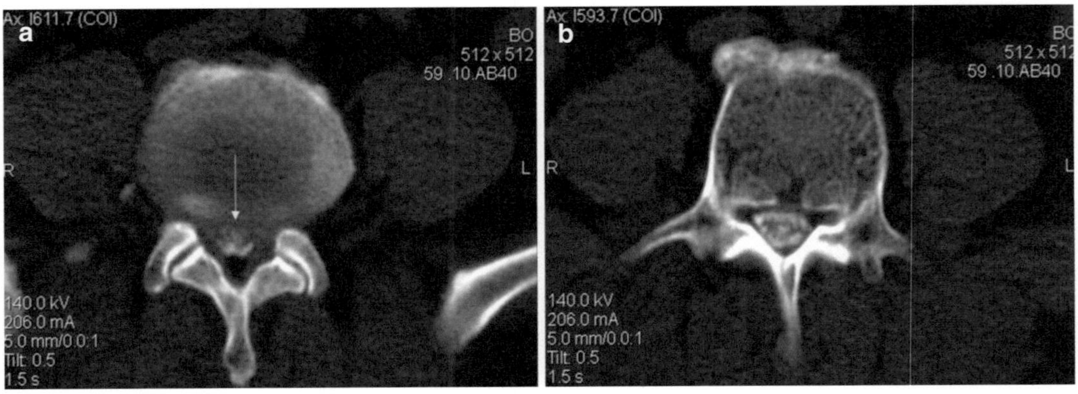

Fig. 1 Axial computed tomography (CT) myelography images obtained from the lumbar level of a 44-year-old male. The spinal canal is markedly narrowed due to the disc-osteophyte complex and ligamentum flavum hypertrophy (arrow, **a**). For comparison, an image of a near region where no spinal stenosis is observed is also given (**b**)

1.1 Isotope Cisternography

Isotope cisternography is a method first introduced by Di Chiro in 1964 to evaluate CSF circulation. It is based on the isotopic representation of gamma activity with the help of external scintillation cameras to evaluate the dynamics of CSF circulation in normal and pathological conditions [16]. After the injection of the radiopharmaceutical agent given in the lumbar region, images are taken in the early and late phases. 99mTcHSA, 169 Yb-DTPA, and 131 I-IHSA are among the agents used. The intracranial area where the tracer is usually first observed after the injection of the agent from the lumbar region is the cisterna magna, and it gradually diffuses to the basal cisterns and parasagittal arachnoid granulations at the level of convexity. Multiplanar evaluations in different axes can be provided with anterior, lateral, posterior, and/or oblique viewing angles [15]. In this examination, focal enlargement in the amount of CSF is the main finding that suggests the AC. On the other hand, Goluboff revealed that the posterior fossa ACs could also be evaluated via isotope cisternography [23].

Isotope cisternography has obvious disadvantages, and it is no longer used today. The success of isotope tracking methods decreases especially in patients with narrow ventricles or small ACs. The Sylvian fissure on lateral images, an interhemispheric fissure on axial and anteroposterior images, and ventricles create superimposed images, making it difficult to evaluate ventricular filling [24]. In addition, repeated or additional isotope cisternography exams cannot be performed due to the high-dose intake at the spinal cord level [24].

1.2 CT Cisternography (CTC)

Due to the disadvantages of radioisotope imaging, in 1974, Greitz and Hindmarsh performed CT cisternography (CTC) for the first time intrathecally using a contrast agent called metrizamide [24]. Metrizamide (Amipaque) and meglumine iocarmate (Dimer-X) were also used for CTC or CT myelography [1, 25].

Generally, low molecular weight contrast agents injected into the subarachnoid space are absorbed by the meningeal membranes, and higher molecular weight agents are absorbed by the arachnoid villi [13]. To demonstrate CSF kinetics, agents that are absorbed by the meningeal membranes were preferred. Metrizamide, a low molecular weight agent, has also been used for this purpose [14]. Metrizamide, which was used in myelography studies, primarily when it was first used in Europe, became the main contrast agent preferred in these studies [54, 55]. CTC or CT myelography with metrizamide can show anatomical compartments better due to its higher resolution than X-ray. It creates a contrast difference in the CSF in the ventricular system and the cisternal spaces.

The first areas of use of CTC were for the evaluation of hydrocephalus and extra-axial tumors, cyst communication, and/or spinal canal. In the evaluation of ACs, this method was used in case series with few participants from the second half of the 1970s to the beginning of the 1980s [27, 28, 51].

Different enhancement patterns were observed in and around the ACs [9, 21] (Figs. 2 and 3). Wang et al. showed contrast enhancement patterns of ACs in CTC images obtained at 1st, 3rd, 6th, 12th, 24th, and 48th hours after intrathecal injection of metrizamide [63]. They especially focused on the type with incomplete communication. According to the classification in this study, ACs that were filled with intrathecal contrast in the first hour were included in the fully communicating group. ACs that filled after the 3rd hour were in the incomplete communicating group, and those that did not fill at the 24th hour later or showed minimal filling were included in the noncommunication group. Complete communicating ACs could be considered as a focal enlargement in the basal cisterns that allows CSF passage to the intra- and extracystic areas [63].

1.3 MR Cisternography (MRC)

ACs are isointense with CSF on all MR sequences. When evaluated together with their morphology and localizations, they can be easily distinguished from other cystic CNS lesions. However, conventional MR sequences are not sufficient to show the communication between ACs and adjacent CSF-containing areas. For this reason, additional

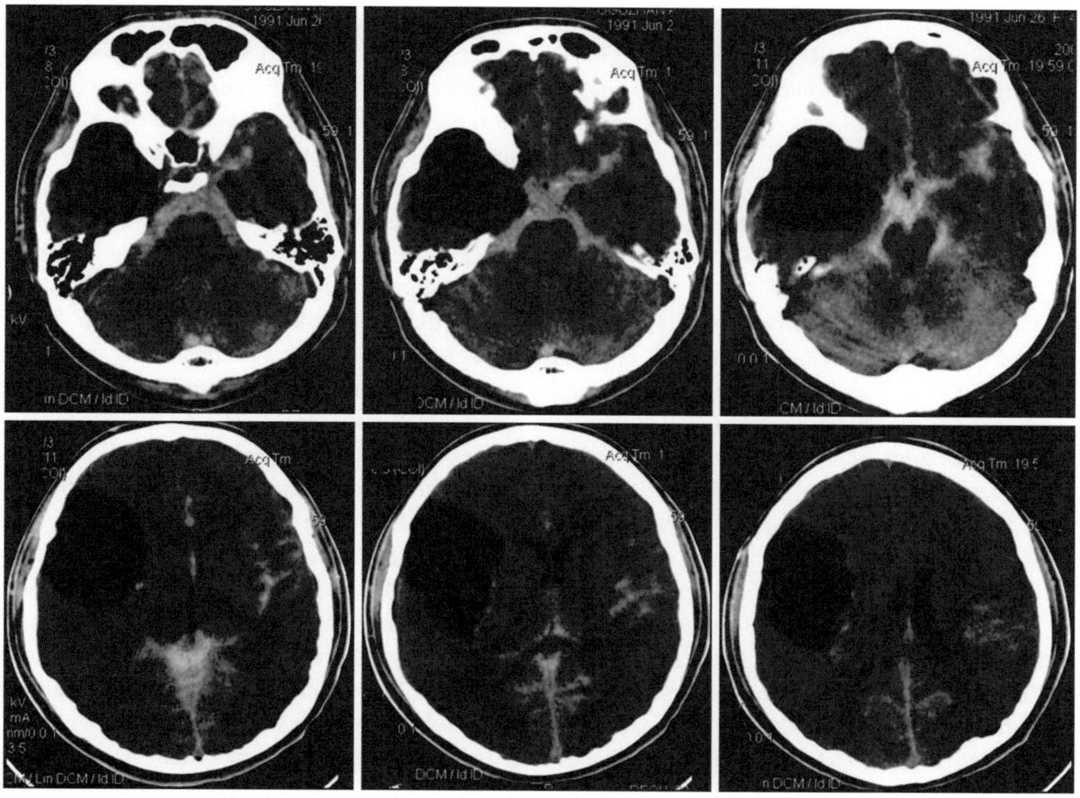

Fig. 2 Early-phase CT cisternography images of a 16-year-old male with right temporal AC. There is no communication between the cyst and surrounding CSF spaces

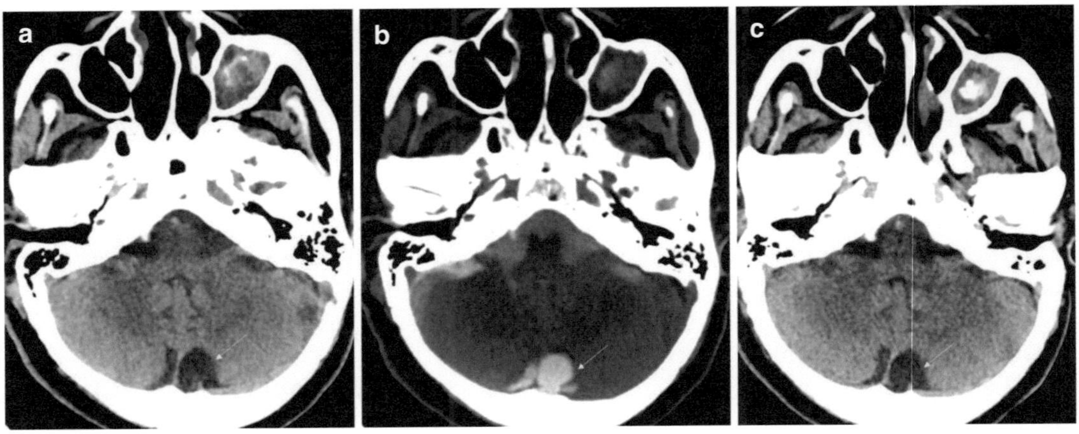

Fig. 3 Axial CT cisternography images of a 57-year-old female with communicating AC. A parasagittal AC was observed in the left posterior fossa on the precontrast image (arrow, **a**). A rapid enhancement was observed in the cyst on the early-phase postcontrast image (arrow, **b**). There is a prominent washout that was observed on the late phase (24th hour) images (arrow, **c**)

MR techniques have been developed to show possible communication.

Compared with radionuclide cisternography and CT cisternography, the main advantages of MR cisternography (MRC) are its high contrast-noise ratio, multiplanar analysis capacity, images with thin section thickness, and not causing radiation exposure [64].

1.3.1 Non-contrast Material-Enhanced MR Cisternography (NCE-MRC)

CTC or radionuclide cisternography is only performed by administering intrathecal contrast material. These tests have invasive natures and rarely serious complication risks (such as meningitis, intracranial hypotension, encephalopathy, and seizures). Therefore, new MR techniques have been developed to evaluate ACs and their communication status [3].

The pathological and physiological processes in structures related to CSF could be demonstrated with cardiac-triggered gradient echo cine MRI [18]. The basic principles determining CSF flow dynamics in MRI modalities were explained by Nitz et al. in 1992 [45]. A "flow void," CSF flow pattern on the PSIF (reversed FISP sequence of MRI) images has been reported as a sign of communicating-type ACs. The "flow-void" pattern has been expressed as the main feature showing the connection between ACs and adjacent CSF-containing areas on MRI. It has been reported that the cardiac-triggered PSIF sequence has a high sensitivity to show the connection between ACs and CSF-containing spaces. The most significant disadvantage of these MR techniques is false-positive results due to turbulent CSF flow [30].

Studies showed that phase-contrast MR imaging (PC-MRI) is superior to conventional images to determine the relationship between ACs and CSF-containing structures [17, 20, 26]. Yildiz et al. found that phase-contrast MRI and CTC results were correlated in 36 of 39 patients [67]. They stated that the "flush-and-fill" CSF flow occurs due to pressure waves of systolic intracerebral arterial inflow in the cardiac cycle [67].

PC-MRI is more sensitive when the flow is laminar. The complex features of CSF and intraventricular AC hydrodynamics compared to ACs in other areas were revealed in 2009 [3]. The turbulent or complex flows due to the mass effect of the AC or narrowing of the adjacent foramina may lead to misdiagnosis on PC-MRI images [3]. 3D-constructive interference into steady state (3D-CISS) and 2D fast imaging with steady-state free precession (FISP) sequences are beneficial for demonstration of the wall structures of ACs and global assessment of the entire ventricular system [4, 10, 57]. In cases with suspicious findings on phase-contrast MRI images, the final decision can be made with contrast material-enhanced MR cisternography (CE-MRC) [3, 67].

Three-dimensional sampling perfection with application-optimized contrasts using different flip-angle evolution (3D-SPACE) is a single-slab turbo-spin-echo (TSE) technique. It allows obtaining T1, T2, proton density, FLAIR, or heavy T2W (HT2W) images with a high SNR within a short time. 3D-SPACE data with isotropic voxel sizes allow high-resolution multiplanar assessment [42, 62]. 3D-SPACE with a variant flip-angle mode (VFAM) approach has a unique capability for evaluating CSF flow. It was successful in showing the communication between ACs and the adjacent CSF-containing areas [6].

Time-spatial labeling inversion pulse (T-SLIP) was used for the first time to evaluate the portal vein [33]. This technique was first tried for CSF flow in 2008 [65]. T-SLIP converts images to the opposite contrast in a predetermined area and shows the contrast difference between unlabeled CSF coming to a selected region. There are also publications in the literature suggesting that it can be used to evaluate spinal ACs [31, 32, 65, 66].

The four-dimensional phase-contrast velocity mapping (4D-flow) method was developed based on time-resolved phase-contrast MRI. In this technique, PC-MRI with three different axes with velocity encoding was obtained. It is mainly used in cardiovascular examinations [56]. This method may also be useful in evaluating complex-type CSF flow [29, 66]. Contrast material-enhanced MR cisternography (CE-MRC) is considered the gold standard in demonstrating the relationship between ACs and CSF-containing spaces [26, 67].

1.3.2 Contrast Material-Enhanced MR Cisternography (CE-MRC)

CE-MRC is a minimally invasive technique, and it can provide both physiological and morphological information about the CSF flow [52].

Multiplanar T1W and 3D heavily T2W images should be obtained before the administration of intrathecal gadolinium-based contrast material for CE-MRC. While T1W images should be fat-suppressed in patients investigated for CSF leakage, there is no such requirement in the examination for ACs [5]. All precontrast and postcontrast T1W series should have the same parameters to make an appropriate evaluation (Figs. 4 and 5).

2D or 3D T1W sequences can be used for CE-MRC. Single isotropic 3D-T1W data is enough for the evaluation of the ACs, but multiplanar acquisitions are necessary for adequate evaluation with 2D-T1W sequences. According to our experiences, 3-T MR units and fat-suppressed isotropic 3D T1W acquisitions are more useful for CE-MRC exams.

In CE-MRC acquisitions, a gadolinium-containing contrast agent (mostly Gd-DTPA) is injected into the subarachnoid space with the help of 20–26-gauge lumbar puncture needles following precontrast T1W and T2W images [5, 34, 68]. After then, postcontrast T1W images should be obtained. Imaging time of the postcontrast T1W series depends on the underlying pathology. By taking the early phase (within the first 2–6 h), it can be understood whether the contrast agent has been successfully injected into the subarachnoid space. In addition, early-phase images are essential in the evaluation of spinal subarachnoid spaces and global CSF circulation.

The lower lumbar region (L4–5 line) is generally preferred for intrathecal GD-DTPA injection. Rarely, the lateral portion of the C1–2 level or other lumbar levels can also be used for intrathecal injection [3]. Fluoroscopy-guided intervention may reduce side effects and complications.

Except for the evaluation of ACs, CE-MRC is also used in the determination of CSF leakage location, investigation of ventricular system patency, evaluation of third ventriculostomy, and assessment of patients with normal pressure hydrocephalus [5].

Contrast material enhancement is found in the communicating-type ACs on postcontrast T1W CE-MRC images, while intensity change is not observed in the noncommunicating-type ACs [58]. Regardless of its size, the pattern of enhancement may affect the surgical plan. Early-

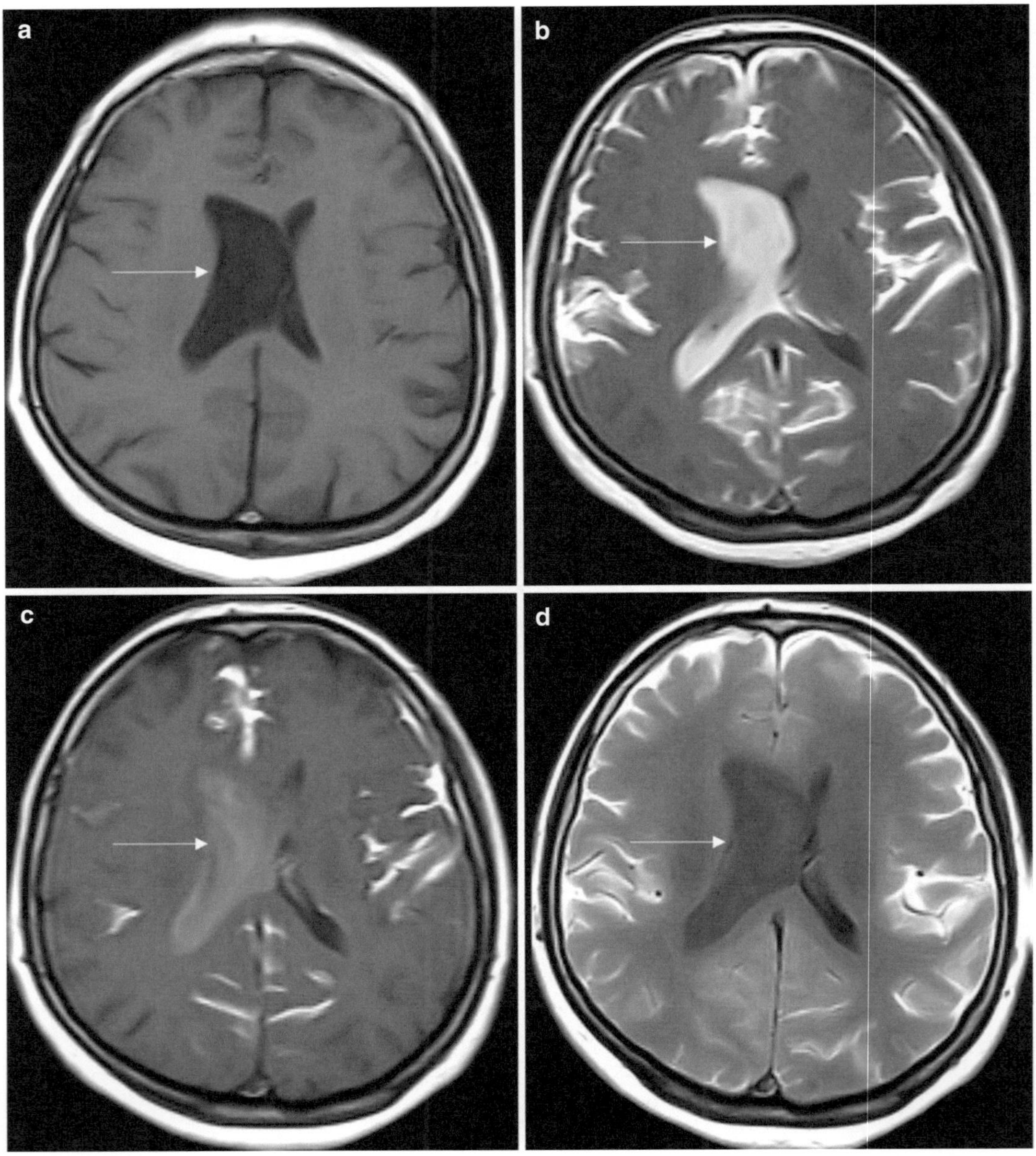

Fig. 4 Axial CE-MRC images of a 59-year-old female. An intraventricular AC (arrow) in the right ventricle was observed on the precontrast image (**a**). In the postcontrast images obtained at the 5th, 12th, and 24th hours, it is observed that the cyst is enhanced in the early phase and begins to wash out at the 24th hour (arrows, **b**–**d**). These findings are consistent with a communicating cyst

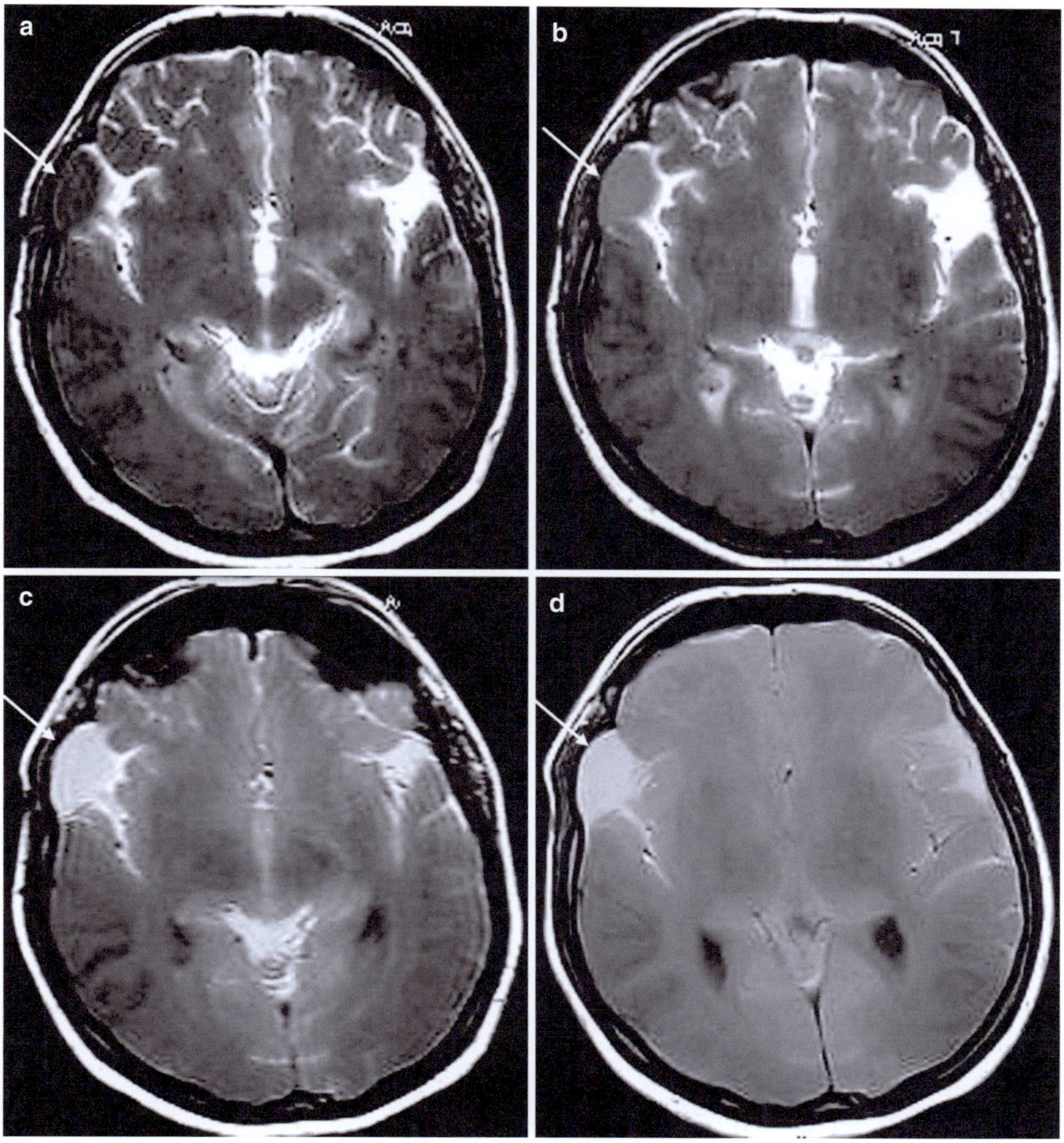

Fig. 5 Axial postcontrast CE-MRC images of a 45-year-old female with right communicating-type temporal AC (arrows). These images were obtained at the 3rd (**a**), 6th (**b**), 12th (**c**), and 24th (**d**) hours after the intrathecal gadolinium DTPA. The cyst was enhanced with intrathecal contrast media in the early and late phases, and it was not cleared of the contrast material afterward

and late-phase postcontrast T1W images should be used together in the differential diagnosis of all ACs [3, 58].

1.4 Safety of Intrathecal Administration of Gadolinium-Based Contrast Agents

Intrathecal gadolinium administration was tested firstly on monkeys in laboratory animals by Di Chiro in 1985 [12]. In the following years, many studies were conducted on laboratory animals to demonstrate dose limits and side-effect profiles [46, 58]. Neurological symptoms (e.g., focal seizures, ataxia, or latent tremor) and histopathological changes (such as loss of oligodendroglia, astrocytic hypertrophy, or eosinophilia) were observed due to high-dose intraventricular gadolinium injection [35, 46, 48, 49, 53]. However, these side effects were not observed if the injected dose was <2 mL or 0.01 mmol [35, 48, 49, 53].

Intrathecal gadolinium reduces T1 and T2 relaxation times. While the effect on T1 is evident at low doses, the T2 effect is more dominant at higher doses [58]. Intrathecally used gadolinium-based contrast agents are gadopentetate dimeglumine, gadodiamide, gadobutrol, and gadoteridol [5]. Gadolinium-based contrast agents are administered into the intrathecal region with the help of different methods (e.g., pure or together with iodine/saline) [7, 8, 43, 58].

Patients given intrathecal gadolinium should ideally be kept under observation in the hospital for 48 h after the procedure. If patients do not show any symptoms during or after the procedure, they can be discharged with bed rest for 2 days. A meta-analysis stated that 13% of the patients developed procedural side effects and these were mostly minor [47]. The most common side effect is postural headache, and it is usually relieved by bed rest and painkillers [47].

Side effects were seen in patients given intrathecal gadolinium at doses higher than 1.0 mmol, usually involving the neurological system [11, 36, 44, 47]. The main side effects are fainting, dysarthria, ataxia, confusion, vertigo, and mental status change. In addition, systemic side effects such as cardiac arrhythmia, respiratory distress, hyperglycemia, and hypertension can be observed at doses above 1.0 mmol [11, 36, 44, 47]. Although gadolinium-based intrathecal contrast agents have not yet been approved for use by the FDA, it has been reported that the use of up to 0.25–1.0 mmol is within the relative safety limits [5, 47]. Randomized controlled trials and prospective multi-participant studies are needed to reveal the dose-dependent side effects of gadolinium-based intrathecal contrast agents.

2 Conclusion

In conclusion, demonstrating the relationship of ACs with adjacent CSF-filled structures is important in making the surgical decision. CTC and CE-MRC play a crucial role in demonstrating this relationship. CE-MRC has many advantages over CTC.

References

1. Ahlgren P. Long term side effects after myelography with water-soluble contrast media: Conturex, Conray Meglumin 282 and Dimer-X. Neuroradiology. 1973;6(4):206–11.
2. Albayram S, Kilic F, Ozer H, Baghaki S, Kocer N, Islak C. Gadolinium-enhanced MR cisternography to evaluate dural leaks in intracranial hypotension syndrome. AJNR Am J Neuroradiol. 2008;29(1):116–21.
3. Algin O, Hakyemez B, Gokalp G, Korfali E, Parlak M. Phase-contrast cine MRI versus MR cisternography on the evaluation of the communication between intraventricular arachnoid cysts and neighboring cerebrospinal fluid spaces. Neuroradiology. 2009;51(5):305–12.
4. Algin O, Hakyemez B, Parlak M. Phase-contrast MRI and 3D-CISS versus contrast-enhanced MR cisternography for the detection of spontaneous third ventriculostomy. J Neuroradiol. 2011;38(2):98–104.
5. Algin O, Turkbey B. Intrathecal gadolinium-enhanced MR cisternography: a comprehensive review. AJNR Am J Neuroradiol. 2013;34(1):14–22.
6. Algin O. Evaluation of the communication between arachnoid cysts and neighboring cerebrospinal fluid spaces by T2W 3D-SPACE with variant flip-angle technique at 3 T. J Comput Assist Tomogr. 2018;42(5):816–21.
7. Arlt S, Cepek L, Rustenbeck HH, Prange H, Reimers CD. Gadolinium encephalopathy due to accidental

intrathecal administration of gadopentetate dimeglumine. J Neurol. 2007;254(6):810–2.
8. Aydin K, Terzibasioglu E, Sencer S, Sencer A, Suoglu Y, Karasu A, et al. Localization of cerebrospinal fluid leaks by gadolinium-enhanced magnetic resonance cisternography: a 5-year single-center experience. Neurosurgery. 2008;62(3):584–9.
9. Banna M. Arachnoid cysts on computed tomography. AJR Am J Roentgenol. 1976;127(6):979–82.
10. Bargalló N, Olondo L, Garcia AI, Capurro S, Caral L, Rumia J. Functional analysis of third ventriculostomy patency by quantification of CSF stroke volume by using cine phase-contrast MR imaging. AJNR Am J Neuroradiol. 2005;26(10):2514–21.
11. Besteher B, Chung HY, Mayer TE, Witte OW, Kirchhof K, Schwab M. Acute encephalopathy and cardiac arrest induced by intrathecal gadolinium administration. Clin Neuroradiol. 2020;30(3):629–31.
12. Di Chiro G, Knop RH, Girton ME, Dwyer AJ, Doppman JL, Patronas NJ, et al. MR cisternography and myelography with Gd-DTPA in monkeys. Radiology. 1985;157(2):373–7.
13. Di Chiro G, Schellinger D. Computed tomography of the spinal cord after lumbar intrathecal introduction of metrizamide (computer-assisted myelography). Radiology. 1976;120(1):101–4.
14. Di Chiro G. Movement of the cerebrospinal fluid in human beings. Nature. 1964;204:290–1.
15. Dichiro G, Reames PM, Matthews WB Jr. RISA-ventriculography and RISA-cisternography. Neurology. 1964;14:185–91.
16. Dichiro G. New radiographic and isotopic procedures in neurological diagnosis. JAMA. 1964;188:524–9.
17. Eguchi T, Taoka T, Nikaido Y, Shiomi K, Fujimoto T, Otsuka H, et al. Cine-magnetic resonance imaging evaluation of communication between middle cranial fossa arachnoid cysts and cisterns. Neurol Med Chir (Tokyo). 1996;36(6):353–7.
18. Enzmann DR, Pelc NJ. Cerebrospinal fluid flow measured by phase-contrast cine MR. AJNR Am J Neuroradiol. 1993;14(6):1301–7; discussion 1309–1310.
19. Feld M, Clement J. Cisternography; technique; indications; results. Presse Med. 1951;59(67):1396–400.
20. Fujimura M, Tominaga T, Koshu K, Shimizu H, Yoshimoto T. Cine-mode magnetic resonance imaging of a thoracic intradural arachnoid cyst: case report. Surg Neurol. 1996;45(6):533–6.
21. Galassi E, Tognetti F, Gaist G, Fagioli L, Frank F, Frank G. CT scan and metrizamide CT cisternography in arachnoid cysts of the middle cranial fossa: classification and pathophysiological aspects. Surg Neurol. 1982;17(5):363–9.
22. Glasauer FE. Isotope cisternography and ventriculography in congenital CNS anomalies. Childs Brain. 1975;1(2-3):116–20.
23. Goluboff LG. Arachnoid cyst of the posterior fossa demonstrated by isotope cisternography. J Nucl Med. 1973;14(1):61–2.
24. Greitz T, Hindmarsh T. Computer-assisted tomography of intracranial CSF circulation using a water-soluble contrast medium. Acta Radiol Diagn (Stockh). 1974;15(5):497–507.
25. Grepe A. Cisternography with the non-ionic water-soluble contrast medium metrizamide. A preliminary report. Acta Radiol Diagn (Stockh). 1975;16(2):146–60.
26. Hakyemez B, Yildiz H, Parlak M. CSF connection of the intracranial cysts and cyst like lesions: analysis with flow sensitive phase-contrast Cine MR imaging. Diagn Interv Radiol. 2003;9(2):152–6.
27. Handa J, Nakano Y, Aii H. CT cisternography with intracranial arachnoidal cysts. Surg Neurol. 1977;8(6):451–4.
28. Hayashi T, Anegawa S, Honda E, Kuramoto S, Mori K, Murata T, et al. Clinical analysis of arachnoid cysts in the middle fossa. Neurochirurgia (Stuttg). 1979;22(6):201–10.
29. Hirayama A, Matsumae M, Yatsushiro S, Abdulla A, Atsumi H, Kuroda K. Visualization of pulsatile CSF motion around membrane-like structures with both 4D velocity mapping and time-SLIP technique. Magn Reson Med Sci. 2015;14(4):263–73.
30. Hoffmann KT, Hosten N, Meyer BU, Röricht S, Sprung C, Oellinger J, et al. CSF flow studies of intracranial cysts and cyst-like lesions achieved using reversed fast imaging with steady-state precession MR sequences. AJNR Am J Neuroradiol. 2000;21(3):493–502.
31. Ishibe T, Senzoku F, Ikeda N, Kamba Y, Mikawa Y. Detection of the communicating hole(s) of spinal extradural arachnoid cysts using time-spatial labeling inversion pulse magnetic resonance imaging. Spine (Phila Pa 1976). 2014;39(23):E1394–7.
32. Ishibe T, Senzoku F, Kamba Y, Ikeda N, Mikawa Y. Time-spatial labeling inversion pulse magnetic resonance imaging of cystic lesions of the spinal cord. World Neurosurg. 2016;88:693.e13–21.
33. Ito K, Koike S, Jo C, Shimizu A, Kanazawa H, Miyazaki M, et al. Intraportal venous flow distribution: evaluation with single breath-hold ECG-triggered three-dimensional half-Fourier fast spin-echo MR imaging and a selective inversion-recovery tagging pulse. AJR Am J Roentgenol. 2002;178(2):343–8.
34. Jinkins JR, Rudwan M, Krumina G, Tali ET. Intrathecal gadolinium-enhanced MR cisternography in the evaluation of clinically suspected cerebrospinal fluid rhinorrhea in humans: early experience. Radiology. 2002;222(2):555–9.
35. Jinkins JR, Williams RF, Xiong L. Evaluation of gadopentetate dimeglumine magnetic resonance cisternography in an animal model: preliminary report. Invest Radiol. 1999;34(2):156–9.
36. Kapoor R, Liu J, Devasenapathy A, Gordin V. Gadolinium encephalopathy after intrathecal gadolinium injection. Pain Physician. 2010;13(5):E321–6.
37. La Torre E, Fortuna A, Occhipinti E. Angiographic differentiation between Dandy-Walker cyst and arachnoid cyst of the posterior fossa in newborn infants and children. J Neurosurg. 1973;38(3):298–308.
38. Leo JS, Pinto RS, Hulvat GF, Epstein F, Kricheff II. Computed tomography of arachnoid cysts. Radiology. 1979;130(3):675–80.

39. Lourie H, Berne AS. Radiological and clinical features of an arachnoid cyst of the quadrigeminal cistern. J Neurol Neurosurg Psychiatry. 1961;24(4):374–8.
40. Maiuri F, Iaconetta G, Gangemi M. Arachnoid cyst of the lateral ventricle. Surg Neurol. 1997;48(4):401–4.
41. Martínez-Lage JF, Pérez-Espejo MA, Almagro MJ, López-Guerrero AL. Hydrocephalus and arachnoid cysts. Childs Nerv Syst. 2011;27(10):1643–52.
42. Mugler JP III. Optimized three-dimensional fast-spin-echo MRI. J Magn Reson Imaging. 2014;39(4):745–67.
43. Nacar Dogan S, Kizilkilic O, Kocak B, Isler C, Islak C, Kocer N. Intrathecal gadolinium-enhanced MR cisternography in patients with otorhinorrhea: 10-year experience of a tertiary referral center. Neuroradiology. 2018;60(5):471–7.
44. Nayak NB, Huang JC, Hathout GM, Shaba W, El-Saden SM. Complex imaging features of accidental cerebral intraventricular gadolinium administration. J Neurosurg. 2013;118(5):1130–4.
45. Nitz WR, Bradley WG Jr, Watanabe AS, Lee RR, Burgoyne B, O'Sullivan RM, et al. Flow dynamics of cerebrospinal fluid: assessment with phase-contrast velocity MR imaging performed with retrospective cardiac gating. Radiology. 1992;183(2):395–405.
46. Park KW, Im SB, Kim BT, Hwang SC, Park JS, Shin WH. Neurotoxic manifestations of an overdose intrathecal injection of gadopentetate dimeglumine. J Korean Med Sci. 2010;25(3):505–8.
47. Patel M, Atyani A, Salameh JP, McInnes M, Chakraborty S. Safety of intrathecal administration of gadolinium-based contrast agents: a systematic review and meta-analysis. Radiology. 2020;297(1):75–83.
48. Ray DE, Cavanagh JB, Nolan CC, Williams SC. Neurotoxic effects of gadopentetate dimeglumine: behavioral disturbance and morphology after intracerebroventricular injection in rats. AJNR Am J Neuroradiol. 1996;17(2):365–73.
49. Ray DE, Holton JL, Nolan CC, Cavanagh JB, Harpur ES. Neurotoxic potential of gadodiamide after injection into the lateral cerebral ventricle of rats. AJNR Am J Neuroradiol. 1998;19(8):1455–62.
50. Robinson RG. The temporal lobe agenesis syndrome. Brain. 1964;87:87–106.
51. Ruscalleda J, Guardia E, dos Santos FM, Carvajal A. Dynamic study of arachnoid cysts with metrizamide. Neuroradiology. 1980;20(4):185–9.
52. Selcuk H, Albayram S, Ozer H, Ulus S, Sanus GZ, Kaynar MY, et al. Intrathecal gadolinium-enhanced MR cisternography in the evaluation of CSF leakage. AJNR Am J Neuroradiol. 2010;31(1):71–5.
53. Siebner HR, Gräfin von Einsiedel H, Conrad B. Magnetic resonance ventriculography with gadolinium DTPA: report of two cases. Neuroradiology. 1997;39(6):418–22; discussion 422.
54. Skalpe IO, Amundsen P. Lumbar radiculography with metrizamide. A nonionic water-soluble contrast medium. Radiology. 1975;115(1):91–5.
55. Skalpe IO, Amundsen P. Thoracic and cervical myelography with metrizamide. Clinical experiences with a water-soluble, non-ionic contrast medium. Radiology. 1975;116(1):101–6.
56. Stankovic Z, Allen BD, Garcia J, Jarvis KB, Markl M. 4D flow imaging with MRI. Cardiovasc Diagn Ther. 2014;4(2):173–92.
57. Stoquart-El Sankari S, Lehmann P, Gondry-Jouet C, Fichten A, Godefroy O, Meyer ME, et al. Phase-contrast MR imaging support for the diagnosis of aqueductal stenosis. AJNR Am J Neuroradiol. 2009;30(1):209–14.
58. Tali ET, Ercan N, Kaymaz M, Pasaoglu A, Jinkins JR. Intrathecal gadolinium (gadopentetate dimeglumine)-enhanced MR cisternography used to determine potential communication between the cerebrospinal fluid pathways and intracranial arachnoid cysts. Neuroradiology. 2004;46(9):744–54.
59. Tamburrini G, D'Angelo L, Paternoster G, Massimi L, Caldarelli M, Di Rocco C. Endoscopic management of intra and paraventricular CSF cysts. Childs Nerv Syst. 2007;23(6):645–51.
60. Tan Z, Li Y, Zhu F, Zang D, Zhao C, Li C, et al. Children with intracranial arachnoid cysts: classification and treatment. Medicine (Baltimore). 2015;94(44):e1749.
61. Tator CH, Murray S. A clinical, pneumoencephalographic and radioisotopic study of normal-pressure communicating hydrocephalus. Can Med Assoc J. 1971;105(6):573–9.
62. Ucar M, Tokgoz N, Koc AM, Kilic K, Borcek AO, Oner AY, et al. Assessment of 3D T2-weighted high-sampling-efficiency technique (SPACE) for detection of cerebellar tonsillar motion: new useful sign for Chiari I malformation. Clin Imaging. 2015;39(1):42–50.
63. Wang X, Chen JX, You C, Jiang S. CT cisternography in intracranial symptomatic arachnoid cysts: classification and treatment. J Neurol Sci. 2012;318(1–2):125–30.
64. Watanabe Y, Makidono A, Nakamura M, Saida Y. 3D MR cisternography to identify distal dural rings: comparison of 3D-CISS and 3D-SPACE sequences. Magn Reson Med Sci. 2011;10(1):29–32.
65. Yamada S, Miyazaki M, Kanazawa H, Higashi M, Morohoshi Y, Bluml S, et al. Visualization of cerebrospinal fluid movement with spin labeling at MR imaging: preliminary results in normal and pathophysiologic conditions. Radiology. 2008;249(2):644–52.
66. Yatsushiro S, Hirayama A, Matsumae M, Kuroda K. Visualization of pulsatile CSF motion separated by membrane-like structure based on four-dimensional phase-contrast (4D-PC) velocity mapping. Annu Int Conf IEEE Eng Med Biol Soc. 2013;2013:6470–3.
67. Yildiz H, Erdogan C, Yalcin R, Yazici Z, Hakyemez B, Parlak M, et al. Evaluation of communication between intracranial arachnoid cysts and cisterns with phase-contrast cine MR imaging. AJNR Am J Neuroradiol. 2005;26(1):145–51.
68. Zeng Q, Xiong L, Jinkins JR, Fan Z, Liu Z. Intrathecal gadolinium-enhanced MR myelography and cisternography: a pilot study in human patients. AJR Am J Roentgenol. 1999;173(4):1109–15.

SPECT Imaging of Arachnoid Cysts

Elias Rizk

1 Introduction

Arachnoid cysts (ACs) are asymptomatic, non-neoplastic, and benign lesions that form within the central nervous system, both in the spinal cord and intracranial regions [4]. These cysts are usually present within the subarachnoid space, containing cerebrospinal fluid (CSF). Most ACs have been reported at or after birth, characterized as head trauma. Large cysts are symptomatic as they compress the structures around them and thus need to be surgically removed [21]. These cysts occur in people of all ages but are more common in children and babies. There are four times a greater chance of ACs developing in males than in females. The prevalence among adults and children is 1.4% and 2.6%, respectively [2]. Clinical symptoms of ACs include dizziness, headache, dyscognition, worsening mood, ataxia, nausea, mental status changes, and seizures [32, 35]. These symptoms occur during the cyst development due to the displacement of neural entities, abnormal local pressure, and obstructions in CSF pathways [8]. It has been proposed that the location of cysts seems to induce symptoms as smaller ACs growing in eloquent regions may result in a presumed clinical diagnosis, as happens with Sylvian suprasellar fissure cysts. ACs do not have a static appearance. They can enlarge and disappear during their progression [16]. Based on the unpredictable behavior of the ACs, patients are treated conservatively and are diagnosed with the appearance of signs and symptoms of cerebral compression and progression [8].

ACs differ in their sites and location. They usually develop in the brain but less often in the spinal cord. ACs in the brain are termed intracranial ACs, while those that develop in the spinal cord are called spinal ACs. In both cases, the ACs develop from the protective membrane around the spinal cord and brain. This membrane is also known as the arachnoid membrane. They have been reported over the cranial axis but occur prominently in the temporal fossa [11]. Some are reported to occur in the suprasellar, cerebellopontine angle, quadrigeminal cisterns, cistern magna, and cerebral convexities (Fig. 1) [2].

Based on clinical reasons and their presentation before surgery, three classes of cysts have been proposed by Choi [5]. The first class includes cysts with intracranial hypertension and hydrocephalus symptoms. The second class contains cysts demonstrating the symptoms of a large head, skull abnormalities, dizziness, seizures, delayed development, strabismus, and headaches. The third group contains cysts with minimal clinical symptoms. It has been proposed

E. Rizk (✉)
Department of Neurosurgery, College of Medicine, The Pennsylvania State University, Hershey, PA, USA

Department of Neurosurgery, Penn State Health Milton S. Hershey Medical Center, Hershey, PA, USA
e-mail: ebr10@psu.edu; erizk@pennstatehealth.psu.edu

M. Turgut et al. (eds.), *Arachnoid Cysts*, https://doi.org/10.1007/978-3-031-22701-1_17

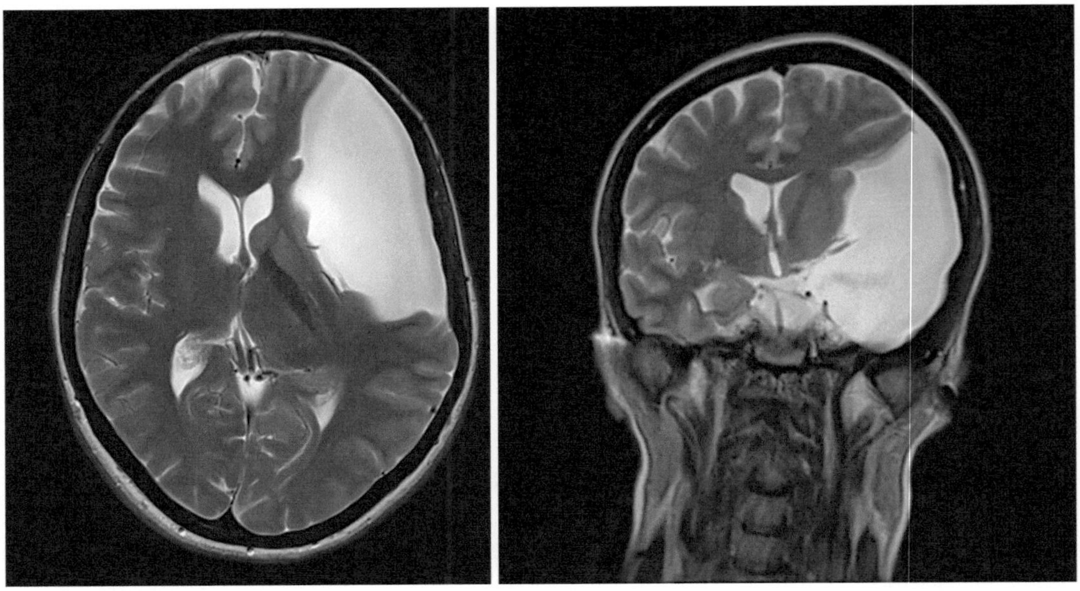

Fig. 1 Magnetic resonance image (MRI) of the brain before operation. The left side shows the axial location, the middle image represents a coronal cyst in the brain

that ACs with smaller sizes possess the potential to remain benign during their lifetime [1]. The diagnosis and treatment of ACs depend on their location and symptoms.

2 Diagnosis of ACs

Initially, the ACs were diagnosed and treated based on their signs and symptoms. However today, the diagnosis of ACs can be made by various means such as ultrasound, computed tomography (CT), magnetic resonance imaging (MRI), and neuroimaging distinguishing them from various lesions such as cystic neurocysticercosis, dermoid tumor, abscess, and epidermoid cysts. CT, MRI, and ultrasound (US) have successfully identified several silent cysts [22]. However, techniques like CT, MRI, and US provide knowledge only regarding the anatomy of the ACs, like location and size [26] using CT-based scans for distinguishing ACs in the middle fossa. ACs exert pressure on the brain tissue, thus restricting the pathways of CSF. It requires further testing to determine the indication of surgical need. Few studies target the CSF-linked indication for the surgical need for treating ACs (Fig. 2) [18].

The cysts require specific pulse sequences to visualize and diagnose the wall of the cysts [12]. On imaging, the ACs are shown as circumscribed cysts having an indistinguishable wall representing linked structures with dense CSF on CT. CT imaging is an established technique with sufficient potential for diagnosis [20]. Dr. Matsuda described the presence of an AC in a 13-year-old person detected by CT imaging. CT imaging is an effective choice for the diagnosis when the location of the cysts can be expected. CT imaging is helpful for the differentiation of non-communicating cysts from communicating cysts. However, the MRI provides a reasonable tool when additional knowledge is required. MRI is a better option to assess cyst location, size, anatomy, and structures. It can help to diagnose differently from CT [33]. The cysts show variations in the signal intensities detected on MRI [12]. All these methods are useful for the morphological identification of ACs. However, these methods do not differentiate those ACs that result in brain malfunctioning [19].

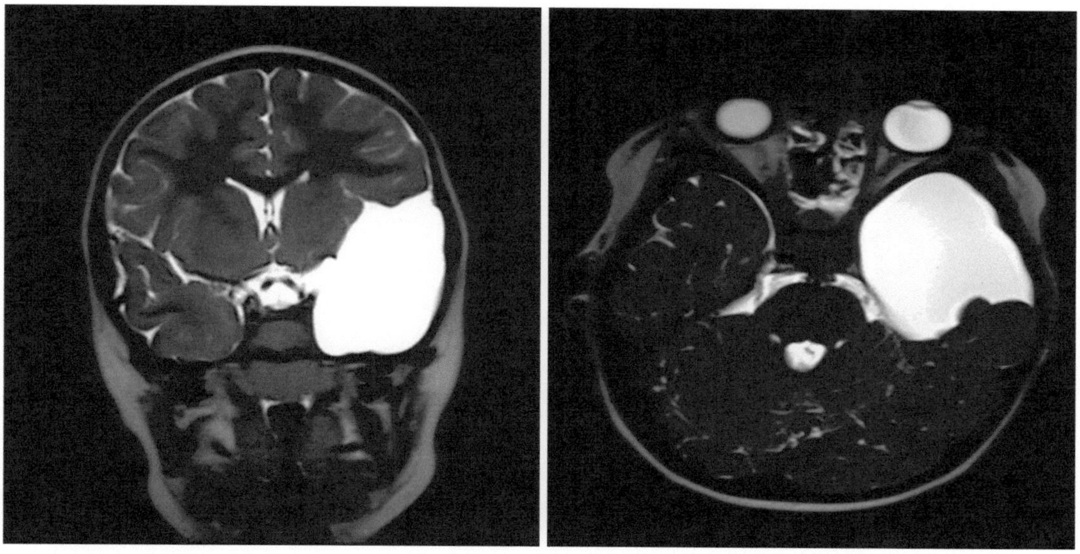

Fig. 2 MRI of a large AC in an adolescent in the frontal temporal region (right side) [14]

3 SPECT Imaging

The development and advancements of single photon emission computed tomography (SPECT) and positron emission tomography (PET) imaging enable researchers to visualize the in vivo and noninvasive biological mechanisms at the cellular and molecular levels. SPECT represents a feasible approach to tracing a number of biological aspects like metabolism, neural transmission, and vascular blood flow [6]. SPECT is a pharmaceutical-based diagnostic method that utilizes pharmaceuticals bound with isotopes to target the regional-cerebral blood flow (rCBF). The improved efficacy of such techniques is based on producing specific molecular probes designed to bind with the specific target with great selectivity [23]. Lena et al. proposed that detecting ACs has become more frequent with the development of neuroimaging [9]. The information necessary for the SPECT is gained by the gamma radiation detector [3]. It has been proposed that a six-fold increase in the image contrast can be achieved with the help of SPECT imaging (Fig. 3) [34].

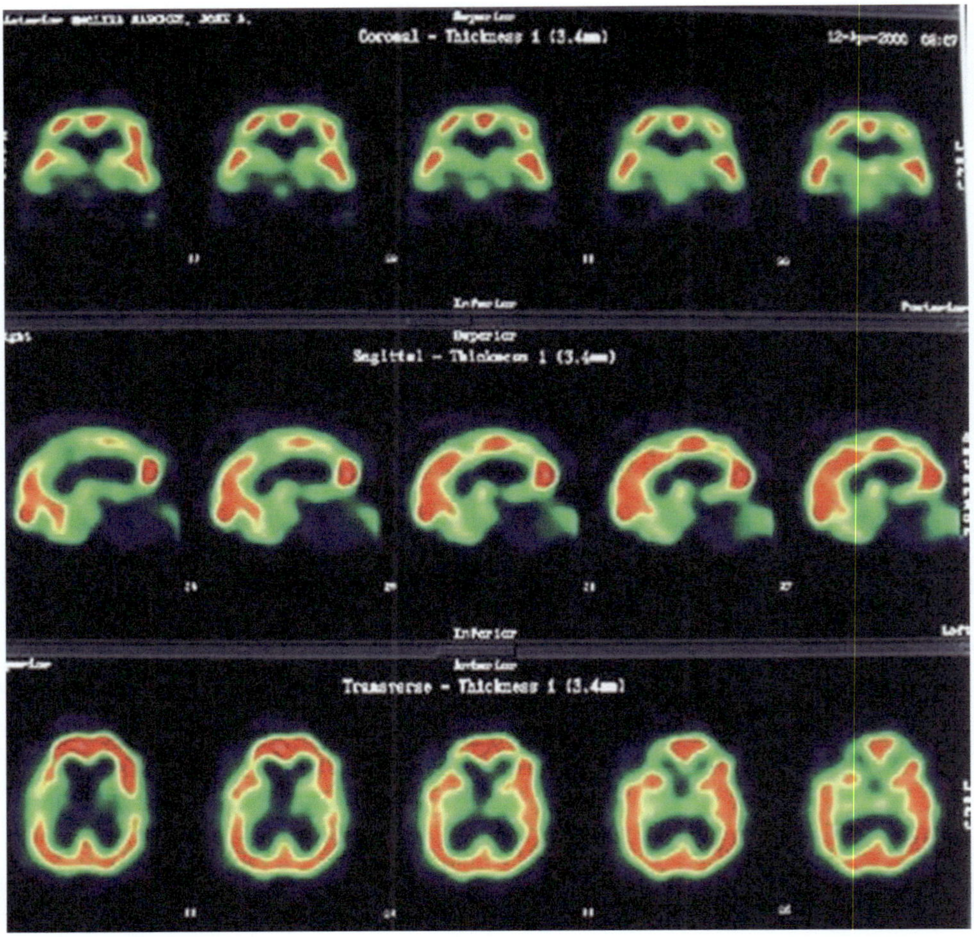

Fig. 3 SPECT results of a patient with an AC [14]

4 Advantages of SPECT Imaging

The advantage of the SPECT imaging technique lies in its ability to identify essential biological mechanisms at the molecular and cellular levels in living entities [31]. Molecular imaging provides a potential tool to predict the disease onset in the earlier stages based on changes in the body. SPECT and PET CT imaging offer advantages over the traditional clinical diagnostic methods of neurological diseases based on their improved sensitivity, resolution, and higher penetration abilities [15]. SPECT imaging is a safe technique as patients can return to their normal routine after the study. The injected tracer will be expelled from the body within 24–72 h through the excretory system. Apart from being safe, the process is painless and requires less time. In comparison with MRI, SPECT imaging has more sensitivity. A brief comparison between the spatial resolution, quantity of probe used, and spatial resolution is given in Table 1 [23].

Table 1 Comparison between the spatial resolution, quantity of probe used, and spatial resolution for SPECT, MRI and PET

Serial No.	Technique	Sensitivity	Quantity of probe used	Spatial resolution
1.	SPECT	10^{-10}–10^{-11}	ng	1–2 mm
2.	MRI	10^{-3}–10^{-5}	μg to mg	25–100 μm
3.	PET	10^{-11}–10^{-12}	ng	1–2 mm

5 SPECT Imaging for the Detection of ACs

Several findings based on SPECT imaging of ACs address the utilization of SPECT imaging to diagnose ACs [19]. Other studies also demonstrate successful research, which report the efficient treatment of ACs (supratentorial) with peritoneal shunting and the use of the Hakim programmable valve [10]. The accurate diagnosis in this study was based on SPECT imaging. In another study, the author performed a cognitive analysis of a male child suffering from congenital-ACs in the left frontal fossa [13]. The neuropsychological analyses documented his cognitive behavior such as memory, language, and frontal functions. The child showed delayed verbal ability. However, the frontal ability was reported as unimpaired. In this analysis, the results from SPECT imaging revealed reduced perfusion in the left temporal lobe. Malfunctioning in the left temporal lobe caused delayed verbal functioning [27]. Hence, the evaluation of cognitive processes based on neuroimaging provided essential evidence for elaborating on the cyst influence and explaining its psychological functioning. Shared research has involved three patients who suffered from ACs of the middle fossa. One patient showed non-specific signs and symptoms and was examined by MRI and SPECT imaging to investigate the effect of the cyst on the blood flow of the cerebral region. In another research, a female (48 years old) showed disturbing behavior. Results on CT represented an AC over the cerebral convexity (left side) [29]. The MRI and SPECT scan results of ACs in the frontal interhemispheric region were obtained in a 10-year-old patient (Fig. 4) [17]. The patient showed severe headache symptoms.

Other researchers reported their findings based on SPECT imaging pre-surgery and post-surgery in seven patients suffering from ACs [10]. The affected patients demonstrated normal cerebral blood flow after shunting the ACs. In addition, some authors have reported their difficulty distinguishing AC symptoms from brain deterioration [16, 25]. They found impaired neural perfusion with ACs in the patients showing symptoms based on SPECT imaging [16]. Patients showing normal rCBF on their SPECT imaging results exhibited asymptomatic conditions during their entire flow-up period. The study reports that the cerebral SPECT scans provide a reasonable tool to correlate with regional brain functions based on the brain anatomy to efficiently diagnose patients suffering from ACs for future clinical or surgical approaches. However, little information is presently based on the rCBF SPECT imaging in the detection of ACs [26]. These authors elaborated on the comparison of MRI images of a 9-year-old patient suffering from ACs in the right Sylvian portion with SPECT image before the surgery (Fig. 5) [19].

They also reported the feasibility of SPECT imaging technique as an effective diagnostic tool in their study [24]. They have precisely elaborated on the comparison of the efficacy of SPECT-CT with the SPECT alone based on the study conducted on 357 patients [28]. They concluded that the SPECT-CT enhanced the radioactive doses given to the patient with the effective dose being due to the combined effect of CT in

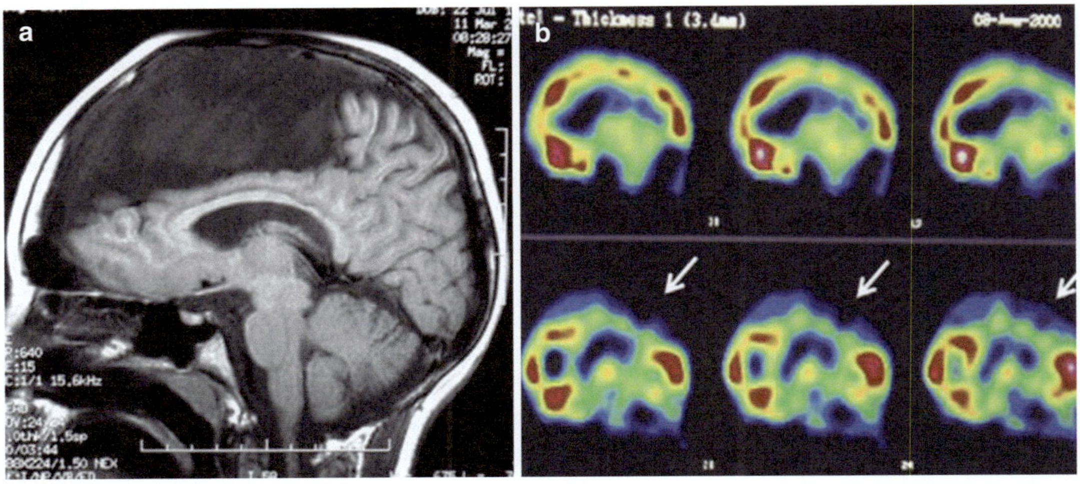

Fig. 4 A comparison between (**a**) MRI scan and (**b**) SPECT scan of a patient having interhemispheric-ACs [26]

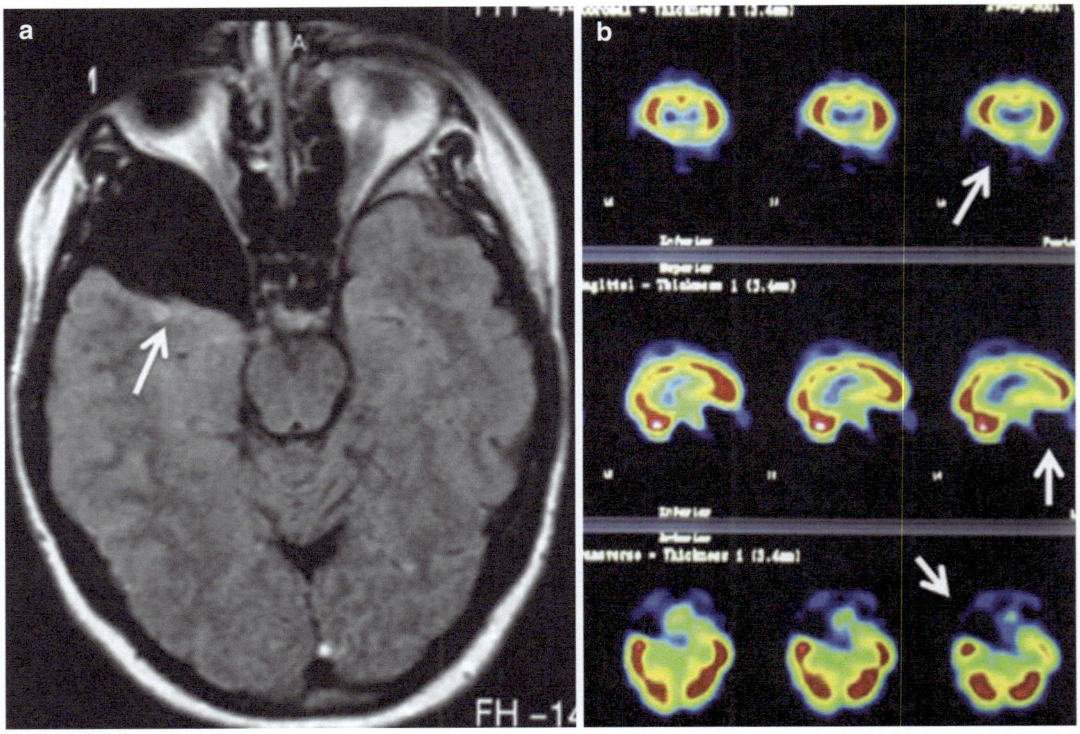

Fig. 5 (**a**) MRI of a 9-year-old patient suffering from the AC in the right Sylvian fissure. (**b**) SPECT image of the AC in the coronal region prior to surgery in the same patient (shown in the upper line), axial region (shown in the lower line), and sagittal region (shown in the middle line). The arrows represent the hypoperfusion near the ACs [14]

many instances. CT combined with SPECT has been used for two decades and offers a more practical approach to localizing and characterizing the findings. The enhanced diagnostic efficacy and accuracy relate to the improved diagnostic specificity and connection [14].

6 Challenges That Need to Be Addressed for SPECT Imaging

Several points need to be addressed while discussing SPECT scans' efficacy in diagnosing ACs. Most of the published literature is based on studies possessing small-size samples with poor controls. Also, the primary concern of SPECT imaging that needs to be addressed is the elevated equipment cost, since there is insufficient knowledge to address this concern. In addition, post-surgery complications, such as cerebral infarction, hemorrhage, neurological infections, and deficits, have been reported. These complications are required to be addressed for better diagnosis and treatments [17]. For most people, SPECT is regarded as safe. Some hurdles reported are pain, bleeding, and swelling during the injection or insertion of the needle. SPECT allergic responses were also noticed [30]. Sometimes this issue is compensated for with the non-multidetector CT scanner. The point needs consideration to compensate for the burden of CT scans it also varies depending on the protocol and system used [7].

7 Conclusion

SPECT has been established as a feasible tool for the in vivo detection and diagnosing diseases, including ACs. Various researchers have shown their results concerning detecting ACs based on SPECT imaging. The technique provides a reasonable approach to visualizing the internal abnormality and offers an effective tool to predict the risk of AC development and its morphological details. However, further investigation and development of novel and more effective radiolabeled substances are required for more accurate disease detection and treatment.

References

1. Adin ME. Hemorrhagic complications of arachnoid cysts: when, why, and who? World Neurosurg. 2018;113:380–2. https://doi.org/10.1016/j.wneu.2018.01.093.
2. Al-Holou WN, Terman S, Kilburg C, Garton HJL, Muraszko KM, Maher CO. Prevalence and natural history of arachnoid cysts in adults. J Neurosurg. 2013;118:222–31. https://doi.org/10.3171/2012.10.JNS12548.
3. Anger H. Scintillation camera. Rev Sci Instrum. 1958;29(1):27–33.
4. Bhatt AS, Mhatre R, Nadeesh BN, Mahadevan A, Yasha TC, Santosh V. Nonneoplastic cystic lesions of the central nervous system-histomorphological spectrum: a study of 538 cases. J Neurosci Rural Pract. 2019;10(3):494–501. https://doi.org/10.1055/S-0039-1698033.
5. Choi JW, Lee JY, Phi JH, Kim S-K, Wang K-C. Stricter indications are recommended for fenestration surgery in intracranial arachnoid cysts of children. Childs Nerv Syst. 2015;31(1):77–86. https://doi.org/10.1007/s00381-014-2525-1.
6. Cuocolo A, Petretta M. PET and SPECT specialty grand challenge. When knowledge travels at the speed of light, photons take to the field. Front Nucl Med. 2021;1:1–3. https://doi.org/10.3389/fnume.2021.671914.
7. Delbeke D, Coleman RE, Guiberteau MJ, et al. Procedure guideline for SPECT/CT imaging 1.0. J Nucl Med. 2006;47(7):1227–34.
8. DiRocco C, Choux M, Raimondi A. Intracranial cyst lesions. Berlin: Springer; 2013.
9. Lena G, Van Calenberg F, Genitori L, Chonx M, et al. Supratentorial interhemispheric cysts associated with callosal agenesis: surgical treatment and outcome in 16 children. Childs Nerv Syst. 1995;11(10):568–73. Springer.
10. Germanò A, Caruso G, Caffo M, et al. The treatment of large supratentorial arachnoid cysts in infants with cyst-peritoneal shunting and Hakim programmable valve. Childs Nerv Syst. 2003;19(3):166–73. https://doi.org/10.1007/s00381-002-0702-0.
11. Helland CA, Lund-Johansen M, Wester K. Location, sidedness, and sex distribution of intracranial arachnoid cysts in a population-based sample. J Neurosurg. 2010;113(5):934–9. https://doi.org/10.3171/2009.11.JNS081663.
12. Hingwala DR, Radhakrishnan N, Kesavadas C, Thomas B, Kapilamoorthy R, Radhakrishnan VV. Neuroenteric cysts of the brain-comprehensive magnetic resonance imaging. Indian J Radiol

Imaging. 2013;23(2):155–63. https://doi.org/10.4103/0971-3026.116579.
13. Horiguchi T, Takeshita K. Cognitive function and language of a child with an arachnoid cyst in the left frontal fossa. World J Biol Psychiatry. 2000;1(3):159–63. https://doi.org/10.3109/15622970009150585.
14. Israel O, Pellet O, Biassoni L, et al. Two decades of SPECT/CT—the coming of age of a technology: an updated review of literature evidence. Eur J Nucl Med Mol Imaging. 2019;46(10):1990–2012. https://doi.org/10.1007/s00259-019-04404-6.
15. Lu F, Yuan Z. PET/SPECT molecular imaging in clinical neuroscience: recent advances in the investigation of CNS diseases. Quant Imaging Med Surg. 2015;5(3):433–47. https://doi.org/10.3978/j.issn.2223-4292.2015.03.16.
16. Martínez-Lage J. Neurosurgical treatment for hydrocephalus, subdural hematomas, and arachnoid cysts in glutaric aciduria type 1. Neuropediatrics. 1996;27(6):335–6.
17. Martínez-Lage JF, Almagro MJ, López-Guerrero AL. SPECT studies in patients with arachnoid cysts. In: Arachnoid cysts: epidemiology, biology, and neuroimaging; 2017. p. 199–214. https://doi.org/10.1016/B978-0-12-809932-2.00016-8.
18. Martínez-Lage JF, Angel Pérez-Espejo M, Almagro M-J, López López-Guerrero A. Hydrocephalus and arachnoid cysts. Childs Nerv Syst. 2011;27:1643. https://doi.org/10.1007/s00381-011-1481-2.
19. Martínez-Lage JF, Valentí JA, Piqueras C, Ruiz-Espejo AM, Román F, Nuño De La Rosa JA. Functional assessment of intracranial arachnoid cysts with TC99 m-HMPAO SPECT: a preliminary report. Childs Nerv Syst. 2006;22:1091–7. https://doi.org/10.1007/s00381-006-0043-5.
20. Matsuda W, Matsuda W, Akutsu H, et al. Apparently asymptomatic arachnoid cyst: postoperative improvement of subtle neuropsychological impediment—case report. Neurol Med Chir (Tokyo). 2010;50(5):430–3.
21. Mustansir F, Bashir S, Darbar A. Management of arachnoid cysts: a comprehensive review. Cureus. 2018;10(4):e2458. https://doi.org/10.7759/cureus.2458.
22. Oberbauer RW, Haase J, Pucher R, et al. Arachnoid cysts in children: a European co-operative study. Childs Nerv Syst. 1992;8(5):281–6.
23. Pimlott SL, Sutherland A. Molecular tracers for the PET and SPECT imaging of disease. Chem Soc Rev. 2011;40:149–62. https://doi.org/10.1039/b922628c.
24. Roach PJ, Schembri GP, Ho Shon IA, Bailey EA, Bailey DL. SPECT/CT imaging using a spiral CT scanner for anatomical localization: impact on diagnostic accuracy and reporter confidence in clinical practice. Nucl Med Commun. 2006;27(12):977–87. https://doi.org/10.1097/01.mnm.0000243372.26507.e7.
25. Santos JMG, Martfnez-Lage J, Gilabert Ubeda A, Alemdn AC, Climent Oltrfi V. Arachnoid cysts of the middle cranial fossa: a consideration of their origins based on imaging. Neuroradiology. 1993;35(5):355–8.
26. Sato H, Sato N, Katayama S, Tamaki N, Matsumoto S. Effective shunt-independent treatment for primary middle fossa arachnoid cyst. Childs Nerv Syst. 1991;7(7):375–81.
27. Sgouros S, Chapman S. Congenital middle fossa arachnoid cysts may cause global brain ischaemia: a study with 99Tc-hexamethylpropyleneamineoxime single photon emission computerised tomography scans. Pediatr Neurosurg. 2001;35(4):188–94. https://doi.org/10.1159/000050420.
28. Sharma P, Sharma S, Ballal S, Bal C, Malhotra A, Kumar R. SPECT-CT in routine clinical practice: increase in patient radiation dose compared with SPECT alone. Nucl Med Commun. 2012;33(9):926–32. https://doi.org/10.1097/MNM.0b013e328355b6d5.
29. Tsurushima H, Harakuni T, Saito A, Tominaga D, Hyodo A, Yoshii Y. Symptomatic arachnoid cyst of the left frontal convexity presenting with memory disturbance—case report. Neurol Med Chir (Tokyo). 2000;40(6):339–41. https://doi.org/10.2176/nmc.40.339.
30. Weiss ME, Bernstein DI, Blessing-Moore J, et al. Drug allergy: an updated practice parameter. Ann Allergy Asthma Immunol. 2010;105(4):259–73.e78. https://doi.org/10.1016/j.anai.2010.08.002.
31. Weissleder R, Mahmood U. Molecular imaging. Radiology. 2001;219(2):316–33. https://doi.org/10.1148/radiology.219.2.r01ma19316.
32. Wester K. Intracranial arachnoid cysts—do they impair mental functions? J Neurol. 2008;255(8):1113–20. https://doi.org/10.1007/s00415-008-0011-y.
33. White M, Das J. Arachnoid cysts. StatPearls; 2021. https://www.ncbi.nlm.nih.gov/books/NBK563272/
34. Whitehead FR. Minimum detectable gray-scale differences in nuclear medicine images. J Nucl Med. 1978;19(1):87–93.
35. Wojcik G. [Intracranial arachnoid cysts in the clinical and radiological aspect]. Wiad Lek. 2016;69(3 pt 2):555–9.

Part IV

Clinical Presentations and Differential Diagnosis of Arachnoid Cysts

Editor's Summary

In this "Part IV: Clinical Presentations and Differential Diagnosis of Arachnoid Cysts," there are a total of six chapters describing the clinical presentations of arachnoid cysts (ACs) in the central nervous system. Interestingly, they can be quite variable and are associated with a broad differential diagnosis when evaluating fluid-containing collections located in the cranial compartment and in the spinal canal. The various clinical symptoms noted at the time of presentation of patients with ACs are described in detail in 18. More complex neurological problems such as hydrocephalus and epilepsy have also been identified concurrently in patients with ACs and will each be addressed in two sequential separate chapters. On rare occasions, psychiatric manifestations have been identified in patients with intracranial ACs as are revealed in 21. As expected, the differential diagnoses for fluid-filled collections that can be localized within the cranium and the spine are extensive. In each of the last two chapters of this part, the differential diagnosis for those intracranial and intraspinal collections will be described and the manner in which their nature can be accurately determined will be discussed by their authors.

Symptomatology of Craniospinal Arachnoid Cysts

Saffet Tüzgen and Barış Küçükyürük

1 Introduction

Arachnoid cysts (ACs) are space-occupying lesions that are benign in nature and filled with cerebrospinal fluid (CSF) [17, 22]. The increasing use of radiological imaging has caused more ACs to be diagnosed incidentally. However, the natural history and behavior of these lesions are not well understood. Furthermore, symptomatology is not clear in many cases as clinical features are mostly nonspecific and does not correlate directly with the location and the size of the AC. In this chapter, clinical signs and symptoms of AC will be reviewed.

2 Intracranial Arachnoid Cysts

Intracranial ACs are rather common, reported to be 1% of all intracranial masses. They are considered as a congenital abnormality of the arachnoid membrane. However, the exact mechanism of their formation has not yet been determined [17]. It is suggested that splitting of the arachnoid may be the pathological mechanism of development. Other theories advocate fluid secretion from the cyst wall or one-way ball valve flow of CSF.

S. Tüzgen (✉) · B. Küçükyürük
Department of Neurosurgery, İstanbul University Cerrahpaşa School of Medicine, Cerrahpaşa, Istanbul, Turkey
e-mail: stuzgen@iuc.edu.tr; baris.kucukyuruk@iuc.edu.tr

ACs are situated in supratentorial space in most of cases. The middle cranial fossa, more specifically anterior to temporal lobes, contains 50–60% of all cases (Figs. 1 and 2). They may also be located in the suprasellar cistern and cerebellopontine angle cistern. Less common locations are in the cisterna magna, the interhemispheric fissure, and the quadrigeminal cistern [17].

ACs are asymptomatic and diagnosed incidentally in most cases; however, some cases may present with neurological signs or symptoms [1, 20]. In many instances, the size of the AC remains stable over time. On the other hand, symptomatic enlargement is a well-known issue, as well as developing clinical signs without evident visual progression in size. On the other hand, it is difficult in most cases to determine whether those symptoms and signs are related to the AC [6]. More specifically, nonspecific symptoms such as headaches are difficult to interpret whether they are caused by the AC.

It is suggested that roughly 5% of cases with an AC present to have symptoms [1, 2]. Leading symptoms are listed as headaches, hydrocephalus, seizures, cranial neuropathy, cognitive complaints, or other focal neurological deficits such as hemiparesis or visual compromise [9, 12, 14, 15]. Specifically, in children, cranial bone deformities accompanied by increasing head size may be the presenting sign [16]. In addition to these, developmental delay and cognitive problems may be detected; however, the relationship of these findings with the AC may be difficult to

M. Turgut et al. (eds.), *Arachnoid Cysts*, https://doi.org/10.1007/978-3-031-22701-1_18

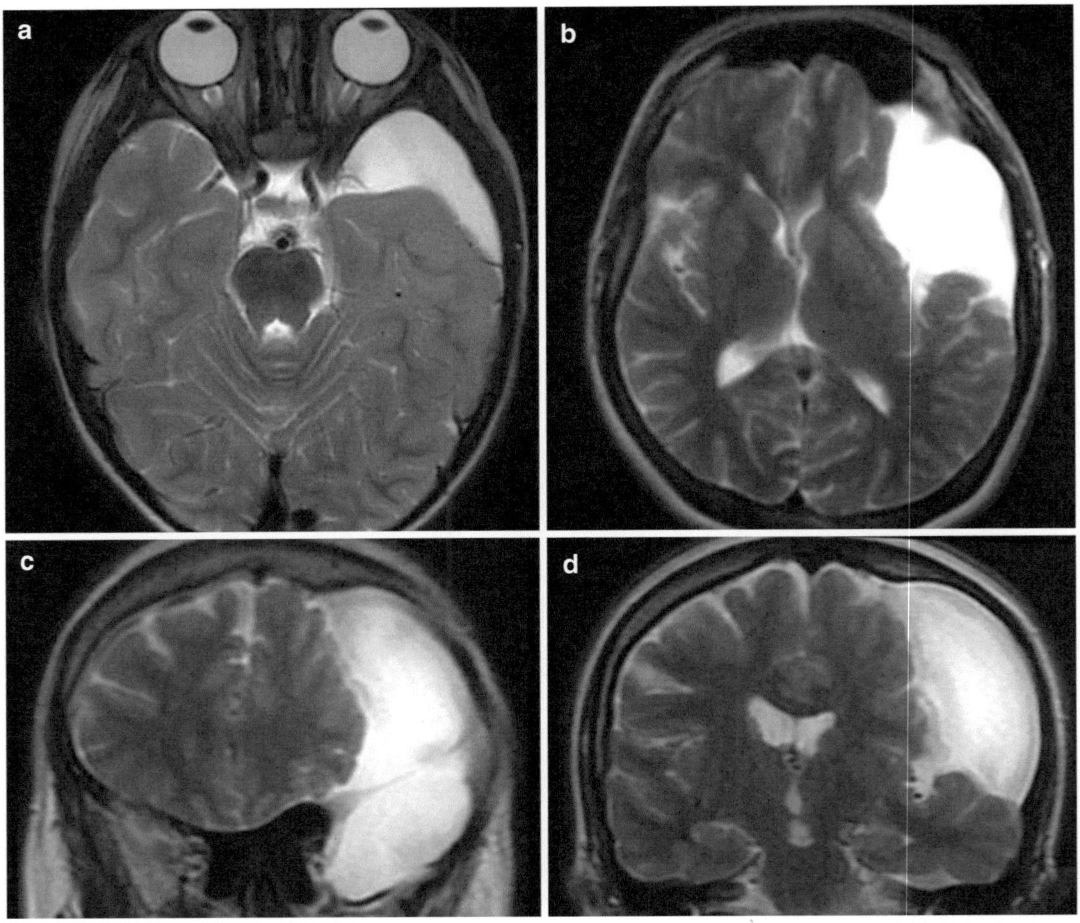

Fig. 1 Magnetic resonance T2-weighted images of a 34-year-old female patient who was admitted with chronic headaches. Axial sections (**a**) and (**b**) show a cystic lesion located in the left hemisphere. The AC is situated anterior to the temporal lobe and extends superiorly to the level of the insula and the frontal operculum. Coronal sections (**c**) and (**d**) show that the AC does not cause significant compression of the cerebrum but has reshaped the overlying calvarium, which confirms the chronic nature of the lesion. The headache, the main complaint, was nonlocalizing and was also present on the right side. Due to minimal compression found on radiological images and nonspecific nature of symptoms, conservative treatment was chosen

prove. On the other hand, some reports suggested that impairment in mental function is likely to improve after surgical treatment [24, 25]. Focal neurological deficits were also reported to benefit from surgery, while headaches and seizures often persist after surgical treatment [14, 23].

ACs situated in the suprasellar, cerebellopontine angle (CPA), ambient, and quadrigeminal cisterns are more prone to cause symptoms compared to cysts in other locations. This finding was statistically significant in the series of Al-Holou et al., which reported that six of nine cases with an AC located in the suprasellar cistern presented with symptoms, most often due to obstructive hydrocephalus [1]. Similarly, 15% of CPA location ACs caused symptoms such as sensorineural hearing loss, tinnitus, or vertigo. On the other hand, more common locations such as the middle fossa or retrocerebellar locations are found to be less likely to cause symptoms, as only 2.1% of patients with middle fossa ACs were considered symptomatic. The pediatric population showed no differences regarding the relation of the location with symptoms as anterior fossa and quadrigeminal plate

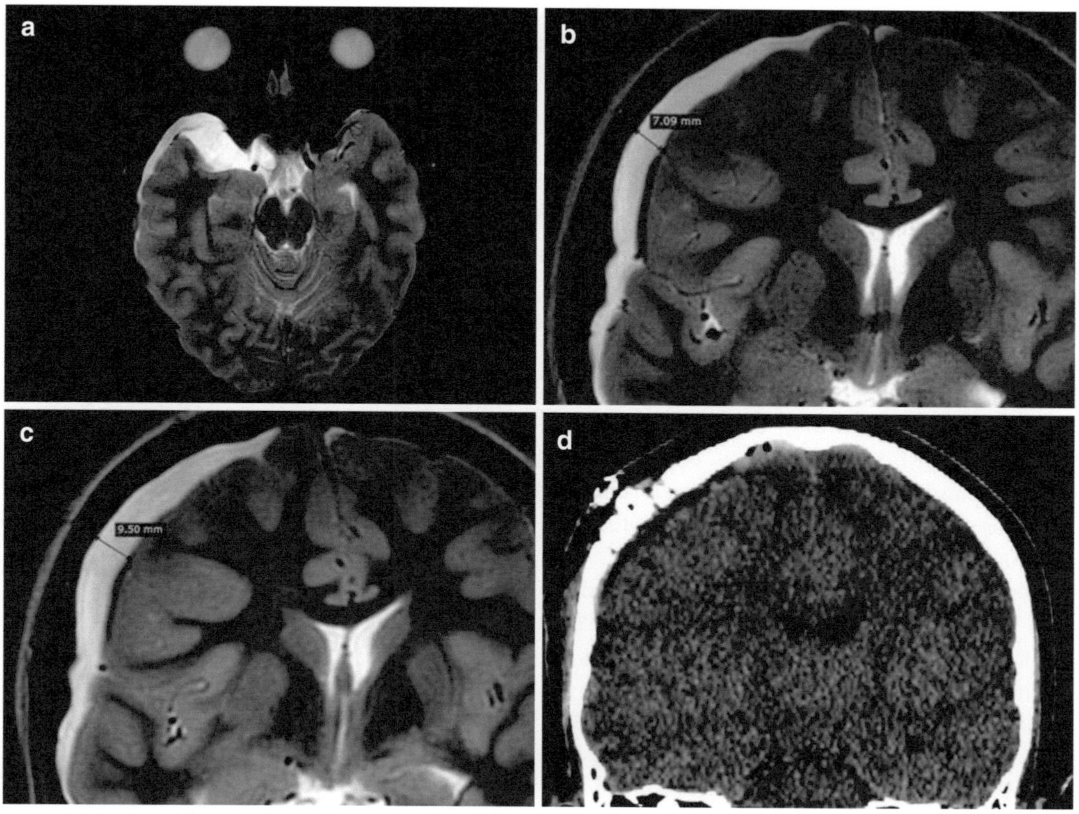

Fig. 2 Magnetic resonance (MR) and computed tomography (CT) images of a 14-year-old male patient who was admitted with the first episode of epileptic seizures and an acute onset headache. Images (**a**) and (**b**) show T2-weighted MR images in axial and coronal sections, respectively. An AC situated anterior to the right temporal lobe and a hygroma extending over the frontal and parietal lobes possibly appearing after the rupture of the cyst were detected. There was no remodeling of the calvarium suggesting an acute nature of the pathology. Additionally, midline shift is present. Image (**c**) shows coronal section of the MR obtained 7 days later, which revealed enlargement of the hygroma. Image (**d**) shows coronal section of CT scan, which was obtained after the patient was operated through a mini-craniotomy to explore the hygroma and placement of a drain

cysts were positively correlated with the presence of neurological symptoms, while the posterior fossa location was not [2].

Another factor for presenting with symptoms is the size of the ACs where larger cysts were positively correlated to cause neurological signs [1, 2].

A difficult clinical determination is to predict if an initially asymptomatic AC will develop new symptoms. It is reported that only around 1% of adult population and 3% of the pediatric population were reported to acquire new symptoms in the midterm follow-up period [1, 2]. Al-Holou et al. reported that all pediatric patients who developed new symptoms were younger than 4 years old, which is a rapid enlargement period for the intracranial contents.

Rupture of an AC into the subarachnoid space causing a hygroma or occurrence of a hemorrhage is a feared but a rare occurrence both in adult and pediatric population [4]. However, surgical intervention after the hemorrhage facilitates a good outcome in many cases, which proves that the risk of hemorrhage should not be an indication for surgical treatment in incidentally discovered cysts [18].

3 Spinal Arachnoid Cysts

Spinal ACs are located mostly in the intradural space but may also be located rarely in the extradural space [3, 5]. Intradural cysts can be grouped as primary and secondary cysts [3]. Primary spinal ACs are idiopathic, and secondary cysts are formed due to inflammatory or traumatic processes [13]. Idiopathic cysts are proposed to arise from the septum posticum, a membrane spanning from the pia to the arachnoid in the dorsum of the spinal canal [19]. A second hypothesis is that these cysts may develop from the growth of entrapped arachnoid granulations [8]. Secondary cysts originate after any inflammatory process affecting the arachnoid, such as subarachnoid hemorrhage, infection, trauma, or intradural surgery [3].

The majority of primary spinal ACs are situated in the thoracic vertebral levels (77.5%), while secondary cysts are formed in locations of the initiating pathology [3, 7].

The most common presentation of spinal ACs were reported to be back pain, which is suggested to be due to nerve root compression [21]. Additionally, myelopathic symptoms such as weakness, numbness, and spastic paraparesis are common findings [13, 21]. These findings can be unilateral or bilateral depending on the position of the cyst. Sphincter dysfunction was also reported as a presenting symptom in a group of patients [11]. Unlike their intracranial counterparts, spinal ACs are reported to show progressively worsening symptoms over time [10].

4 Conclusion

Intracranial and spinal ACs have different characteristics. Intracranial cysts are common lesions, but they rarely produce lesion-specific symptoms. Moreover, it is difficult to identify if a more common but nonspecific symptom such as headache is related with the lesion. Therefore, surgical treatment at first is an option for discussion since even acutely presenting symptoms respond well to timely surgery. On the other hand, spinal ACs may present with signs and symptoms directly related to nerve compression in many cases. Often, the thoracic location of these lesions should be kept in mind when searching for lower spinal pathologies.

References

1. Al-Holou WN, Terman S, Kilburg C, Garton HJ, Muraszko KM, Maher CO. Prevalence and natural history of arachnoid cysts in adults. J Neurosurg. 2013;118(2):222–31.
2. Al-Holou WN, Yew AY, Boomsaad ZE, Garton HJ, Muraszko KM, Maher CO. Prevalence and natural history of arachnoid cysts in children. J Neurosurg Pediatr. 2010;5(6):578–85.
3. Baig Mirza A, Bartram J, Vastani A, Gebreyohanes A, Al Banna Q, Lavrador JP, et al. Systematic review of surgical management of spinal intradural arachnoid cysts. World Neurosurg. 2022;158:e298–309.
4. Bilginer B, Onal MB, Oguz KK, Akalan N. Arachnoid cyst associated with subdural hematoma: report of three cases and review of the literature. Childs Nerv Syst. 2009;25(1):119–24.
5. Cai Z, Hong X, Huang J, Hu H, Lu C, Ding X, et al. Microsurgical treatment of symptomatic spinal extradural arachnoid cyst: a consecutive case series of 34 patients and literature review. Clin Neurol Neurosurg. 2021;210:107000.
6. Di Rocco C. Sylvian fissure arachnoid cysts: we do operate on them but should it be done? Childs Nerv Syst. 2010;26(2):173–5.
7. Fam MD, Woodroffe RW, Helland L, Noeller J, Dahdaleh NS, Menezes AH, et al. Spinal arachnoid cysts in adults: diagnosis and management. A single-center experience. J Neurosurg Spine. 2018;29(6):711–9.
8. Fortuna A, Mercuri S. Intradural spinal cysts. Acta Neurochir (Wien). 1983;68(3–4):289–314.
9. Galassi E, Tognetti F, Frank F, Fagioli L, Nasi MT, Gaist G. Infratentorial arachnoid cysts. J Neurosurg. 1985;63(2):210–7.
10. Galzio RJ, Zenobii M, Lucantoni D, Cristuib-Grizzi L. Spinal intradural arachnoid cyst. Surg Neurol. 1982;17(5):388–91.
11. Garg K, Borkar SA, Kale SS, Sharma BS. Spinal arachnoid cysts—our experience and review of literature. Br J Neurosurg. 2017;31(2):172–8.
12. Kang JK, Lee KS, Lee IW, Jeun SS, Son BC, Jung CK, et al. Shunt-independent surgical treatment of middle cranial fossa arachnoid cysts in children. Childs Nerv Syst. 2000;16(2):111–6.
13. Klekamp J. A new classification for pathologies of spinal meninges-part 2: primary and secondary intradural arachnoid cysts. Neurosurgery. 2017;81(2):217–29.
14. Levy ML, Wang M, Aryan HE, Yoo K, Meltzer H. Microsurgical keyhole approach for middle fossa arachnoid cyst fenestration. Neurosurgery. 2003;53(5):1138–44; discussion 44–5.

15. Maher CO, Goumnerova L. The effectiveness of ventriculocystocisternostomy for suprasellar arachnoid cysts. J Neurosurg Pediatr. 2011;7(1):64–72.
16. Oberbauer RW, Haase J, Pucher R. Arachnoid cysts in children: a European co-operative study. Childs Nerv Syst. 1992;8(5):281–6.
17. Osborn AG, Preece MT. Intracranial cysts: radiologic-pathologic correlation and imaging approach. Radiology. 2006;239(3):650–64.
18. Parsch CS, Krauss J, Hofmann E, Meixensberger J, Roosen K. Arachnoid cysts associated with subdural hematomas and hygromas: analysis of 16 cases, long-term follow-up, and review of the literature. Neurosurgery. 1997;40(3):483–90.
19. Perret G, Green D, Keller J. Diagnosis and treatment of intradural arachnoid cysts of the thoracic spine. Radiology. 1962;79:425–9.
20. Pradilla G, Jallo G. Arachnoid cysts: case series and review of the literature. Neurosurg Focus. 2007;22(2):E7.
21. Sadek AR, Nader-Sepahi A. Spinal arachnoid cysts: presentation, management and pathophysiology. Clin Neurol Neurosurg. 2019;180:87–96.
22. Santamarta D, Aguas J, Ferrer E. The natural history of arachnoid cysts: endoscopic and cine-mode MRI evidence of a slit-valve mechanism. Minim Invasive Neurosurg. 1995;38(4):133–7.
23. Shim KW, Lee YH, Park EK, Park YS, Choi JU, Kim DS. Treatment option for arachnoid cysts. Childs Nerv Syst. 2009;25(11):1459–66.
24. Wester K, Hugdahl K. Arachnoid cysts of the left temporal fossa: impaired preoperative cognition and postoperative improvement. J Neurol Neurosurg Psychiatry. 1995;59(3):293–8.
25. Wester K. Intracranial arachnoid cysts—do they impair mental functions? J Neurol. 2008;255(8):1113–20.

Arachnoid Cysts Associated with Hydrocephalus

Nikolaos Syrmos, Vaitsa Giannouli, Sotirios Kottas, and Mehmet Turgut

1 Introduction

Intracranial arachnoid cysts (ACs) are benign, liquid formations, inside the arachnoid brain matter [1–4]. The combination of ACs with hydrocephalus is presented both in adult and pediatric age patients [5–10]. According to statistical data, intracranial ACs are about 1% of all brain space-occupying lesions and a little less than 1% of all the brain lesions treated worldwide by neurosurgeons and pediatric neurosurgeons [4–6, 11, 12]. Their prevalence in the adult population (>16 years old) is approximately 1.5%, with more cases in females than in males [4–6, 13, 14]. In children (<12 years old), the prevalence is a little more than 2.5% for some authors and between 1% and 3% for others [7–10, 15, 16].

If the ACs are large enough, they may influence the cerebrospinal fluid (CSF) pathways causing often the hydrocephalus phenomenon and also marked midline shift, as a notable radiological sign [10–13, 17–19]. The close association between ACs and hydrocephalus has been commonly described by various authors as related to a mass effect, but also closely to brain ventricular abnormalities [13–16, 19–22].

2 Etiological and Pathogenetic Features

The true etiological and pathogenetic factors closely related to the formation of ACs are still unclear and mainly controversial, according to the literature [1, 5, 13, 16, 20–22]. Through the passing of the years, various theoretical models have been proposed in order to explain the origin of the genesis/formation of the ACs [2, 5, 13, 17, 18, 22–24] (Table 1).

Usually, the ACs arise close to the CSF cisterns with a mass quantity of arachnoid [3, 5, 13, 19, 22–26] (Table 2).

Table 1 Theoretical models about the genesis of arachnoids cysts

• Partial brain agenesis
• Splitting or duplication of arachnoid membrane
• Mesenchymal deficits closely related to CSF flow

N. Syrmos (✉)
Arsitotle University of Thessaloniki,
Thessaloniki, Macedonia, Greece

Human Performance and Health, Master Science Program, Aristotle University of Thessaloniki,
Thessaloniki, Macedonia, Greece

V. Giannouli
Arsitotle University of Thessaloniki,
Thessaloniki, Macedonia, Greece

S. Kottas
Papanikolou General Hospital,
Thessaloniki, Macedonia, Greece

M. Turgut
Department of Neurosurgery, Aydın Adnan Menderes University School of Medicine, Aydın, Turkey

Department of Histology and Embryology, Aydın Adnan Menderes University Health Sciences, Aydin, Turkey

M. Turgut et al. (eds.), *Arachnoid Cysts*, https://doi.org/10.1007/978-3-031-22701-1_19

This close relationship with CSF is most likely the main genesis factor for hydrocephalus [1, 6, 11, 22–28]. Basically, ACs can be divided into two main types [1–4, 19, 22, 28–30]:

- Congenital (true), as a result of primary embryologic development, more common
- Secondary (acquired), less common

The secondary often occurred after traumatic brain situations and as result of [7–10, 20–22, 30–32] inflammatory factors, tumors, various chemical reactions, and hemorrhages.

Another classification option was also proposed, depending on the surrounding CSF dynamics and on the size of the cyst or cysts during opening [7–10, 22, 25–27]:

- Communicating
- Non-communicating

The surrounding CSF dynamics can lead, sooner or later, to hydrocephalus [7–10, 22, 24, 26]. This classification is always in concordance with the relation to the subarachnoid compartments [7–10, 22, 25, 28].

The expansion of ACs is related to various mechanisms according to various studies [7–10, 22, 28–30] (Table 3).

Table 2 CSF cisterns with mass quantity of arachnoid

(a) Posterior infratentorial midline
(b) Sylvian fissures
(c) Quadrigeminal
(d) Cerebellopontine
(e) Suprasellar

Table 3 Expansion theories of ACs

Ball-valve phenomenon	Permits the CSF entrance into the cyst but also prevents egress
Fluid movement	Provocated by osmotic factors
Intracystic fluid	Production by secretion of cyst wall cells

3 Clinical Signs-Symptoms and Location

Clinical signs and symptoms are related to the particular location of the ACs [5, 13, 22, 25, 27, 29]. They are mainly supratentorial, found in the middle fossa in nine of ten cases, but there is a possibility to be also infratentorial, in the posterior fossa in one of ten cases [5, 13, 22, 26, 28, 30]. In the supratentorial location, six of ten cases are localized in the temporal lobe [5, 6, 13, 22, 27, 29, 31]. In the posterior fossa, the signs and symptoms are as follows: headache, vomiting, and various cerebral disorders all closely related to the obstructive hydrocephalus phenomenon [5, 7, 13, 22, 30, 32].

In supratentorial location, there are a variety of symptoms [5, 8, 13, 15, 17, 22, 29] (Table 4). Headache is the most common symptom, present in around 66% of all cases [5, 9, 10, 13, 20, 22, 26]. Other general symptoms are as follows [5, 9, 10, 13, 19, 21, 22, 26] (Table 5): dizziness, nausea, vomiting, and ataxia.

In quadrigeminal ACs, symptoms include [5, 11, 13, 20, 22, 27] (Table 6): Concezio di Rocco, a pioneer Italian pediatric neurosurgeon from Rome, in the middle 1990s was the first to describe this entity in the scientific literature [6, 7, 10–12, 22] (Fig. 1). Quadrigeminal ACs are in unusual topography brain location (5–10% of the whole AC appearance) [6–12, 22–28].

Endoscopy procedures for better and safer removal of ACs were proposed since the middle 1990s, first by American pediatric neurosurgeon John R. Ruge and later by other authors [26] (Fig. 2).

Another reported entity is the appearance of acquired hydrocephalus, in preexisting ACs forming after aneurysmal subarachnoid hemorrhage (SAH) [26–30].

For better clinical evaluation and management of ACs in combination with hydrocephalus, the neu-

Table 4 Supratentorial location of ACs

Temporal lobe	Suprasellar region	Pineal region	Convexity area
Asymptomatic headaches in case of enlargement Bleeding in case of vascular wall	Headaches, vomiting Endocrine disorders Hydrocephalus	Failure of upward gaze Obstructive hydrocephalus	Seizures neurological deficits

Table 5 Other general symptoms of ACs

- Dizziness
- Nausea
- Vomiting
- Mood changes
- Mental changes
- Ataxia
- Balance disorders
- Urinary deficits
- Seizures
- Hearing alterations

Table 6 Symptoms of quadrigeminal ACs

- Macrocrania
- Headaches
- Vomiting
- Lethargy
- Papilledema
- Ocular disorders
- Impairment of upward gaze

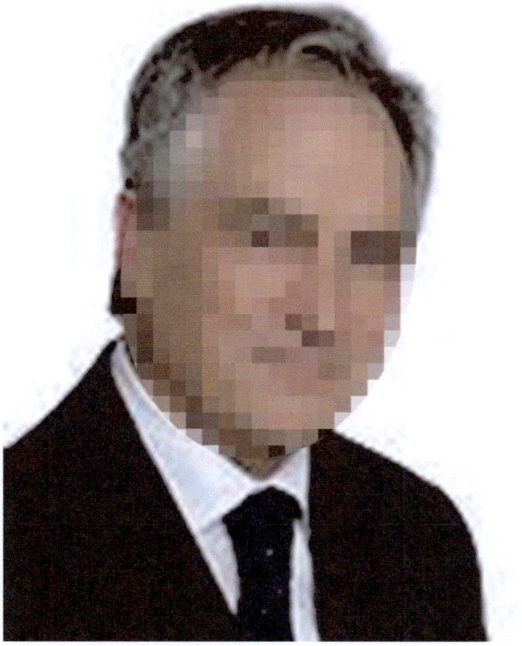

Fig. 1 Concezio Di Rocco, an Italian pediatric neurosurgeon

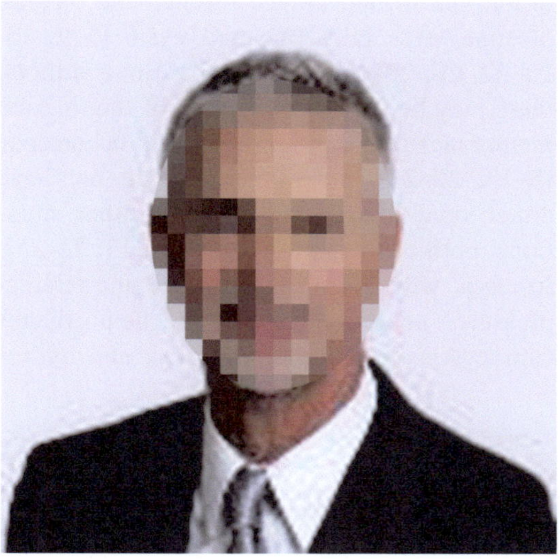

Fig. 2 John R. Ruge, an American pediatric neurosurgeon

rosurgeon and the pediatric neurosurgeon should collaborate with other medical disciplines such as neurologists, neuroradiologists, orthopedics, otorhinolaryngologists, pediatricians, pediatric neurologists, neonatologists, urologists, cardiologists, geriatricians, internal medicine physicians, intensive care physicians, pediatric intensive care physicians, neurorehabilitation physicians, psychiatrists, etc. [6–12, 22, 30–32].

This multidisciplinary approach through collaboration and scientific dialogue can lead to the optimal evaluation and better decision-making in cases in order to optimally treat both the AC and the hydrocephalus [6, 12, 22, 30, 31]. In pediatric cases, it is also very important to consider the role played by the parents and the family [6, 12, 22, 30, 31]. The final decisions remain up to neurosurgery and also pediatric neurosurgery which is still a considerable challenge nowadays [1, 6, 11, 12, 20, 24, 30, 31].

4 Differential Diagnosis and Natural Evolution

ACs need to be differentiated from various others central nervous system compartmental enlargements [2, 5, 12, 13, 17–19, 22] (Table 7).

In the majority of the cases, we have involution and disappearance through the passing of time, especially in small cysts [5–9, 13, 20–22, 28, 29]. According to various authors, there may be a possible rupture of the internal membranes that can facilitate this occurrence [5–13, 20–23]. Sometimes, we do not have either symptoms or signs, but in other situations, both of them are present [5, 13, 22–25]. In cases with seizures, increased intracranial pressure, neurological deficits, hemorrhages (intracystic or subdural or both), and hydrocephalus, we may have to act immediately [2, 5, 13, 14, 22, 27–30].

Table 7 Differential diagnosis of ACs

• Colloid cysts
• Various parasitic cystic infections
• Cystic metastases
• Porencephalic cysts
• Agenesis of the corpus callosum
• Various neurodevelopment disorders
• Dandy-Walker syndrome

Imaging and neuroimaging both in adults and in the pediatric population with the CT scan (Figs. 3 and 4) and MRI scan are really useful for the clinical neurosurgeon and pediatric neurosurgeon. Also, other imaging techniques have been proposed such as [5, 13–17, 22–26] diffusion tensor imaging (DTI), which is common in recent reports, and sometimes also carotid angiography in complex cases.

Optimal and accurate imaging remains essential in order to validate the particular situations of a combination of hydrocephalus and ACs and to help in order to plan an appropriate treatment [5–8, 13, 22–26].

The new upcoming neuroimaging techniques allow for the recognition of small, asymptomatic, incidental posterior fossa ACs in order to prevent enlargement at an early stage and hydrocephalus with progression through the advancement of age and consequent symptom appearance [9–12, 22–26].

When there is hydrocephalus, these cysts may be decompressed successfully by shunting or fenestration or neuroendoscopic techniques [5, 13–16, 26–29].

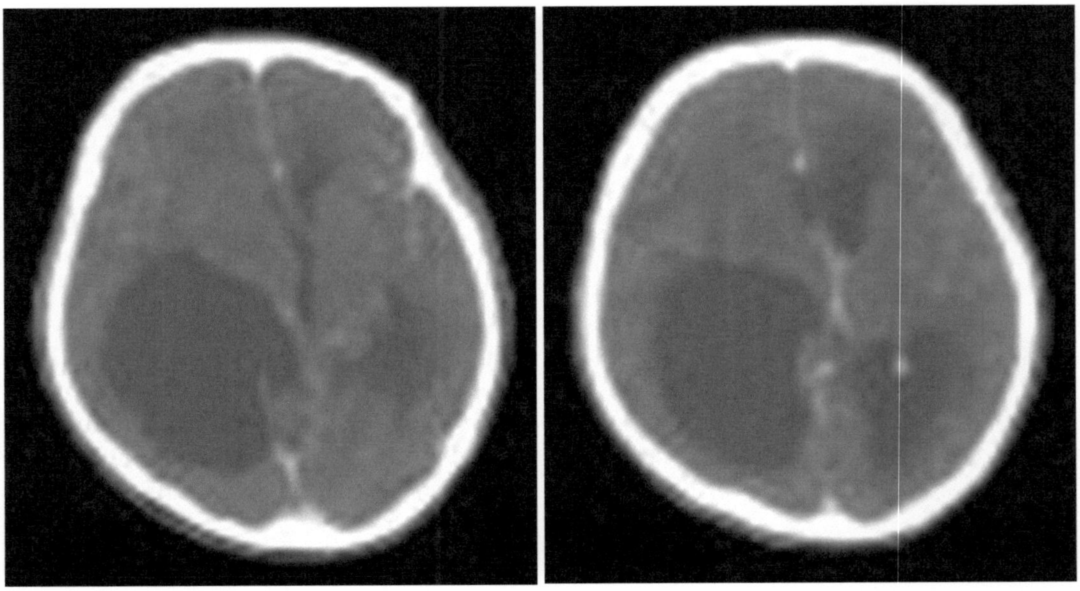

Figs. 3 and 4 Large middle fossa AC with hydrocephalus in an 80-year-old woman

Table 8 Galassi classification system

Type I Small cysts	Type II Middle cysts	Type III Large cysts
• Mainly spindle-shaped located into the anterior part of the middle cranial fossa • Free communication with subarachnoid space	• Superior extent along the Sylvian fissure located into the temporal lobe • Slow communication with subarachnoid space	• Fills the hole middle cranial fossa located into temporal, frontal and parietal lobes • Little communication with subarachnoid space

Various radiology models have been proposed [5, 13, 17–19, 25, 26]. For the middle fossa ACs, the Galassi classification system (small cysts, middle cysts, large cysts) is widely used with optimal results [5, 13, 20, 21, 27–29] (Table 8).

Accurate neuroimaging in combination with the clinical examination can lead to optimal decision-making in order to choose the most appropriable surgical approach which are classical techniques such as shunting and newer upcoming techniques such as neuroendoscopy, etc. [16–18, 28–32].

In infants with midline posterior fossa ACs, obstructive hydrocephalus is a very frequent associated phenomenon together with the appearance of intracranial hypertension due to size-related obstruction of the aqueduct [6–9, 17, 18, 30–32]. This situation leads to head enlargement without other lateralizing signs [10–12, 17–21]. In adults, this association may remain occult for a long time period and lead to normal pressure hydrocephalus (NPH) [22–26].

In the appearance of NPH, an important contribution was also the provocation by various factors such as defective CSF absorption, a long duration of signs, an episodic course of symptoms, and postural influences [15–18, 26–29].

5 Surgical Management

Many operative techniques have been proposed [5–8, 19–22, 29] (Table 9). The location of ACs determines both the surgical approach and also the final clinical outcome [5–7, 13, 16–20].

The final outcome and the degree of relief (partial or complete) of the symptoms due to the AC appearance, after surgical intervention for treating them, both in adult and pediatric patients, are still a controversial subject in the literature [2, 5, 11, 12]. This situation still remains controversial or even more so in the case of the combination of these two entities, hydrocephalus and ACs [3, 5, 13–15].

In middle fossa ACs and hydrocephalus, shunting, microsurgery and neuroendoscopy are effective surgical options [5, 13, 18, 21–23]. In cases with a suprasellar location, we have a close relation to the ventricular system (third ventricle) and associated hydrocephalus [5, 13, 22–26]. Neuroendoscopic fenestration seems to be the best choice in these situations [1, 2, 5, 13, 24, 25, 30].

Suprasellar ACs are basal midline formations, and they present a rare entity for surgically treatable hydrocephalus and other neurological deficits [5, 13, 22, 23, 31, 32].

The differential diagnosis for cystic midline neoplasms depends on various factors such as [5, 13, 22–29] (Table 10). The differential diagnosis for other third ventricular enlargements due to obstructive hydrocephalus and from third ventricular ependymal cysts can be made through specific criteria [5, 13, 22–28] (Table 11).

The interhemispheric ACs present as follows [3–7, 11–13, 26]: (a) midline, mainly without agenesis of the corpus callosum, and (b) parasagittal, associated with agenesis of the corpus callosum. Both types do not present with hydrocephalus [4–7, 11–13, 16, 27]. The quadri-

Table 9 Types of surgical management

- Microsurgery
- Shunts
- Various neuroendoscopic techniques
- Various stereotactic techniques

Table 10 Differential diagnosis between ACs and cystic midline neoplasms

- Density
- Homogeneity
- Lack of fat
- Lack of calcification
- Absence of contrast enhancement

geminal ACs are associated with hydrocephalus when symptomatic [6–13, 16, 17, 28]. They are divided into three types [8–11, 29, 30] (Table 12). Intraventricular or intracisternal ACs are located deep inside the brain, near or inside the ventricular system, and are difficult to treat [11–13, 25–29]. The surgical approach can provoke various complications [11, 16–18, 22, 25–29] (Table 13).

Other disadvantages regarding the appropriate management are reported by various authors [10, 19, 22, 23, 27–29]. These are long durations of surgery, long and complex anesthesia procedures, and high morbidity [6–11, 13, 22, 27–29]. All these risks lead more neurosurgeons and pediatric neurosurgeons toward minimally invasive approaches [10–14, 22, 27–29]. The surgical results, worldwide, confirm the gained surgical experience through the passing of the years [2–6, 13–15, 19, 21].

The classical shunting seems to have efficacy and safety but can sometimes demonstrate the classic problems, which are the same as those encountered by the standard hydrocephalus shunting options (infection, reoperation after shunt malfunction over the years, etc.) [2, 13–17, 19, 20].

Microsurgery, which requires appropriate technical support and also experience in this field, remains a very good option [6–10, 17, 18, 21]. The most appropriate choice is still a controversial topic, but it seems that minimally invasive techniques will be the only choice in the near future, especially in young age patients [1–9, 20–24].

Table 11 Differential diagnosis criteria between ACs and third ventricular ependymal cysts

- Basal cisternal expansion
- Instinctive (?) mass effect
- Displacement at the foramen of Monro

Table 12 Types of quadrigeminal ACs

Type I	Type II	Type III
Supratentorial and infratentorial extension	Infratentorial extension (supracerebellar or supraretrocerebellar)	Large extension to the temporal bone

Table 13 Complications of surgical approaches to intraventricular AC

• Seizures
• Various neuroparesis
• Cranial nerve injuries
• Subdural hematomas
• CSF leak
• Infections
• Death

6 Conclusions

Based on results of our review, it is concluded that:

1. The appropriate resolution, management, and treatment of ACs are still controversial.
2. Additional problems are resulting from the combination of hydrocephalus associated with ACs.
3. Hydrocephalus is generally observed in cases with midline and posterior fossa ACs.
4. Ventriculomegaly or hydrocephalus is encountered in many cases with interhemispheric lesions, but it is rarely seen in cases with middle fossa lesions.
5. Patients' age, location, and size of the ACs, macrocephaly, and altered CSF dynamics are important factors in the development of hydrocephalus in cases with AC.
6. Neuroendoscopic techniques have become, over the years, a very good treatment option as also are cystoperitoneal shunting and open fenestration with optimal results.
7. A multidisciplinary approach and collaboration with other medical disciplines lead to better patient management and optimal clinical results.

References

1. Abbott R. The endoscopic management of arachnoidal cysts. Neurosurg Clin N Am. 2004;15(1):9–17.
2. Akgun B, Ozturk S, Hergunsel OB, Erol FS, Demir F. Endoscopic third ventriculostomy for obstructive hydrocephalus and ventriculocystostomy for intraventricular arachnoid cysts. Acta Med. 2021;64:29–35.

3. Akutagawa K, Tamura G, Tsurubuchi T, Ishikawa E, Matsumura A, Inagaki T. Quadrigeminal arachnoid cyst with perinatal encephalocele. Childs Nerv Syst. 2020;36(7):1393–7.
4. Ali ZS, Lang S-S, Bakar D, Storm PB, Stein SC. Pediatric intracranial arachnoid cysts: comparative effectiveness of surgical treatment options. Childs Nerv Syst. 2014;30(3):461–9.
5. Benton JA, Dominguez J, Ng C, et al. Acute communicating hydrocephalus after intracranial arachnoid cyst decompression: a report of two cases. Surg Neurol Int. 2021;12:533.
6. Caldarelli M, Di Rocco C. Surgical options in the treatment of interhemispheric arachnoid cysts. Surg Neurol. 1996;46(3):212–21.
7. Caldarelli M, Novegno F, Di Rocco C. A late complication of CSF shunting: acquired Chiari I malformation. Childs Nerv Syst. 2009;25(4):443–52.
8. Choi JY, Cha SH, Cho WH, Ko JK. Communicating hydrocephalus accompanied by arachnoid cyst in aneurismal subarachnoid hemorrhage. J Cerebrovasc Endovasc Neurosurg. 2013;15(4):311–5.
9. Cincu R, Agrawal A, Eiras J. Intracranial arachnoid cysts: current concepts and treatment alternatives. Clin Neurol Neurosurg. 2007;109(10):837–43.
10. Di Rocco C. Sylvian fissure arachnoid cysts: we do operate on them but should it be done? Childs Nerv Syst. 2010;26(2):173–5.
11. Di Rocco C, Caldarelli M. Supratentorial interhemispheric and pineal region cysts. In: Raimondi AJ, Choux M, Di Rocco C, editors. Intracranial cyst lesions. Principles of pediatric neurosurgery. New York: Springer; 1993. p. 153–68.
12. Dishman G, Fliss DM, Benjamin S, Margalit N, Gil Z, Derowe A, Constantini S, Beni-Adani L. Multidisciplinary surgical approach for cerebrospinal fluid leak in children with complex head trauma. Childs Nerv Syst. 2009;25(8):915–23.
13. El-Ghandour NM. Endoscopic treatment of quadrigeminal arachnoid cysts in children. J Neurosurg Pediatr. 2013;12:521–8.
14. Erşahin Y, Kesikçi H. Endoscopic management of quadrigeminal arachnoid cysts. Childs Nerv Syst. 2009;25:569–76.
15. Feletti A, Alicandri-Ciufelli M, Pavesi G. Transaqueductal trans-magendie fenestration of arachnoid cyst in the posterior fossa. Acta Neurochir. 2016;158(4):655–62.
16. Fujio S, Bunyamin J, Hirano H, Oyoshi T, Sadamura Y, Bohara M, Arita K. A novel bilateral approach for suprasellar arachnoid cysts: a case report. Pediatr Neurosurg. 2016;51(1):30–4.
17. García-Conde M, Martín-Viota L. Quistes aracnoideos: embriología y anatomía patológica. Neurocirugia. 2015;26(3):137–42.
18. Gui S, Bai J, Wang X, Zong X, Li C, Cao L, Zhang Y. Assessment of endoscopic treatment for quadrigeminal cistern arachnoid cysts: a 7-year experience with 28 cases. Childs Nerv Syst. 2016;32(4):647–54.
19. Hinojosa J, Esparza J, Muñoz MJ, Valencia J. Tratamiento endoscópico de los quistes aracnoideos supraselares. Neurocirugia. 2001;12(6):482–8.
20. Law M. Neurological complications. Cancer Imaging. 2009;9 Spec No A(Special issue A):S71–4.
21. López R, Bienvenido ÁMG, Moroño SI. Quistes aracnoideos del sistema nervioso central. Algoritmos y recomendaciones generales de manejo. Neurocirugia. 2016;27(2):67–74.
22. Martínez-Lage JF, Pérez-Espejo MA, Almagro M-J, López-Guerrero AL. Hydrocephalus and arachnoid cysts. Childs Nerv Syst. 2011;27(10):1643–52.
23. Mustansir F, Bashir S, Darbar A. Management of arachnoid cysts: a comprehensive review. Cureus. 2018;10(4):e2458.
24. Özek MM, Urgun K. Neuroendoscopic management of suprasellar arachnoid cysts. World Neurosurg. 2013;79(2):S19.e13–8.
25. Reganchary SS, Watanabe I. Ultrastructure and pathogenesis of intracranial arachnoid cysts. J Neuropathol Exp Neurol. 1981;40:61–83.
26. Ruge JR, Johnson RF, Bauer J. Burr hole neuroendoscopic fenestration of quadrigeminal cistern arachnoid cyst: technical case report. Neurosurgery. 1996;38(4):830–7.
27. Sengul G, Tuzun Y, Cakir M, Duman S, Colak A, Kadioglu HH, Aydin IH. Neuroendoscopic approach to quadrigeminal cistern arachnoid cysts. Eurasian J Med. 2012;44:18–21.
28. Shou X, Zhao Y, Li S, Wang Y. Ventriculoscopic surgery for arachnoid cysts in the lateral ventricle: a comparative study of 21 consecutive cases. Int J Clin Exp Med. 2015;8(11):20787–95.
29. Spacca B, Kandasamy J, Mallucci CL, Genitori L. Endoscopic treatment of middle fossa arachnoid cysts: a series of 40 patients treated endoscopically in two centres. Childs Nerv Syst. 2010;26(2):163–72.
30. Spennato P, Ruggiero C, Aliberti F, Buonocore MC, Trischitta V, Cinalli G. Interhemispheric and quadrigeminal cysts. World Neurosurg. 2013;79(2):S20.e1–7.
31. Topsakal C, Kaplan M, Erol F, Cetin H, Ozercan I. Unusual arachnoid cyst of the quadrigeminal cistern in an adult presenting with apneic spells and normal pressure hydrocephalus—case report. Neurol Med Chir (Tokyo). 2002;42(1):44–50.
32. Zanini MA, Rondinelli G, Fernandes AY. Endoscopic supracerebellar infratentorial parapineal approach for third ventricular colloid cyst in a patient with quadrigeminal cistern arachnoid cyst. Case report. Clin Neurol Neurosurg. 2013;115:751–5.

Epilepsy and Arachnoid Cysts

Amal Satte

1 Introduction

With the development of intracranial imaging techniques, their widespread availability, and affordability, incidental arachnoid cysts (ACs) are being increasingly discovered. Only a few patients are considered to be symptomatic. Epilepsy is the second most frequent symptom associated with AC after headache. However, the relationship between ACs and seizures is controversial. Moreover, few studies report specifically on the type of seizures or syndrome, electroencephalographic data, and the correlation between the seizure focus and the localization of the cyst. From a practical standpoint, there is currently no consensus regarding the diagnostic workup, and treatment modalities are still debated. Large studies evaluating the relationship between AC and epilepsy; clinical, electroencephalographic, and imaging correlations; as well as treatment modalities and outcomes are of utmost importance to reach standardized consensus and optimize the management.

2 Epidemiology

The overall incidence of ACs in the general population remains difficult to estimate because of their minimal or absent symptomatic nature. Epilepsy is the second most frequent associated symptom after headache in up to one-third of patients with AC [37]. The incidence of the association of epilepsy with AC has been reported to be between 3.6% and 40.9% [50]. However, the true prevalence and incidence can't be determined because radiodiagnostic tools are not always available in all countries. On the other hand, even when available, imaging is not systematically performed in all epileptic syndromes. For instance, in absence epilepsy, it has been traditionally known that there are no radiological abnormalities; however, Ventura found two cases of ACs among a cohort of 22 patients with absence epilepsy [47].

The frequency of seizures is reported to be greater in children compared to adults with AC [8]. In a survey, Wester studied the literature, including a total of 1526 patients from published patients' series of at least 20 cases. He found that there were either slight differences or no differences between the prevalence in adults and children with AC [50].

A. Satte (✉)
Department of Neurophysiology, Mohamed V Teaching Military Hospital, Mohamed V University in Rabat, Rabat, Morocco

M. Turgut et al. (eds.), *Arachnoid Cysts*, https://doi.org/10.1007/978-3-031-22701-1_20

3 Pathophysiology

The relationship between epilepsy and ACs remains a matter of debate. Some authors highlight the lack of an association between seizures and ACs. In a study on 1157 adults, Del Brutto et al. attempted to assess the prevalence of supratentorial AC and whether they were associated with seizures. They found no significant difference in the prevalence of seizures between the group of patients with ACs (4%) and the group without ACs (2.7%) ($p = 0.508$) [7]. Similar conclusions were achieved by Rabiei et al. in a study of 1235 individuals that showed no differences in the frequency of seizures between AC cases and controls [39].

Other authors suggest a possible relationship between ACs and epilepsy [35]. Koch and colleagues reviewed the world's medical literature dealing with surgically treated ACs. Their study included 76 patients, aged from 2 months to 70 years. They found that seizure outcome correlated directly with postoperative AC size reduction [23]. This finding was consistent with the results of the Helland et al.'s study in a pediatric population [16]. Other authors reported cases of dramatic improvement of refractory epilepsies after AC surgery [13, 41]. The improvement of epileptic seizures after surgical treatment could be an argument in favor of a causal or at least an aggravating relationship. However, the exact mechanisms of epileptogenesis remain unknown. Compression on the adjacent cortex can be suspected. However, Okada found that the volume of ACs in nonepileptic patients was significantly larger than that in epileptic patients [36]. Hajek suggested an increased level of excitatory amino acids in the cystic fluid found in two patients as a possible mechanism of epileptogenesis [15]. But this wasn't confirmed in Wieser's study that included 22 patients and concluded that there was a lack of evidence for a close correlation between excitatory amino acids in cyst fluid and epilepsy [51]. Another proposed mechanism is cerebral blood perfusion of the surrounding brain cortex where studies using single-photon emission computed tomography (SPECT) in patients with epilepsy showed hypoperfusion around ACs that may form an epileptogenic focus [36, 43]. Finally, ACs can be associated with brain parenchymal lesions that are known to cause seizures such as neurofibromatosis, polymicrogyria, Sturge-Weber, cortical dysplasia, heterotopia, and hippocampal sclerosis [3, 4, 9, 11, 21, 29]. Nikolic suggests that "More likely, focal epilepsy and AC share a common etiological (possibly genetic) ancestor but represent distant and distinct entities" [35].

4 Electroclinical and Imaging Features

Most of the studies don't indicate the type of seizure or epileptic syndrome that is present, and few of them used video EEG to better localize the seizure focus. Different types of seizures have been reported in association with ACs. Most of seizures were focal: frontal, temporal, or occipital [2, 12, 13, 20, 35, 41, 53]. Generalized seizures have also been reported [47, 52]. Based on the type of seizures and EEG abnormalities, studies have reported various epileptic syndromes: absence epilepsy, juvenile myoclonic epilepsy, and other idiopathic generalized epilepsies. In a case report, Ventura suggests a possible link between absence epilepsy and ACs based on the theory of the role of a cortical focus in primary generalized epilepsies [32, 47, 52]. Other studies reported associations to benign rolandic epilepsy, Panayiotopoulos syndrome, epileptic encephalopathy, and epilepsia partialis continua [34, 46, 47, 52, 53].

Based on MRI or CT, the majority of ACs associated with epilepsy were located within the middle cranial fossa. Other less commonly reported locations included the interhemispheric fissure, cerebral convexity, and even the posterior fossa, which according to the authors was explained by the role of the cerebellum as a modulator on seizure activity [8, 13, 40, 50].

Studies have tried to investigate the correlation between electroclinical features of epilepsies and AC locations. Arroyo reported that among 12 epileptic patients with temporal AC, only three had temporal seizures, and among four cases with frontal cysts, only one had frontal seizures ipsilateral to the cyst. There was also a patient with a cerebellopontine angle cyst who presented with frontal seizures. He concluded that AC locations do not necessarily reflect the seizure focus [2]. Yalcin studied a series of 20 patients with AC and epilepsy. Eight patients had idiopathic focal or generalized epilepsy. Epilepsy couldn't be classified in two cases, and ten had epilepsy with focal seizures. He found agreement between electroclinical and cyst locations in only one patient. Thus, he suggested that ACs may not be related to specific seizure type and EEG focus [52]. More recently, Martínez came to similar conclusions. In his study from 1990 to 2019, 25 patients with epilepsy and at least one AC were included. Congruence between electroclinical features and cyst location was found in only two patients [30]. Yet, the agreement between clinical, electroencephalographic, and imaging features is crucial when surgical treatment is considered.

5 Diagnostic Workup

The current data in the literature do not allow for the establishment of a clear consensus for treatment. The studies available include few or isolated cases, and most of them lack clinical and electroencephalographic details. From a practical standpoint, case series do not support a correlation between radiological and clinical data. On the other hand, the reported cases of dramatic improvement after cyst surgery cannot be ignored.

When AC and epilepsy are associated, the first step should be to classify as accurately as possible the type of epilepsy according to the ILAE classifications [38, 42]. This should take into account adequate semiology description, neurological and neuropsychological examination, electroencephalography, imaging, and genetic or metabolic testings if needed [10, 38, 42]. The patients may be then be classified into three groups:

1. Patients with syndromes that are typically not associated with lesions such as idiopathic generalized epilepsies and self-limited focal epilepsies. The AC in these cases is more likely to be incidental. This situation is illustrated by the first case: a patient with juvenile myoclonic epilepsy where the MRI shows a right temporal AC (Fig. 1a, b).
2. Patients with AC and structural abnormalities that are known to be epileptogenic. Abnormalities can be acquired, such as stroke and trauma, or genetic, such as malformations of cortical development and tuberous sclerosis complex. In these cases, structural abnormalities might more likely cause seizures than AC [2]. Yet, electroclinical and imaging correlation should be checked to confirm which of the AC or cortical abnormality causes the seizures. Video EEG plays an important role, especially if a seizure is recorded. If EEG or video EEG is inconclusive, positron emission tomography (PET) or single-photon emission computed tomography (SPECT) can be performed to detect the epileptogenic focus [8]. A case reported by Martinez-Luna illustrates this situation: a 6-year-old child with a temporal AC and an ipsilateral frontal dysembryoplastic neuroepithelial tumor was revealed by refractory focal seizures. Seizure semiology was analyzed and concluded to have a frontotemporal pattern. Then an EEG was performed and showed frontotemporal abnormalities. Neuropsychological assessment found frontal region alterations. Thus, the frontal lesion was operated on, and the patient became seizure-free without medication [27]. The situation can be more complex when the two lesions are adjacent as in case 2 (Fig. 2) which shows an AC adjacent

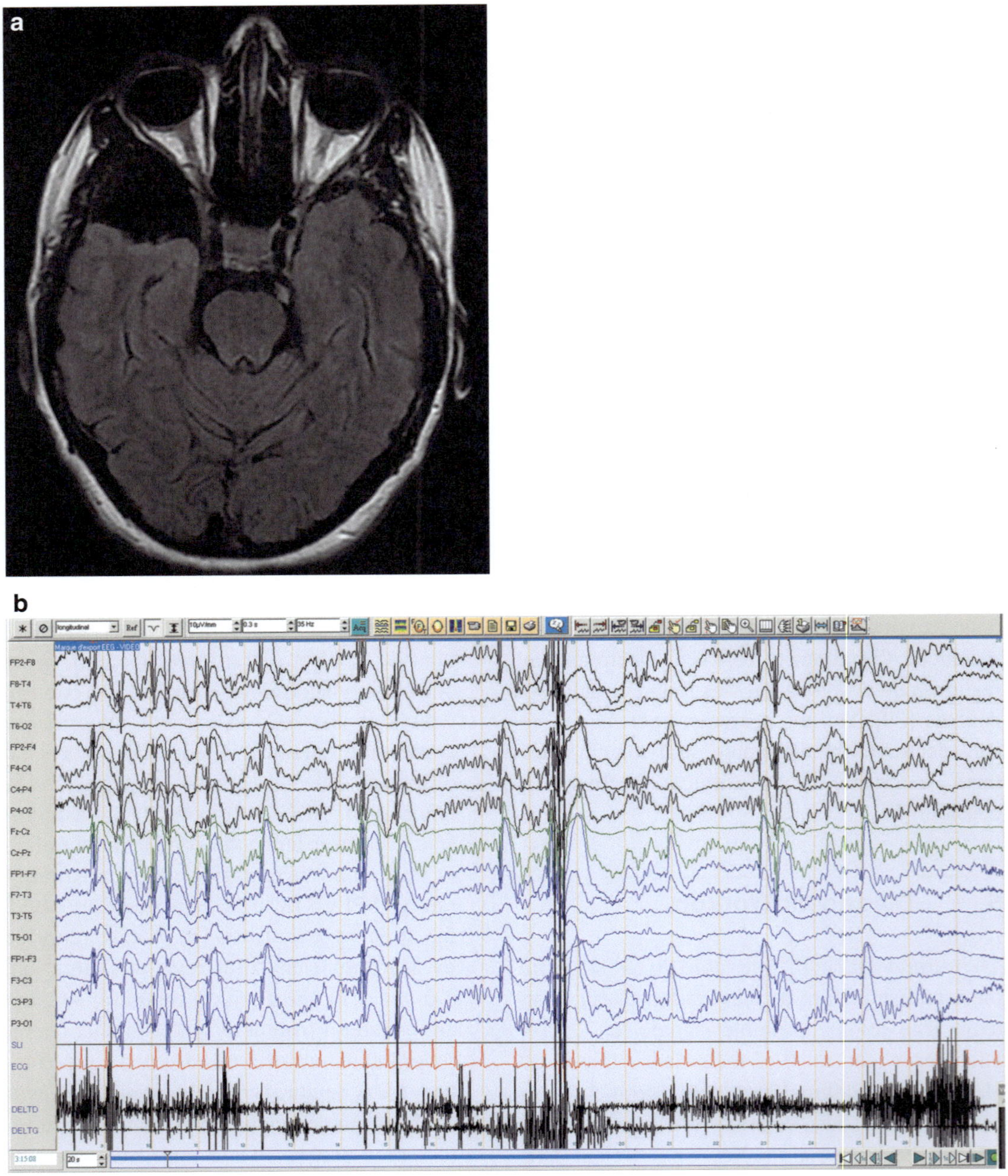

Fig. 1 (**a** and **b**) Case 1—a 7-year-old boy with no medical history presented with a generalized tonic-clonic seizure while falling asleep. Neurological examination was unremarkable. Basic neuropsychological assessment was normal. (**a**) T2-weighted FLAIR axial MRI shows a right temporal AC. (Courtesy of Dr. Rachida Saouab). (**b**) EEG shows a normal background with rapid generalized polyspike and wave associated with myoclonia

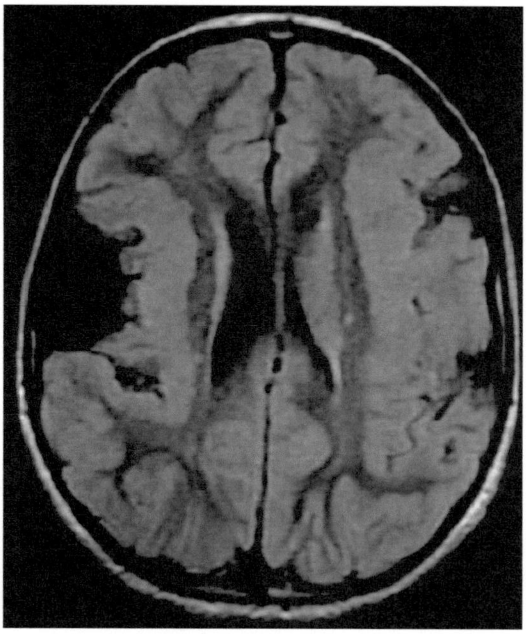

Fig. 2 Case 2—a 6-year-old boy presents with focal clonic seizures of the right limbs. T2-weighted FLAIR axial MRI showing left insular polymicrogyria with adjacent AC. (Courtesy of Dr. Meriem Edderai)

to polymicrogyria of the insular cortex. Polymicrogyria is known to cause seizures more frequently than ACs [28].

3. Patients with ACs with neither associated brain lesions on MRI nor criteria for nonlesional epileptic syndrome. As for the second group, the correlation between clinical features, EEG, and anatomy is important. Video EEG, PET, or SPECT may help better localize the focus. If inconclusive, intracranial EEG recording may be performed. When the assessment finds a focus far from the AC, then the cyst is likely incidental, as in case 3 (Fig. 3a, b). However, when the focus is located near the cyst, a structural abnormality in the surrounding cortex cannot be ruled out. Intraoperative corticography or intracranial EEG recording may be required. However, the placement of subdural electrode grids is challenging when the surface is not convex. Kushien and Frim reported two cases on whom they placed subdural grids in the concave cyst cavity and held them in place with rolled gelatin foam padding. This allowed for good electrode contact and thus focused localization. The padding and electrode grids were removed before resecting the seizure focus [25]. Hoyt used fibrin sealant to fix the grids on the concave cortical surface within a decompressed AC. There was no loss of signal from any of the grid electrodes which allowed for accurate focus localization. Electrodes were easily removed without underlying brain injury, before resection of the frontal pole sparing the inferior frontal gyrus. The patient became seizure-free without medication [18]. Based on the available literature data, we summarize the "ideal" diagnostic workup in an algorithm (Fig. 4). The main limit of this approach is the availability of the different tools, mainly, PET, SPECT, intracranial EEG, and electrocorticography.

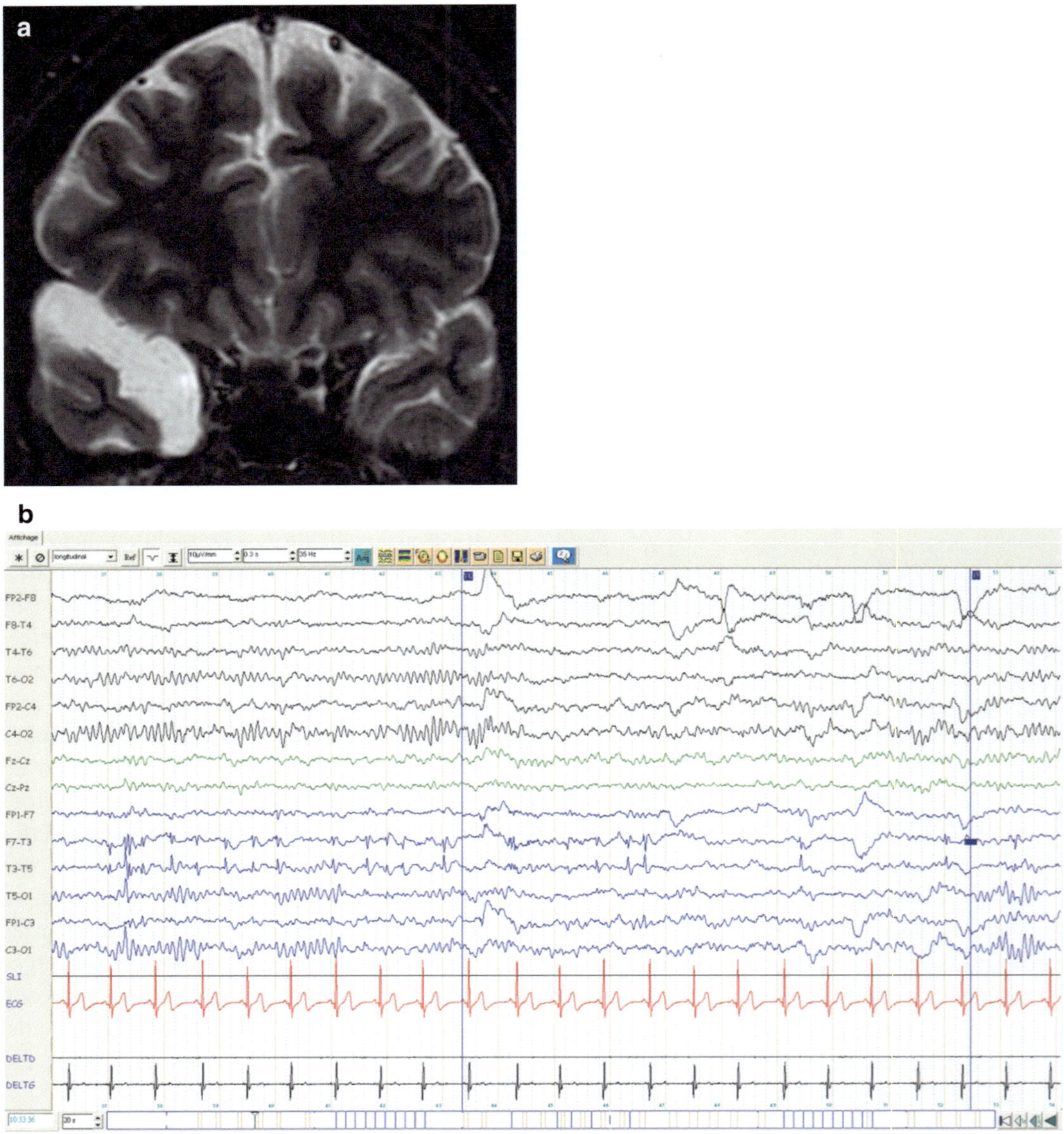

Fig. 3 (**a** and **b**) Case 3—a 12-year-old girl with focal temporal seizures, abnormal epigastric sensations followed by clonic movements of the right limbs and then bilateral tonic-clonic movements. MRI shows a right temporal AC (**a**), while clinical semiology and EEG (**b**) are consistent with a left temporal focus. (Courtesy of Dr. Jamal Fenni)

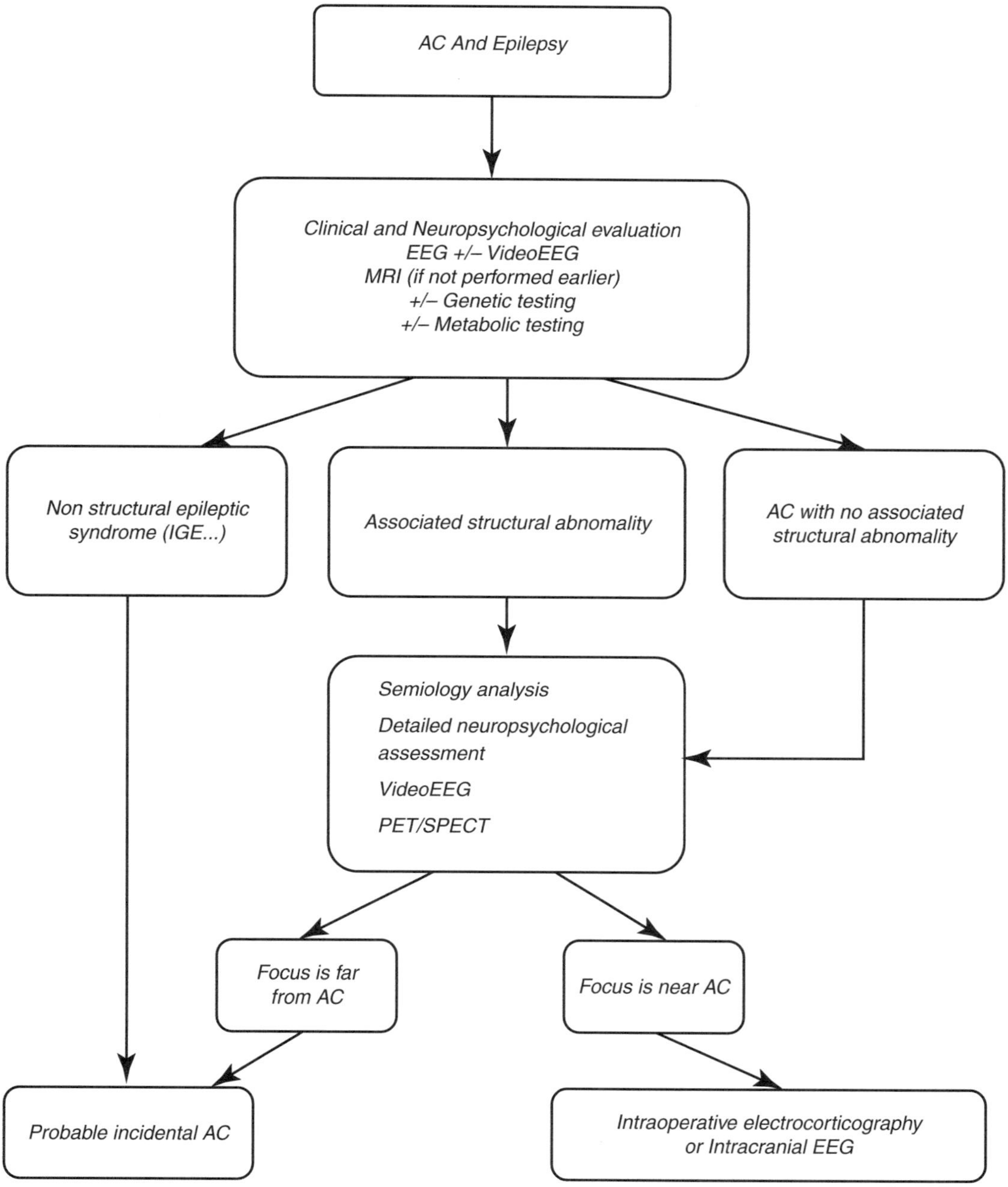

Fig. 4 Algorithm summarizing the proposed diagnosis workup for AC associated with epilepsy (*ACs* arachnoid cyst, *EEG* elecroencephalography, *video EEG* video electroencephalography, *MRI* magnetic resonance imaging, *IGE* idiopathic generalized epilepsy, *PET* positron emission tomography, *SPECT* single-photon emission computed tomography)

6 Management of the Association of Arachnoid Cyst with Epilepsy

There is no consensus regarding the treatment choices in cases of AC with associated epilepsy [33, 50]. In a survey, including 45 pediatric neurosurgery centers, one-fourth of the participants considered seizures as a primary indication for surgery [45].

As in almost all epilepsies, antiseizure medication should be attempted. The choice of the drug depends on the type of seizure, the epileptic syndrome, and the patient's background [22], in addition to the availability, affordability, and tolerability of antiseizure medications.

Surgical treatment may be considered in patients with refractory seizures when presurgical evaluation reveals a strong correlation between cyst localization and the clinic-encephalographic features [33, 48]. There are no recommendations regarding the type of surgery to choose when AC is associated with epilepsy [33]. Surgical technique is usually chosen based on cyst localization rather than its association or not to seizures [31]. According to Wang, microsurgical craniotomy is the technique of choice in the case of cyst-related epilepsy [48]. Holst and colleagues highlight that microsurgical decompression through craniotomy allowed the best results in their study [17]. According to Murthy, the favorable outcome in both studies may be explained by the associated surgical resection that was guided by intraoperative electrocorticography [33]. The approach we propose in the diagnostic workup would be useful to assess the extent of surgical resection.

Regarding the effect of surgery, few studies report specifically on the results of epilepsy. On the other hand, as Wester highlighted, terms such as "improved" and "good outcome" used remain vague as it is impossible to find out whether patients were seizure-free or had a reduction of seizure frequency and whether the medication was maintained, reduced, or discontinued after surgery [50]. Some studies failed to demonstrate a difference in outcome between operated and non-operated patients [14, 24, 30, 49]. Other studies report favorable outcome on seizure control [5, 6, 17, 44, 48]. Children particularly may experience marked improvement after surgery [19, 49, 50]. The improvement was correlated to cyst reduction in size and, probably as in all lesional epilepsy, to the correlation between clinic-electroencephalographic features with the localization [1, 24, 33]. This highlights once again the utmost importance of the presurgical evaluation. Finally, patients with no history of epilepsy may experience seizures in the immediate postoperative phase and even in the long term that might be associated with the increase in the perfusion of the hypoperfused cortex [26, 50]. Thus, when considering a surgical treatment in patients without epilepsy, the risk-benefit balance should be adequately assessed.

7 Conclusion

Managing AC associated with epilepsy should be performed by a multidisciplinary team including not only neurosurgeons but also neurologists, neuropediatricians, neuropsychologists, neurophysiologists, neuroradiologists, and anesthesiologists. Thorough multimodality evaluation is needed before deciding whether the patient requires medical treatment, surgical treatment, or both. When surgery is considered, an accurate presurgical evaluation is necessary to confirm the clinico-electroencephalography and imaging correlation which will guide the choice of the correct technique and weigh its risks and benefits. There is an urgent need for prospective multicentric studies pooling compiled data from multiple institutions to obtain a large sample size that would allow the study of the relationship of AC to epilepsy, treatment indications, the most appropriate surgical technique when surgery is considered, and the short- and long-term outcome.

References

1. Armon C, Radtke RA, Friedman AH, Dawson DV. Predictors of outcome of epilepsy surgery: multivariate analysis with validation. Epilepsia. 1996;37(9):814–21. https://doi.org/10.1111/j.1528-1157.1996.tb00033.x.
2. Arroyo S, Santamaria J. What is the relationship between arachnoid cysts and seizure foci? Epilepsia. 1997;38(10):1098–102. https://doi.org/10.1111/j.1528-1157.1997.tb01199.x.
3. Blauen A, Stutterd CA, Stouffs K, Dumitriu D, Deggouj N, et al. Chudley-McCullough syndrome: a recognizable clinical entity characterized by deafness and typical brain malformations. J Child Neurol. 2021;36(2):152–8. https://doi.org/10.1177/0883073820960314.
4. Boronat S, Barber I. Less common manifestations in TSC. Am J Med Genet C Semin Med Genet. 2018;178(3):348–54. https://doi.org/10.1002/ajmg.c.31648.
5. Couvreur T, Hallaert G, Van Der Heggen T, Baert E, Dewaele F, et al. Endoscopic treatment of temporal arachnoid cysts in 34 patients. World Neurosurg. 2015;84(3):734–40. https://doi.org/10.1016/j.wneu.2015.04.053.
6. D'Angelo V, Gorgoglione L, Catapano G. Treatment of symptomatic intracranial arachnoid cysts by stereotactic cyst-ventricular shunting. Stereotact Funct Neurosurg. 1999;72(1):62–9. https://doi.org/10.1159/000029672.
7. Del Brutto OH, Mera RM, Kiernan J, Castle P, Zambrano M, Sedler MJ. Supratentorial arachnoid cysts and seizures/epilepsy: a population study in community dwellers aged ≥20 years. Epilepsia. 2019;60(8):e83–7. https://doi.org/10.1111/epi.16287.
8. Di Rocco C, Tamburrini G. Arachnoid cysts. In: Shorvon SD, Andermann F, Guerrini R, editors. The causes of epilepsy: common and uncommon causes in adults and children. Cambridge: Cambridge University Press; 2019. p. 341–5. https://doi.org/10.1017/CBO9780511921001.053.
9. Ergün R, Ökten Aİ, Gezercan Y, Gezici AR. Sturge-Weber syndrome accompanied with multiple congenital intracranial lesions. Acta Neurochir. 2007;149(8):829–30. https://doi.org/10.1007/s00701-007-1224-z.
10. Fisher RS, Cross JH, French JA, Higurashi N, Hirsch E, et al. Operational classification of seizure types by the International League Against Epilepsy: position paper of the ILAE Commission for Classification and Terminology. Epilepsia. 2017;58(4):522–30. https://doi.org/10.1111/epi.13670.
11. Fuchs F, Moutard ML, Blin G, Sonigo P, Mandelbrot L. Prenatal and postnatal follow-up of a fetal interhemispheric arachnoid cyst with partial corpus callosum agenesis, asymmetric ventriculomegaly and localized polymicrogyria. Fetal Diagn Ther. 2008;24(4):385–8. https://doi.org/10.1159/000165511.
12. Furune S, Negoro T, Maehara M, Nomura K, Miura K, et al. Magnetic resonance imaging in complex partial seizures. Psychiatry Clin Neurosci. 1989;43(3):361–7. https://doi.org/10.1111/j.1440-1819.1989.tb02927.x.
13. Gan YC, Connolly MBC, Steinbok P. Epilepsy associated with a cerebellar arachnoid cyst: seizure control following fenestration of the cyst. Childs Nerv Syst. 2008;24(1):125–34. https://doi.org/10.1007/s00381-007-0439-x.
14. Gosalakkal JA. Intracranial arachnoid cysts in children: a review of pathogenesis, clinical features, and management. Pediatr Neurol. 2002;26(2):93–8. https://doi.org/10.1016/s0887-8994(01)00329-0.
15. Hajek M, Do KQ, Duc C, Boesiger P, Wieser HG. Increased excitatory amino acid levels in brain cysts of epileptic patients. Epilepsy Res. 1997;28(3):245–54. https://doi.org/10.1016/s0920-1211(97)00050-8.
16. Helland CA, Wester K. A population-based study of intracranial arachnoid cysts: clinical and neuroimaging outcomes following surgical cyst decompression in children. J Neurosurg Pediatr. 2006;105(5):385–90. https://doi.org/10.3171/ped.2006.105.5.385.
17. Holst AV, Danielsen PL, Juhler M. Treatment options for intracranial arachnoid cysts: a retrospective study of 69 patients. Acta Neurochir Suppl. 2012;114:267–70. https://doi.org/10.1007/978-3-7091-0956-4_52.
18. Hoyt AT, LaViolette PS, Lew SM. Fibrin sealant to prevent subdural electrode migration during intracranial electroencephalographic monitoring in a patient with a large arachnoid cyst. J Neurosurg Pediatr. 2014;14(1):115–9. https://doi.org/10.3171/2014.3.PEDS13489.
19. Huang YH, Yang TM, Lin YJ, Tsai NW, Lin WC, et al. Risk factors and outcome of seizures after chronic subdural hematoma. Neurocrit Care. 2011;14(2):253–9. https://doi.org/10.1007/s12028-011-9509-8.
20. Jiménez-Genchi A, Díaz-Galviz JL, García-Reyna JC, Avila-Ordoñez MU. Coexistence of epileptic nocturnal wanderings and an arachnoid cyst. J Clin Sleep Med. 2007;3(4):399–401.
21. Kawamura T, Morioka T, Nishio S, Fukui K, Yamasaki R, Matsuo M. Temporal lobe epilepsy associated with hippocampal sclerosis and a contralateral middle fossa arachnoid cyst. Seizure. 2002;11(1):60–2. https://doi.org/10.1053/seiz.2001.0564.
22. Kim H, Kim DW, Lee ST, Byun JI, Seo JG, et al. Antiepileptic drug selection according to seizure type in adult patients with epilepsy. J Clin Neurol. 2020;16(4):547–55. https://doi.org/10.3988/jcn.2020.16.4.547.
23. Koch CA, Moore JL, Voth D. Arachnoid cysts: how do postsurgical cyst size and seizure outcome correlate? Neurosurg Rev. 1998;21(1):14–22. https://doi.org/10.1007/BF01111480.

24. Koch CA, Voth D, Kraemer G, Schwarz M. Arachnoid cysts: does surgery improve epileptic seizures and headaches? Neurosurg Rev. 1995;18(3):173–81. https://doi.org/10.1007/BF00383722.
25. Kushen MC, Frim D. Placement of subdural electrode grids for seizure focus localization in patients with a large arachnoid cyst. Neurosurg Focus. 2007;22(2):1–3. https://doi.org/10.3171/foc.2007.22.2.5.
26. Kwiatkowska K, Milczarek O, Dębicka M, Baliga Z, Maryniak A, Kwiatkowski S. Epilepsy and cognitive deterioration as postoperative complications of the arachnoid cyst fenestration. Clin Neuropsychol. 2020;26:1–11. https://doi.org/10.1080/13854046.2020.1837959.
27. Landgrave-Gómez J, Mercado-Gómez OF, Vázquez-García M, Rodríguez-Molina V, Córdova-Dávalos L, et al. Anticonvulsant effect of time-restricted feeding in a pilocarpine-induced seizure model: metabolic and epigenetic implications. Front Cell Neurosci. 2016;10:1–12. https://doi.org/10.3389/fncel.2016.00007.
28. Leventer RJ, Jansen A, Pilz DT, Stoodley N, Marini C, et al. Clinical and imaging heterogeneity of polymicrogyria: a study of 328 patients. Brain. 2010;133(Pt 5):1415–27. https://doi.org/10.1093/brain/awq078.
29. Martínez-Lage JF, Poza M, Rodriguez Costa T. Bilateral temporal arachnoid cysts in neurofibromatosis. J Child Neurol. 1993;8(4):383–5. https://doi.org/10.1177/088307389300800417.
30. Martínez JO, Pisón JL, Simón BC, García-Iñiguez JP, Villagrasa PS, Hidalgo ML. Intracranial arachnoid cysts and epilepsy in children: should this be treated surgically? Our 29-year experience and review of the literature. Neurocirugia. 2021;16:S1130-1473(21)00033-6. https://doi.org/10.1016/j.neucir.2021.03.003.
31. Masoudi M, Yousefi O, Azami P. Results of surgical treatment in patients with intracranial arachnoid cyst during last 5 years in a referral center in a developing country: Shiraz, Iran. World Neurosurg. 2021;150:e420–6. https://doi.org/10.1016/j.wneu.2021.03.038.
32. Meeren H, van Luijtelaar G, Lopes da Silva F, Coenen A. Evolving concepts on the pathophysiology of absence seizures. Arch Neurol. 2005;62(3):371. https://doi.org/10.1001/archneur.62.3.371.
33. Murthy JMK. Intracranial arachnoid cysts: epileptic seizures. Neurol India. 2013;61(4):343. https://doi.org/10.4103/0028-3886.117580.
34. Nasr MJ, Zohrevand AH, Khatir AA. Late onset epilepsia partialis continua in a middle-aged patient with huge arachnoid cyst. Casp J Intern Med. 2021;12(Suppl 2):464–6. https://doi.org/10.22088/cjim.12.0.464.
35. Nikolić I, Ristić A, Vojvodić N, Baščarević V, Ilanković A, et al. The association of arachnoid cysts and focal epilepsy: hospital based case control study. Clin Neurol Neurosurg. 2017;159:39–41. https://doi.org/10.1016/j.clineuro.2017.05.014.
36. Okada Y, Hamano K, Iwasaki N, Horigome Y, Enomoto T, et al. Epilepsy accompanied by intracranial arachnoid cysts: Studies on volume and regional cerebral blood perfusion using MRI and SPECT. J Epilepsy. 1998;11(4):195–201. https://doi.org/10.1016/S0896-6974(98)00017-6.
37. Pain M, Ghatan S. Arachnoid cysts in childhood. Neurological surgery, vol. 2. New York: Elsevier Saunders; 2017. p. 1524–30.
38. Pressler RM, Cilio MR, Mizrahi EM, Moshé SL, Nunes ML, et al. The ILAE classification of seizures and the epilepsies: modification for seizures in the neonate. Position paper by the ILAE Task Force on Neonatal Seizures. Epilepsia. 2021;62(3):615–28. https://doi.org/10.1111/epi.16815.
39. Rabiei K, Jaraj D, Marlow T, Jensen C, Skoog I, Wikkelsø C. Prevalence and symptoms of intracranial arachnoid cysts: a population-based study. J Neurol. 2016;263(4):689–94. https://doi.org/10.1007/s00415-016-8035-1.
40. Recio MV, Gallagher MJ, McLean MJ, Abou-Khalil B. Clinical features of epilepsy in patients with cerebellar structural abnormalities in a referral center. Epilepsy Res. 2007;76(1):1–5. https://doi.org/10.1016/j.eplepsyres.2007.05.006.
41. Sajko T, Hećimović H, Borić M, Sesar N, Rotim K. Complete resolution of medically refractory temporal lobe epilepsy after arachnoid cyst fenestration. Acta Clin Croat. 2011;50(4):589–93. PMID: 22649891.
42. Scheffer IE, Berkovic S, Capovilla G, Connolly MB, French J, et al. Classification of the epilepsies: position paper of the Commission for Classification and Terminology. Epilepsia. 2017;58(4):512–21. https://doi.org/10.1111/epi.13670.
43. Sgouros S, Chamilos C. Pathophysiology of intracranial arachnoid cysts. In: Arachnoid cysts. Elsevier; 2018. p. 67–74. https://doi.org/10.1016/B978-0-12-809932-2.00006-5.
44. Spacca B, Kandasamy J, Mallucci CL, Genitori L. Endoscopic treatment of middle fossa arachnoid cysts: a series of 40 patients treated endoscopically in two centres. Childs Nerv Syst. 2010;26(2):163–72. https://doi.org/10.1007/s00381-009-0952-1.
45. Tamburrini G, Del Fabbro M, Di Rocco C. Sylvian fissure arachnoid cysts: a survey on their diagnostic workout and practical management. Childs Nerv Syst. 2008;24(5):593–604. https://doi.org/10.1007/s00381-008-0585-9.
46. Vaquerizo-Madrid J. Sylvian arachnoid cysts, temporal lobe hypoplasia and epileptic encephalopathy. Rev Neurol. 1999;29(12):1188–9. PMID: 10652748.
47. Ventura N, D'Andrea I, Cardoso MFBS, Alves-Leon SV, Gasparetto EL. Arachnoid cysts and absence epilepsy an evidence or a coincidence? Arq Neuropsiquiatr. 2011;69(2 A):262–3. https://doi.org/10.1590/S0004-282X2011000200024.
48. Wang C, Liu C, Xiong Y, Han G, Yang H, et al. Surgical treatment of intracranial arachnoid cyst in

adult patients. Neurol India. 2013;61(1):60. https://doi.org/10.4103/0028-3886.108013.
49. Wang P-J, Lin H-C, Liu H-M, Tseng C-L, Shen Y-Z. Intracranial arachnoid cysts in children: related signs and associated anomalies. Pediatr Neurol. 1998;19(2):100–4. https://doi.org/10.1016/S0887-8994(98)00020-4.
50. Wester K. Intracranial arachnoid cysts and epilepsy. Elsevier Inc.; 2017. p. 23–8. https://doi.org/10.1016/B978-0-12-814378-0.00003-0.
51. Wieser H-G, Rudolph U, Blau N, Boison D, Imhof H-G, et al. Amino acid composition of brain cysts: levels of excitatory amino acids in cyst fluid fail to predict seizures. Epilepsy Res. 2013;55(3):191–9. https://doi.org/10.1016/S0920-1211(03)00106-2.
52. Yalçın AD, Öncel Ç, Kaymaz A, Kuloğlu N, Forta H. Evidence against association between arachnoid cysts and epilepsy. Epilepsy Res. 2002;49(3):255–60. https://doi.org/10.1016/S0920-1211(02)00050-5.
53. Yalçın AD, Toydemir HE, Çelebi LG, Forta H. Panayiotopoulos syndrome with coincidental brain lesions. Epileptic Disord. 2009;11(3):270–6. https://doi.org/10.1684/epd.2009.0267.

Psychiatric Manifestations of Arachnoid Cysts

Osman Vırıt, Öykü Özçelik, and Volkan Dizman

1 Introduction

Arachnoid cysts (ACs) are often congenital and present at birth. Head injury or trauma can also result in a secondary AC. The most common location for ACs is the middle cranial fossa, followed by a retrocerebellar location and over the cerebral convexity or rarely other anatomic localizations such as interhemispheric region [1, 29, 42, 62]. Radiologically, most ACs appear to be expansive lesions, and functional imaging has shown that ACs may cause a reorganization of cortical functions and reduced cortical thickness of the adjacent cerebral cortex [26]. It has been reported that ACs reduce perfusion and metabolism in the surrounding cortical regions [13, 49]. Symptomatic ACs are most often associated with a degree of intracystic pressure [22], and there are also results reporting that the occurrence of symptoms is not related to the intracystic pressure [40]. The nature of the neurological and psychiatric symptoms is generally related to the location of the cyst, its size, the intracystic pressure, and patient age [51, 67].

O. Vırıt (✉) · Ö. Özçelik · V. Dizman
Department of Psychiatry, Muğla Sıtkı Koçman University School of Medicine, Muğla, Turkey

2 Psychiatric Symptoms or Disorders Related to ACs

Many reports, either case studies or studies where groups of patients with neuropsychiatric disorders have been radiologically examined, suggest that ACs may indeed affect mental functions [17, 27, 29, 66]. Psychiatric disorders or symptoms that include alexithymia [5], attention deficit hyperactivity disorder [14, 42], delirium [7], depression and anxiety [6, 15, 18, 53, 63, 70], insomnia and irritability [61], organic dementia syndrome [8, 28], schizophrenia-like symptoms or other psychotic disorders [4, 5, 10–12, 16, 17, 21, 30, 34, 63, 69, 70], anorexia nervosa with delusions of guilt and catatonia [68], obsessive-compulsive disorder [20], developmental delay [20], autistic condition [20], suicide attempts [28], aggressive behavior [12, 44], and homicide [39, 48] have been reported.

It has been reported that very few of these patients were operated on for their ACs [66]. Also, AC case series have reported that there were patients with psychiatric diagnoses [18, 28, 35, 49, 55, 66]. It has been reported that most of the patients who were operated on, albeit a small number, showed improvement in their symptoms [66]. However, no postoperative improvement in behavioral problems was found [3]. Standard cognitive tests were used in all case series [3, 28, 33, 35, 49, 50, 55]. It has been concluded that ACs can sometimes complicate the diagnosis of psychiatric conditions [56, 65].

M. Turgut et al. (eds.), *Arachnoid Cysts*, https://doi.org/10.1007/978-3-031-22701-1_21

There is a case report in the literature describing negative psychotic symptoms. In a 28-year-old male patient with a posterior fossa AC, negative symptoms such as shallowing of the affect, avolition, and catatonic symptoms such as staying in the same poster for a long time were described. It was noted that the patient did not have a depressive mood. The patient had surgery. However, the surgical outcome was not mentioned in the article [54].

3 Cognition in ACs

Recently, there has been an increase in the number of studies testing cognition in individuals with ACs. Dyscognition has also been demonstrated in several case reports and case series on AC patients. Some of these patients had clinically overt cognitive problems [7, 13, 14, 40, 46, 57, 58, 60, 62]; in others the dyscognition was revealed only after neuropsychological testing [25, 32, 33, 35, 36, 49, 50, 61, 72] in adults and in children. Very few patients received surgical treatment, and most of them recovered after surgery [35, 49, 66]. Several aspects of dyscognition have been reported: agraphia [24], dementia [8, 9, 23, 45], mental retardation [13, 25, 38, 40, 43, 59], delayed language development and learning problems in children [7, 12, 25, 57, 64], verbal learning, visual perception, constructional skills, conceptual shifting, psychomotor speed [53], and memory deficits [25, 53, 57, 61, 72]. However, very few of these articles report on the functional results after cyst decompression although they all describe normalization of the cognition, including developmental delays [14, 25, 43, 53, 61], even with only minimal reduction of the volume of the decompressed cyst [53]. However, well-established mental retardation seems to be irreversible [3].

Currently, many surgeons prefer not to perform surgery on the basis of relatively little evidence of psychiatric disorders and cognitive deficits associated with ACs [56, 66]. In this regard, the team that contributed the most to the literature, Wester et al., emphasized that the available evidence is sufficient to recommend a surgical procedure [66]. In children with cysts, even in the absence of obvious symptoms, brain development in children continues with external stimuli. Accounting for the growth nature of the cysts, and considering that most of the cysts are located in the temporal region where there are very dense neural networks, the child should be protected from irreversible injury. Reports suggest that it is more reasonable and necessary to consider surgery to protect neural development in children [56, 66].

In addition to the decision to have the operation, especially in children, when the operation should be performed is another matter for discussion. The question of waiting for the brain tissue to continue to develop in asymptomatic children and/or those with mild to moderate symptoms or whether it is preferable to resort to earlier surgery in order not to miss the so-called treatment window still remains important [41, 56, 64, 66].

Almost all authors emphasize that a standard examination and neuroimaging alone are not sufficient to evaluate for cognitive impairment and that neuropsychological cognitive tests should be used to fully understand the degree of impairment and to indicate whether an operation should be considered. It has been reported that testing should be performed after the operation as well as before the operation [33, 49, 50, 66]. Kwiatkowska et al. stated that apart from the requirements mentioned above, it is important to use tests and to provide school support to children in following their school performance, and they suggested neuropsychological testing should be a routine part of case management in pediatric patients with cysts [33].

In the decision to operate, the degree of evidence for the surgery should be well explained to the patients and their families, and that in some cases, not having surgery may result in the deprivation of the opportunity for full improvement. The decision for a surgical operation should be made with the consensus of the patient, family, neurosurgeon, and psychiatrist, and it was stated that it would also be prudent to include a neurologist, a neuropsychologist, and an ethicist in the decision process [56, 66].

As a result of their review, Wester et al. stated that surgeons should no longer wait for dramatic signs to decide on whether to operate and that almost all cases and case series that were operated on showed significant improvement indicating that the available evidence was sufficient to favor performance of the operation [66]. In the decision to operate, neuroimaging, the examination, test results, activities reflected in the daily life of the patient, and their quality of life should also be taken into consideration [66].

4 Physiopathology

There may not be a direct parallel between the neuroimaging findings and the progressing symptoms. A possible explanation for this apparent discrepancy between the radiological studies and the clinical manifestations may be the fact that the AC has created its own intracranial cavity. In childhood, the neurocranium takes its shape after the growing neural contents, which is primarily the brain in normal people. An AC, by its pure presence during the growth of the skull, will create an increase in the intracranial space. This excess space may allow for the cyst to be present without producing dramatic symptoms as expected from its radiological appearance. There is also substantial evidence that cysts can grow significantly in children. This indicates an increased intracystic pressure that develops over time [31, 47, 67].

There appears to be a relationship between the intracystic pressure and subjective patient complaints [19]. Therefore, it seems reasonable to assume that the patient's symptoms are due to the pressure exerted by the cyst on its surroundings. However, the presence of symptoms may not always be due to the intracystic pressure [19]. Most ACs are considered congenital and often remain clinically silent [2]. This finding shows that although the effects of the cyst on the adjacent brain tissue have lasted for a lifetime, the pressure of the cyst on the surrounding brain parenchyma does not necessarily cause permanent damage, but rather reversible suppression of brain functions. The complete remission of symptoms, even after decompression of very large ACs, reveals the particularly impressive neuroplasticity of the brain [66].

5 ACs in Patient Populations with Psychiatric Disorders

There are few studies investigating the prevalence of ACs in patients with psychiatric disorders. One of them by Zeegers et al. reported that 8.5% of children under 3 years of age with developmental disorders had ACs [73]. However, Lingam et al. found a smaller fraction of cysts in a computed tomography study of 76 mentally abnormal children, most of whom were severely retarded [37]. Another study reported that only 3 of 168 adult psychotic patients had ACs. Kohn et al. reported eight patients with ACs who were diagnosed with a primary psychiatric disorder and two of their patients underwent surgical decompression that was resulted in improvement of the psychiatric symptoms in both patients [28].

6 Psychiatric Treatments

In the treatment of psychiatric symptoms, the treatment is determined based on the existing symptoms. Antipsychotic drugs, mood stabilizers, antidepressants, and benzodiazepines are used in psychiatric situations. Outpatient or inpatient treatment options should be considered according to the degree of psychiatric symptoms [52, 56, 71]. In case reports, it has been described that electroconvulsive therapy (ECT) can be used safely in patients who need that treatment [50]. These treatments should be evaluated in conjunction with a neurosurgery consultation. If symptoms resist pharmacological treatment in patients for whom primary surgery was not considered, the surgical option should be readdressed. It is difficult to distinguish whether the psychiatric condition is due to a primary source or an AC [56, 65]. The atypicality, complexity, and course of the symptoms are important in the evaluation of treatment options. There are reports that psychiatric symptoms completely resolved with only cyst decompression [66].

7 Conclusion

It is reported in the literature that patients with ACs may have psychiatric disorders or symptoms related to the ACs, some of which completely resolve with surgical operations, or the procedure contributes positively to the treatment process. It should be kept in mind that in cases of atypical psychiatric symptoms and resistance to standard treatments, there may be an AC, apart from other factors. In the treatment of psychiatric symptoms and disorders, psychotropic drugs are used in pharmacotherapy according to the diagnosis and the symptoms, and ECT can be performed if necessary. In the evaluation and treatment management process of ACs in children, additional sensitive thinking is very important in order to prevent irreversible injury. The use of neuropsychological tests should definitely be a part of the evaluation process. The potential need for school support in children should also be considered.

References

1. Al-Holou WN, Terman S, Kilburg C, Garton HJL, Muraszko KM, Maher CO. Prevalence and natural history of arachnoid cysts in adults. J Neurosurg. 2013;118:222–31.
2. Alkadhi H, Crelier GR, Imhof HG, Kollias SS. Somatomotor functional MRI in a large congenital arachnoid cyst. Neuroradiology. 2003;45:153–6.
3. Arai H, Sato K, Wachi A, Okuda O, Takeda N. Arachnoid cysts of the middle cranial fossa: experience with 77 patients who were treated with cystoperitoneal shunting. Neurosurgery. 1996;39:1108–12.
4. Bahk WM, Pae CU, Chae JH, Jun TY, Kim KS. A case of brief psychosis associated with an arachnoid cyst. Psychiatry Clin Neurosci. 2002;56:203–5.
5. Blackshaw S, Bowen RC. A case of atypical psychosis associated with alexithymia and a left fronto-temporal lesion: possible correlations. Can J Psychiatry. 1987;32:688–92.
6. Bulbul F, Demir B, Aksoy I, Alpak G, Unal A, Savas H. Electroconvulsive therapy in a major depression patient with arachnoid cyst. Düşünen Adam. 2013;26:392–4.
7. Caldarelli M, DiRocco C. Surgical options in the treatment of interhemispheric arachnoid cysts. Surg Neurol. 1996;46:212–21.
8. Clavel M, Taborga FG, Onzain I. Arachnoid cysts as a cause of dementia in the elderly. Acta Neurochir. 1985;78:28–32.
9. Cohen AJ. Localized neuropsychiatric symptoms of an intracranial cyst. J Neuropsychiatry Clin Neurosci. 1989;1:445–6.
10. Colameco S, DiTomasso RA. Arachnoid cyst associated with psychological disturbance. J Med Soc N J. 1982;79:209–10.
11. Cullum CM, Heaton RK, Harris MJ, Jeste DV. Neurobehavioral and neurodiagnostic aspects of late-onset psychosis. Arch Clin Neuropsychol. 1994;9:371–82.
12. da Silva JA, Alves A, Talina M, Carreiro S, Guimaraes J, Xavier M. Arachnoid cyst in a patient with psychosis: case report. Ann Ger Psychiatry. 2007;6:16.
13. De Volder AG, Michel C, Thauvoy C, Willems G, Ferrire G. Brain glucose utilisation in acquired childhood aphasia associated with a sylvian arachnoid cyst: recovery after shunting as demonstrated by PET. J Neurol Neurosurg Psychiatry. 1994;57(3):296–300.
14. Deonna T, Davidoff V, Maeder-Ingvar M, Zesiger P, Marcoz JP. The spectrum of acquired cognitive disturbances in children with partial epilepsy and continuous spike-waves during sleep. A 4-year follow-up case study with prolonged reversible learning arrest and dysfluency. Eur J Paediatr Neurol. 1997;1:19–29.
15. Escalona PR, Coffey CE, Maus-Feldman J. Electroconvulsive therapy in a depressed patient with an intracranial arachnoid cyst: a brain magnetic resonance imaging study. Convuls Ther. 1991;7:133–8.
16. Fontana M, Di Fonzo T, Aliquo C, Hadjichristos A. A case of schizophrenia-like psychosis in a patient with temporal arachnoid cyst. Eur Neuropsychopharmacol. 2003;13:S328.
17. Gewirtz G, Squires-Wheeler E, Sharif Z, Honer WG. Results of computerized tomography during first admission for psychosis. Br J Psychiatry. 1994;164:789–95.
18. Gjerde PB, Litleskare S, Lura NG, Tangen T, Helland CA, Wester K. Anxiety and depression in patients with intracranial arachnoid cysts—a prospective study. World Neurosurg. 2019;132:e645–53.
19. Golaz J, Bouras C. Frontal arachnoid cyst. A case of bilateral frontal arachnoid cyst without clinical signs. Clin Neuropathol. 1993;12:73–8.
20. Guell X, Anteraper SA, Ghosh SS, Gabrieli JDE, Schmahmann JD. Neurodevelopmental and psychiatric symptoms in patients with a cyst compressing the cerebellum: an ongoing enigma. Cerebellum. 2020;19(1):16–29.
21. Gulsun M, Sabanci U, Ozdemir B. Neurological signs in a case with arachnoid cyst, localized in the left temporal region, and psychotic disorder: a case report. Turkiye Klinikleri Tip Bilimleri Dergisi. 2007;27:615–7.
22. Helland CA, Wester K. Intracystic pressure in patients with temporal arachnoid cysts. A prospective study of preoperative complaints and post-operative outcome. J Neurol Neurosurg Psychiatry. 2007;78:620–3.
23. Hishikawa T, Chikama M, Tsuboi M, Yabuno N. Two cases of symptomatic arachnoid cysts in elderly

patients—a comparison and analysis with child cases. No Shinkei Geka. 2002;30:959–65.
24. Hodges JR. Pure apraxic agraphia with recovery after drainage of a left frontal cyst. Cortex. 1991;27:469–73.
25. Horiguchi T, Takeshita K. Cognitive function and language of a child with an arachnoid cyst in the left frontal fossa. World J Biol Psychiatry. 2000;1:159–63.
26. Hund-Georgiadis M, Yves von Cramon D, Kruggel F, Preul C. Do quiescent arachnoid cysts alter CNS functional organization? A fMRI and morphometric study. Neurology. 2002;59:1935–9.
27. Koch CA, Voth D, Kraemer G, Schwarz M. Arachnoid cysts: does surgery improve epileptic seizures and headaches? Neurosurg Rev. 1995;18:173–81.
28. Kohn R, Lilly RB, Sokol MS, Malloy PF. Psychiatric presentations of intracranial cysts. J Neuropsychiatry Clin Neurosci. 1989;1(1):60–6.
29. Kotil K, Balci N, Bilge T. Intracranial symptomatic giant arachnoid cyst of the interhemispheric fissure presenting with frontal lobe syndrome. Turk Neurosurg. 2007;17:147–15.
30. Kuhnley EJ, White DH, Granoff AL. Psychiatric presentation of an arachnoid cyst. Clin Psychiatry. 1981;42(4):167–8.
31. Kumagai M, Sakai N, Yamada H, Shinoda J, Nakashima T, Iwama T, et al. Postnatal development and enlargement of primary middle cranial fossa arachnoid cyst recognized on repeat CT scans. Childs Nerv Syst. 1986;2:211–5.
32. Kuntzer T, Assal G, de Tribolet N. Supratentorial intracranial arachnoid cysts. Neurochirurgie. 1986;32:235–41.
33. Kwiatkowska K, Milczarek O, Dębicka M, Baliga Z, Maryniak A, Kwiatkowski S. Are arachnoid cysts actually clinically mute in relation to neuropsychological symptoms? Cognitive functioning in children with AC of middle and cranial fossa. Neurol Neurosurg. 2021;208:106825.
34. Lanczik M, Fritze J, Classen W, Ihl R, Maurer K. Schizophrenia-like psychosis associated with an arachnoid cyst visualized by mapping of EEG and P300. Psychiatry Res. 1989;29:421–3.
35. Lang W, Lang M, Kornhuber A, Gallwitz A, Kriebel J. Neuropsychological and neuroendocrinological disturbances associated with extracerebral cysts of the anterior and middle cranial fossa. Eur Arch Psychiatry Neurol Sci. 1985;235:38–41.
36. Lebowitz BK, Schefft BK, Marc Testa S, Patton JA, Yeh HS. Neurocognitive sequelae of a giant arachnoid cyst: case study. Neurocase. 2006;12:339–45.
37. Lingam S, Read S, Holland IM, Wilson J, Brett EM, Hoare RD. Value of computerised tomography in children with non-specific mental subnormally. Arch Dis Child. 1982;57:381–3.
38. Locatelli D, Bonfanti N, Sfogliarini R, Gajno TM, Pezzotta S. Arachnoid cysts: diagnosis and treatment. Childs Nerv Syst. 1987;3:121–4.
39. Margetic B, Zarkovic Palijan T, Kovacevic D. Homicide and subsequent catatonia associated with a large arachnoid cyst: case report. Acta Clin Croat. 2013;52(4):497–505.
40. Martinez-Lage JF, Poza M, Sola J, Puche A. Congenital arachnoid cyst of the lateral ventricles in children. Childs Nerv Syst. 1992;8:203–6.
41. Massimi L, Izzo A, Paternoster G, Frassanito P, Di Rocco C. Arachnoid cyst: a further anomaly associated with Kallmann syndrome? Childs Nerv Syst. 2016;32(9):1607–14.
42. Millichap JG. Temporal lobe arachnoid cyst-attention deficit disorder syndrome: role of the electroencephalogram in diagnosis. Neurology. 1997;48(5):1435–9.
43. Oka Y, Kumon Y, Kohno K, Saitoh M, Sakaki S. Treatment of suprasellar arachnoid cyst-two case reports. Neurol Med Chir. 1996;36:721–4.
44. Paradis CM, Horn L, Lazar RM, Schwartz DW. Brain dysfunction and violent behavior in a man with a congenital subarachnoid cyst. Hosp Community Psychiatry. 1994;45:714–6.
45. Park SW, Cho KH, Shin YS, Kim SH, Ahn YH, Cho KG, et al. Helmet like skull deformity with a large arachnoid cyst. Surg Neurol. 2006;65:95–8.
46. Ramtahal J. Arachnoid cyst mimicking normal pressure hydrocephalus. A case report and review of the literature. J Neurosurg Sci. 2006;50:79–81.
47. Rao G, Anderson RC, Feldstein NA, Brockmeyer DL. Expansion of arachnoid cysts in children: report of two cases and review of the literature. J Neurosurg. 2005;102:314–7.
48. Relkin N, Plum F, Mattis S, Eidelberg D, Tranel D. Impulsive homicide associated with an arachnoid cyst and unilateral frontotemporal cerebral dysfunction. Semin Clin Neuropsychiatry. 1996;1:172–83.
49. Sandvik U, Adolfsson T, Jacobson DN, Tedroff K. Cognition in children with arachnoid cysts. J Clin Med. 2020;9(3):850.
50. Schertz M, Constantini S, Eshel R, Sela AH, Roth J, Fattal-Valevski A. Neurodevelopmental outcomes in children with large temporal arachnoid cysts. J Neurosurg Pediatr. 2018;21(6):578–86.
51. Sgouros S, Chapman S. Congenital middle fossa arachnoid cysts may cause global brain ischaemia: a study with 99Tc-hexamethylpropyleneamineoximesingle photon emission computerised tomography scans. Pediatr Neurosurg. 2001 Oct;35(4):188–94.
52. Skaric M, Margetic BA, Dijakovic AB, Karlovic D. Cognitive and psychotic symptoms in a patient with infratentorial arachnoid cyst: a case report. Acta Clin Croat. 2021;60(2):304–8.
53. Soukup VM, Patterson J, Trier TT, Chen JW. Cognitive improvement despite minimal arachnoid cyst decompression. Brain Dev. 1998;20:589–93.
54. Soumitra DAS. Posterior fossa arachnoid cyst presenting as negative symptoms of psychosis. Arch Psychiatry. 2018;30(3):202–3.
55. Spansdahl T, Solheim O. Quality of life in adult patients with primary intracranial arachnoid cysts. Acta Neurochir. 2007;149:1025–32.
56. Steyn PJ, Van den Heuvel LL. Cut it out or wait it out? Case series of middle fossa arachnoid cysts present-

ing with psychiatric symptoms and a discussion of the ethics of neurosurgical management. Gen Psychiatry. 2021;34:e100523.
57. Stracciari A, Ciucci G, Bissi G. Transient global amnesia associated with a large arachnoid cyst of the middle cranial fossa of the non dominant hemisphere. Ital J Neurol Sci. 1987;8:609–61.
58. Sztriha L, Gururaj A. Hippocampal dysgenesis associated with temporal lobe hypoplasia and arachnoid cyst of the middle cranial fossa. J Child Neurol. 2005;20:926–30.
59. Takaesu E, Watanabe K, Inokuma K, Matsumoto A, Sugiura M, Negoro T. EEG topography in porencephaly and arachnoid cyst. Clin Electroencephalogr. 1985;16:21–9.
60. Tolmie JL, Day R, Fredericks B, Galea P, Moffett AW. Dominantly inherited cerebral dysplasia: arachnoid cyst associated with mild mental handicap in a mother and her son. J Med Genet. 1997;34:1018–20.
61. Tsurushima H, Harakuni T, Saito A, Tominaga D, Hyodo A, Yoshii Y. Symptomatic arachnoid cyst of the left frontal convexity presenting with memory disturbance-case report. Neurol Med Chir. 2000;40:339–41.
62. Ure J, Giudice F, Videla H, Ollari J, Diez M, Delembert W, et al. Partial agenesis of the temporal lobe—behavioral correlations. Int J Neuroradiol. 1999;5:225–31.
63. Vidrih B, Karlovic D, Bosnjak Pasic M. Arachnoid cyst as the cause of bipolar affective disorder: case report. Acta Clin Croat. 2012;51:655–9.
64. von Gontard A, Muller U. Psychiatric and neuropsychological symptoms in children with arachnoid cysts—a case report. Z Kinder Jugendpsychiatr. 1991;19:30–7.
65. Wahl AS, Löffler M, Hausner L, Ruttorf M, Nees F, Frölich L. Case report: a giant arachnoid cyst masking Alzheimer's disease. BMC Psychiatry. 2019;19:274.
66. Wester K. Intracranial arachnoid cysts—do they impair mental functions? J Neurol. 2008;255:1113–20.
67. Wester K, Moen G. Documented growth of a temporal arachnoid cyst. J Neurol Neurosurg Psychiatry. 2000;69:699–700.
68. Wolanczyk T, Komender J, Brzozowska A. Catatonic syndrome preceded by symptoms of anorexia nervosa in a 14-year-old boy with arachnoid cyst. Eur Child Adolesc Psychiatry. 1997;6:166–9.
69. Wong CW, Ko SF, Wai YY. Arachnoid cyst of the lateral ventricle manifesting positional psychosis. Neurosurgery. 1993;32:841–3.
70. Wu YY, Shen YC. Delusions of control in a case of schizophrenia coexisting with a large cerebellar arachnoid cyst. Ci Ji Yi Xue Za Zhi. 2017;29:115–7.
71. Yang C, Zhang J, Zhang X, Feng N, Hao L, Gaonkar S. Anxiety, phobia, and depression in patients with temporal arachnoid cyst—a case report. MOJ Clin Med Case Rep. 2020;10(5):119–21.
72. Zaatreh MM, Bates ER, Hooper SR, Palmer G, Elmenshawi EE, Courvoisie HE, et al. Morphometric and neuropsychologic studies in children with arachnoid cysts. Pediatr Neurol. 2002;26:134–8.
73. Zeegers M, Van Der Grond J, Durston S, Nievelstein RJ, Witkamp T, VanDaalen E, et al. Radiological findings in autistic and developmentally delayed children. Brain Dev. 2006;28:495–9.

Differential Diagnosis of Intracranial Arachnoid Cysts

Ali Akhaddar

1 Introduction

Intracranial arachnoid cysts (ACs) are an uncommon heterogeneous pathologic entity that are more complex than they were considered in the past. These cystic lesions may present with variable clinical signs and symptoms as well as neuroimaging appearances which depend principally on their anatomic localizations, cyst sizes, etiological forms, and the patient's age. Some of the cysts are asymptomatic (known as incidental imaging findings), while others manifest as a space-occupying lesion or mass [5, 16, 52]. ACs may be confused with many intracranial cysts of different etiologies [28, 56, 59]. Both neurosurgeons and radiologists must be prepared to recognize all possible considerations in preoperative images, during the therapeutic planning process and even throughout the patient's care. Consequently, a high index of suspicion needs to be kept in mind in order to achieve an appropriate analysis of ACs and to develop a list of the possible intracranial cyst-mimicking lesions.

A summary of the most common imaging differential diagnoses for intracranial ACs is given in this chapter according to the anatomic localizations and origin of the cysts. Moreover, chapter "Differential Diagnosis of Intraspinal Arachnoid Cysts" provides a review of the differential diagnosis for intraspinal ACs.

A. Akhaddar (✉)
Department of Neurosurgery, Avicenne Military Hospital of Marrakech, Mohammed V University in Rabat, Rabat, Morocco

2 Subdural Hygromas

Subdural hygromas (SHG) refer to the accumulation of fluid in the subdural space usually after trauma. Other underlying causes may exist such as spontaneous intracranial hypotension and secondary to intracranial surgery. SHG are encountered in all age-groups but are generally most common among the elderly [49]. Some cases called "idiopathics" are seen in pediatric patients. SHG differ from ACs in many aspects such as the content of the subdural fluid collection, neuroimaging appearance, and clinical manifestations [49, 50]. The vast majority of patients are asymptomatic. However, some symptoms, unusually reported, consist of headaches, nausea/vomiting, changes in mental status, focal neurological deficits, and seizures. Most SHG develop around the Sylvian fissure and the frontal lobe convexities without significant mass effect on the surrounding structures. The posterior fossa is rarely involved.

On both the computed tomography scan (CT scan) and magnetic resonance (MR) imaging, classic subdural hygromas manifest as "crescentic" subdural collections that do not extend into the sulci [2, 49]. The density and signal characteristics are similar to those of cerebrospinal fluid (CSF) (Fig. 1). However, in some atypical cases, there is an increased density within the hygroma on CT scan as well as a heterogeneous signal on MR imaging (primarily hyperintense on the fluid attenuated inversion recovery sequence (FLAIR))

M. Turgut et al. (eds.), *Arachnoid Cysts*, https://doi.org/10.1007/978-3-031-22701-1_22

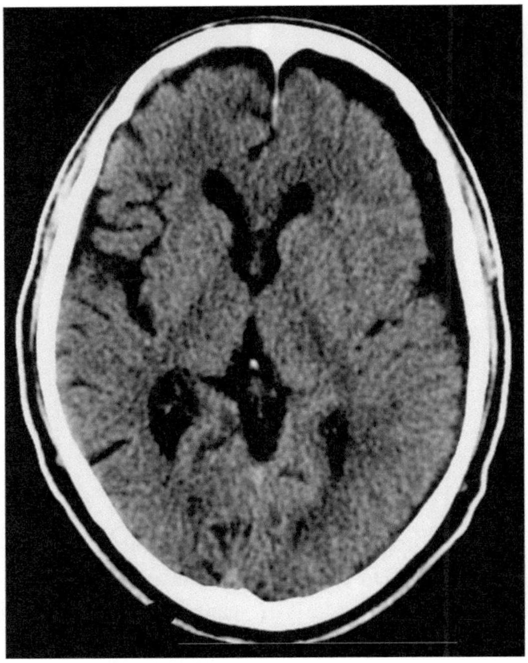

Fig. 1 Axial CT scan image showing a left frontal subdural hygroma

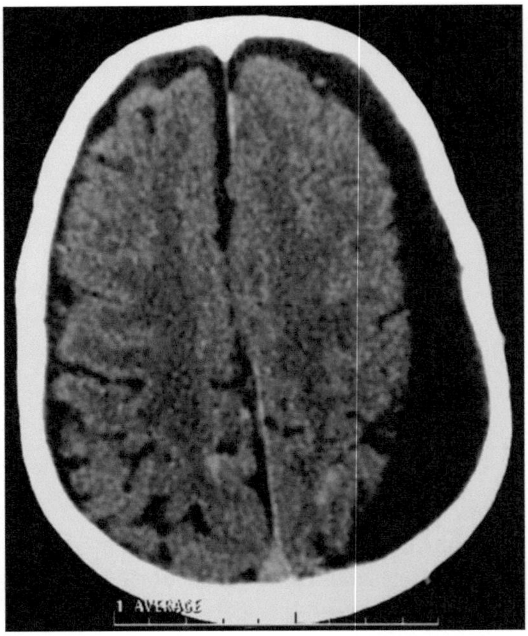

Fig. 2 Axial CT scan image revealing a left hemispheric chronic subdural hematoma

related to a mixture of CSF and blood [49, 50]. Also, hygromas are frequently seen bilaterally, but bilaterality is not sufficient to differentiate SHG from ACs.

3 Chronic Subdural Hematomas

Chronic subdural hematoma (CSDH) is a collection of blood accumulating in the subdural space which is the potential space between the dura and arachnoid mater of the meninges. CSDH can appear among any age group, particularly in the aging population [13]. This type of hematoma is mainly due to head trauma which occurred at least 3 weeks previously. CT scans without contrast injection are usually sufficient to make the proper diagnosis. Clinical signs and symptoms vary widely depending on the volume and chronicity of the bleeding. Often, the diagnosis may be inconclusive prior to obtaining a neuroimaging study [13, 34].

The majority of CSDH is unilateral in adults, mainly seen over the frontoparietal convexities and in the middle cranial fossa (Fig. 2). However, isolated interhemispheric/parafalcine CSDH is encountered more frequently among children than in adults and is common in cases without injury.

CSDH is usually crescentic, not rounded or scalloped, and may have similar CT attenuation as ACs. Whereas with MR imaging, the signal appearance is never completely identical. CSDH shows evidence of prior bleeding, especially on T2* and FLAIR sequences, and can have enhancing membranes following contrast administration [2, 13].

4 Epidermoid and Dermoid Cysts

Epidermoid and dermoid cysts are congenital lesions occurring due to the inclusion of ectodermal elements during neural tube closure. The two cysts are often grouped together but epidermoids are lined with only stratified squamous epithelium, whereas dermoids contain additional skin appendages such as hair, sebaceous, and sweat glands. Both epidermoids and dermoids have been confused pathologically for a long time. Epidermoid cysts are known to occur in the cerebellar pontine angle, in the quadrigeminal cistern, para/suprasellar region, and the temporal fossa. They engulf blood vessels and nerves, insinuating themselves along CSF cisterns [56, 65]. While dermoids are typically located in the midline [71]. Some intracranial dermoid and epidermoid cysts are asymptomatic and are only found fortuitously. Often, patients may present with unclear nonspecific clinical symptoms such as headache, dizziness, or blurred vision. More unusually, there are symptoms of aseptic chemical meningitis caused by cyst rupture within the subarachnoid spaces [48].

Epidermoids are by far the most common diagnostic differential of ACs especially those that develop in the posterior fossa. Both ACs and epidermoid cysts may have similar characteristics on CT scan and on T1/T2-weighted images and neither show gadolinium enhancement. However, the two cystic lesions present differences on FLAIR sequences and on diffusion-weighted imaging (DWI) [81]. FLAIR demonstrates a heterogeneous/dirty signal for epidermoids that is opposite of the low (suppressed) signal in the case of ACs. In addition, epidermoids have a typically elevated signal on DWI with corresponding dark signal on the apparent diffusion coefficient (ADC) scan (due to presence of fat epithelial keratin inside the cyst); whereas ACs have unrestricted diffusion and low signal on the ADC scan [26, 56, 65].

On imaging, dermoid cysts are usually well-defined lobulated midline masses that have low attenuation (fat density due to sebum) on CT scan and high signal intensity on T1-weighted MR images. Instead, dermoids can be differentiated on CT or MR imaging with signal intensities that are similar to fat not CSF (Fig. 3) [48]. Typically, dermoid cysts do not enhance after contrast administration. In ruptured cysts, the most common finding is that of foci with high signals on T1-weighted MR images, throughout the sub-

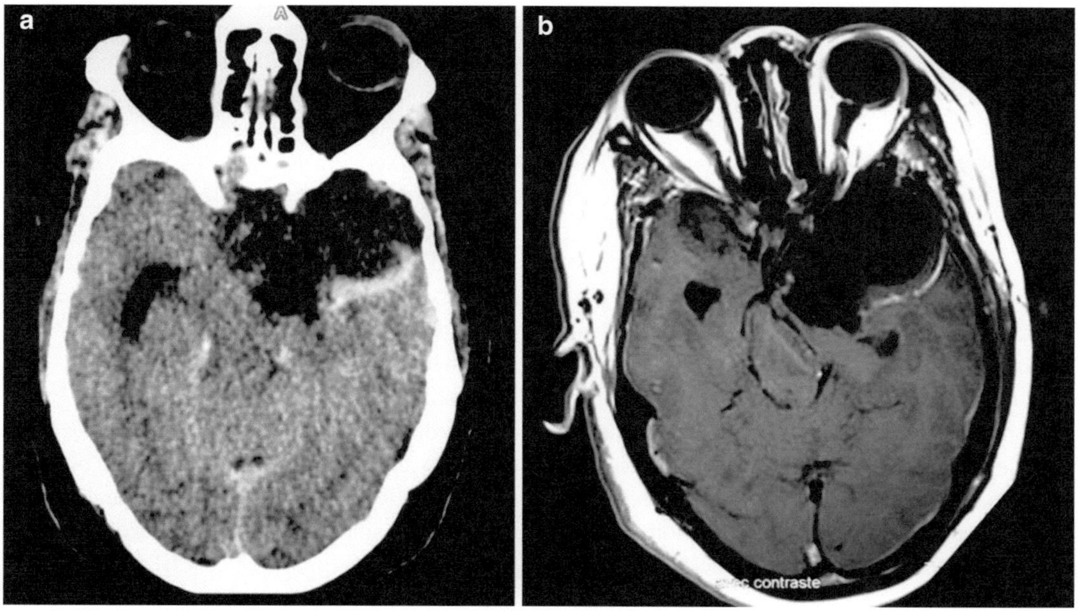

Fig. 3 Temporo-parasellar dermoid cyst on the left side. Axial CT scan (**a**), post-gadolinium T1- (**b**) and T2-weighted MR images (**c**). Coronal on FLAIR sequence (**d**)

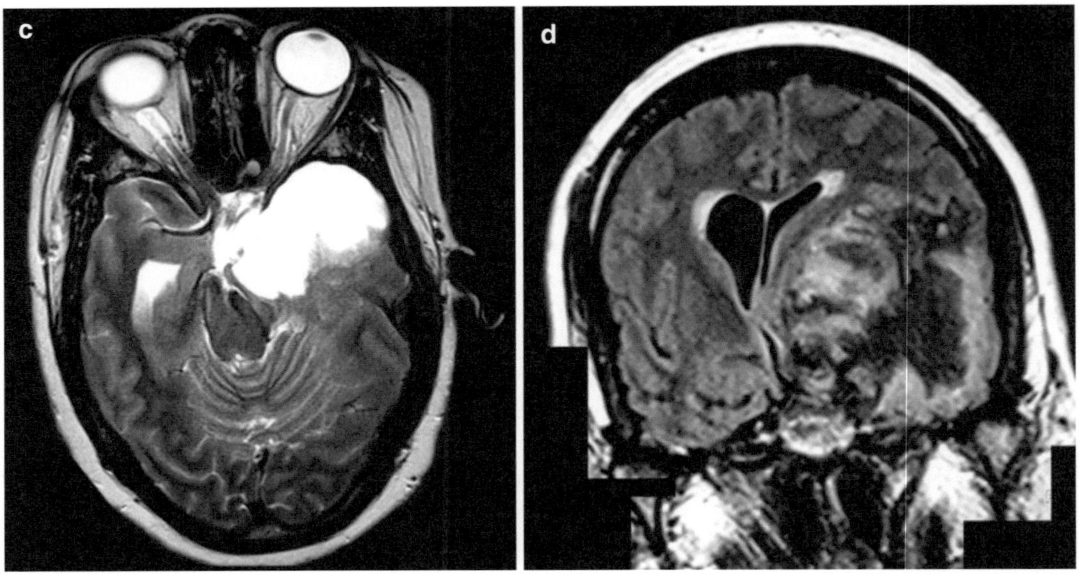

Fig. 3 (continued)

arachnoid space and occasionally within the ventricles [71].

Lastly, it is useful to add that some epidermoid and dermoid cysts demonstrate calcifications within the cysts on the CT scan. Likewise, partial enhancement may be seen around the cystic margin of some unusual forms of dermoids and epidermoids [48, 65, 71].

5 Cystic Tumors

5.1 Pilocytic Astrocytomas

Pilocytic astrocytomas (also known as juvenile pilocytic astrocytomas) are well circumscribed astrocytic gliomas that usually occur in the pediatric population, especially at the end of the first decade of life. More than half of pediatric pilocytic astrocytomas are found in the cerebellum. These benign tumors may involve both the vermis and the cerebellar hemisphere. Brainstem sites are rare. Pilocytic astrocytomas represent the single most frequent pediatric central nervous system (CNS) tumor [53]. The majority of cases are sporadic but they may be seen among children with type I neurofibromatosis. Clinical presentation depends on tumor location. In the posterior fossa, there is most often mass effect with signs of increased intracranial pressure, especially when hydrocephalus is present. Cerebellar signs with or without bulbar symptoms may also be present.

These tumors have a range of imaging appearances [53, 56], with the majority presenting as a large cystic lesion with a brightly enhancing mural nodule (Figs. 4 and 5). Calcification can be identified in about 20% of cases.

Cystic collections are often slightly hyperdense compared to CSF on the CT scan with an intensely enhancing mural nodule on both CT scan and MRI (Fig. 4). Cyst wall enhancement is inconsistent and is principally seen in higher grade gliomas (Figs. 6 and 7) [56].

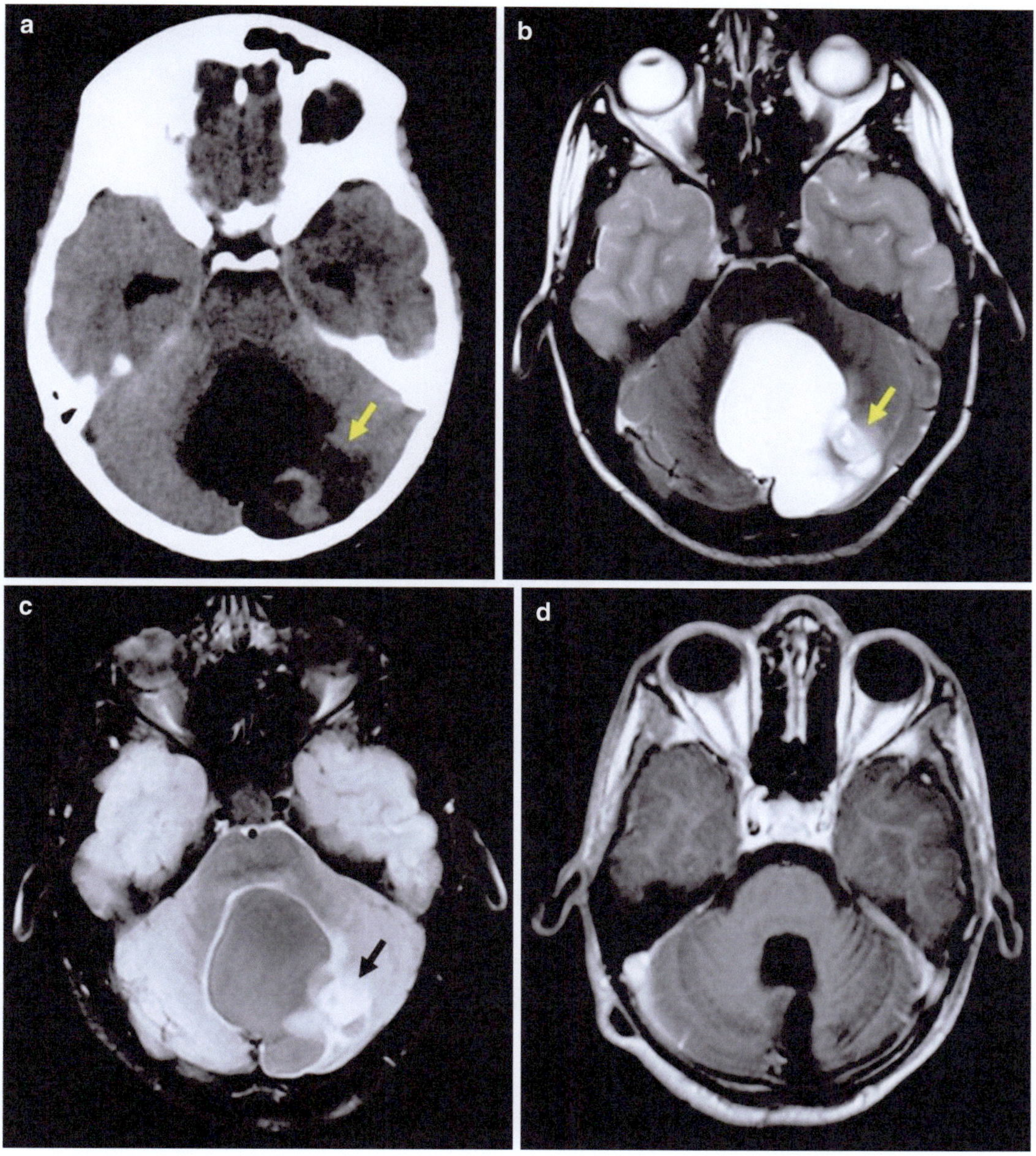

Fig. 4 Cerebellar pilocytic astrocytoma presenting as a large cystic lesion with a mural nodule (arrows). Axial CT scan (**a**), T2-weighted MR image (**b**), and FLAIR sequence (**c**). Post-operative axial post-gadolinium T1-weighted MR image (**d**)

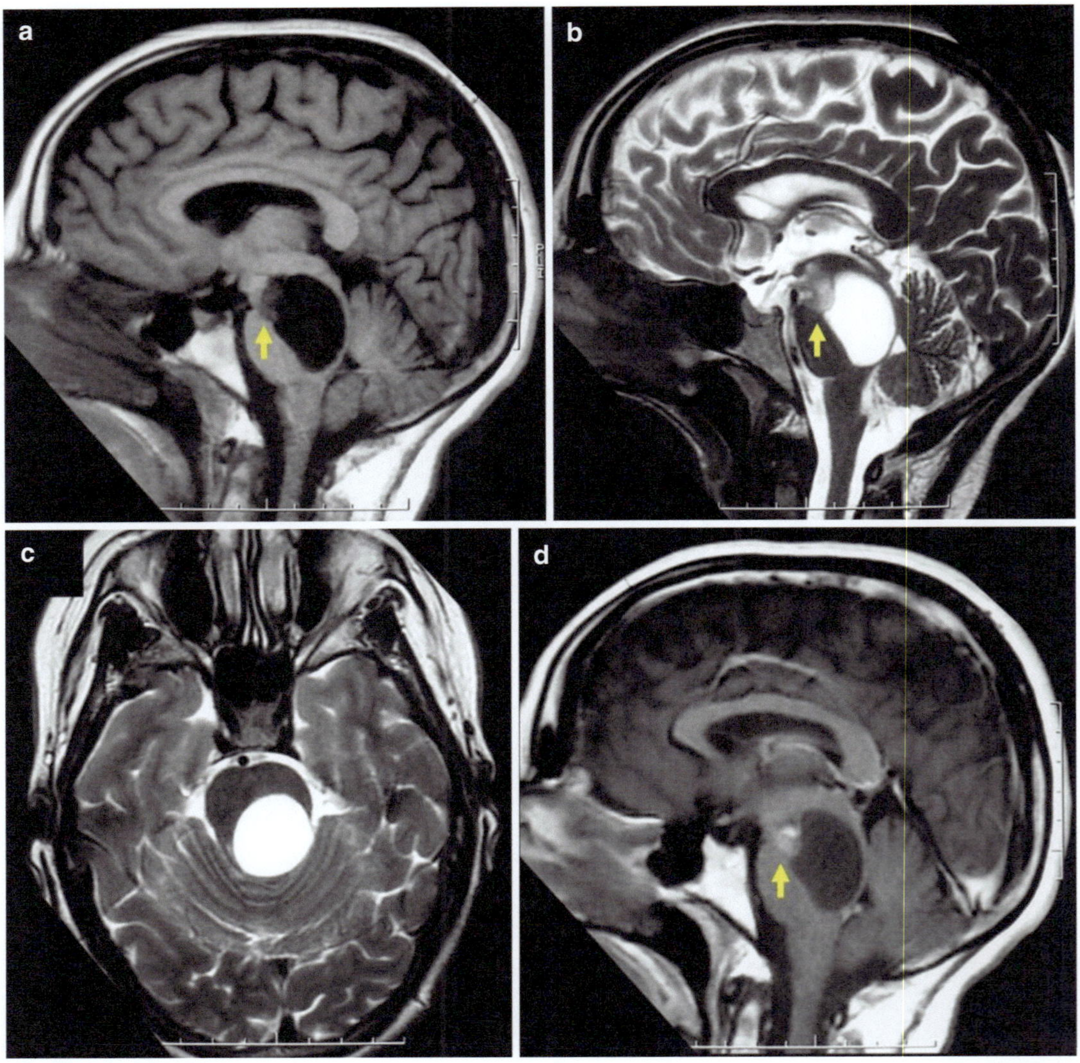

Fig. 5 Ponto-mesencephalic pilocytic astrocytoma with a mural nodule (arrows). Sagittal T1-(**a**), T2- (**b**), and axial T2-weighted MR images (**c**). Note the enhancing mural nodule on sagittal T1-weighted MR image following gadolinium injection (**d**)

5.2 Hemangioblastomas

Hemangioblastomas are rare vascular tumors that occur both sporadically and among patients with von Hippel Lindau disease [83]. They are benign tumors that can arise in the central nervous system (CNS) (particularly in the posterior fossa), or elsewhere in the body, including in the retina, kidneys, and liver. Hemangioblastomas typically occur in young and middle-aged adults with a slight male predilection [47]. Patients may have headaches, nausea/vomiting, vertigo/dizziness, and walking difficulties due to balance problem. Hemangioblastomas may be solid but most cases are associated with formation of intratumoral cysts as a consequence of vascular leakage [33].

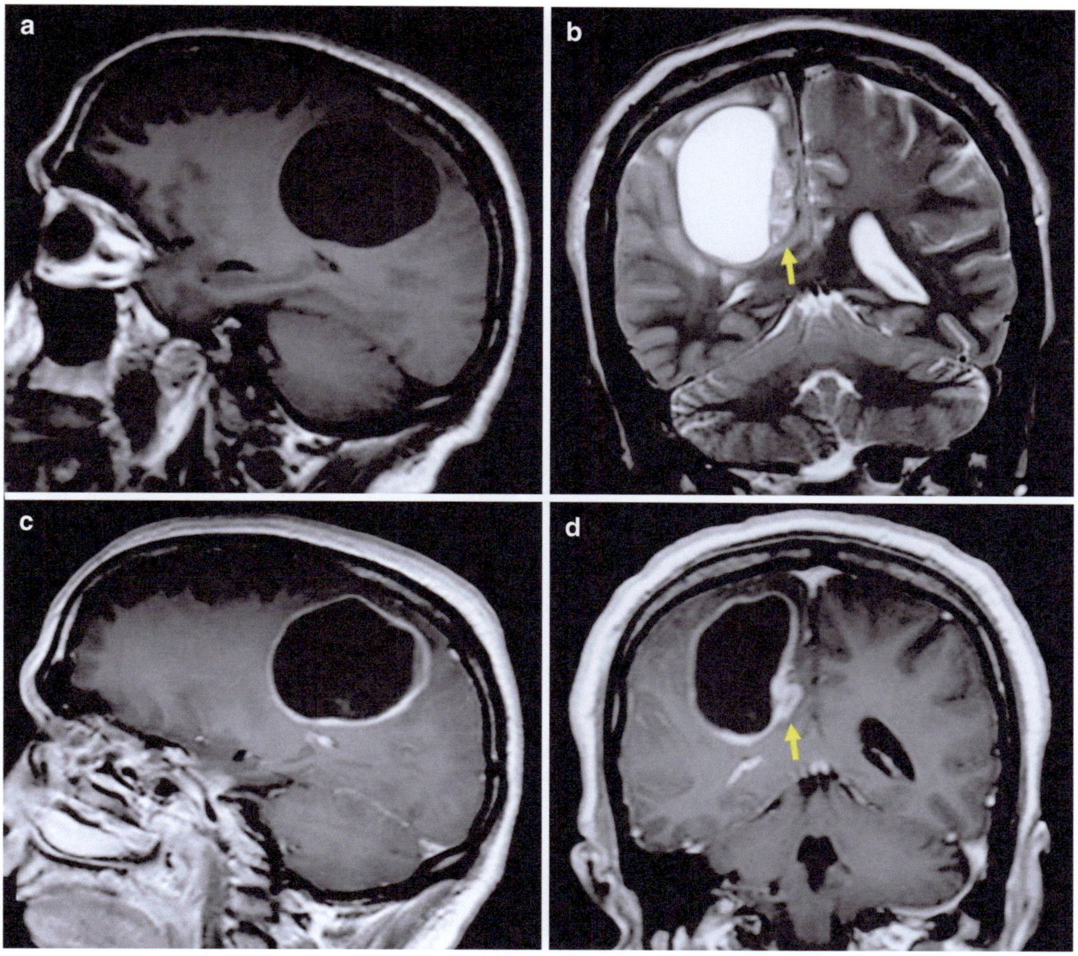

Fig. 6 Right parietal cystic glioblastoma with a mural nodule (arrows). Sagittal T1- (**a**) and T2-weighted MR images (**b**). Post-gadolinium sagittal (**c**) and coronal (**d**) T1-weighted MR images showing both mural nodule (arrow) and cyst wall enhancement

These tumors generally appear on imaging as demarcated homogeneous masses composed of a fluid-filled cyst (similar to CSF) with non-enhancing walls and a mural nodule which strongly enhances (Fig. 8). Interestingly, the majority of mural nodules have prominent serpentine flow voids due to enlarged vessels. On cerebral angiography, hemangioblastomas appear with enlarged feeding arteries and often dilated draining veins with an important central tumor blush [82]. In addition, diffusion weights images (DWI) and apparent diffusion coefficient (ADC) scans may be useful for differentiating hemangioblastomas from other intraaxial enhancing tumors occurring in the posterior fossa [63, 81].

5.3 Gangliogliomas

Gangliogliomas are another uncommon, usually low-grade, brain tumor that may contain a fluid-filled cystic collection. They have been described everywhere in the CNS but are generally found

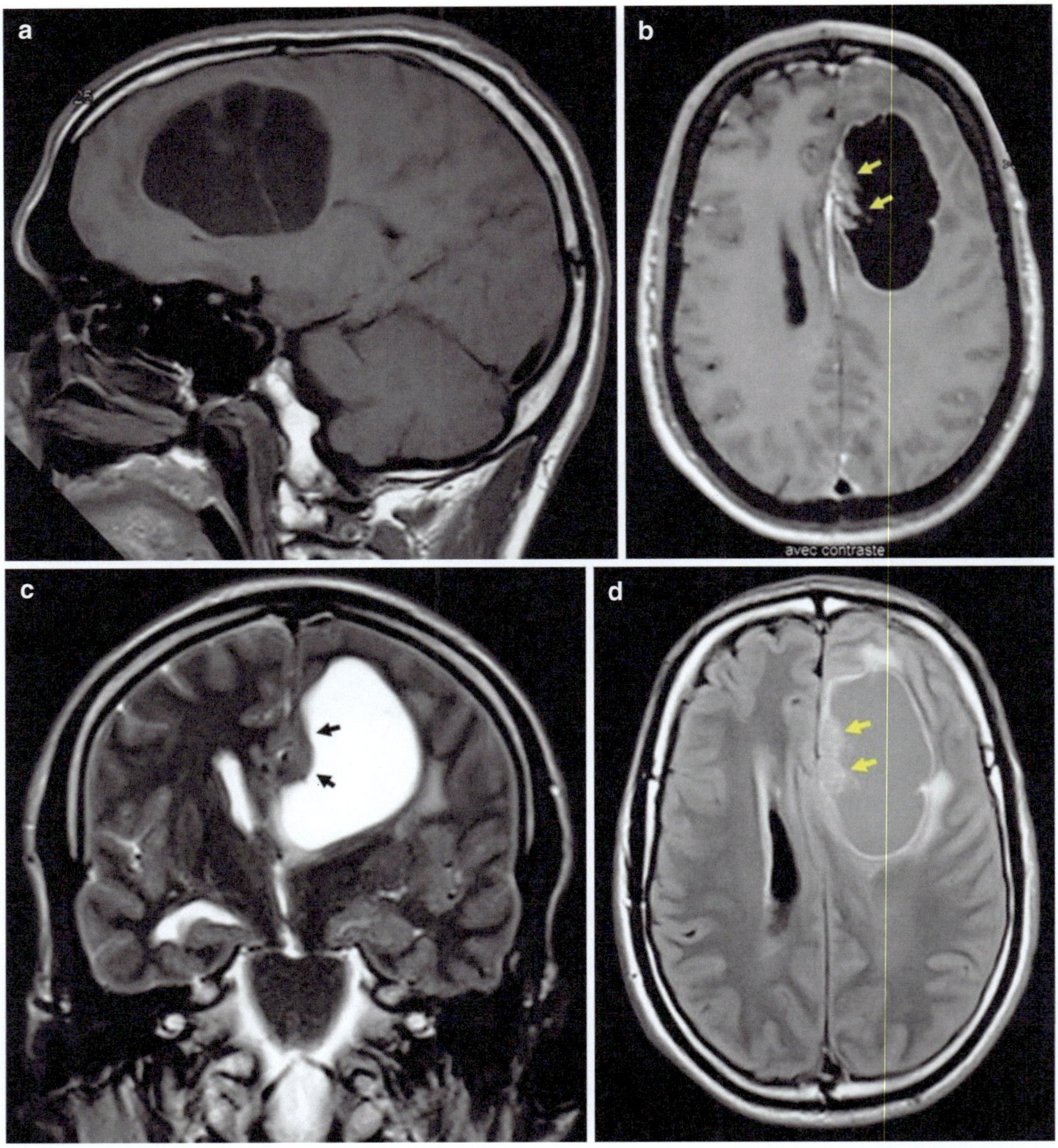

Fig. 7 Left frontal anaplastic astrocytoma with a mural nodule (arrows). Sagittal (**a**) and axial (**b**) post-gadolinium T1-weighted MR images. Coronal T2-weighted MR image (**c**) and axial FLAIR sequence (**d**)

in the temporal lobes [51]. Children and young adults are frequently affected without a gender predominance [39]. Temporal lobe epilepsy is the most common clinical presentation with or without symptoms of raised intracranial pressure or focal neurologic deficits. Their appearance on neuroimaging varies from a partially cystic mass with an enhancing mural nodule to a solid mass infiltrating adjacent temporal gyri [51]. Contrast enhancement is inconsistent and often nonspecific involving the solid tumoral component [39].

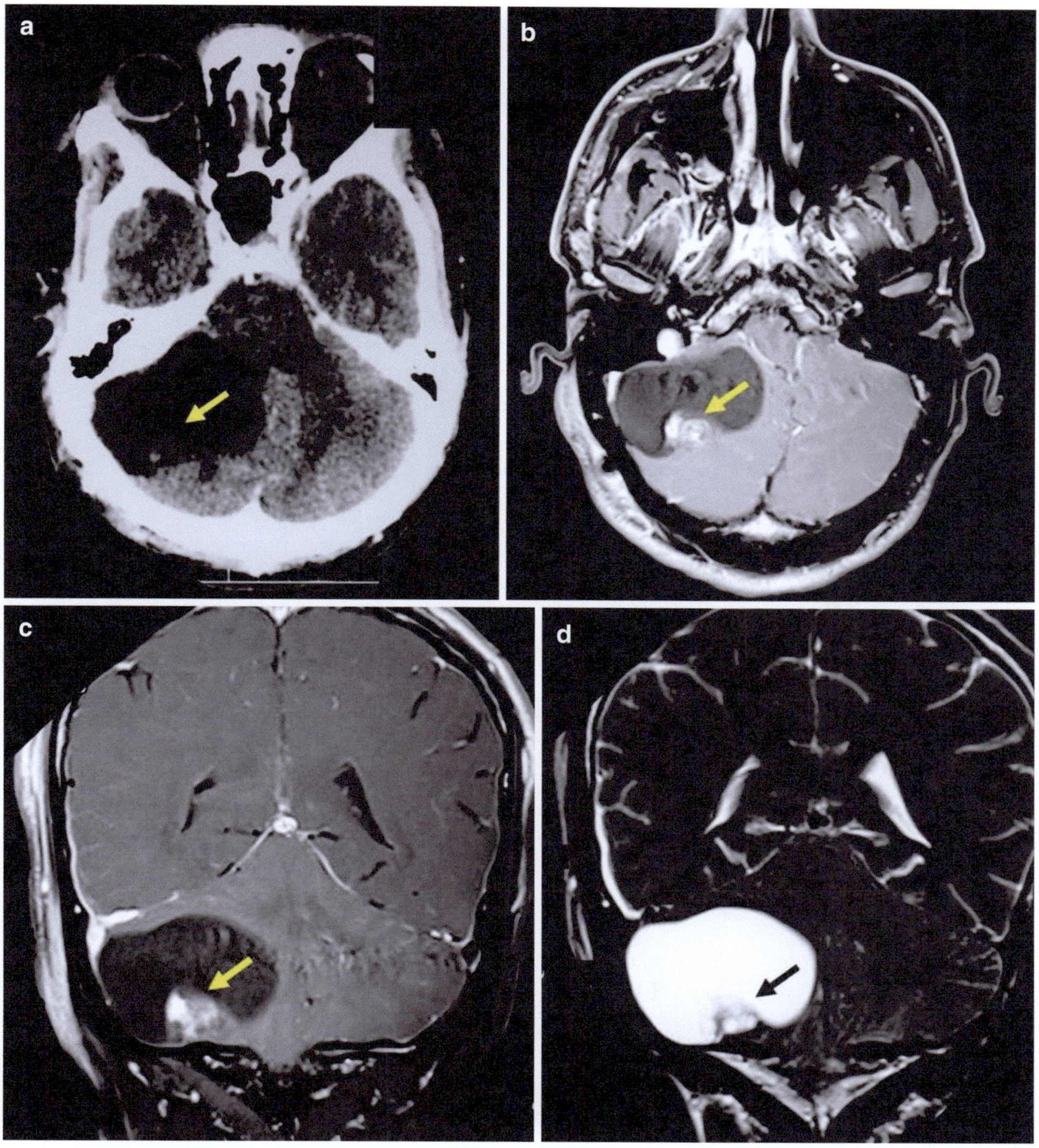

Fig. 8 Right hemispheric cerebellar hemangioblastoma presenting as a large cystic lesion with a mural nodule (arrows). Axial post-contrast CT scan (**a**), axial (**b**) and coronal (**c**) post-gadolinium T1-weighted MR images, and coronal T2-weighted MR image (**d**)

5.4 Tumors Developed in the Subarachnoid Space

Some other cystic tumors are extra-axial and develop in the subarachnoid space. These include meningiomas (Fig. 9), schwannomas, and brain metastases. In 1979, Nauta classified cystic meningiomas into four types: central tumoral cyst, peripheral intratumoral cyst, peritumoral cyst in the adjacent brain parenchyma, and cyst between the tumor and the adjacent brain parenchyma [55]. Indeed, some associated cysts correspond to a trapped encysted accumulation of CSF contiguous with large extra-axial tumors.

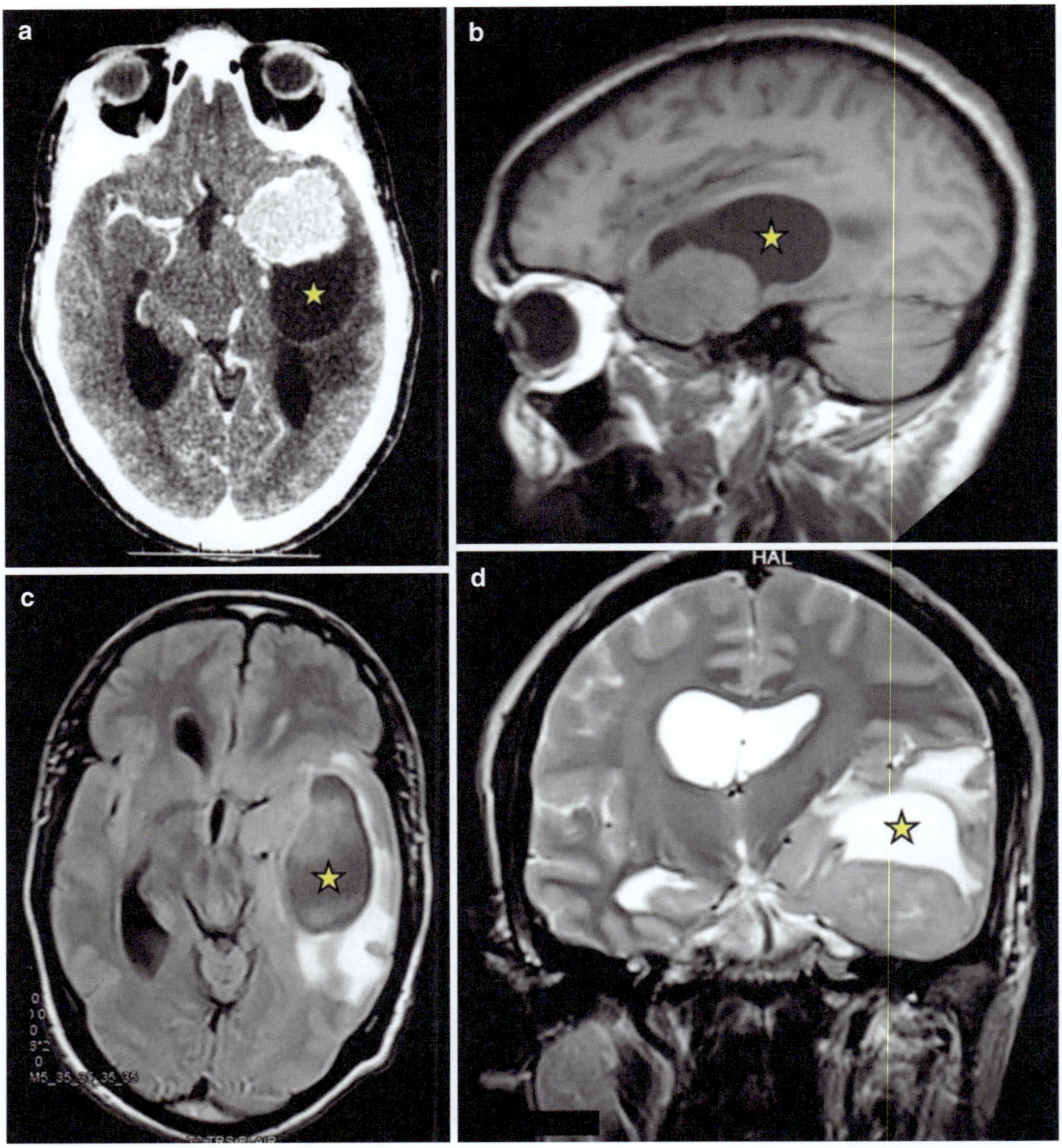

Fig. 9 Left temporal cystic meningioma (stars). Axial post-contrast CT scan (**a**), sagittal T1-weighted MR image (**b**), axial FLAIR sequence (**c**), and coronal T2-weighted MR image (**d**)

When a neoplasm develops it traps the CSF between itself and the bordering brain parenchyma. On the contrary, an intratumoral cyst may be secondary to a degenerative phenomenon, ischemic necrosis, bleeding, tumor cell secretion, or adjacent white matter demyelination [29, 58, 79].

The majority of these cystic tumors are easy to differentiate from ACs due to their solid components. Contrast/gadolinium injection can differentiate between similar lesions where an enhancing portion is typical in fleshy tumors but not in ACs [64]. Entirely cystic tumors were previously described but are rare [25, 42].

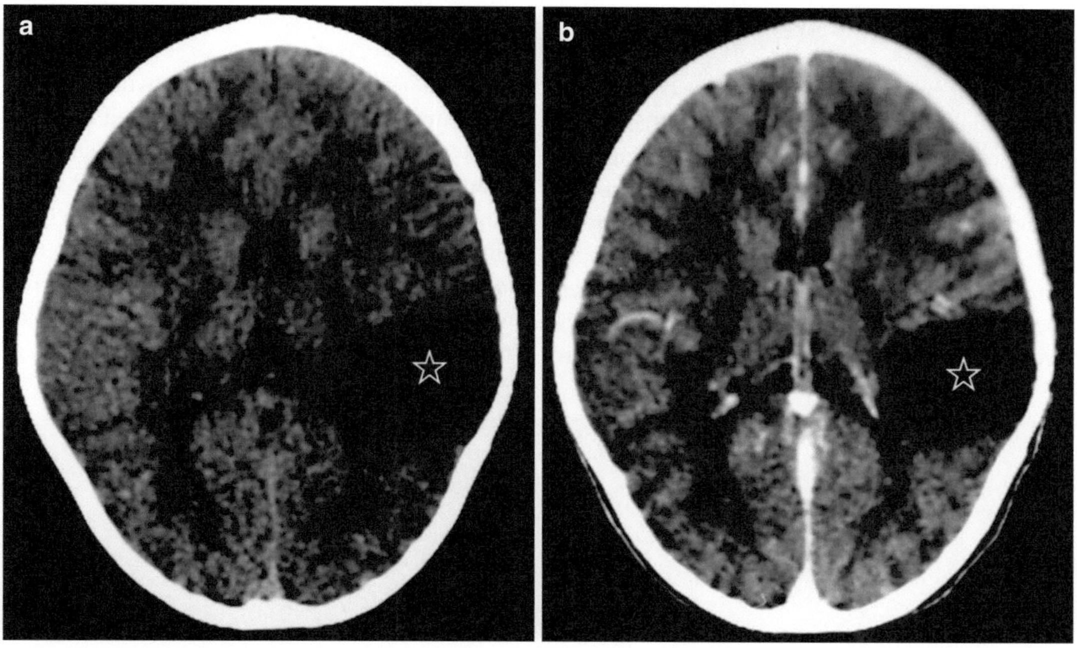

Fig. 10 Axial CT scan before (**a**) and after (**b**) contrast injection showing a hypodense low-grade glioma in the left parietal region (stars)

5.5 Low-Density Tumors

Conversely, some homogeneous low-density tumors (e.g. low-grade gliomas) on CT scan may be confused with ACs (Fig. 10). However, development of advanced MR imaging techniques, especially using multiples sequences and gadolinium administration, facilitates the differentiation between both types of lesion. Careful inspection of the solid component within the suspected lesion, examination of its relationship to surrounding structures, and evaluation of the enhancement effect after gadolinium injection will help to avoid this error.

6 Non-neoplastic Cysts

6.1 Neurenteric Cysts

Neurenteric cysts (also known as enterogenous cyst) are rare, benign, congenital, endodermal lesions resulting from incomplete resorption of the neurenteric canal. The cyst content is generally mucoid in nature, with a variable protein composition [19]. These extra-axial cystic lesions are more commonly located in the spine rather than in the brain. Most cysts are intradural, extramedullary, and anterior to the spinal cord in the thoracic spine. Association with anterior spinal dysraphism and Klippel-Feil anomalies is highly suggestive.

Patients with neurenteric cysts may present variable clinical symptoms such as headache, vertigo, focal neurologic deficits, seizures, or cranial nerve deficits (particularly third, fifth, and eighth cranial nerve dysfunction) [19, 60].

On CT scan, neurenteric cysts are iso/hypodense lesions. They can be similar to ACs although most of them are iso-/slightly hyperintense compared to CSF on T1-weighted and typically hyperintense on T2-weighted MR imaging sequences. The imagery appearances may vary depending on protein content. Peripheral rim enhancement is rare following contrast injection. An important fact should be considered according to Preece et al., all neurenteric cysts are hyperintense compared to CSF on FLAIR sequences [60].

6.2 Ependymal Cysts

Intracranial ependymal cysts are rare benign neuroepithelial cysts lined by ependymal cells that produce a clear serous liquid. They occur less frequently than ACs. The cysts are most frequently located deep in the brain parenchyma (Fig. 11), but other locations can be involved such as intraventricular, periventricular, brainstem, cerebellopontine area, and suprasellar and subarachnoid spaces [27, 61]. Most ependymal cysts are small and asymptomatic. Conversely, symptomatic cases are correlated with large sizes that manifest with headache or obstructive hydrocephalus.

On imaging, these cysts are difficult to differentiate from ACs. The lesions are isodense and isointense with CSF on CT scan and MR imaging, respectively, without peripheral wall enhancement. Sometimes, the cyst content may be hyperintense compared to CSF if there is a high protein concentration. The lack of diffusion restriction should be underlined [56, 61].

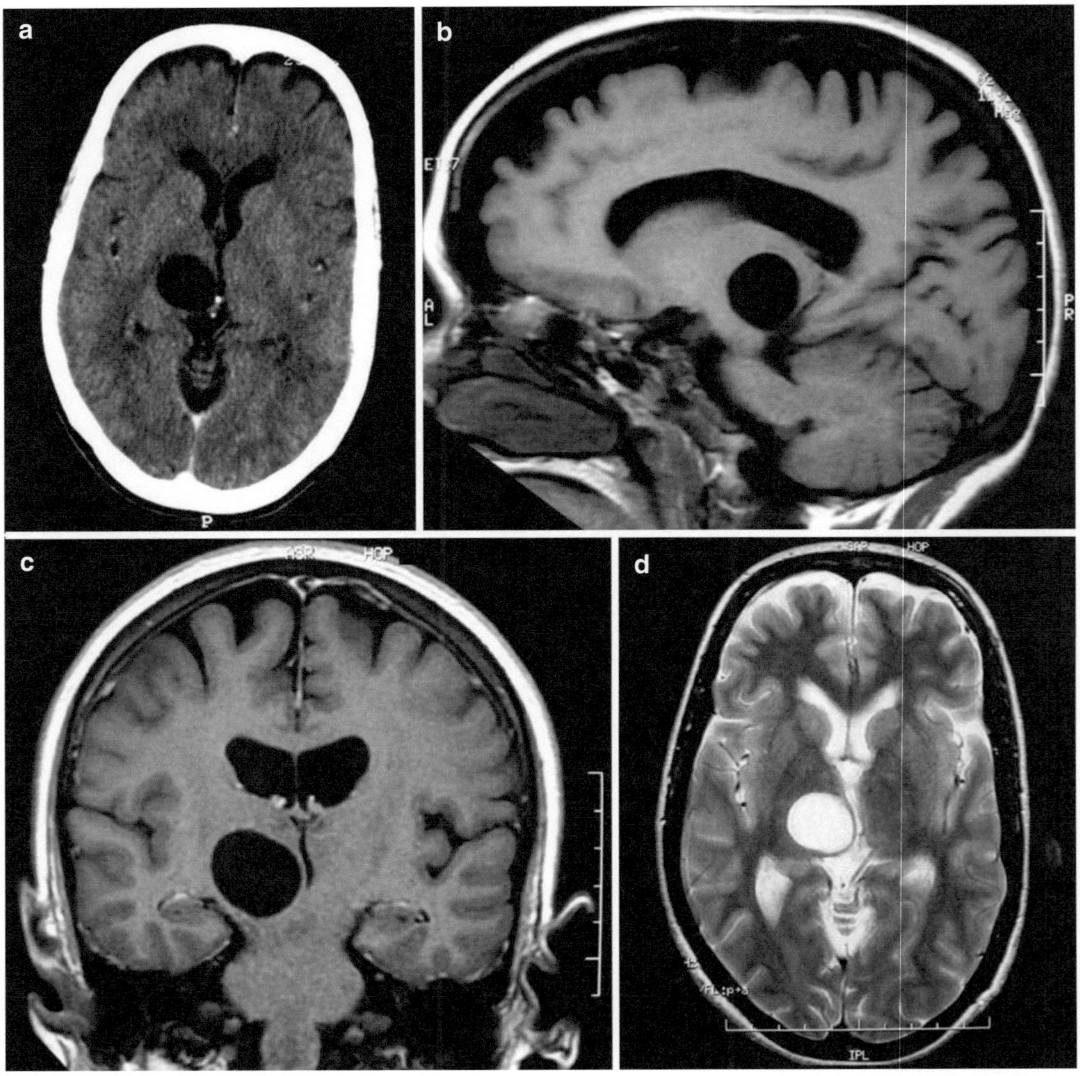

Fig. 11 Thalamo-mesencephalic neuroepithelial cyst mimicking an AC. Axial CT scan with contrast injection (**a**), sagittal (**b**) and coronal T1-weighted MRI (**c**), and axial T2-weighted MRI (**d**). (Reproduced from Akhaddar A. (2017) Brain Hydatid Disease. In: Atlas of Infections in Neurosurgery and Spinal Surgery. Springer, Cham. https://doi.org/10.1007/978-3-319-60086-4_26; with permission)

6.3 Neuroglial Cysts

Neuroglial cysts (also known as glial cysts or glioependymal cysts) are rare, benign congenital glial-lined cystic lesions developing within the brain white matter. These cysts are often erroneously named and confused with other non-neoplastic cysts particularly ependymal cysts [4, 66].

Neuroglial cysts are classically unilocular with rounded and well-defined borders. They can be intra- or extra-axial and mainly develop in the frontal lobes [Osborn]. On neuroimaging, glial cysts are not easy to differentiate from ACs. Hence, they are characterized as CSF-like parenchymal cystic collections without surrounding edema. Neuroglial cysts do not show calcifications on CT scan and they do not enhance with gadolinium on MR imaging [4]. The cyst content is usually suppressed on T2 FLAIR sequences [66].

7 Dandy-Walker Malformations

Dandy-Walker malformation (DWM) is the most common posterior fossa malformation, characterized by a triad of the following congenital anomalies [11]:

1. Agenesis or hypoplasia of the vermis and cephalad rotation of the vermian remnant
2. Dilatation of the fourth ventricle extending posteriorly with an enlarged posterior fossa
3. Supratentorial hydrocephalus

The Dandy-Walker variant is a less severe form of DWM in which there is less noticeable vermian hypoplasia, partial obstruction to the fourth ventricle but without enlargement of the posterior fossa (or only moderate enlargement). Supratentorial hydrocephalus may or may not be present.

Classically, retrocerebellar ACs may be confused with DWM or its variant.

The majority of cases of DWM manifest during the first year of life (rarely among adults) with symptoms of hydrocephalus and various associated neurological symptoms. Macrocephaly is the most common manifestation in about 80% of patients but older children may present with symptoms of elevated intracranial pressure [15, 23]. Many CNS and systemic anomalies may be associated with DWM.

MR imaging is the modality of choice for the assessment of DWM, although both CT scan and ultrasound will demonstrate significant findings (Figs. 12 and 13). Communication between the third and the fourth ventricles is important to know because some cases of DWM may be associated with an aqueductal stenosis (sometimes called triventricular hydrocephalus). CSF flow study on Cine MRI is recommended to better assess this communication [15, 23].

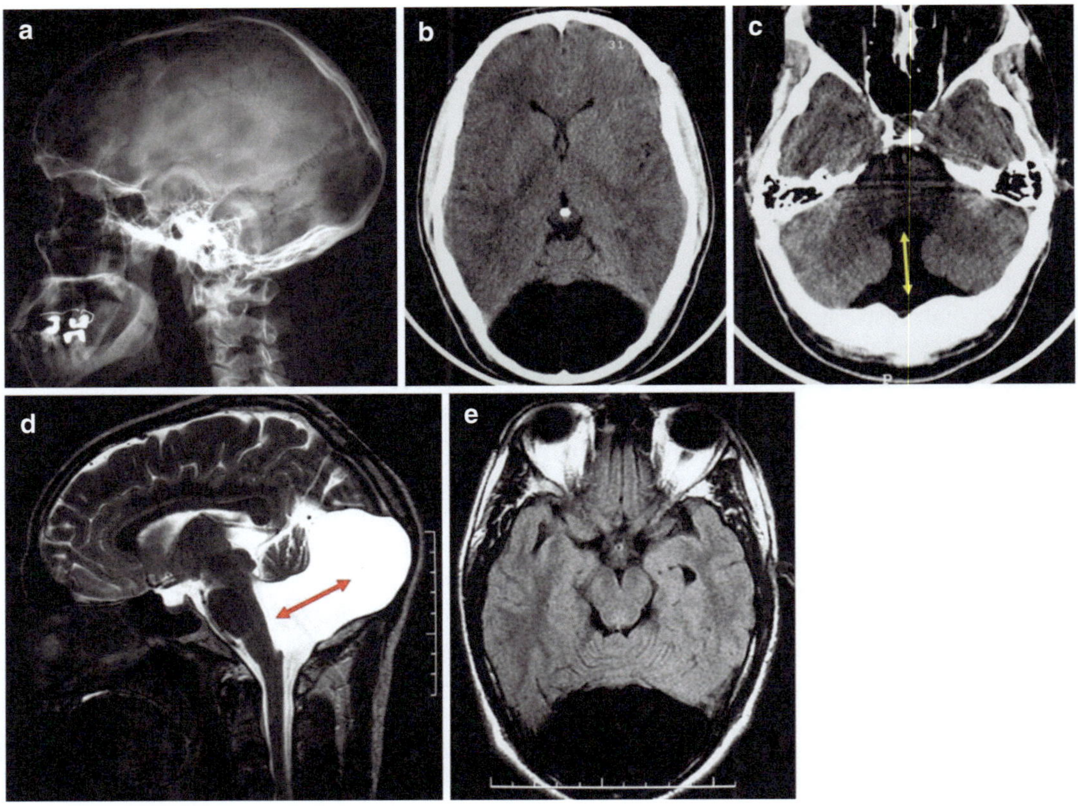

Fig. 12 Dandy-Walker malformation in an adult. Lateral skull plain radiography (**a**), axial CT scan (**b** and **c**), sagittal T2-weighted MR image (**d**), and axial FLAIR sequence (**e**), and coronal T2-weighted MR image (**d**) showing the dilatation of the fourth ventricle extending posteriorly (double arrows) with an enlarged posterior fossa but without any hydrocephalus

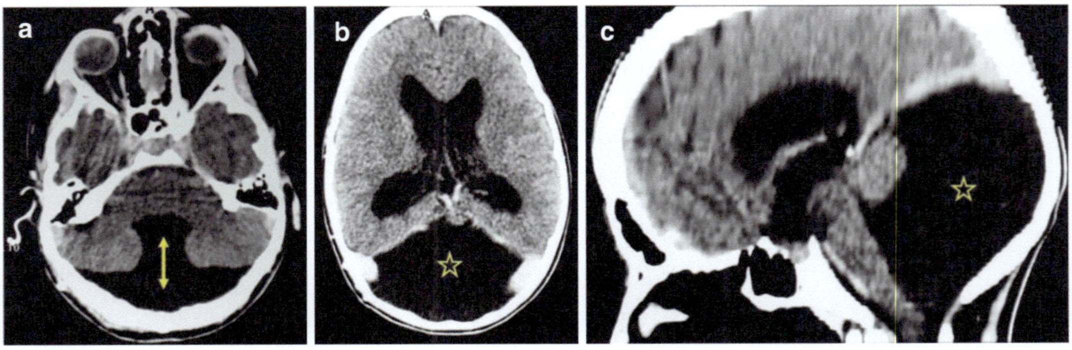

Fig. 13 Dandy-Walker malformation in a child. Axial (**a** and **b**) and sagittal reconstruction CT scan (**c**) showing the dilatation of the fourth ventricle extending posteriorly (double arrows) with an enlarged posterior fossa (stars) and a supratentorial hydrocephalus

8 Schizencephaly

Schizencephaly is a rare congenital disorder of the brain cortical development that is characterized by a CSF-filled cleft which is lined by gray matter and extends from the pial surface of the cortex to the ependyma of the lateral ventricle [17, 36]. This defect allows direct communication between the lateral ventricle and the subarachnoid space. Unilateral or bilateral, the majority of schizencephaly involves the posterior frontal or parietal lobes (perisylvian region). This congenital affection is frequently associated with other cerebral anomalies such as cortical dysplasia, heterotopic gray matter, absent septum pellucidum, or dysgenesis of the corpus callosum [17, 31, 36].

Identification of gray matter lining the cleft is the pathognomonic finding in differentiating schizencephaly from both ACs and porencephaly. This disorder is best demonstrated on MRI [17, 36].

9 Neonatal Hypoxic-Ischemic Encephalopathy

Neonatal hypoxic-ischemic encephalopathy refers to the perinatal asphyxia secondary to the brain hypoxic-ischemic injury with complex and severe neurodevelopmental sequelae [9]. Hypoxic-ischemic encephalopathy is one of the most common causes of cerebral palsy and other severe neurological deficits in children.

It results from the destruction of a previously normal brain by an in-utero vascular accident, infection, or maternal exposure to drugs, smoking, or radiation [72]. This can manifest in different ways, depending on the severity/time of hypoxia and age of the patient [9, 18, 78]. The typical patterns, in terms of the timing of the insult, are expected as follows:

- **Hydranencephaly and porencephaly** as illustrated in Fig. 14, in patients born before 28 weeks of gestation.
- **Periventricular leukomalacia**, in those born between 32 and 36 weeks of gestation.
- **Multicystic encephalomalacia** as illustrated in Fig. 15, in those born at 39 or 40 weeks of gestation.

On neuroimaging, CT scan is the least sensitive modality for evaluation of hypoxic-ischemic encephalopathy because of reduced parenchymal contrast resolution in the neonatal brain. MRI is the most sensitive and specific imaging technique for examining infants with suspected hypoxic-ischemic brain injury [9, 78]. In addition, conventional pulse sequences can help to eliminate other etiologies of encephalopathy such as congenital malformations, bleeding, cerebral infarction, or tumors.

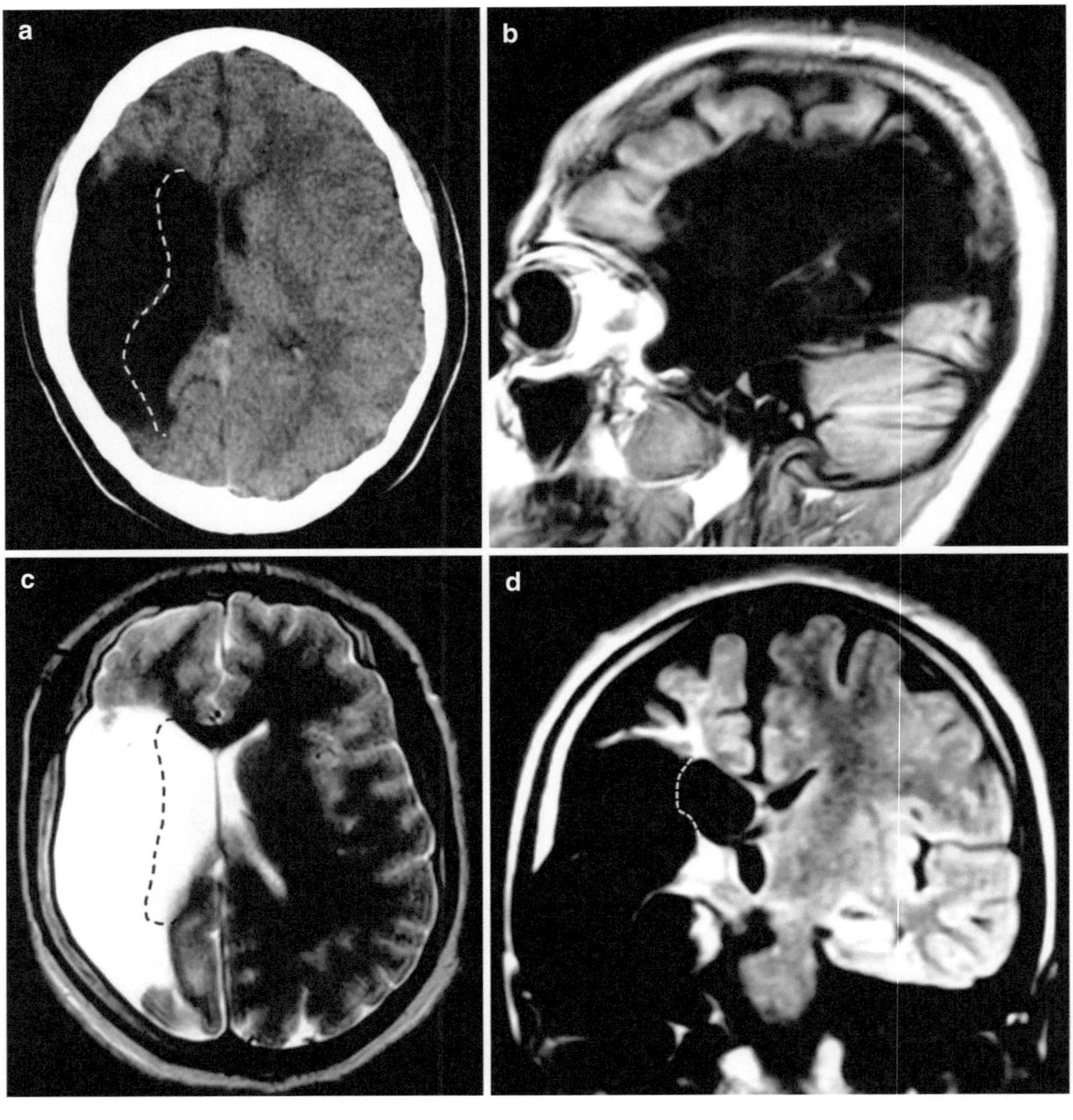

Fig. 14 Hypoxic-ischemic encephalopathy in a child presenting with a right cerebral palsy. Axial CT scan (**a**), sagittal T1- (**b**) and axial T2-weighted MR images (**c**), and coronal FLAIR sequence (**d**) showing resorption of the area corresponding to the right middle cerebral artery that was replaced with CSF mimicking a congenital AC. Note the adjacent sulcal and ventricular enlargement without mass effect

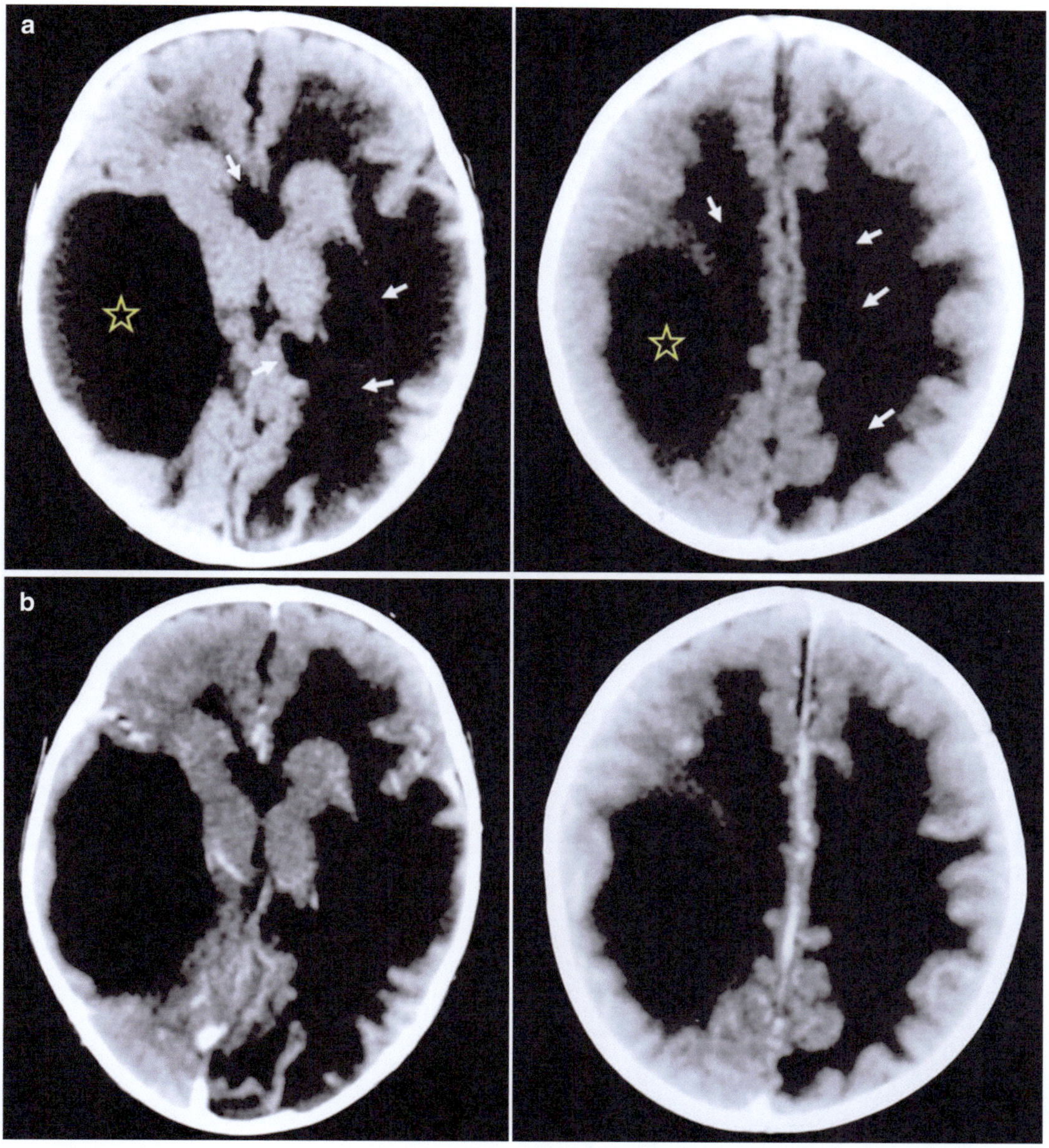

Fig. 15 Multicystic encephalomalacia (stars and arrows) in a child secondary to a severe meningoencephalitis. Axial CT scan before (**a**) and after (**b**) contrast injection

10 Encephalomalacia

Encephalomalacia is a "nonspecific name" of the end result of liquefactive necrosis of brain parenchyma which corresponds to a tissue loss. This condition usually occurs after cerebral ischemia, cerebral infection, inflammation, toxins, hemorrhagic stroke, traumatic brain injury, or surgery [32, 43, 62]. Encephalomalacia is often surrounded by an area of brain gliosis, which is the proliferation of glial cells in response to an injury.

All age categories may be involved, even for patients in utero (please refer to *Multicystic Encephalomalacia* in Sect. 9) [9, 78]. The majority of encephalomalacias are either asymptomatic, or manifest as motor or sensory deficits, or represent a focus of seizure.

On CT scan, areas of encephalomalacia are hypodense or somewhat higher than CSF. A key finding in encephalomalacia is adjacent sulcal or ventricular enlargement without mass effect (Figs. 16 and 17).

On MRI, the cavity is typically isointense to CSF on all sequences (because the cavity is filled

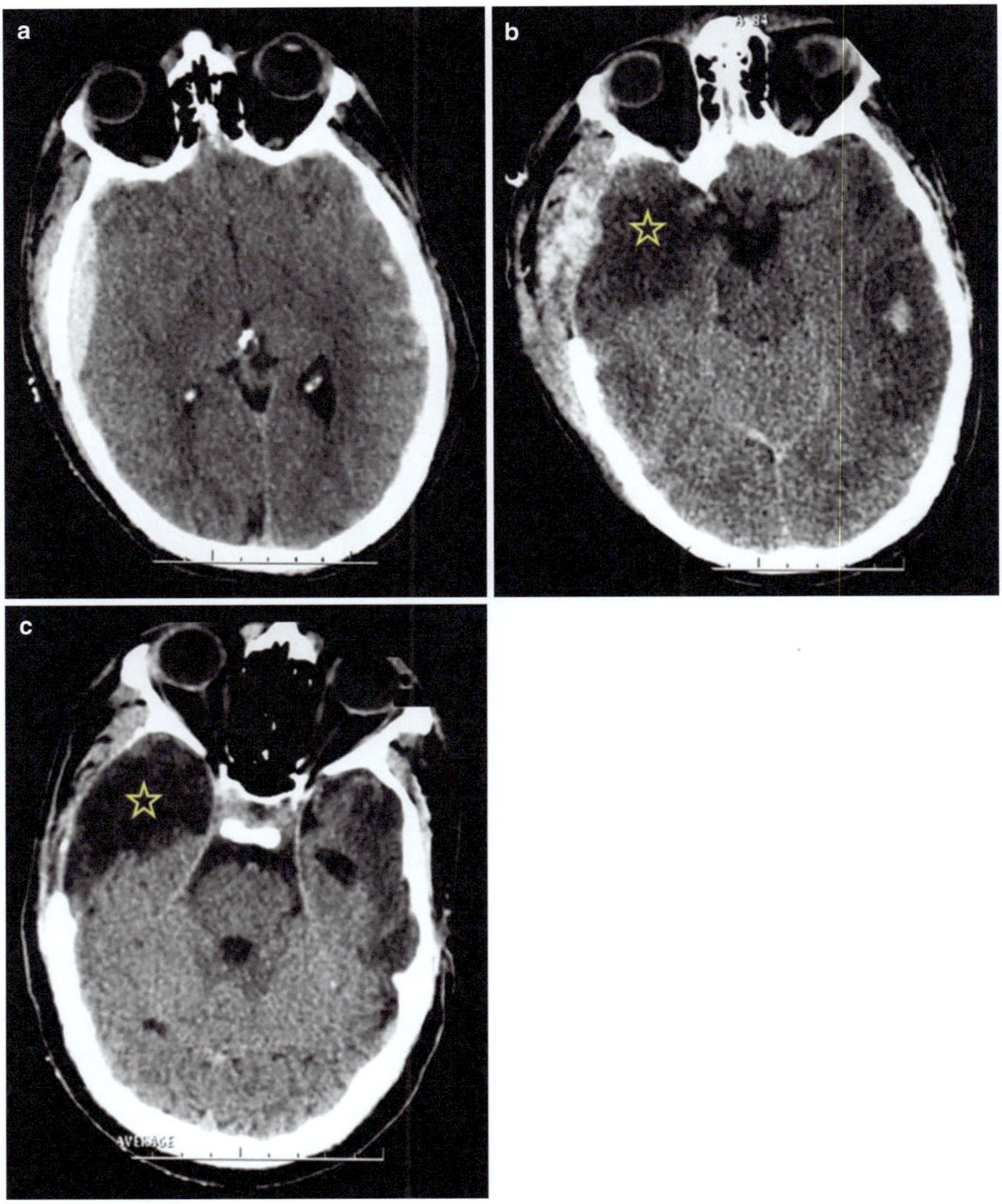

Fig. 16 Post-traumatic encephalomalacia (stars). Axial CT scan showing a right temporal acute extradural hematoma following a head injury (**a**). Post-operative CT scan 4 days (**b**) and 12 months later (**c**)

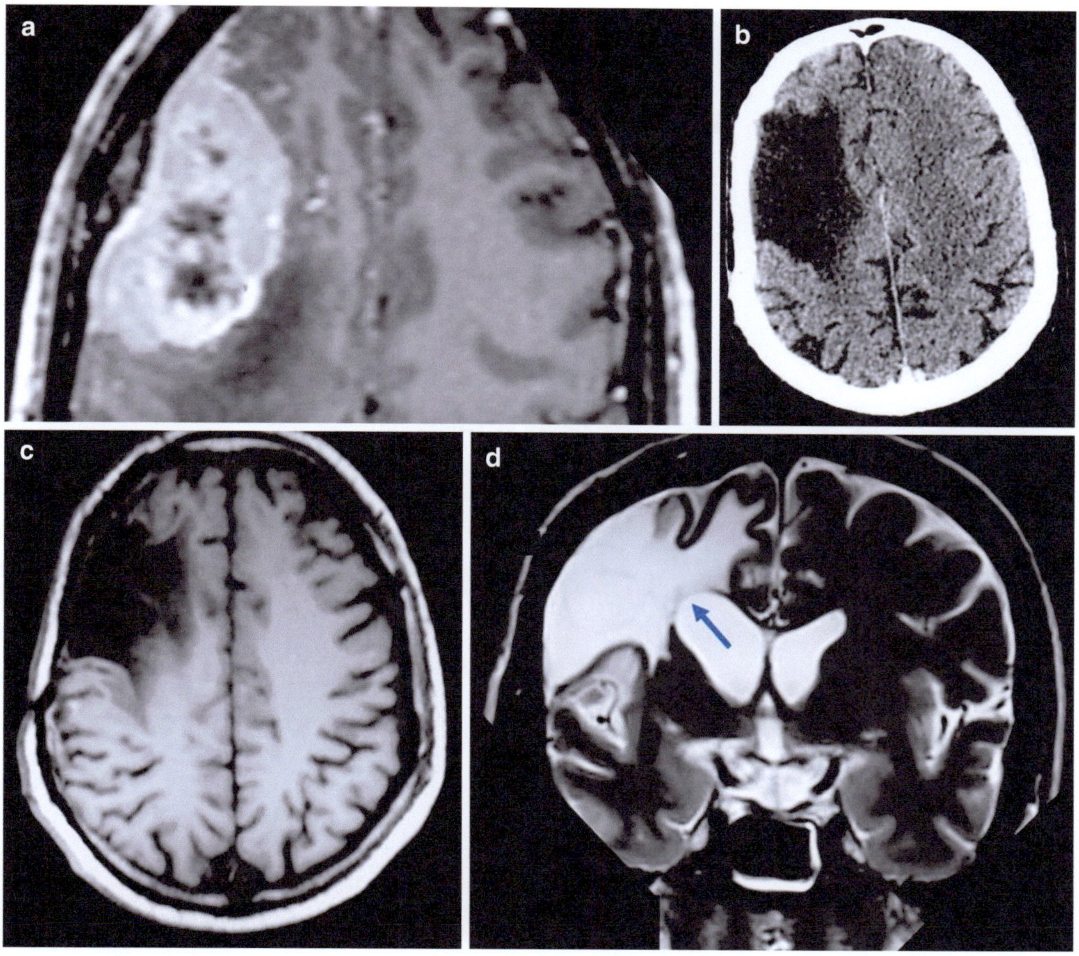

Fig. 17 Preoperative axial T1-weighted image showing a meningioma of the right frontal convexity (**a**). Postopearative axial CT scan (**b**), on axial T1- (**c**) and on coronal T2-weighted images (**d**) revealing frontal area of encephalomalacia (resection cavity). Note enlargement of the right frontal ventricular horn (arrow) without mass effect

with CSF): T1 hypointense, T2 hyperintense, and FLAIR hypointense with brain parenchyma volume loss (Figs. 17, 18, and 19) [32, 43]. However, encephalomalacia is very often associated with adjacent gliosis which is hyperintense on FLAIR images.

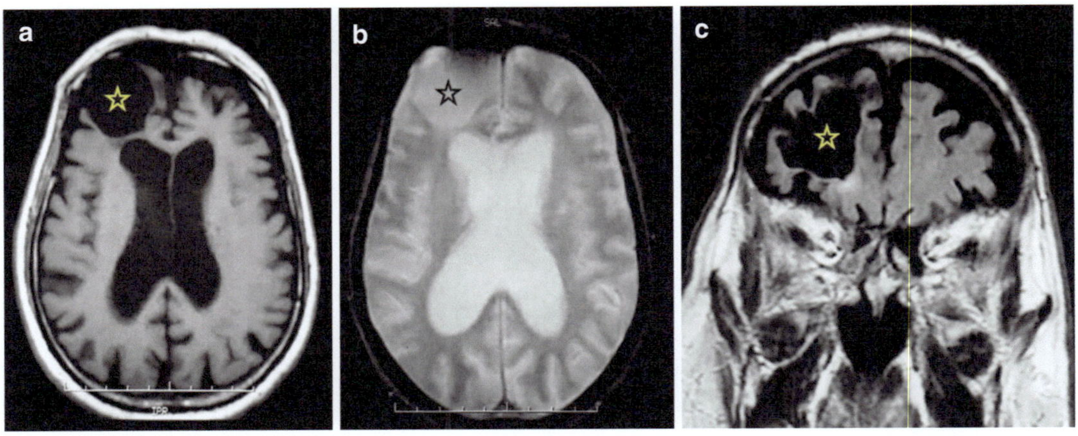

Fig. 18 Post-traumatic encephalomalacia on the right frontal area (stars). Axial T1- (**a**) and T2-weighted MR images (**b**) and coronal FLAIR sequence (**c**)

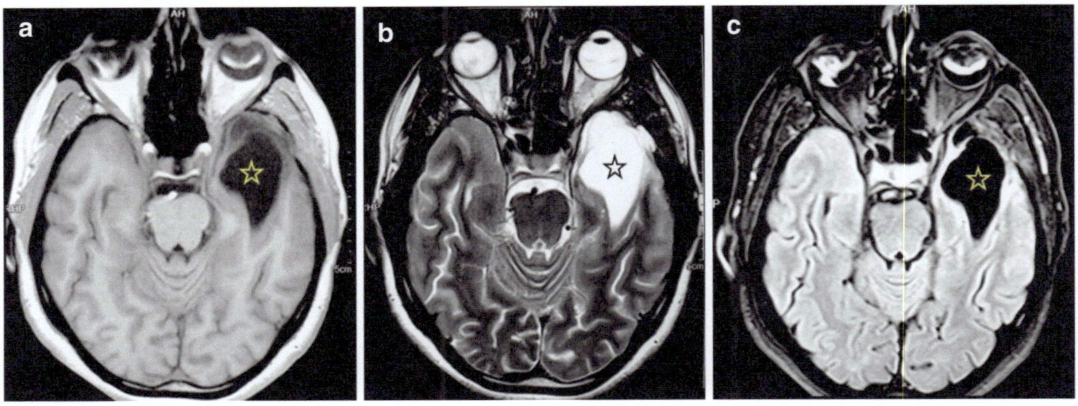

Fig. 19 Post-traumatic encephalomalacia on the left temporal area (stars). Axial T1- (**a**) and T2-weighted MR images (**b**) and on FLAIR sequence (**c**)

11 Infectious Lesions

11.1 Subdural Empyemas

Intracranial subdural empyema is a pyogenic collection that developed in the subdural space. ENT and oral cavity infections are the most common contiguous sources of subdural empyema. Other forms may be secondary to meningitis, cranial bone osteomyelitis, post-operative/traumatic infections, or hematogenous spreading from a distant cause of sepsis. More subdural empyemas are located over the convexity, in the parafalcine region or in the posterior fossa near the mastoids. The diagnosis should be considered in any patient who presents with fever, meningitis, or focal neurological deficits with or without seizures. Inflammatory biomarkers and the white blood cell count may help in the diagnosis but they are not specific and changeable in their expression [1, 30].

On CT scan, subdural empyema usually is visible as an isodense or low-density crescentic subdural lesion compared with adjacent brain edema [30]. The peripheral margins of the suppurative collections are better demonstrated after contrast medium injection (Fig. 20). Association with paranasal sinusitis or mastoiditis is not rare. On MRI, the majority of subdural empyemas seen on

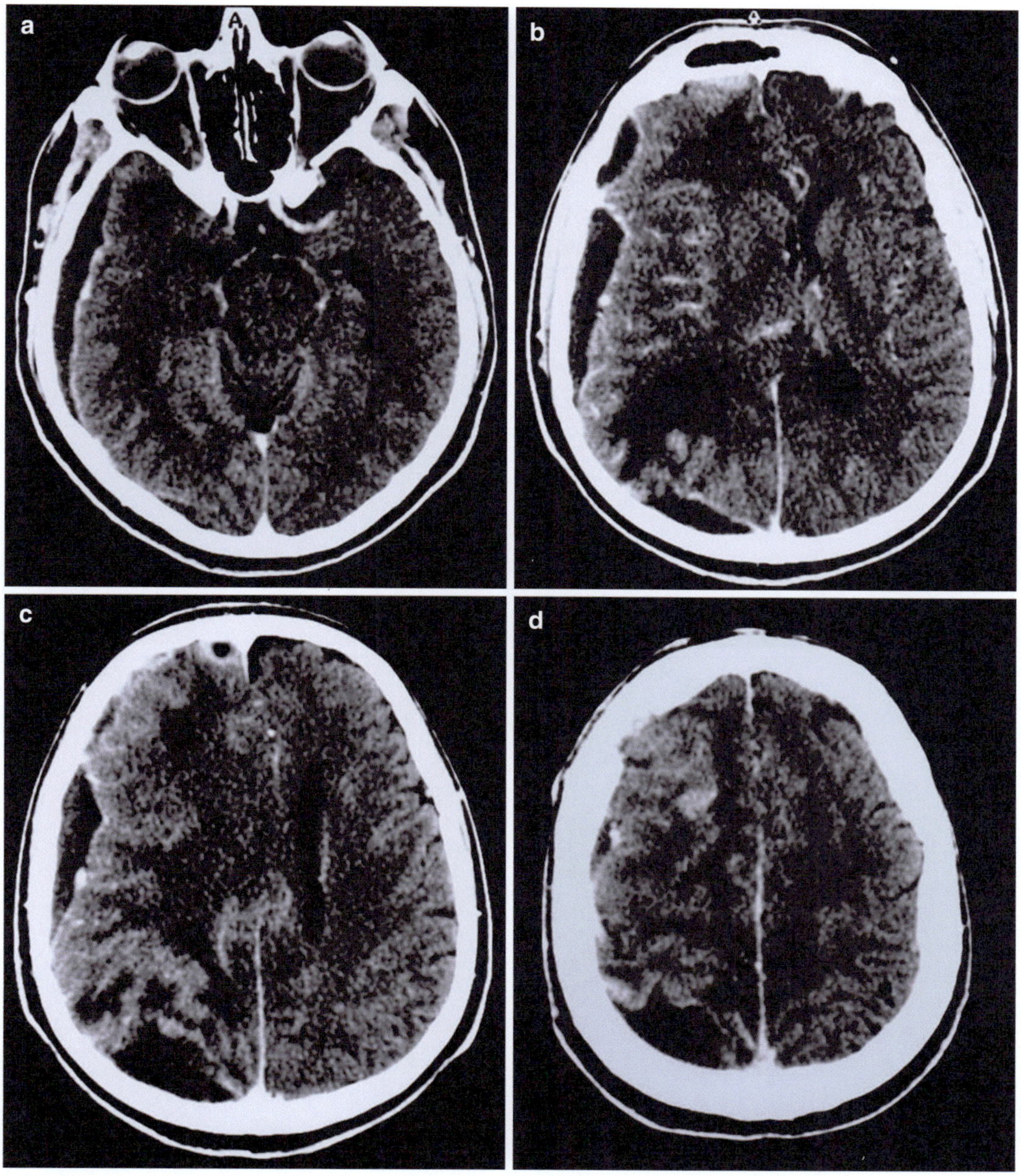

Fig. 20 Case 1. Axial cranial enhanced CT scan showing multiple subdural empyemas in the right side (**a**–**d**). (Reproduced from Akhaddar A. (2017) Cranial Subdural Empyemas. In: Atlas of Infections in Neurosurgery and Spinal Surgery. Springer, Cham. https://doi.org/10.1007/978-3-319-60086-4_6; with permission)

T1-weighted imaging are isointense due to their proteinaceous content, while the empyema appears isointense to low signal and high signal on T2-weighted images. After gadolinium injection, the contiguous dura matter appears markedly enhanced. Also, there is restricted DWI (Fig. 21) and hypointensity on ADC images [1]. Different sources of infection can be seen in adjacent structures that support the diagnosis. In severe clinical presentations, extensive cerebral edema, encephalitis, brain abscess, thrombophlebitis, and venous infarction are encountered.

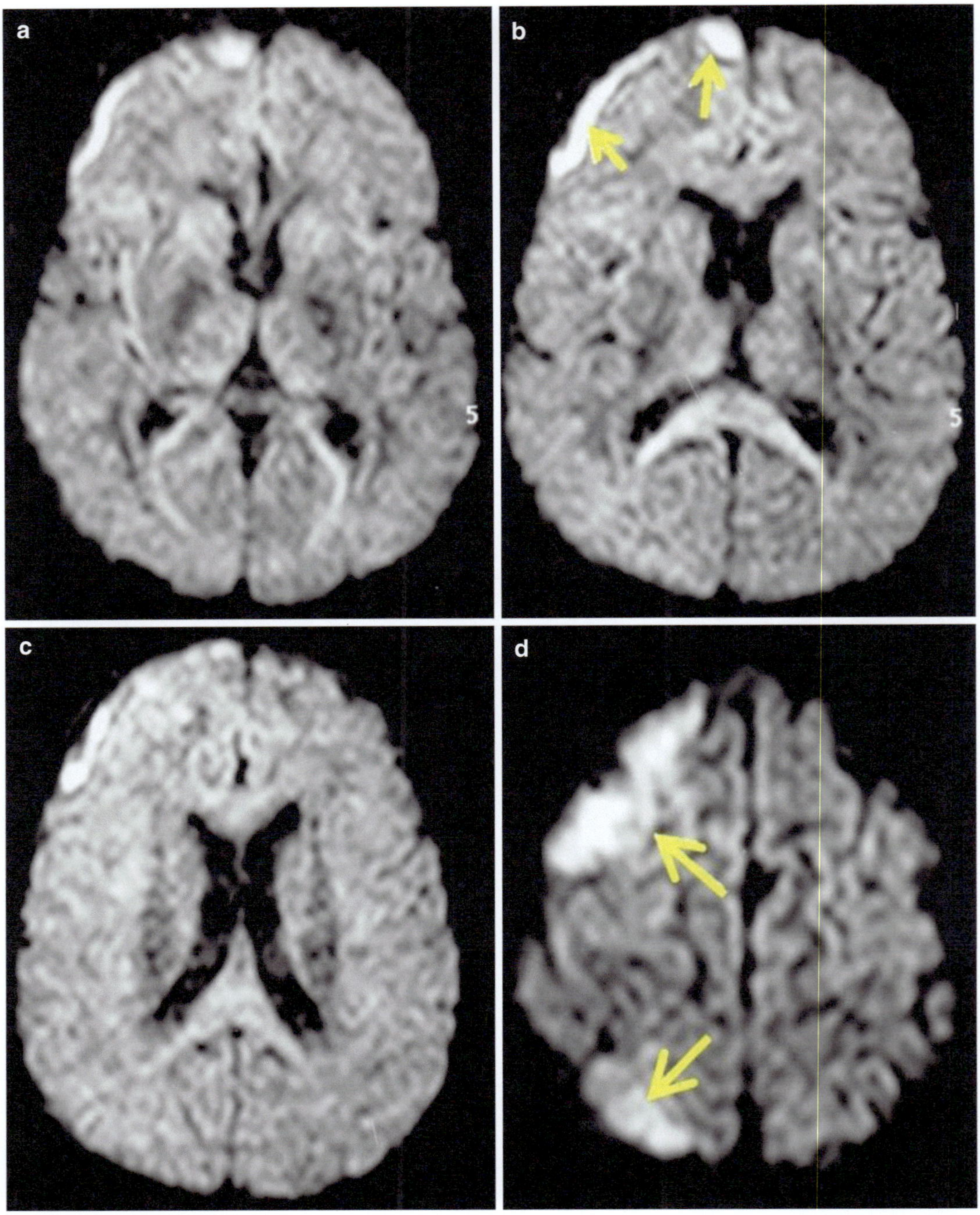

Fig. 21 Case 1. Axial cranial diffusion-weighted MRI (**a**–**d**). Subdural empyemas have high signal indicating restricted diffusion (bright signal) (arrows). (Reproduced from Akhaddar A. (2017) Cranial Subdural Empyemas. In: Atlas of Infections in Neurosurgery and Spinal Surgery. Springer, Cham. https://doi.org/10.1007/978-3-319-60086-4_6; with permission)

11.2 Neurocysticercosis

The most common parasitic infection of the CNS is neurocysticercosis which is caused by the larva of the tapeworm *Taenia solium*. This infection represents the leading cause of epilepsy in developing countries. Two forms of cysts tend to develop in the brain: simple cysts (Cysticercus cellulosae) and multiples cysts (Cysticercus racemosus). Both cystic forms may involve brain parenchyma and subarachnoid spaces as well as the intracerebral ventricles [44].

Most neurocysticercosis cysts are similar in appearance to an AC with a signal similar to that of the CSF on T1- and T2-weighted images, without restricted diffusion and without significant enhancement by gadolinium [59]. It is well known that the individual scolex is difficult to detect on MR imaging. However, the cystic parasites are very likely to be multiloculated. In addition, there are other findings that suggest this parasitic lesion on brain imaging: medical history and byimmunology workup (enzyme-linked immunosorbent assay and electroimmunotransfer blot assay) [54]. Conversely, these cystic lesions may be associated with cerebral calcifications that are best detected on CT scan.

11.3 Hydatid Cysts

Hydatidosis is the larval stage of the tapeworm *Echinococcus granulosus*. This parasitic disease often happens in the liver and lungs. Cerebral cysts are rare, seen in only 2% of cases, and are usually solitary, spherical, unilocular, subcortical, and supratentorial (Fig. 22). Other rare sites may be involved such as posterior fossa, subarachnoid spaces, and ventricular system (Fig. 23). Presenting symptoms depends on the area involved and the cystic size. However, the most common signs and symptoms are those of intracranial hypertension, neurologic deficits, seizures, and mental changes [69, 81].

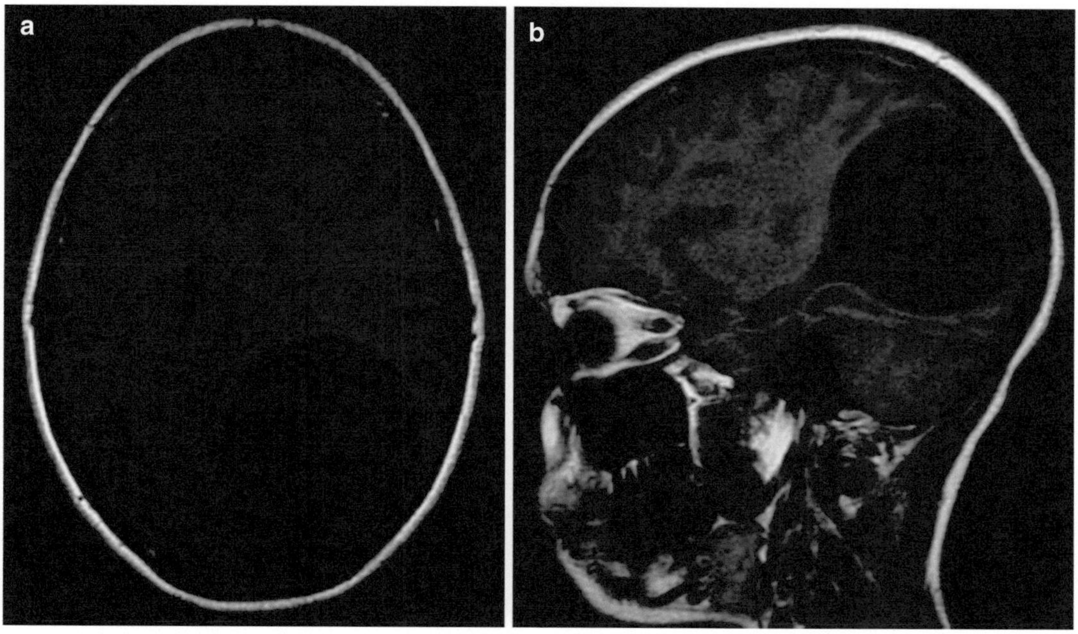

Fig. 22 Brain hydatid cyst. Large well-defined unilocular cystic lesion in the left parieto-occipital region without marginal edema on axial (**a**) and sagittal (**b**) T1-weighted MRI, axial T2-weighted MRI (**c**), and coronal FLAIR sequence (**d**). (Reproduced from Akhaddar A. (2017) Brain Hydatid Disease. In: Atlas of Infections in Neurosurgery and Spinal Surgery. Springer, Cham. https://doi.org/10.1007/978-3-319-60086-4_26; with permission)

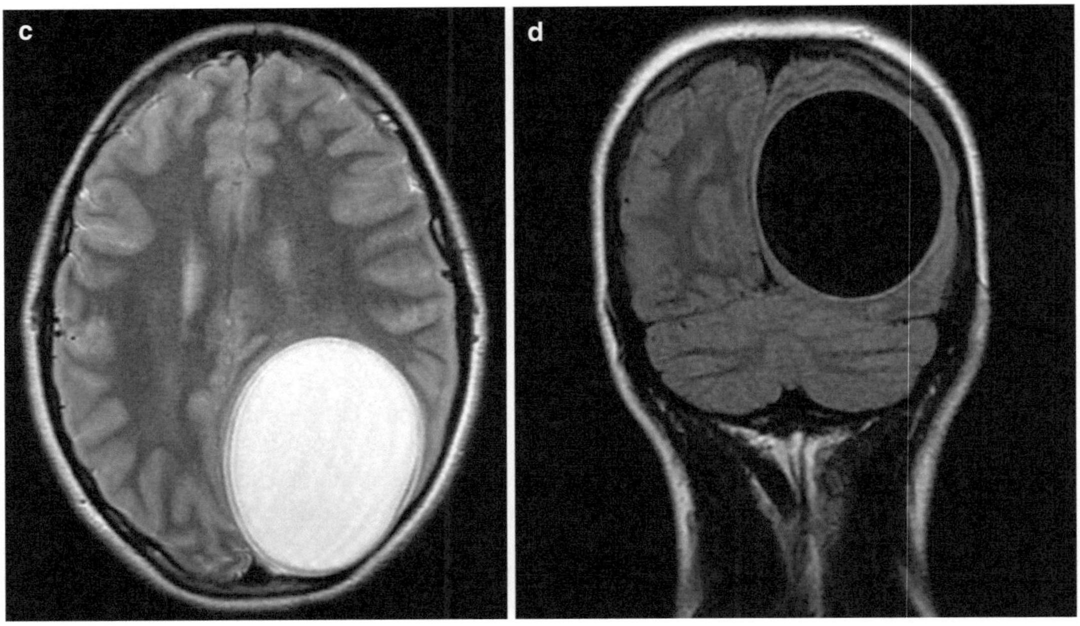

Fig. 22 (continued)

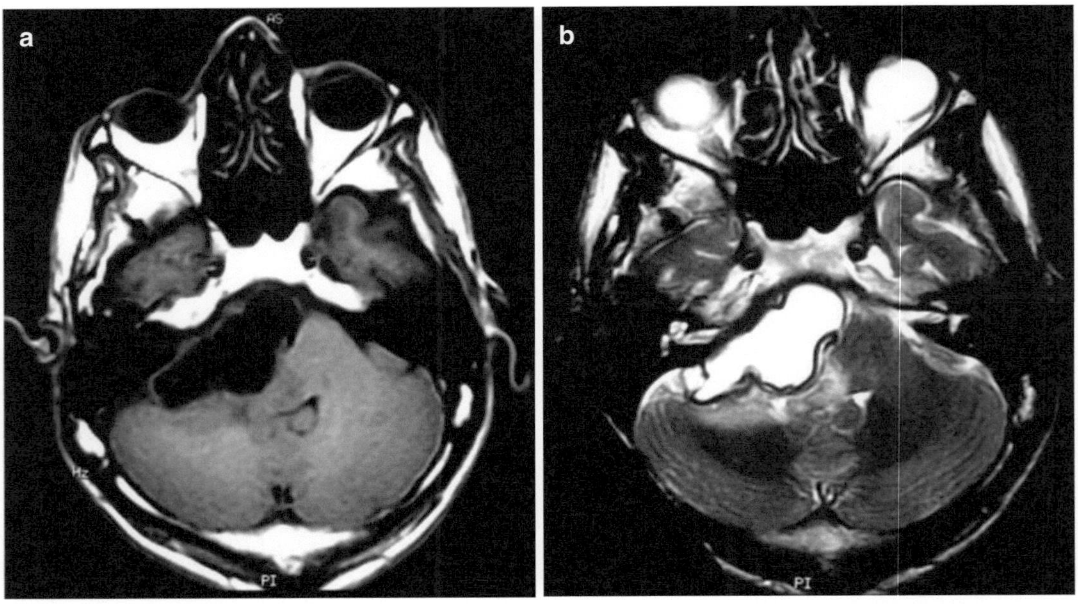

Fig. 23 Intracranial hydatid cyst of the right cerebellopontine angle with brainstem compression. Axial T1-weighted MRI (**a**), FLAIR sequence (**b**), T2-weighted MRI (**c**), and apparent diffusion coefficient map (**d**). (Reproduced from Akhaddar A. (2017) Brain Hydatid Disease. In: Atlas of Infections in Neurosurgery and Spinal Surgery. Springer, Cham. https://doi.org/10.1007/978-3-319-60086-4_26; with permission)

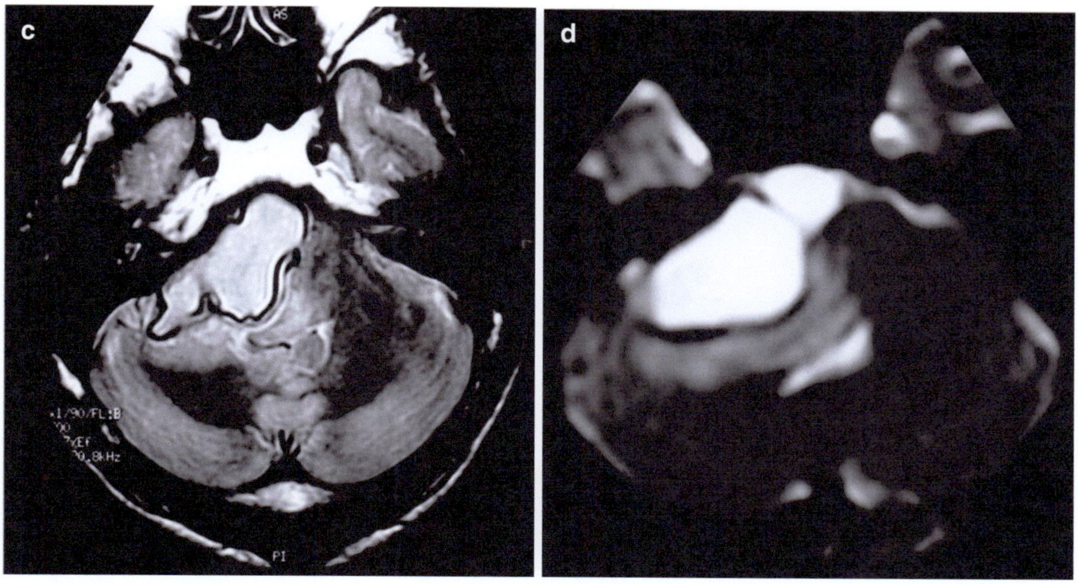

Fig. 23 (continued)

On CT scan or MR imaging examination, the hydatid lesions have a characteristic appearance: large, spherical, unilocular cystic masses that are well limited from the contiguous brain parenchyma. Typically, the cyst fluid is isodense with CSF on CT scans and isointense with CSF on MR imaging studies without surrounding edema or contrast enhancement (Fig. 22) [69, 81]. We have recently reported a rare case of unsuspected hydatid cyst in the cerebellopontine area [12]. Proton MR spectroscopy may be used to identify the metabolic contents of the cystic collection. Occasionally, some forms with internal septations suggest "daughter cysts" inside the unilocular mass. In infected forms, the cystic contents may be heterogeneous with ring enhancement. Calcifications of the cyst wall are rare and better identified on CT imaging.

12 Giant Intracranial Aneurysms

Although rare, some giant intracranial aneurysms may be confused with various intracranial cystic lesions including parasellar AC and hydatid cysts [21, 75]. The possibility of such aneurysms should always be considered in evaluating cyst-mimicking lesions, especially in the peri-sellar region, to avoid potentially disastrous consequences. Preoperative angiographic studies will rapidly help correct this differential diagnosis (Fig. 24).

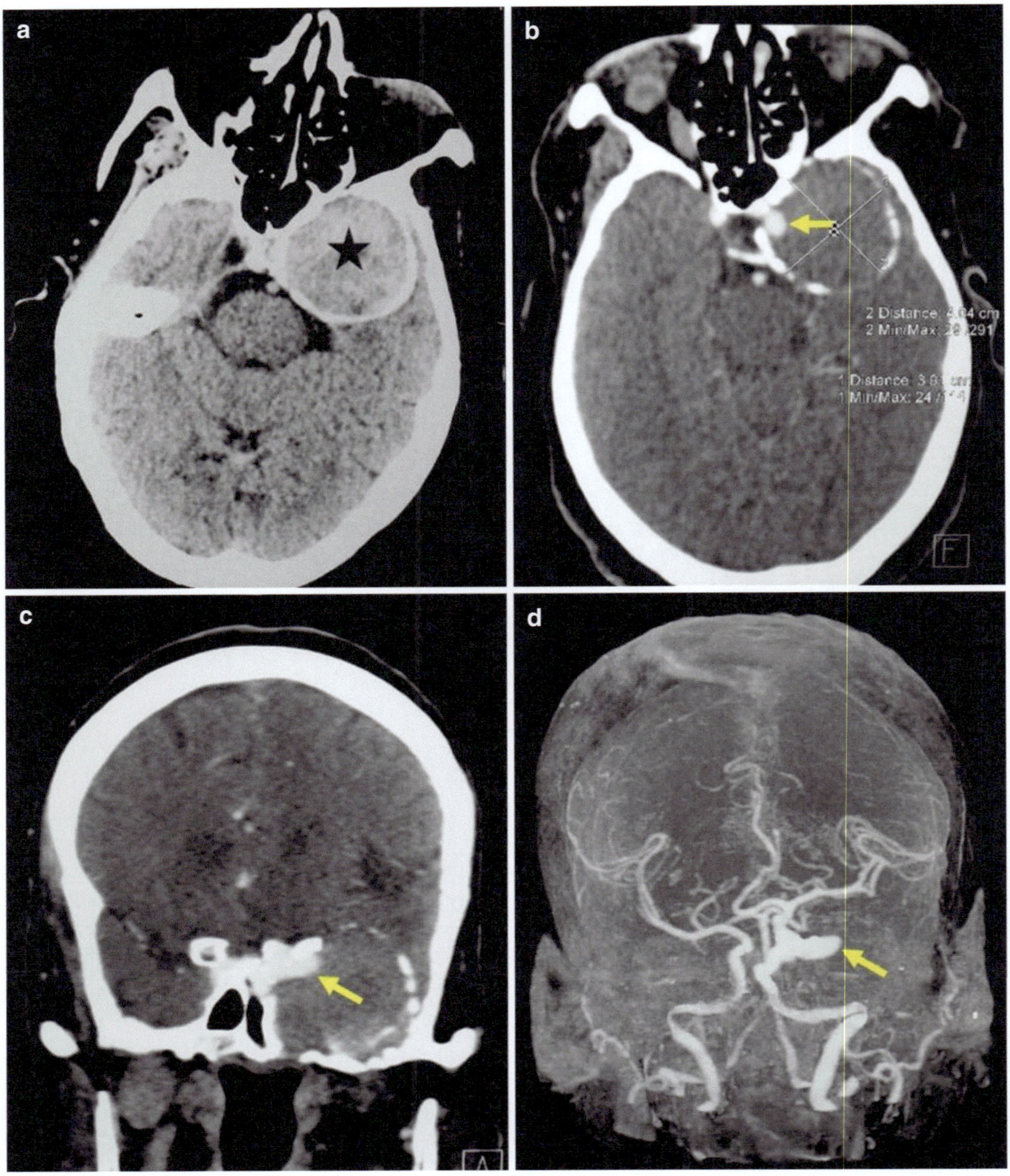

Fig. 24 Giant intracranial carotid artery aneurysm on the left parasellar side. Axial CT scan (**a**), axial (**b**) and coronal (**c**) CT-angiography, and angio-MR image (**d**) showing the endoluminal circulating part of the aneurysm (arrows)

13 Intraventricular Cysts

Intraventricular ACs are very rare. Other intraventricular cystic lesions include colloid cysts, subependymal cysts, and choroid plexus cysts. A colloid cyst is most often located at the foramen of Monro and usually has a characteristically high CT attenuation.

13.1 Colloid Cysts

Colloid cysts are benign neuroepithelial lined cysts that commonly occur in the antero-superior part of the third ventricle, near the foramen of Monro. The cyst content is frequently composed of fragments of necrotic inflammatory cells with occasional lipid droplets (rich in proteins and cholesterol). Although usually asymptomatic due to their small size, these cysts can occasionally present with various neurological signs and symptoms if they rich a large size [20]. Classically, rapid neurological deterioration is related to the sudden development of obstructive hydrocephalus. On the CT scan, these cysts are usually hyperdense, but some of them may be iso- or hypodense compared to CSF attenuation. On MR imaging, colloid cysts are often hyperintense on T1- and iso/hypointense on T2-weighted images (low signal intensity on T2 predicts a difficult surgical aspiration) (Fig. 25). Generally, the MR imaging appearance has a lack of specificities because some forms may be confused with intraventricular ACs. Interestingly, most colloid cysts show increased signal intensity on FLAIR sequences and demonstrate decreased signal intensity on diffusion-weighted sequences. Peripheral rim enhancement is unusual and calcifications are rare [20, 38].

13.2 Choroid Fissure Cysts

Choroid or choroidal fissure cysts (CFC) are benign congenital intracranial cysts occurring within the choroidal fissure just medial to the temporal horn of the lateral ventricle, between the fornix and thalamus. For many authors, CFC are not a true distinct neuropathological entity but are considered as a subtype of ACs [7, 24]. CFC are true CSF-containing cysts that can develop anywhere along the choroid fissure. These cysts are frequently small between 10 and 20 mm in size. Most CFC are asymptomatic and discovered incidentally. However, a rare proportion of them may cause seizures due to mass effect within the temporal lobe [6].

The CT scans and MR imaging characteristics are similar with respect to CSF density/signal without calcification, surrounding cerebral edema or contrast enhancement. The coronal images are superior to other imaging projections to demonstrate the relationship between the cystic lesion and the choroid fissure [6, 24]. Typically,

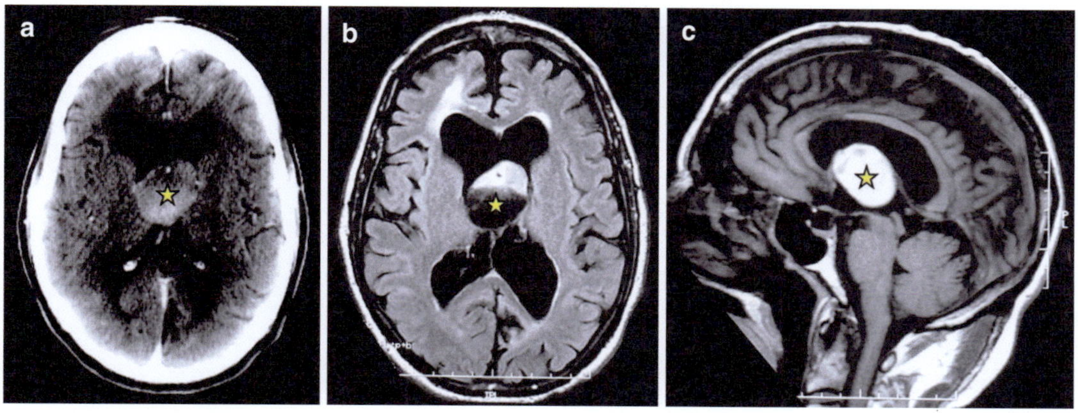

Fig. 25 Colloid cyst of the third ventricle (stars). Axial CT scan (**a**), axial FLAIR sequence (**b**), and (**c**) sagittal T1-weighted MR image

the choroid plexus is medially displaced in the case of an "intraventricular" choroid **plexus** cyst and laterally displaced in the case of "arachnoid" choroid **fissure** cyst [7, 56].

13.3 Choroid Plexus Cysts

Choroid plexus cysts (CPC) are CSF fluid-filled collections found associated with the choroid plexus of the intracranial ventricular system. They are typically less than 10 mm in diameter and are commonly located within the body of choroid plexus cysts, especially in the atrium, but they can develop throughout the ventricular system. They are among the most common intracranial cysts occurring at both ends of the age spectrum [56]. They can be congenital, diagnosed in the prenatal/neonatal period, or acquired (degenerative) seen at autopsy in the elderly. CPC are almost always asymptomatic and are found incidentally on neuroimaging studies. The majority of isolated congenital CPC have a benign course and regress during the third trimester or shortly after birth. Rarely, CPC may be associated with other anomalies, particularly in trisomic patients [57]. Some rare symptomatic patients with very large cysts may require surgery [41].

On imaging, differentiation between ACs and CPC is difficult. The lesions are isodense and isointense with CSF on CT scan and MR imaging, respectively, with no contrast enhancement [41]. As cited previously, ventricular CPC displace the choroid plexus medially.

13.4 Ventricular Diverticula

Ventricular diverticula are rare cystic subpial collections of CSF resulting from rupture of the ependymal wall of the intracranial ventricular system in cases of severe long standing obstructive hydrocephalus. These cystic herniations can occur at any point in the four cavities of the ventricular system; however, most cases originate from the atrium or the posterior wall of the third ventricle [3, 40]. Because of their rarity, ventricular diverticula could be overlooked or misdiagnosed as another cystic lesion such as an AC. Both types of cystic lesions have similar attenuation and MR imaging signal appearance. Typically, there is an obvious communication between the diverticulum and the ventricular system on MRI (Fig. 26). Nevertheless, in some complex or ambiguous forms, post-contrast ventriculography may be useful for diagnostic confirmation as suggested by Jabaudon et al. [40]. Surgical management of the obstructive hydrocephalus might be helpful in reducing the ventricular dilatation and improving the clinical symptoms (Fig. 26) [3]. A direct surgical approach to the diverticulum itself is therefore generally of no benefit.

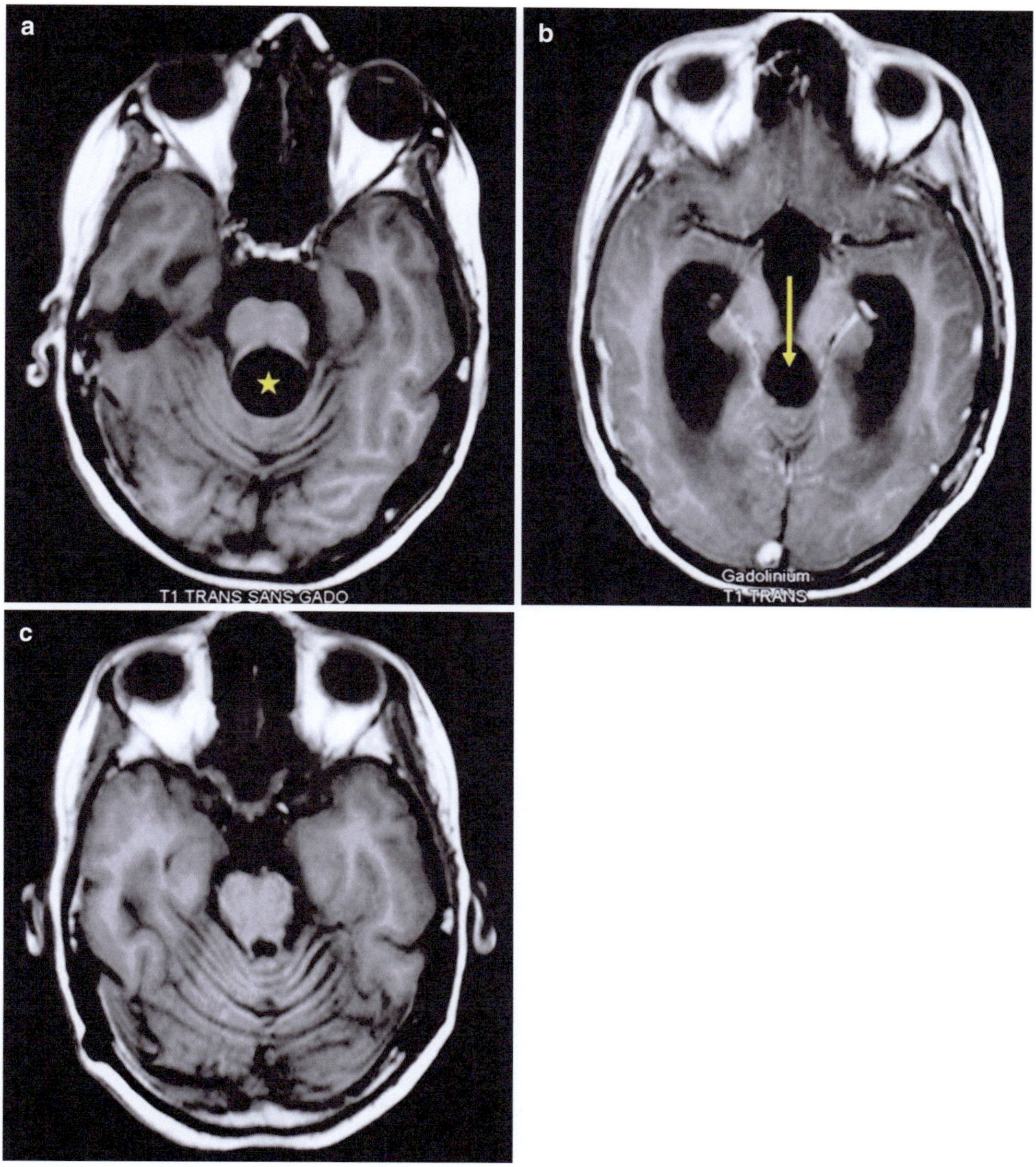

Fig. 26 Ventricular diverticulum of the posterior wall of the third ventricle (star). Preoperative axial T1-weighted MR images (**a**, **b**) showing the communication between the diverticulum and the third ventricle (arrow). Postoperative axial T1-weighted MR image revealing complete resolution of the diverticulum following surgical management of the obstructive hydrocephalus (**c**)

14 Pineal Cysts

Pineal cysts are common on routine imaging and correspond to a benign non-neoplastic cystic lesion. Typically, they manifest as an unilocular cyst within the pineal gland with an MRI signal similar to that of the CSF. The majority of pineal cysts are asymptomatic and smaller than 10 mm [74]. Generally, only large pineal cysts (larger than 15 mm in size) may be symptomatic and cause hydrocephalus, secondary to compression of the aqueduct of Sylvius, or Parinaud syndrome, due to brainstem compression [52]. However, even larger pineal cysts can be asymptomatic and require no neurosurgical intervention [22, 52]. Some authors suggest follow-up based only on clinical indications.

In most cases, pineal cysts present with ring contrast enhancement of the pineal parenchyma, and some contain calcifications. However, cysts involving the pineal region may mimic tumors rather than ACs [22].

15 Cystic Suprasellar Lesions

15.1 Dilated Third Ventricle

An enlarged third ventricle secondary to obstructive hydrocephalus (especially due to congenital aqueductal stenosis between the third and the fourth ventricles) may be misdiagnosed as a suprasellar AC. In patients where the obstruction is partial, there may be no symptoms despite considerable ventricular dilatation. However, the majority of patients with complete aqueductal obstruction present symptoms of increased intracranial pressure such as headaches, nausea, and/or vomiting. Then, fundus examination reveals papilledema (swelling of the optic disk due to increased intracranial pressure).

On neuroimaging, differentiation between suprasellar ACs and a dilated third ventricle may be difficult (Fig. 27). Nevertheless, some distinct features can be definitive. For SAC, the optic chiasm is vertically displaced, the mammillary bod-

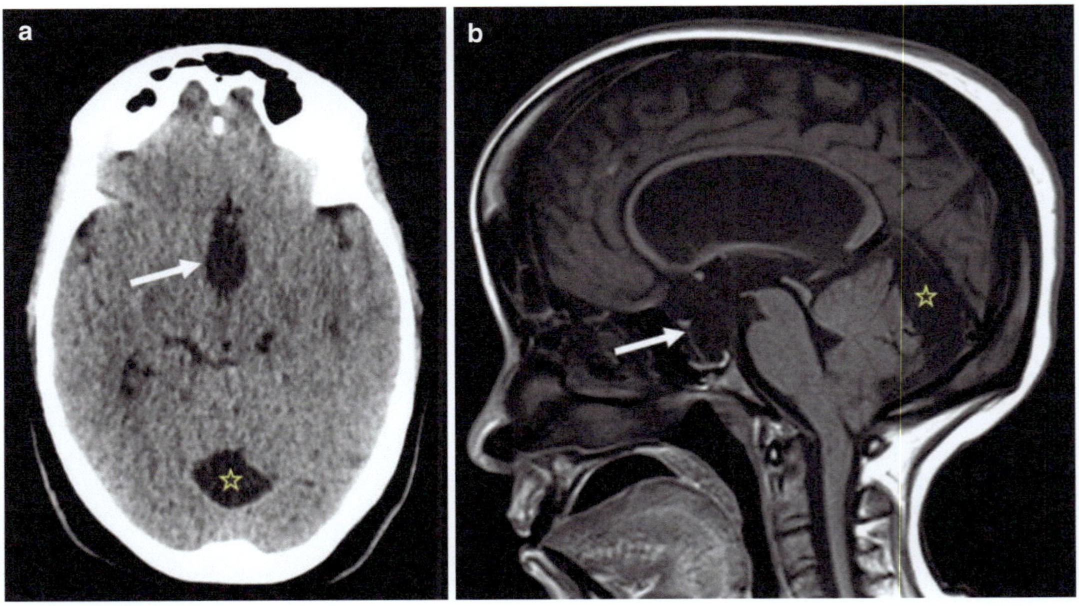

Fig. 27 Axial CT scan (**a**) and sagittal T1-weighted MR image (**b**) showing a hydrocephalus with a dilated third ventricle (arrows) which it was difficult to differentiate from a suprasellar AC. There is also a retrocerebellar AC (stars) in this patient

ies are displaced upwards, and the middle portion of the brainstem is bowed forward. In comparison, the mammillary bodies and the floor of the third ventricle are somewhat displaced down in patients with an enlarged third ventricle [35, 80].

15.2 Rathke's Cleft Cysts

Rathke's cleft cysts (RCC) are congenital collections arising from the embryological remnants of Rathke's pouch. RCC are primarily intrasellar and develop between the anterior and intermediate lobes of the pituitary gland, but can also be found in the suprasellar region [10]. The majority of RCC do not exceed 1 or 2 cm in diameter, they are lined by a single layer of cuboidal epithelium, and the cyst collection is mainly mucoid material. Although most cases are asymptomatic, some patients can present with neurological signs and symptoms due to compression of the optic chiasm, pituitary gland, or hypothalamic system. Classically, there is a female predominance [8].

On MR imaging, the intensity of the signal is variable, depending on cyst content, but without calcification or gadolinium enhancement. Some cases may be associated with a small non-enhancing intracystic nodule. The most suggestive appearance for the diagnosis of RCC is as the following: cystic collection with low to iso signal intensity on T1-weighted and with iso to high signal intensity on T2-weighted MR images. Nevertheless, the intracystic nodule presents high signal intensity on T1-weighted and low signal intensity on T2-weighted MR images [8, 10]. In addition to AC, diagnosis of RCC is often discussed with that of craniopharyngiomas.

15.3 Craniopharyngiomas

Craniopharyngiomas are benign epithelial neoplasms that typically extend above the pituitary gland into the suprasellar area. They are encountered in both children and adults. Children with craniopharyngiomas usually present with hydrocephalus, growth retardation, and obesity, while adults present with visual symptoms. Adamantinomatous and papillary are two well-known distinct histological subtypes of craniopharyngioma. These tumors are predominately solid but almost always have a cystic component, especially with the adamantinomatous subtype. Classically, the lesion has calcified areas and the solid parts enhance on neuroimaging. Associated calcifications are best detected by CT scan, which is key evidence for their diagnosis. Craniopharyngiomas have a predisposition to being large, extending superiorly into the third ventricle, encompassing blood vessels, and even adhering to adjacent neurologic structures [70]. Cystic component may be unilocular or multilocular with iso to high signal intensity on T1-weighted images (highlighting the importance of their protein content) and with variable signal intensity on T2-weighted MR images (Figs. 28, 29, 30, and 31). However, most adamantinomatous cysts are totally or partly hyperintense on T2-weighted images [56].

One of the main differential diagnoses for craniopharyngioma is pituitary macroadenoma with cystic degeneration or necrosis. However, a pituitary adenoma habitually has an intrasellar epicenter with pituitary fossa enlargement rather than the suprasellar extension or epicenter. Even with the irregular presence of T1 hyperintense cystic areas on MR imaging which is the case for most adamantinomatous craniopharyngiomas, calcifications are rare, compared with most adamantinomatous craniopharyngiomas which are calcified.

More rarely, other types of cystic lesions may also occur in parasellar and suprasellar regions. These lesion types may be misdiagnosed as ACs such as epidermoid/dermoid cysts, giant saccular aneurysm, neurocysticercosis [54], and pilocytic astrocytoma, which have already been discussed. Also, true intrasellar ACs without suprasellar extension are an unusual condition that is sometimes confused or associated with cases of empty sella syndrome (Fig. 32) [37].

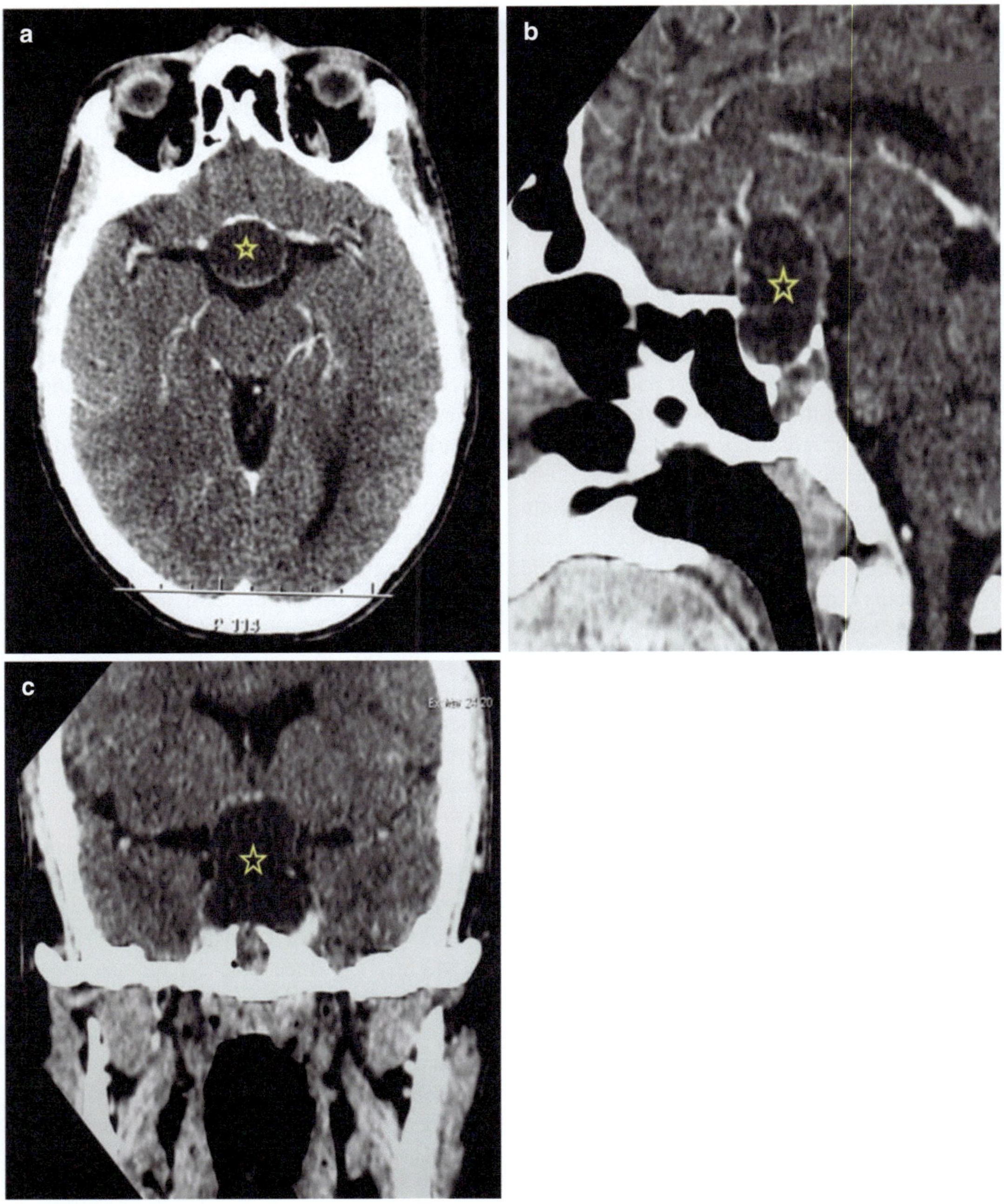

Fig. 28 Case 2. Intra- and suprasellar cystic craniopharyngioma (stars). Axial (**a**), coronal (**b**), and sagittal (**c**) post-contrast CT scan

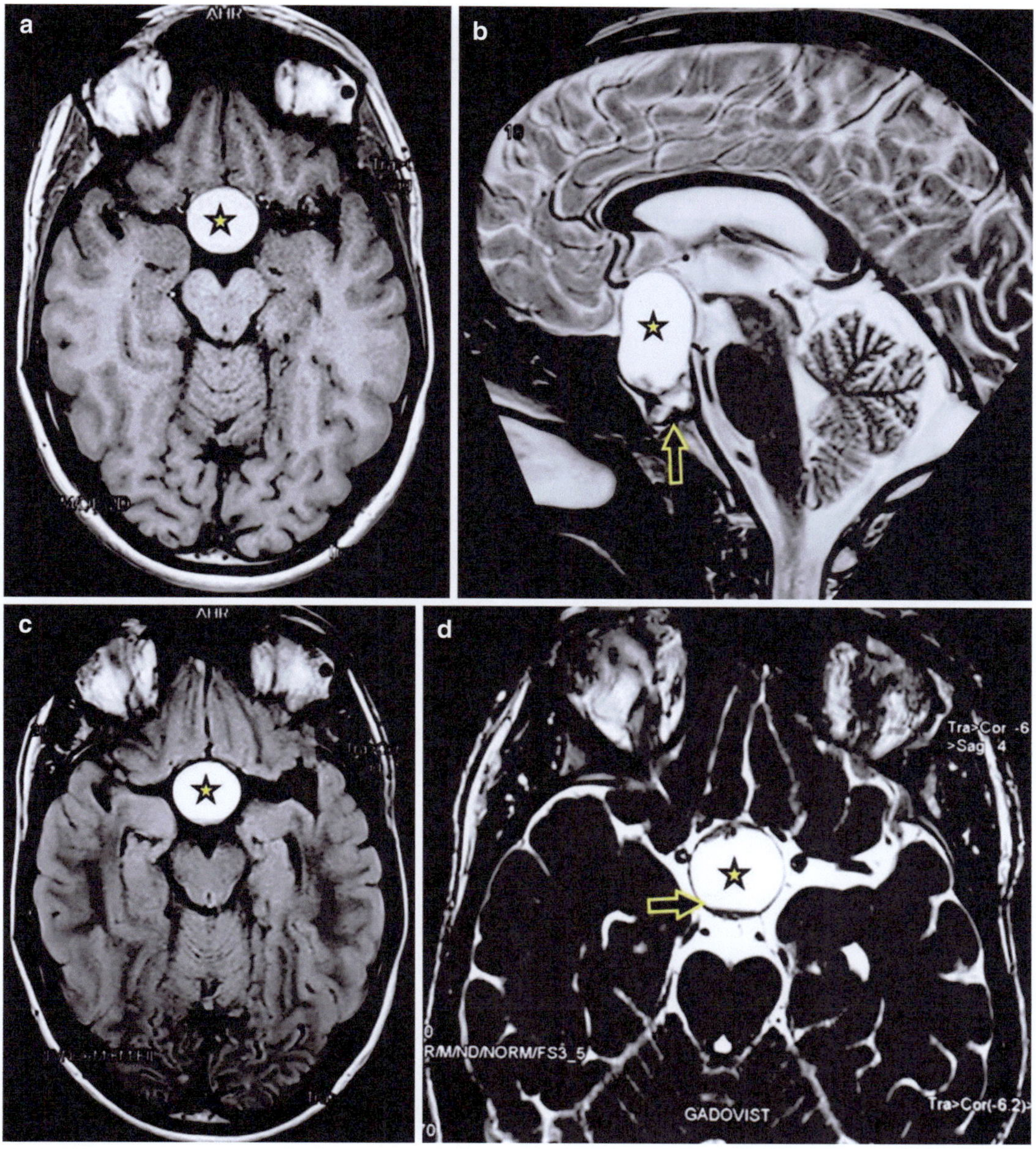

Fig. 29 Case 2. Intra- and suprasellar cystic craniopharyngioma (stars). Axial T1- (**a**) and sagittal T2-weighted MR images (**b**). Axial FLAIR sequence (**c**) and 3D-CISS MR image (**d**)

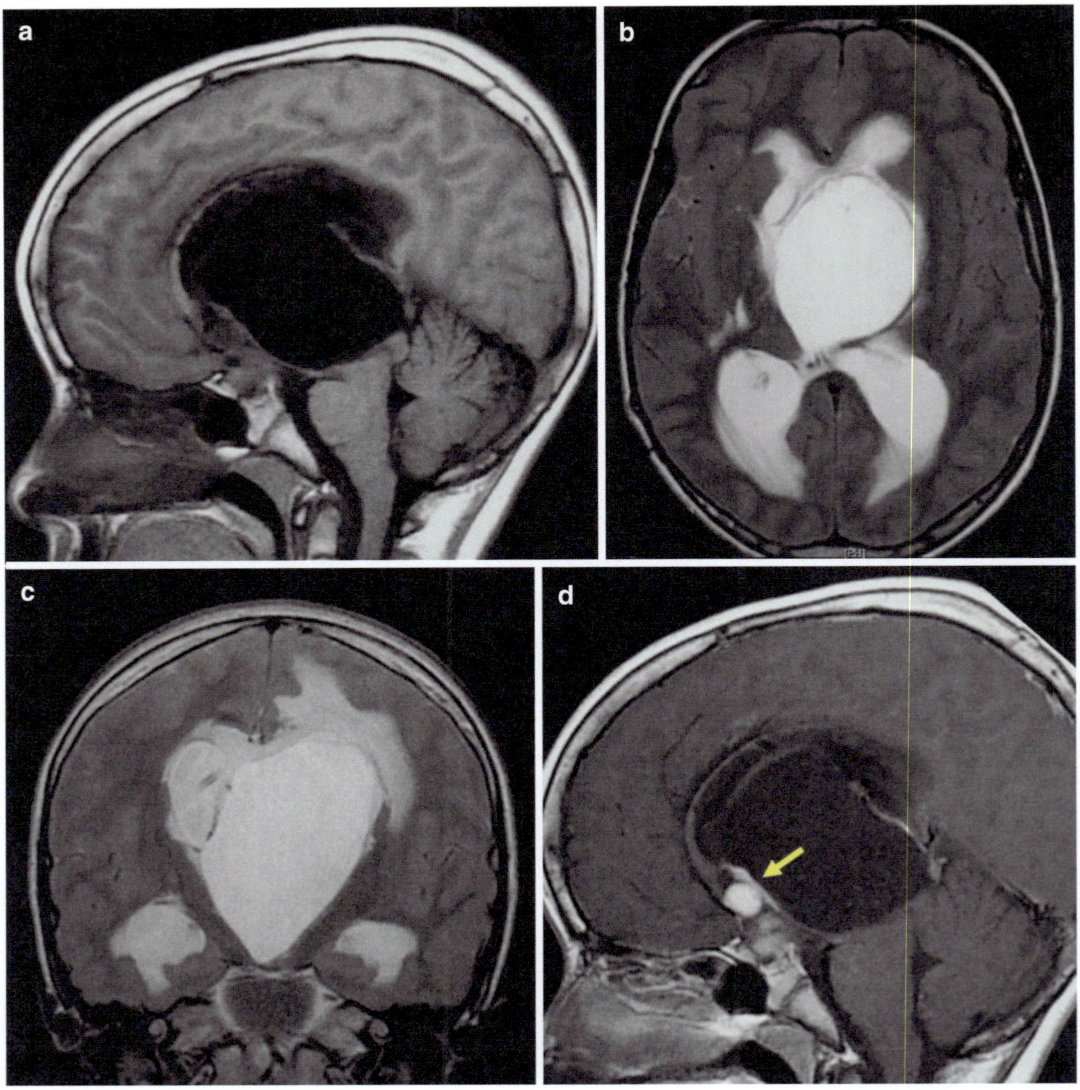

Fig. 30 Giant cystic craniopharyngioma of the diencephalon. Sagittal T1- (**a**) and axial (**b**) and coronal (**c**) T2-weighted MR images. Note the enhancing solid part (arrow) on post-gadolinium sagittal T1-weighted MR image (**d**)

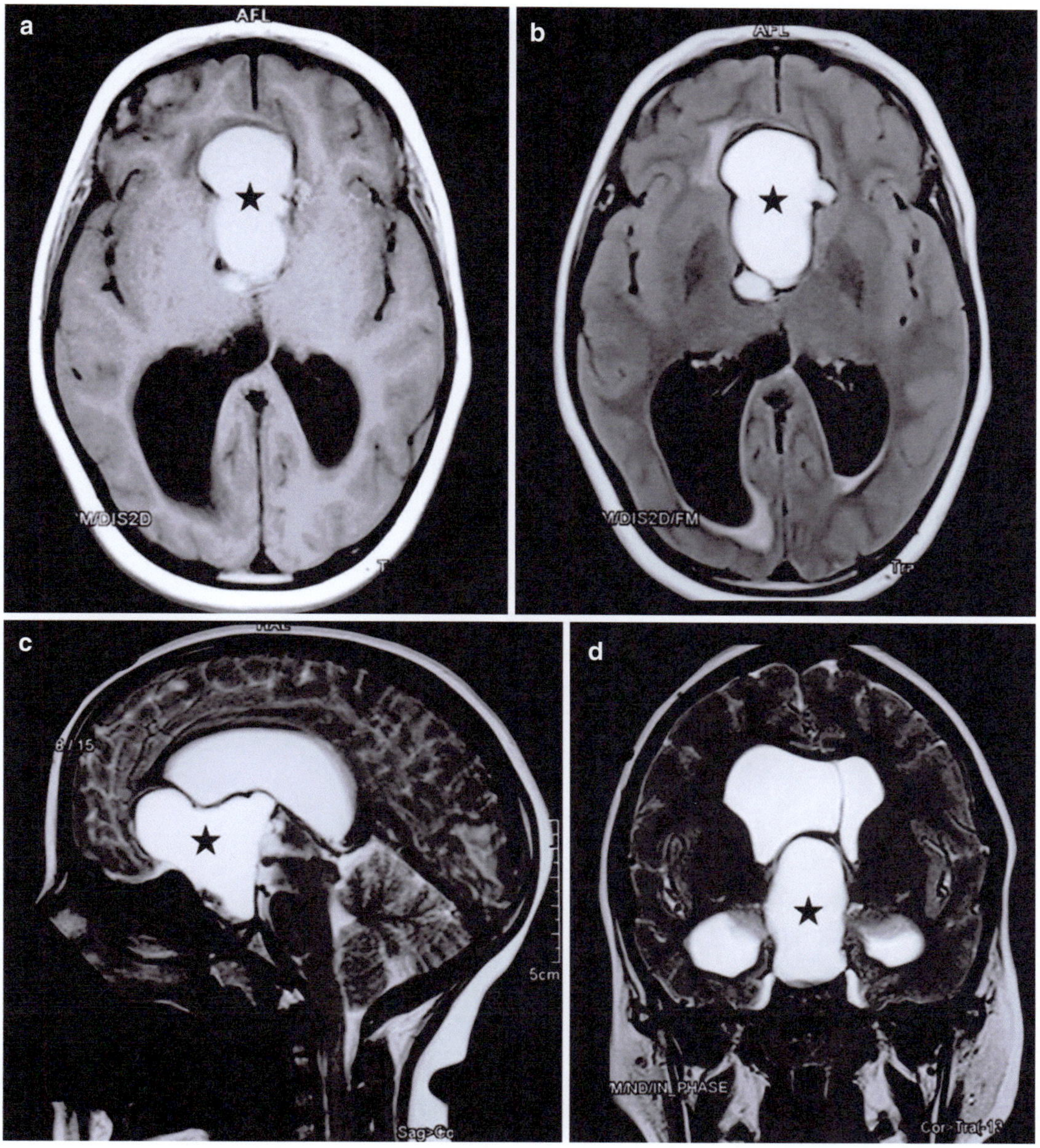

Fig. 31 Cystic craniopharyngioma (stars) with suprasellar, subfrontal, and midbrain involvement. Axial T1-weighted MR image (**a**) and axial FLAIR sequence (**b**). Sagittal (**c**) and coronal (**d**) T2-weighted MR images

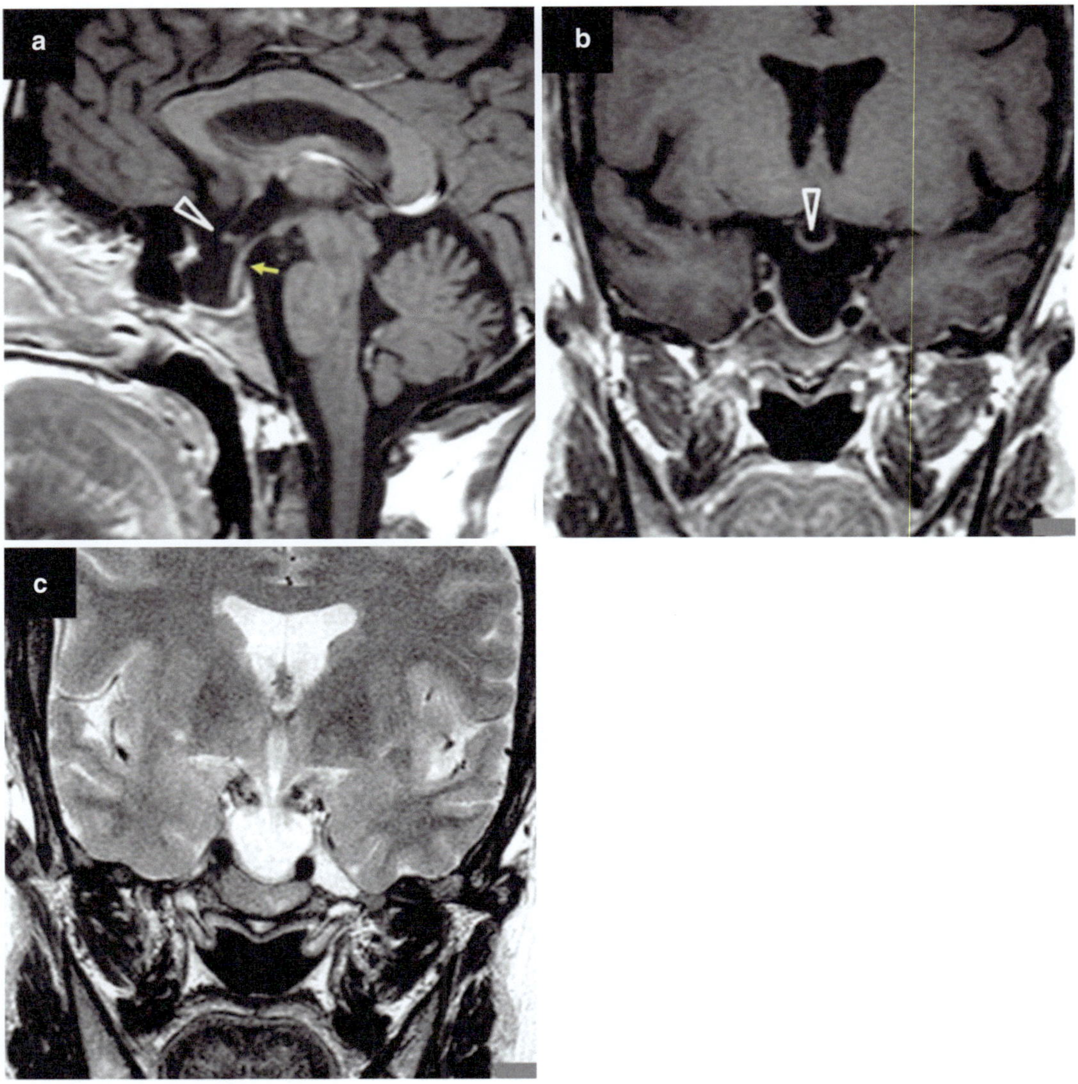

Fig. 32 Empty sella turcica. Sagittal (**a**) and coronal (**b**) T1-weighted MR images and coronal T2-weighted MR image (**c**). The optic chiasm (arrowheads) is pulled down into the empty and enlarged sella turcica. Note that the infundibulum (arrow) can be seen to traverse the intrasellar CSF space, in that way excluding a cystic mass

16 Common Anatomical Variants

Various normal intracranial structures can mimic cystic lesions on both CT scan and MR imaging. Among them, mega cistern magna, tumefactive perivascular spaces, and cavum septum pellucidum may be misdiagnosed as true ACs and constitute a diagnostic challenge for both neurosurgeons and radiologists.

16.1 Mega Cisterna Magna

A large cisterna magna is a normal variant characterized by a truly focal enlargement of the CSF-filled subarachnoid space in the postero-inferior part of the posterior cranial fossa. When the cisterna magna measures more than 10 mm on the midsagittal images, it may be confused with the presence of a retrocerebellar AC [15]. Absence of mass effect on the cerebellum, a normal morpho-

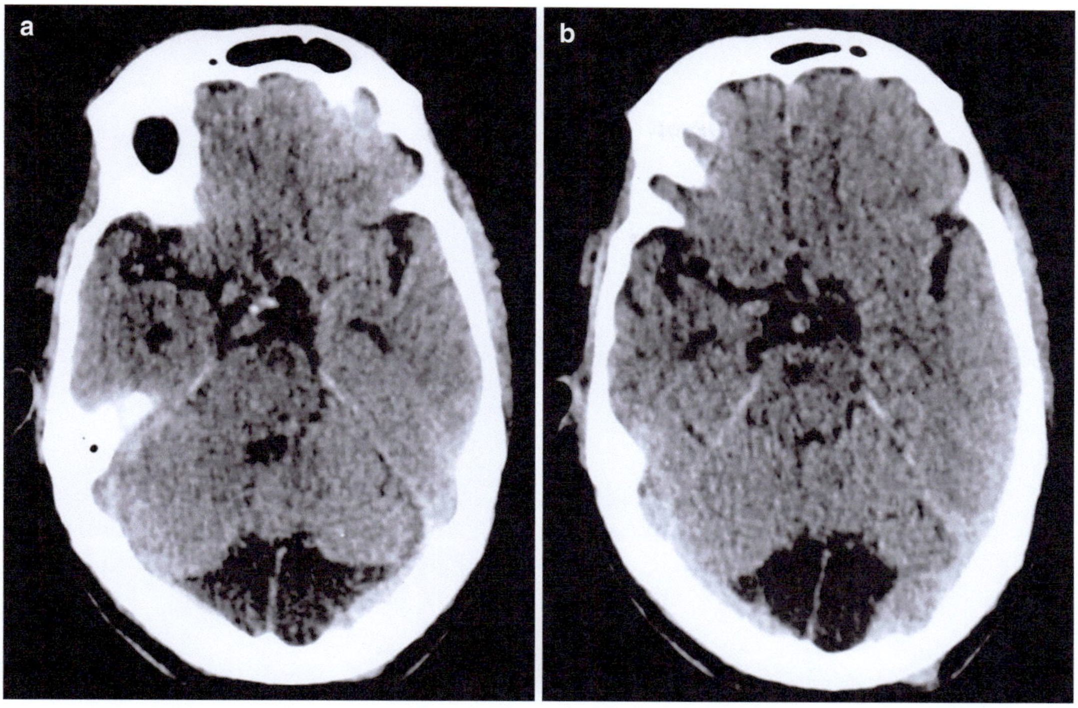

Fig. 33 Mega cisterna magna appearance on axial CT scan (**a**, **b**)

logical appearance of the vermis and fourth ventricle as well as free communication with the contiguous subarachnoid space suggest the diagnosis of a mega cisterna magna rather than AC (Figs. 33 and 34). Sometimes a mega cisterna magna can be asymmetric with apparent mass effect, mimicking an AC. When this happens, some authors suggest performing CT cisternography (lumbar intrathecal injection of *contrast* material followed by an immediate CT scan with the patient positioned on his back) which reveals communication of the enlarged cistern with the adjacent subarachnoid space [45].

16.2 Tumefactive Perivascular Spaces

Perivascular spaces also recognized as "Virchow-Robin spaces" are anatomic structures lined by pia mater, which encircles the penetrating arterioles on their way from the subarachnoid space into inside the brain parenchyma for variable distances [46]. Sometimes, these perivascular spaces can be enlarged and are also called "tumefactive," which can cause relative mass effect on the surrounding brain structures [67]. Enlarged perivascular spaces have been described in many encephalic areas and at a variety of anatomical levels that include the thalamus, basal ganglia, subcortical white matter, midbrain, and the anterior temporal lobe, rarely involving the posterior fossa [68].

The cystic appearance may be regular or variable in size with CSF signal intensity on all MR imaging pulse sequences. The orientation of the tumefactive perivascular spaces may follow a radial pattern that is oriented in the direction of the perforating arterioles, particularly on frontal images. Some cases may be associated with surrounding white matter gliosis that appears as slightly increased signal intensity on T2 or FLAIR sequences; however, no gadolinium enhancement can be identified [46, 68].

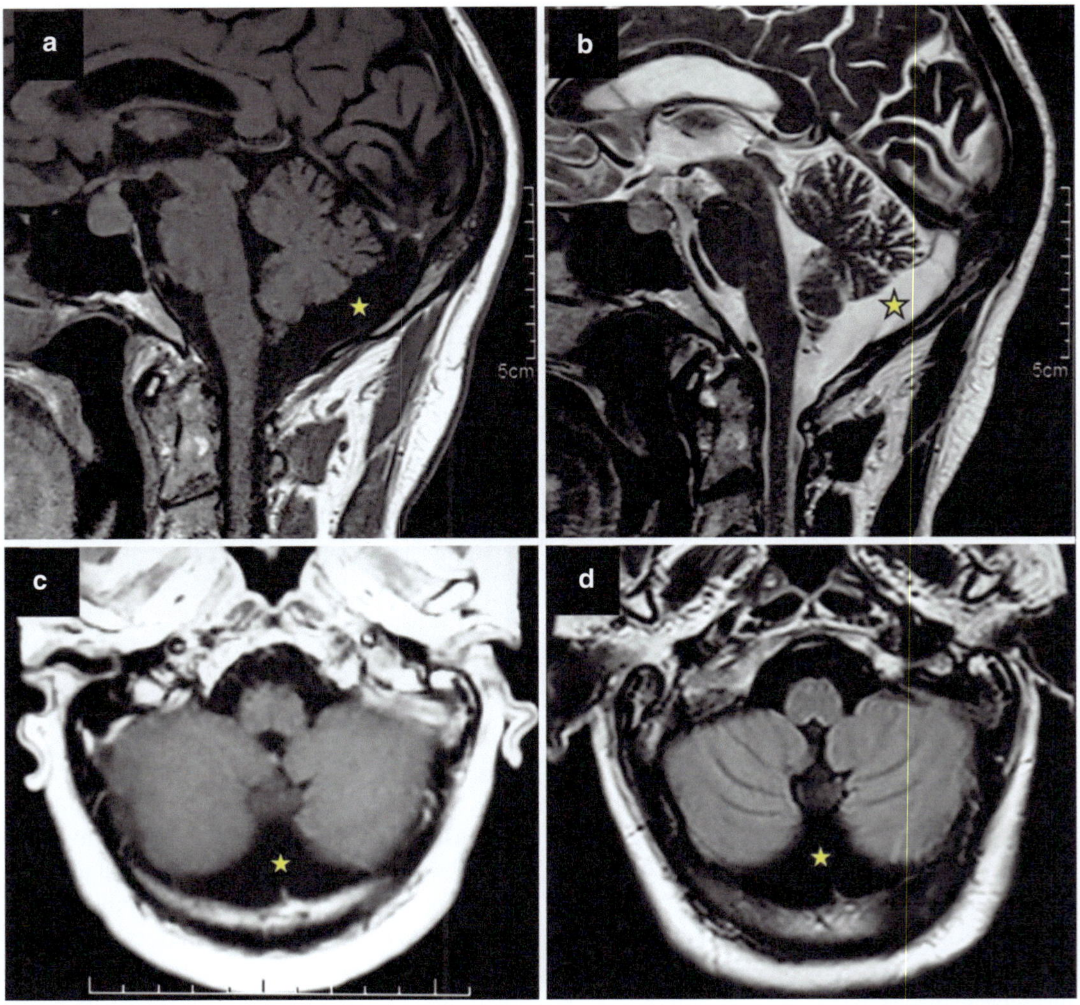

Fig. 34 Mega cisterna magna appearance on MR imaging (stars). Sagittal T1- (**a**) and T2-weighted MR images (**b**) and axial T1-weighted MR image (**c**) and on FLAIR sequence (**d**)

16.3 Cavum Septum Pellucidum

The septum pellucidum which means transparent fence in Latin is a thin triangular double vertical membrane separating the two frontal horns of the lateral ventricles. This structure extends between the anterior segment of the corpus callosum and the body of the fornix [14, 77]. A cavity (cavum in Latin) is present between the leaflets of the septum pellucidum in the normal fetus, but this space fuses together by the first year of age. However, a cavum septum pellucidum persists in about 10% of the adult population (Fig. 35), commonly representing an asymptomatic normal anatomical variation [73, 77]. In the past, it has also been called the fifth ventricle, but this term has fallen out of favor because of the lack of any direct communication between the cavum and the ventricular system [73, 77]. Sometimes, cavum septum pellucidum may communicate with a more posterior cavity named "cavum Vergae" [14, 73, 76, 77]. For some authors, association of a cavum septum pellucidum with a cavum vergae is referred to as cavum septum pellucidum and Vergae [14] (Fig. 36). Tsutsumi et al. proposed using the constructive interference in steady state (CISS) sequences when managing lesions that involve these cavities [76].

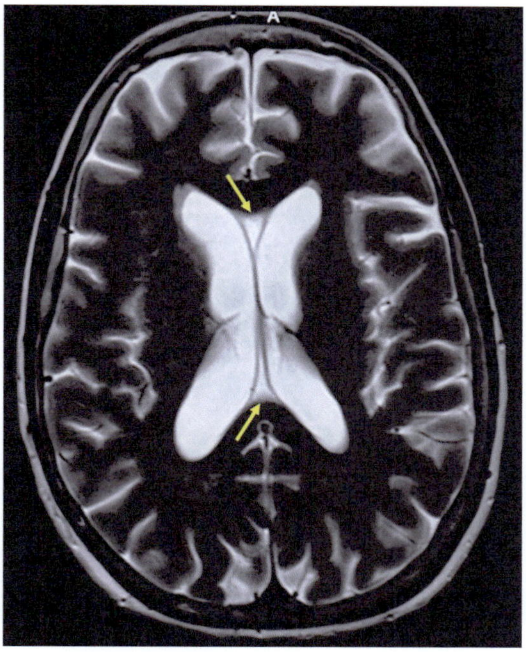

Fig. 35 Cavum of the septum pellucidum (arrows) on axial T2-weighted MR image

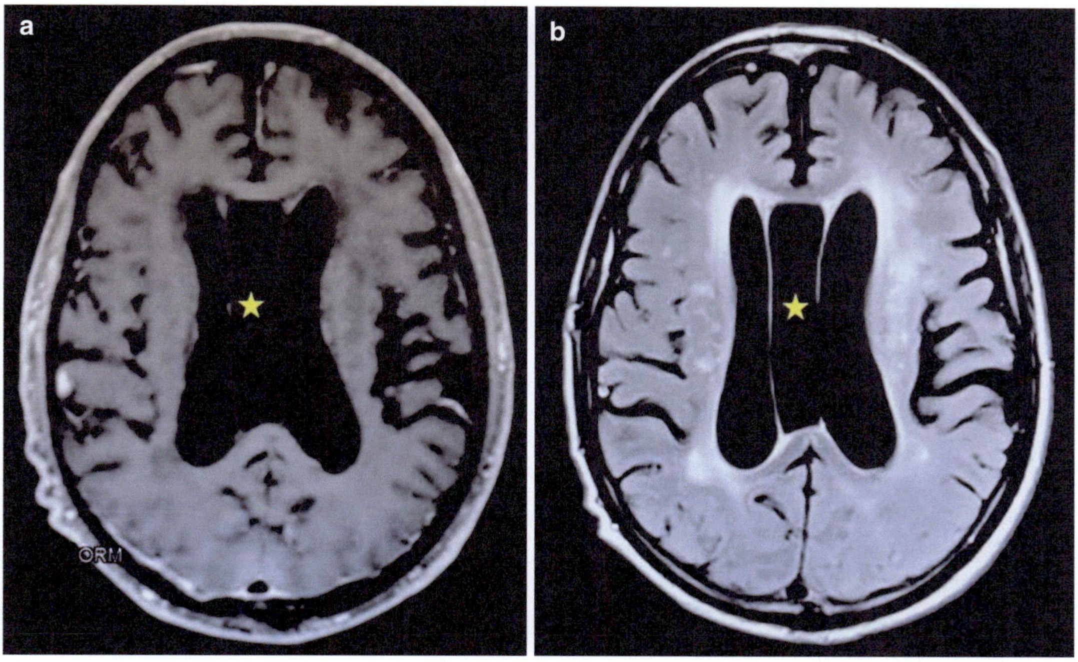

Fig. 36 Cavum septum pellucidum and Vergae (stars) on axial T1-weighted MR image (**a**), FLAIR sequence (**b**), and DWI sequence (**c**). Coronal T2-weighted MR image (**d**)

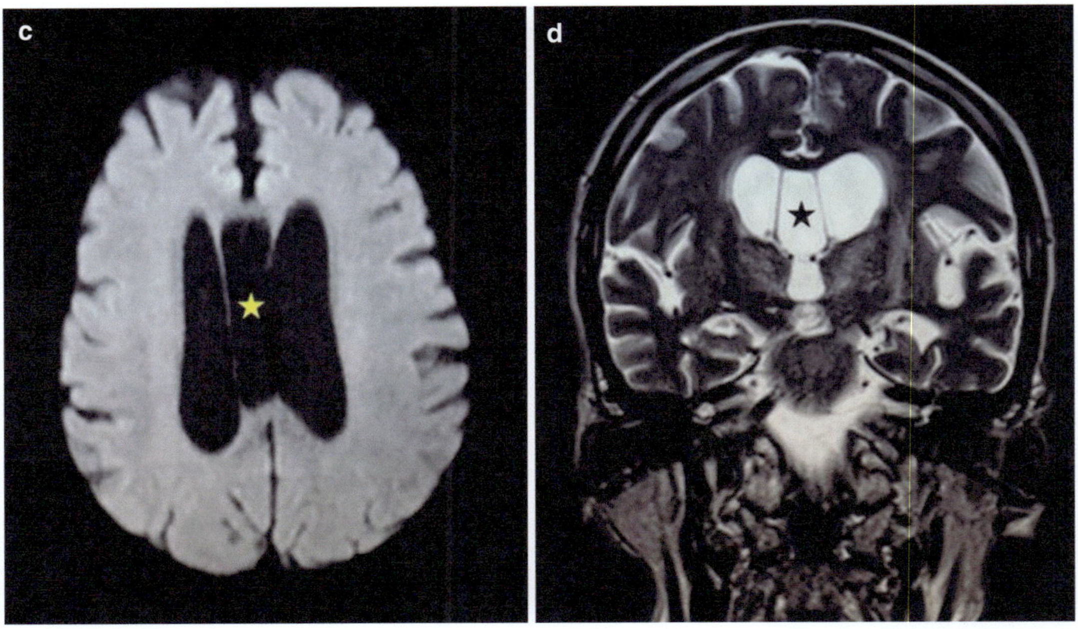

Fig. 36 (continued)

17 Meningoceles and Pseudomeningoceles

Pseudomeningocele is an abnormal collection of CSF that communicate with the subarachnoid space surrounding the brain in the skull base or cranial convexity. They are mainly seen as a result of a traumatic injury or a surgical procedure. The CSF collection has no surrounding membrane, but it is contained in a cavity within the soft tissues [32, 56, 62]. In contrast, for a "real meningocele," the CSF is contained within an extension of the meningeal layers. ***Meningoceles*** are typically classified as "congenital." They result from herniation of the meninges through a defect in the cranium usually involving the soft tissues under the scalp or skin surface [11, 15, 45]. In the opposite, the majority of cranial pseudomeningoceles are "iatrogenic" and mainly occur in the posterior fossa following cranial surgery (Fig. 37).

Pseudomeningoceles are frequently asymptomatic, but some patients may present recurrent headache, motor weakness, cranial nerve abnormality, seizure, subcutaneous swelling, or symptoms of intracranial hypotension. CSF leakage from the wound may be the cause of severe subarachnoid and CNS infections (Fig. 37). On CT scan, pseudomeningocele appears as a low-density collection that extends to the dura with no or minimal peripheral contrast enhancement. Both on MRI and CT scan, the cyst content has similar features to CSF. MRI remains the neurodiagnostic procedure of choice. Suspected fluid can be examined for detecting Beta2 transferrin which is a sensitive and specific method for the diagnosis of a CSF leak. Unlike the majority of intracranial ACs, pseudomeningoceles are extradural and the diagnosis will be highly evocative when there is a previous history of cranial surgery or traumatic injury. Also, congenital meningoceles are defects of the neural tube, mostly associated in neuroimaging with an anterior or posterior bone defect in the cranium [11, 15, 56].

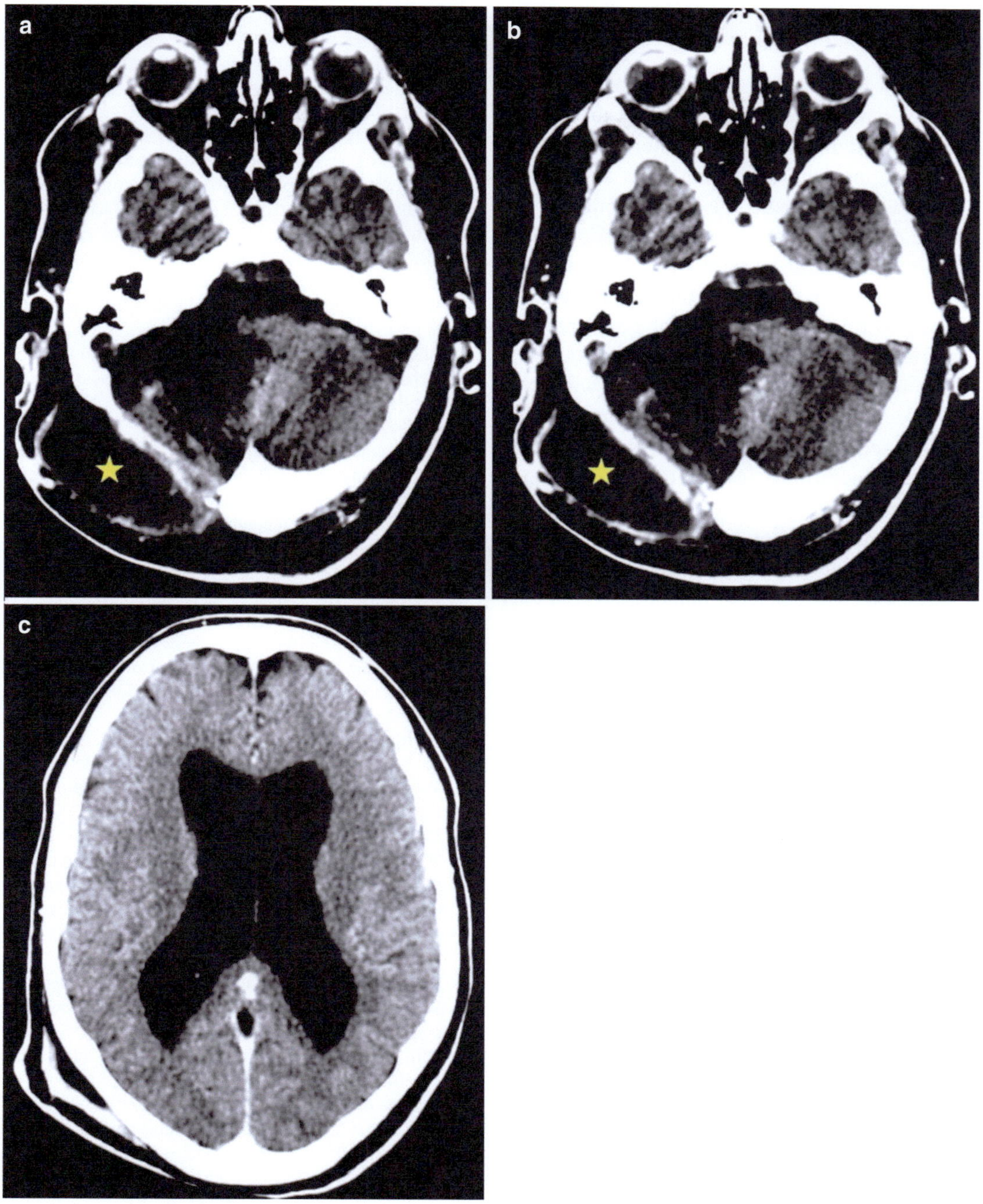

Fig. 37 Axial cranial CT scan without (**a**) and with contrast administration (**b**, **c**) showing a large right suboccipital pseudomeningocele (star) in a patient operated on 3 weeks ago for a giant vestibular schwannoma of the cerebellopontine angle. This patient has also a bacterial meningitis. Note the peripheral enhancement of the pseudomeningocele (**b**) and the concomitant hydrocephalus (**c**). (Reproduced from Akhaddar A. (2017) Surgical Site Infections in Cranial Surgery. In: Atlas of Infections in Neurosurgery and Spinal Surgery. Springer, Cham. https://doi.org/10.1007/978-3-319-60086-4_21; with permission)

18 Conclusion

Although intracranial ACs have been recognized as rare entities for a long time, these cysts are more and more often encountered on routine neuroimaging studies currently. In asymptomatic and symptomatic cases, the practitioner should consider other intracranial cystic lesions or normal anatomic variants that can sometimes be confused with an "authentic" AC. In the case of diagnostic doubt or atypical neuroimaging features, additional and/or better magnetic resonance imaging should be requested whenever possible such as CT or MRI cisternography, FLAIR sequences, DWI, and phase-contrast MRI. This additional information may demonstrate the exact topography of the cysts and their internal structures, defining the precise margins of the fluid collections, and determining their relationship with adjacent anatomic formations as well as any communication between cyst and adjacent subarachnoid spaces. Such information, the clinical presentation and sometimes biological data, will be crucial to enhance the ability to discuss the best therapeutic option for each case.

References

1. Akhaddar A. Cranial subdural empyemas. In: Akhaddar A, editor. Atlas of infections in neurosurgery and spinal surgery. Cham: Springer; 2017. p. 51–64. https://doi.org/10.1007/978-3-319-60086-4_6.
2. Akhaddar A. Neuroimaging differential diagnosis (imaging mimicking conditions) of cranial chronic subdural hematoma. In: Turgut M, Akhaddar A, Hall WA, Turgut AT, editors. Subdural hematoma. Cham: Springer; 2021. p. 311–26. https://doi.org/10.1007/978-3-030-79371-5_26.
3. Akhaddar A, Baallal H. Suprapineal ventricular diverticula secondary to hydrocephalus shunt malfunction. Childs Nerv Syst. 2020;36:15–6. https://doi.org/10.1007/s00381-019-04379-7.
4. Akhaddar A, Mahi M, Amarti A, el Quessar A, el Hassani MY, Chakir N, et al. Kyste simple du cervelet. A propos d'un cas [Simple cyst of the cerebellum. Report of a case]. J Neuroradiol. 2001;28:209–14.
5. Al-Holou WN, Terman S, Kilburg C, Garton HJ, Muraszko KM, Maher CO. Prevalence and natural history of arachnoid cysts in adults. J Neurosurg. 2013;118:222–31. https://doi.org/10.3171/2012.10.JNS12548.
6. Al-Saadi T. The dilemma of choroidal fissure cyst and seizure. J Epilepsy Res. 2020;10:1–2. https://doi.org/10.14581/jer.20001.
7. Altafulla JJ, Suh S, Bordes S, Prickett J, Iwanaga J, Loukas M, et al. Choroidal fissure and choroidal fissure cysts: a comprehensive review. Anat Cell Biol. 2020;53:121–5. https://doi.org/10.5115/acb.20.040.
8. Altuwaijri N, Cote DJ, Lamba N, Albenayan W, Ren SP, Zaghloul I, et al. Headache resolution after Rathke cleft cyst resection: a meta-analysis. World Neurosurg. 2018;111:e764–72. https://doi.org/10.1016/j.wneu.2017.12.170.
9. Bano S, Chaudhary V, Garga UC. Neonatal hypoxic-ischemic encephalopathy: a radiological review. J Pediatr Neurosci. 2017;12:1–6. https://doi.org/10.4103/1817-1745.205646.
10. Barkhoudarian G, Palejwala SK, Ansari S, Eisenberg AA, Huang X, Griffiths CF, et al. Rathke's cleft cysts: a 6-year experience of surgery vs. observation with comparative volumetric analysis. Pituitary. 2019;22:362–71. https://doi.org/10.1007/s11102-019-00962-y.
11. Barkovich AJ, Kjos BO, Norman D, Edwards MS. Revised classification of posterior fossa cysts and cystlike malformations based on the results of multiplanar MR imaging. AJR Am J Roentgenol. 1989;153:1289–300. https://doi.org/10.2214/ajr.153.6.1289.
12. Belfquih H, Azami MA, Akhaddar A. Rare case of hydatid cyst in the cerebellopontine cistern. World Neurosurg. 2021;145:48–50. https://doi.org/10.1016/j.wneu.2020.09.004.
13. Borger V, Vatter H, Oszvald Á, Marquardt G, Seifert V, Güresir E. Chronic subdural haematoma in elderly patients: a retrospective analysis of 322 patients between the ages of 65-94 years. Acta Neurochir (Wien). 2012;154:1549–54. https://doi.org/10.1007/s00701-012-1434-x.
14. Born CM, Meisenzahl EM, Frodl T, Pfluger T, Reiser M, Möller HJ, et al. The septum pellucidum and its variants. An MRI study. Eur Arch Psychiatry Clin Neurosci. 2004;254:295–302. https://doi.org/10.1007/s00406-004-0496-z.
15. Bosemani T, Orman G, Boltshauser E, Tekes A, Huisman TA, Poretti A. Congenital abnormalities of the posterior fossa. Radiographics. 2015;35:200–20. https://doi.org/10.1148/rg.351140038.
16. Boutarbouch M, El Ouahabi A, Rifi L, Arkha Y, Derraz S, El Khamlichi A. Management of intracranial arachnoid cysts: institutional experience with initial 32 cases and review of the literature. Clin Neurol Neurosurg. 2008;110:1–7. https://doi.org/10.1016/j.clineuro.2007.08.009.
17. Braga VL, da Costa MDS, Riera R, Dos Santos Rocha LP, de Oliveira Santos BF, Matsumura Hondo TT, de Oliveira Chagas M, Cavalheiro S. Schizencephaly: a review of 734 patients. Pediatr Neurol. 2018;87:23–9. https://doi.org/10.1016/j.pediatrneurol.2018.08.001.

18. Cabaj A, Bekiesińska-Figatowska M, Mądzik J. MRI patterns of hypoxic-ischemic brain injury in preterm and full term infants—classical and less common MR findings. Pol J Radiol. 2012;77:71–6. https://doi.org/10.12659/pjr.883379.
19. Chakraborty S, Priamo F, Loven T, Li J, Insinga S, Schulder M. Supratentorial neurenteric cysts: case series and review of pathology, imaging, and clinical management. World Neurosurg. 2016;85:143–52. https://doi.org/10.1016/j.wneu.2015.08.057.
20. Chibbaro S, Champeaux C, Poczos P, Cardarelli M, Di Rocco F, Iaccarino C, et al. Anterior trans-frontal endoscopic management of colloid cyst: an effective, safe, and elegant way of treatment. Case series and technical note from a multicenter prospective study. Neurosurg Rev. 2014;37:235–41. https://doi.org/10.1007/s10143-013-0508-4.
21. Chihi M, Jabbarli R, Gembruch O, Teuber-Hanselmann S, Darkwah Oppong M, Pierscianek D, et al. A rare case of a completely thrombosed bilobed giant intracranial aneurysm of the anterior cerebral artery with spontaneous parent vessel thrombosis: case report. BMC Neurol. 2019;19:297. https://doi.org/10.1186/s12883-019-1529-6.
22. Choque-Velasquez J, Colasanti R, Baluszek S, Resendiz-Nieves J, Muhammad S, Ludtka C, et al. Systematic review of pineal cysts surgery in pediatric patients. Childs Nerv Syst. 2020;36:2927–38. https://doi.org/10.1007/s00381-020-04792-3.
23. Correa GG, Amaral LF, Vedolin LM. Neuroimaging of Dandy-Walker malformation: new concepts. Top Magn Reson Imaging. 2011;22:303–12. https://doi.org/10.1097/RMR.0b013e3182a2ca77.
24. de Jong L, Thewissen L, van Loon J, Van Calenbergh F. Choroidal fissure cerebrospinal fluid-containing cysts: case series, anatomical consideration, and review of the literature. World Neurosurg. 2011;75:704–8. https://doi.org/10.1016/j.wneu.2010.12.056.
25. De La Peña NM, Amrami KK, Spinner RJ. Totally cystic schwannoma: a misnomer. World Neurosurg. 2021;157:21–9. https://doi.org/10.1016/j.wneu.2021.09.098.
26. Dutt SN, Mirza S, Chavda SV, Irving RM. Radiologic differentiation of intracranial epidermoids from arachnoid cysts. Otol Neurotol. 2002;23:84–92. https://doi.org/10.1097/00129492-200201000-00019.
27. El-Ghandour NMF. Endoscopic treatment of intraventricular ependymal cysts in children: personal experience and review of literature. Childs Nerv Syst. 2018;34:2441–8. https://doi.org/10.1007/s00381-018-3965-9.
28. Epelman M, Daneman A, Blaser SI, Ortiz-Neira C, Konen O, Jarrín J, et al. Differential diagnosis of intracranial cystic lesions at head US: correlation with CT and MR imaging. Radiographics. 2006;26:173–96. https://doi.org/10.1148/rg.261055033.
29. Fortuna A, Ferrante L, Acqui M, Guglielmi G, Mastronardi L. Cystic meningiomas. Acta Neurochir (Wien). 1988;90:23–30. https://doi.org/10.1007/BF01541262.
30. French H, Schaefer N, Keijzers G, Barison D, Olson S. Intracranial subdural empyema: a 10-year case series. Ochsner J. 2014;14:188–94.
31. Ghosn Y, Kamareddine MH, Adem C, Jabbour R. A patient with schizencephaly and agenesis of corpus callosum with no neurological deficits. J Neurosci Rural Pract. 2018;9:404–5. https://doi.org/10.4103/jnrp.jnrp_564_17.
32. Ginat D, Westesson PA, editors. Atlas of postsurgical neuroradiology. Heidelberg: Springer; 2012. 653pp
33. Gläsker S, Vortmeyer AO, Lonser RR, Lubensky IA, Okamoto H, Xia JB, et al. Proteomic analysis of hemangioblastoma cyst fluid. Cancer Biol Ther. 2006;5:549–53. https://doi.org/10.4161/cbt.5.5.2657.
34. Guénot M. Chronic subdural hematoma: diagnostic imaging studies. Neurochirurgie. 2001;47:473–8.
35. Gui SB, Wang XS, Zong XY, Zhang YZ, Li CZ. Suprasellar cysts: clinical presentation, surgical indications, and optimal surgical treatment. BMC Neurol. 2011;11:52. https://doi.org/10.1186/1471-2377-11-52.
36. Halabuda A, Klasa L, Kwiatkowski S, Wyrobek L, Milczarek O, Gergont A. Schizencephaly-diagnostics and clinical dilemmas. Childs Nerv Syst. 2015;31:551–6. https://doi.org/10.1007/s00381-015-2638-1.
37. Hatipoğlu HG, Cetin MA, Gürses MA, Dağlioğlu E, Sakman B, Yüksel E. Petrous apex cephalocele and empty sella/arachnoid cyst coexistence: a clue for cerebrospinal fluid pressure imbalance? Diagn Interv Radiol. 2010;16:7–9. https://doi.org/10.4261/1305-3825.DIR.2650-09.2.
38. Hoffman CE, Savage NJ, Souweidane MM. The significance of cyst remnants after endoscopic colloid cyst resection: a retrospective clinical case series. Neurosurgery. 2013;73:233–7. https://doi.org/10.1227/01.neu.0000430300.10338.71.
39. Imperato A, Spennato P, Mazio F, Arcas E, Ozgural O, Quaglietta L, et al. Desmoplastic infantile astrocytoma and ganglioglioma: a series of 12 patients treated at a single institution. Childs Nerv Syst. 2021;37:2187–95. https://doi.org/10.1007/s00381-021-05057-3.
40. Jabaudon D, Charest D, Porchet F. Pathogenesis and diagnostic pitfalls of ventricular diverticula: case report and review of the literature. Neurosurgery. 2003;52:209–12. https://doi.org/10.1097/00006123-200301000-00026.
41. Jeon JH, Lee SW, Ko JK, Choi BG, Cha SH, Song GS, et al. Neuroendoscopic removal of large choroid plexus cyst: a case report. J Korean Med Sci. 2005;20:335–9. https://doi.org/10.3346/jkms.2005.20.2.335.
42. Jorge D, Nadia G, Claudio V, Carlos M, Eduardo GT. Cystic meningioma simulating arachnoid cyst: report of an unusual case. Case Rep Radiol. 2014:371969. https://doi.org/10.1155/2014/371969.
43. Karaman E, Isildak H, Yilmaz M, Enver O, Albayram S. Encephalomalacia in the frontal lobe: complication of the endoscopic sinus surgery. J Craniofac

Surg. 2011;22:2374–5. https://doi.org/10.1097/SCS.0b013e318231e511.
44. Kimura-Hayama ET, Higuera JA, Corona-Cedillo R, Chávez-Macías L, Perochena A, Quiroz-Rojas LY, et al. Neurocysticercosis: radiologic-pathologic correlation. Radiographics. 2010;30:1705–19. https://doi.org/10.1148/rg.306105522.
45. Kollias SS, Ball WS Jr, Prenger EC. Cystic malformations of the posterior fossa: differential diagnosis clarified through embryologic analysis. Radiographics. 1993;13:1211–31. https://doi.org/10.1148/radiographics.13.6.8031352.
46. Kwee RM, Kwee TC. Tumefactive Virchow-Robin spaces. Eur J Radiol. 2019;111:21–33. https://doi.org/10.1016/j.ejrad.2018.12.011.
47. Kuharic M, Jankovic D, Splavski B, Boop FA, Arnautovic KI. Hemangioblastomas of the posterior cranial fossa in adults: demographics, clinical, morphologic, pathologic, surgical features, and outcomes. A systematic review. World Neurosurg. 2018;110:e1049–62. https://doi.org/10.1016/j.wneu.2017.11.173.
48. Kumaran SP, Srinivasa R, Ghosal N. Unusual radiological presentation of intracranial dermoid cyst: a case series. Asian J Neurosurg. 2019;14:269–71. https://doi.org/10.4103/ajns.AJNS_304_17.
49. Lee HC, Chong S, Lee JY, Cheon JE, Phi JH, Kim SK, et al. Benign extracerebral fluid collection complicated by subdural hematoma and fluid collection: clinical characteristics and management. Childs Nerv Syst. 2018;34:235–45. https://doi.org/10.1007/s00381-017-3583-y.
50. Liu Y, Gong J, Li F, Wang H, Zhu S, Wu C. Traumatic subdural hydroma: clinical characteristics and classification. Injury. 2009;40:968–72. https://doi.org/10.1016/j.injury.2009.01.006.
51. Lou X, Gui QP, Sun L, Wu NZ, Lyu JH, Ma L. Comparisons of MR findings between supratentorial and infratentorial gangliogliomas. Clin Neuroradiol. 2016;26:65–71. https://doi.org/10.1007/s00062-014-0333-3.
52. Muhlestein WE, Maher CO. Incidental intracranial cysts in children. Pediatr Clin North Am. 2021;68:775–82. https://doi.org/10.1016/j.pcl.2021.04.005.
53. Murray RD, Penar PL, Filippi CG, Tarasiewicz I. Radiographically distinct variant of pilocytic astrocytoma: a case series. J Comput Assist Tomogr. 2011;35:495–7. https://doi.org/10.1097/RCT.0b013e3182237cbf.
54. Musara A, Soko N, Shamu S. Suprasellar cysticercosis cyst with optic nerve compression masquerading as an arachnoid cyst. Middle East Afr J Ophthalmol. 2019;26:114–6. https://doi.org/10.4103/meajo.MEAJO_142_18.
55. Nauta HJ, Tucker WS, Horsey WJ, Bilbao JM, Gonsalves C. Xanthochromic cysts associated with meningioma. J Neurol Neurosurg Psychiatry. 1979;42:529–35. https://doi.org/10.1136/jnnp.42.6.529.
56. Osborn AG, Preece MT. Intracranial cysts: radiologic-pathologic correlation and imaging approach. Radiology. 2006;239:650–64. https://doi.org/10.1148/radiol.2393050823.
57. Ostlere SJ, Irving HC, Lilford RJ. Fetal choroid plexus cysts: a report of 100 cases. Radiology. 1990;175:753–5. https://doi.org/10.1148/radiology.175.3.2188298.
58. Parisi G, Tropea R, Giuffrida S, Lombardo M, Giuffrè F. Cystic meningiomas. Report of seven cases. J Neurosurg. 1986;64:35–8. https://doi.org/10.3171/jns.1986.64.1.0035.
59. Pereira RG, Ribeiro BNF, Hollanda RTL, de Almeida LB, Simeão TB, et al. Non-neoplastic intracranial cystic lesions: not everything is an arachnoid cyst. Radiol Bras. 2021;54:49–55. https://doi.org/10.1590/0100-3984.2019.0144.
60. Preece MT, Osborn AG, Chin SS, Smirniotopoulos JG. Intracranial neurenteric cysts: imaging and pathology spectrum. AJNR Am J Neuroradiol. 2006;27:1211–6.
61. Prieto R, Subhi-Issa I, Pascual JM. Ependymal cyst of the midbrain. Clin Neuropathol. 2013;32:183–8. https://doi.org/10.5414/NP300563.
62. Provenzale JM. Imaging of traumatic brain injury: a review of the recent medical literature. AJR Am J Roentgenol. 2010;194:16–9. https://doi.org/10.2214/AJR.09.3687.
63. Quadery FA, Okamoto K. Diffusion-weighted MRI of haemangioblastomas and other cerebellar tumours. Neuroradiology. 2003;45:212–9. https://doi.org/10.1007/s00234-003-0951-y.
64. Raz E, Zagzag D, Saba L, Mannelli L, Di Paolo PL, D'Ambrosio F, et al. Cyst with a mural nodule tumor of the brain. Cancer Imaging. 2012;12:237–44. https://doi.org/10.1102/1470-7330.2012.0028.
65. Ren X, Lin S, Wang Z, Luo L, Jiang Z, Sui D, et al. Clinical, radiological, and pathological features of 24 atypical intracranial epidermoid cysts. J Neurosurg. 2012;116:611–21. https://doi.org/10.3171/2011.10.JNS111462.
66. Robles LA, Paez JM, Ayala D, Boleaga-Duran B. Intracranial glioependymal (neuroglial) cysts: a systematic review. Acta Neurochir (Wien). 2018;160:1439–49. https://doi.org/10.1007/s00701-018-3566-0.
67. Rudie JD, Rauschecker AM, Nabavizadeh SA, Mohan S. Neuroimaging of dilated perivascular spaces: from benign and pathologic causes to mimics. J Neuroimaging. 2018;28:139–49. https://doi.org/10.1111/jon.12493.
68. Salzman KL, Osborn AG, House P, Jinkins JR, Ditchfield A, Cooper JA, et al. Giant tumefactive perivascular spaces. AJNR Am J Neuroradiol. 2005;26:298–305.
69. Sanlı AM, Türkoğlu E, Kertmen H, Gürer B. Hydatid cyst of the ambient cistern radiologically mimicking an arachnoid cyst. J Neurosurg Pediatr. 2012;10:186–8. https://doi.org/10.3171/2012.6.PEDS11562.
70. Sartoretti-Schefer S, Wichmann W, Aguzzi A, Valavanis A. MR differentiation of adamantinous and

squamous-papillary craniopharyngiomas. AJNR Am J Neuroradiol. 1997;18:77–87.

71. Schneider UC, Koch A, Stenzel W, Thomale UW. Intracranial, supratentorial dermoid cysts in paediatric patients—two cases and a review of the literature. Childs Nerv Syst. 2012;28:185–90. https://doi.org/10.1007/s00381-011-1646-z.
72. Sherer DM, Anyaegbunam A, Onyeije C. Antepartum fetal intracranial hemorrhage, predisposing factors and prenatal sonography: a review. Am J Perinatol. 1998;15:431–41. https://doi.org/10.1055/s-2007-993971.
73. Simonin A, Lind CRP. Surgical management of symptomatic cavum septum pellucidum cysts: systematic review of the literature. Neurosurg Rev. 2021;44:2425–32. https://doi.org/10.1007/s10143-020-01447-4.
74. Storey M, Lilimpakis K, Grandal NS, Rajaraman C, Achawal S, Hussain M. Pineal cyst surveillance in adults—a review of 10 years' experience. Br J Neurosurg. 2020;34(5):565–8. https://doi.org/10.1080/02688697.2019.1635989.
75. Tempel ZJ, Johnson SA, Richard PS, Friedlander RM, Rothfus WE, Hamilton RL. Parasellar arachnoid cyst presenting with a nonpupil sparing third nerve palsy mimicking a posterior communicating artery aneurysm in an adult. Surg Neurol Int. 2013;4:87. https://doi.org/10.4103/2152-7806.114799.
76. Tsutsumi S, Ishii H, Ono H, Yasumoto Y. Visualization of the cavum septi pellucidi, cavum Vergae, and cavum veli interpositi using magnetic resonance imaging. Surg Radiol Anat. 2018;40:159–64. https://doi.org/10.1007/s00276-017-1935-7.
77. Tubbs RS, Krishnamurthy S, Verma K, Shoja MM, Loukas M, Mortazavi MM, et al. Cavum velum interpositum, cavum septum pellucidum, and cavum vergae: a review. Childs Nerv Syst. 2011;27:1927–30. https://doi.org/10.1007/s00381-011-1457-2.
78. Varghese B, Xavier R, Manoj VC, Aneesh MK, Priya PS, Kumar A, Sreenivasan VK. Magnetic resonance imaging spectrum of perinatal hypoxic-ischemic brain injury. Indian J Radiol Imaging. 2016;26:316–27. https://doi.org/10.4103/0971-3026.190421.
79. Vassilouthis J, Ambrose J. Computerized tomography scanning appearances of intracranial meningiomas. An attempt to predict the histological features. J Neurosurg. 1979;50:320–7. https://doi.org/10.3171/jns.1979.50.3.0320.
80. Wang JC, Heier L, Souweidane MM. Advances in the endoscopic management of suprasellar arachnoid cysts in children. J Neurosurg. 2004;100(5 Suppl Pediatrics):418–26. https://doi.org/10.3171/ped.2004.100.5.0418.
81. Yikilmaz A, Durak AC, Mavili E, Donmez H, Kurtsoy A, Kontas O. The role of diffusion-weighted magnetic resonance imaging in intracranial cystic lesions. Neuroradiol J. 2009;21:781–90. https://doi.org/10.1177/197140090802100605.
82. Yoshino M, Nakatomi H, Kin T, Saito T, Shono N, Nomura S, et al. Usefulness of high-resolution 3D multifusion medical imaging for preoperative planning in patients with posterior fossa hemangioblastoma: technical note. J Neurosurg. 2017;127:139–47. https://doi.org/10.3171/2016.5.JNS152646.
83. Yousef A, Rutkowski MJ, Yalcin CE, Eren OC, Caliskan I, Tihan T. Sporadic and Von-Hippel Lindau disease-associated spinal hemangioblastomas: institutional experience on their similarities and differences. J Neurooncol. 2019;143:547–52. https://doi.org/10.1007/s11060-019-03189-w.

Differential Diagnosis of Intraspinal Arachnoid Cysts

Ali Akhaddar

1 Introduction

The incidence of spinal arachnoid cysts (ACs) is much lower than that of cranial ACs probably because of the lack of intraspinal arachnoid cisterns which could represent the site of their development.

Intraspinal ACs are an unusual heterogeneous pathologic lesion that is more complex than was previously thought. These cystic lesions may present with variable clinical signs and symptoms as well as neuroimaging features which depend above all on the anatomic locations, cyst dimensions, etiological forms, and the patient's age. Some of them are asymptomatic and are considered incidental on imaging, while others present simply with rachialgia or even complete paraplegia/quadriplegia. Spinal ACs can manifest with atypical clinical findings such as radicular pain, isolated gait difficulty, isolated urinary urgency, non-cardiac chest pain or even abdominal pain, or recurrent neurological symptoms mimicking multiple sclerosis [1, 34, 47]. Some other cases with chronic spinal cord compression may be associated with muscle changes mimicking a primary myopathy [61].

Intraspinal ACs may be confused with many spinal and intraspinal cysts that differ by their origins and locations. Magnetic resonance (MR) with sensitivity imaging represents the gold standard for differentiating between the majority of these cystic entities essentially because of their diverse contents. Both neurosurgeons/spinal surgeons and radiologists must be prepared to recognize all possible considerations on preoperative images, during the therapeutic planning process and even throughout the patient's care. Consequently, a high index of suspicion needs to be kept in mind to achieve an appropriate analysis of intraspinal ACs and to define the list of possible intraspinal cyst-mimicking lesions.

A summary of the most common imaging differential diagnoses of spinal ACs is provided in this chapter according to the anatomic locations and origins of the cysts. Moreover, chapter "Differential Diagnosis of Intracranial Arachnoid Cysts" provides a review of the main differential diagnosis of intracranial ACs.

2 Hydro-Syringomyelia

The use of the general term "hydro-syringomyelia" or "syrinx" has been proposed because of difficulty in distinguishing between "syringomyelia" and "hydromyelia" in current neuroimaging studies. Hydromyelia refers to a cystic collection or dilatation of the central spinal canal, for that reason the ependyma line the cavity wall. Whereas syringomyelia refers to a cystic cavitation within spinal cord parenchyma that can be primary or secondary to any etiology, situated adjacent to the

A. Akhaddar (✉)
Department of Neurosurgery, Avicenne Military Hospital of Marrakech, Mohammed V University in Rabat, Rabat, Morocco

M. Turgut et al. (eds.), *Arachnoid Cysts*, https://doi.org/10.1007/978-3-031-22701-1_23

central ependymal canal, such that this cyst is not lined by ependymal cells [55]. The majority of hydro-syringomyelia is located in the cervicothoracic cord, especially between the C2 and T9 vertebral levels; however, the cystic cavitation can span the entire length of the spinal cord. Typically, syrinx fluid has the same characteristics as CSF which explains why hydro-syringomyelia may be confused with a true intramedullary spinal AC.

Patients with hydro-syringomyelia present with a wide variety of neurological symptoms depending on the size, level, and chronicity of the syrinx, but classically, there is a mix of motor and sensory features, with both acute and chronic findings. Most patients present with cervico-occipital pain, a suspended "cape" dissociated sensory loss, and lower motor neuron weakness of the hand and arm. This motor and sensory damage can eventually cause atrophy and severe hand deformities.

On neuroimaging, the syrinx has the same radiographic characteristics on all imaging modalities as an intramedullary AC (Fig. 1). However, on T2-weighted MR imaging, the hydro-syringomyelia may be hypointense areas representing a flow artifact. Recent advances in dynamic MRI sequencing propose more accurate techniques for detecting intradural spinal ACs and differentiating it from hydro-syringomyelia. Recently, cine-mode balanced steady-state free precession MR imaging emerges as a new useful technique to differentiate intradural spinal cystic lesions, especially those containing CSF [30, 81].

In any case, when a significant intramedullary cyst is identified, it is important to screen for other potential neurologic congenital malformations, particularly craniocervical junction abnormalities (e.g. Chiari malformations).

Interestingly, some syringomyelia may be associated with intradural spinal ACs probably due to alterations in normal CSF circulation [32, 76]. Recognition of this association can be challenging on MRI because these ACs can be fenestrated or webbed. Careful assessment of the MRI can reveal subtle indentation of the spinal cord at the superior or inferior extent of the syrinx cavity [76].

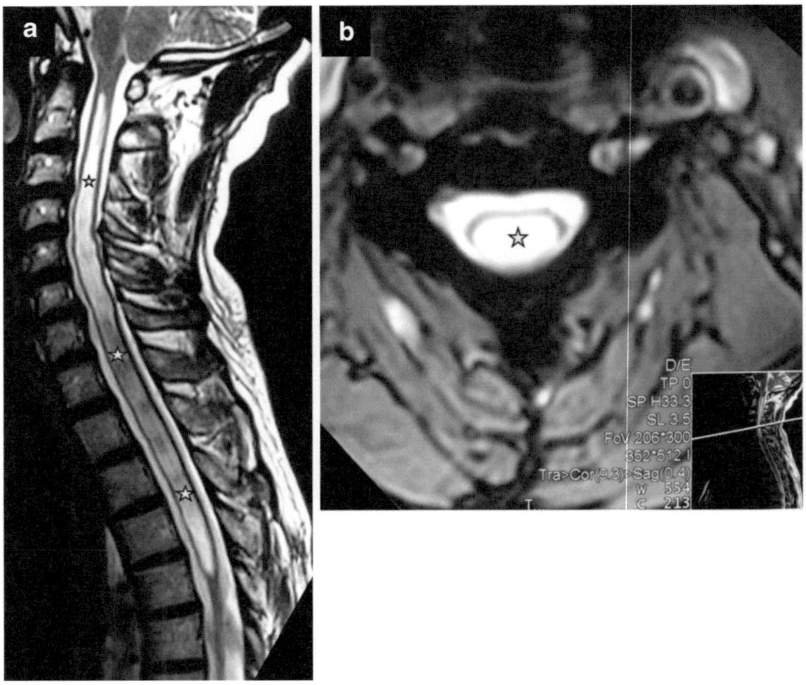

Fig. 1 Sagittal (**a**) and axial (**b**) T2-weighted MR images showing an extensive intramedullary syrinx from C2 to T5 vertebral level (stars). This hydro-syringomyelia is associated with type I Chiari malformation

3 Spinal Hygromas

A spinal hygroma refers to the accumulation of CSF in the subdural space along the spine [50]. Some spinal hygromas can be extradural, but this is a very rare condition [66]. Classically, spinal subdural hygromas appear after trauma [25, 67]. However, other underlying causes may exist such as iatrogenic interventions (including spinal surgery), spontaneous intracranial hypotension, and possibly, following meningeal inflammation [75]. Spinal hygromas are encountered in all age groups from children to aging adults.

Intraspinal hygroma differs from intraspinal ACs in many aspects such as the content of subdural fluid collection, neuroimaging appearance, and clinical manifestations. The vast majority of patients are asymptomatic. However, some symptoms that are unusually reported consist of back pain, postural headaches, nausea/vomiting, blurred vision, vestibulocochlear manifestations, symptoms of spinal cord or cauda equina compression as well as symptoms associated with the underlying etiology. On neuroimaging, most spinal hygromas have a crescent or spindle-shaped appearance and can typically cover several spinal levels, from the cervical spine to the lumbosacral region. On CT scan without intrathecal contrast injection, it is not possible to differentiate hygroma from ACs. However, both MR with T2-weignted imaging and CT-myelography are good initial choices for diagnosis and can further detect the CSF leak site [75]. Also, some authors have reported the usefulness of MR myelography with intrathecal gadolinium or radionuclide cisternography [44]. In the axial plane, intraspinal hygromas can have a tent shape due to the meningovertebral ligaments around the spinal cord. Subdural hygromas can also have a tri-radiate pattern called an "inverted Mercedes Benz sign" in the lumbar area due to the position of the spinal nerve roots. In contrast, spinal ACs have a well-defined scalloped or round margin and do not often extend over several spinal levels. Some large spinal hygromas can show MRI features of craniospinal hypotension such as engorgement of the venous sinuses, enhancement of the pachymeninges, pituitary hyperemia, and a decreased pontomesencephalic angle [16, 44, 83].

Signal contents are similar to those of CSF on MRI. However, in some atypical cases, there is a heterogeneous signal on MR imaging especially hyperintensity on the fluid attenuated inversion recovery sequence related to a mixture of CSF and blood.

4 Spinal Subdural Hematomas

A spinal subdural hematoma (SDH) is a collection of blood in the intraspinal subdural space which is the potential space between the arachnoid mater and the dura mater of the meninges that envelop the spinal cord and the cauda equina. There are several different conditions or etiologies that can cause spinal SDH, including bleeding disorders, hematologic disease, anticoagulation therapy, traumatic injury, iatrogenic injury, intraspinal vascular malformations, and intraspinal tumors [53]. Sometimes, the exact cause of the bleeding is not known and the intraspinal SDH is then considered "idiopathic" [41].

The incidence of intraspinal SDH is much lower than that of the cranial subdural hematoma because the intraspinal subdural space lacks the same number of blood vessels or bridging veins which could be a cause of subdural bleeding [33, 53]. Also, subdural hematomas are among the most unusual types of intraspinal hematomas [33, 40].

Clinical signs and symptoms of spinal SDH are diverse and vary depending on the size, level, and cause of the hematomas. Except for post-traumatic forms, the majority of cases will present with back pain and varying degrees of spinal cord compression or cauda equina syndrome. Often, the diagnosis may be unpredictable prior to an imaging study.

Often a long standing unrecognized pathology, spinal SDH has greatly benefited from the contribution of magnetic resonance (MR) imaging that is now the imaging modality of choice for obtaining a diagnosis [60]. MR imaging can demonstrate both the subdural hematoma, its location and may reveal the underlying tumoral or vascular etiology. The hematoma itself has a variable T1 and T2 signal depending on the chronicity of the bleeding. The axial view is particularly important for differentiating between subdural and epidural hematomas. Spinal epidural hematoma has a convex lens-like shape and is typically located dorsal to the spinal cord, while a subdural hematoma is usually found ventral and lateral to and around the spinal cord with a semi-circular "cap sign" pattern, or in a tri-radiate pattern called "inverted Mercedes Benz sign" in the lumbar area [40, 45]. It is primarily chronic forms of spinal SDH that may be confused with an intraspinal AraC when the collection demonstrates CSF signal intensity on all MR imaging pulse sequences. However, spinal SDH is usually crescentic, not round or scalloped, and the signal appearance is never exactly identical. Subdural hematomas show evidence of prior hemorrhage, especially on T2* and fluid attenuated inversion recovery (FLAIR) sequences, and can have enhancing membranes following gadolinium injection [41, 45, 60].

5 Cystic Tumors

Some spinal extradural cystic tumors on CT scan may be confused with other cystic lesions such as spinal ACs. However, the development of advanced MR imaging techniques, especially using multiple sequences and gadolinium administration, facilitates the differentiation between both lesions. Careful inspection of solid/cystic components within the suspected lesion, examination of its relationship to surrounding structures, evaluation of the enhancement pattern after gadolinium injection, will help in avoiding this confusion. Indeed, the majority of these tumors arise in the vertebrae with limited epidural extension as seen with aneurysmal bone cysts, giant cell tumors, and lymphangiomas [19, 26, 35, 87]. Intraspinal ACs do not cause bone damage although occasionally large epidural ACs will cause only moderate bony indentation without real spinal osteolysis.

Most intradural-extramedullary spinal tumors are meningiomas and schwannomas, and both may be associated with a cystic component [78, 85]. An intratumoral cyst may be secondary to a degenerative process, ischemic necrosis, bleeding, and/or tumor cell secretion [28, 57, 80]. Tumor cyst fluid has generally *a high level of protein* in its composition. In addition, some tumor associated cysts represent a trapped encysted accumulation of CSF contiguous with large intradural-extramedullary tumors. When a neoplasm develops within the subarachnoid space, it traps the CSF between itself and the adjacent spinal cord parenchyma.

The majority of these cystic tumors are easy to differentiate from intraspinal ACs due to their solid parts. In addition, post-gadolinium injection images can differentiate between similar lesions where an enhancing component is typical in fleshy tumors but is not present in intradural ACs [65]. It is important to remember that some schwannomas are intra/extradural and even intra/extraspinal dumbbell-shaped tumors [20]. Pure cystic tumors that developed entirely within the subarachnoid space are rare [3, 37].

Although intramedullary ACs are rare, various spinal cord tumors such as astrocytoma, ependymoma (Fig. 2), hemangioblastoma, and even ganglioglioma can show both solid and cystic areas mimicking a "true" spinal cord AC especially when the cystic collection is predominant. Cyst fluids that will eventually coalesce have a different consistency than CSF. Nevertheless, the majority of these tumors have adjacent edema. Additionally, these cystic tumors will demonstrate enhancement of the solid component after gadolinium administration on MR imaging [41, 62, 72, 82].

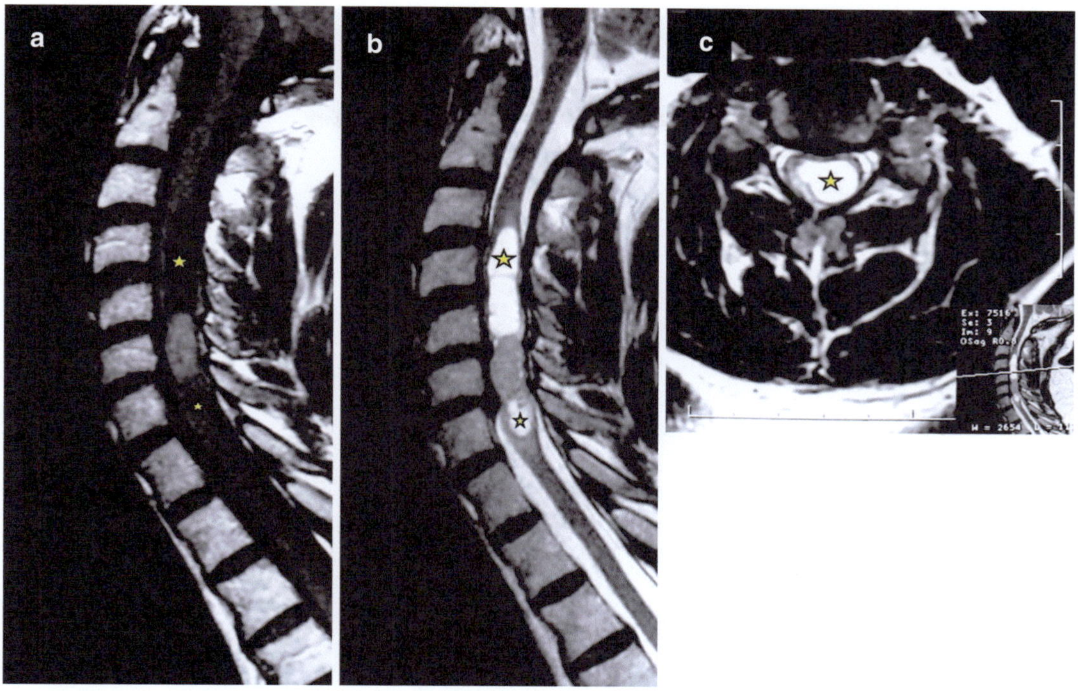

Fig. 2 Sagittal T1- (**a**) and sagittal (**b**) and axial (**c**) T2-weighted MR images revealing a cervical C4–C7 spinal cord ependymoma with both solid and cystic (stars) areas

6 Non-Neoplastic Cysts

Non-neoplastic cysts are relatively unusual lesions, rarely seen in the spinal canal. These cystic lesions encompass a wide variety of diseases usually congenital in nature. They include ACs, dermoid cysts and epidermoid cysts, enterogenous cysts, teratomatous cysts (cystic teratomas) (Fig. 3), neurenteric cysts, ependymal cysts, and bronchogenic cysts [54]. All these non-neoplastic cysts may mimic other intraspinal cystic lesions of various etiologies. Although MRI is considered the diagnostic procedure of choice, some non-epithelial cysts have been reported to be confused with intraspinal ACs due to their similar shape, topographic location, and even the signal intensity of the cyst contents. Therefore, the definitive diagnosis is obtained only through histopathological evaluation.

6.1 Epidermoid and Dermoid Cysts

Epidermoid and dermoid cysts are congenital lesions that occur due to the inclusion of ectodermal elements during neural tube closure. The two cyst types are often grouped together, but epidermoid cysts are lined only with stratified squamous epithelium, whereas dermoid cysts contain additional skin appendages, such as hair, sebaceous glands, and sweat glands. Both epidermoid and dermoid cysts have been confused pathologically for many years [54].

Most spinal epidermoid and dermoid cysts are thought to be congenital in origin but acquired cases have also been reported as a result of intraspinal lumbar needle puncture or following surgery due to epidermal cell implantation into the spinal canal [79]. These cysts usually develop in

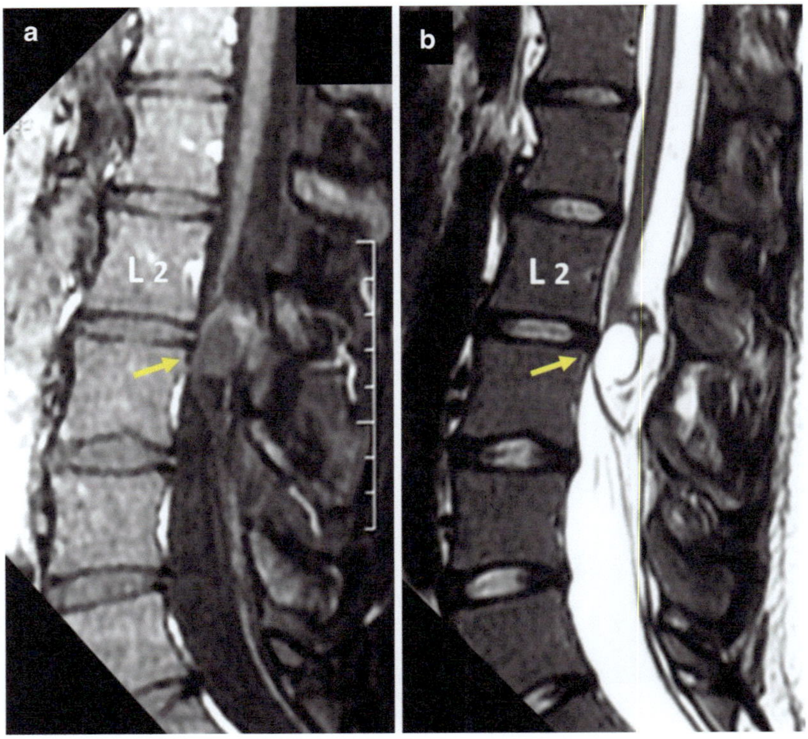

Fig. 3 Sagittal T1- following gadolinium injection (**a**) and T2-weighted (**b**) MR images showing a cystic teratoma of the conus medullaris

the subarachnoid space of the lumbosacral area and are less often located in the cervical/thoracic spinal column or within the spinal cord [5]. Epidermoid cysts have a strong association with concomitant spinal dysraphism and a dermal sinus tract [63]. Because of the slow-growing nature of these cysts, presentation in the adult is most common. Usually patients will present with nonspecific clinical symptoms similar to those of any other intradural spinal lesion. Uncommonly, there are clinical symptoms suggesting aseptic chemical meningitis caused by cyst rupture within the subarachnoid space [79].

Both epidermoid cysts and spinal ACs may have similar characteristics on T1/T2-weighted images and neither demonstrates gadolinium enhancement. However, the two cystic lesions present with differences visible on diffusion-weighted imaging (DWI): epidermoid cysts typically have an elevated signal on DWI due to the presence of fat and epithelial keratin inside the cyst, whereas ACs have unrestricted diffusion and a low signal in imaging [77].

Conversely, it is difficult to differentiate between epidermoid and dermoid cysts on MRI. Dermoid cysts are usually well-defined lobulated masses that have low attenuation from fat density due to sebum on CT scan and high signal intensity on T1-weighted MR images. In contrast, dermoids can be differentiated on MR imaging by signal intensities that follow that of fat not CSF [5, 54]. Lastly, it is useful to add that some epidermoid and dermoid cysts can demonstrate calcifications within the cysts on CT scan and enhancement may be seen around the cystic margin of some unusual forms of dermoid and epidermoid cysts.

6.2 Neurenteric Cysts

Neurenteric cysts which are also known as enterogenous cysts are rare, benign, congenital, endodermal lesions, resulting from incomplete resorption of the neurenteric canal between the notochord and the foregut. The cyst content is generally mucoid in nature, with a variable protein composition [18]. These extra-axial cystic lesions are more commonly seen in the spine than in the brain. They develop anterior to the neural axis and are frequently associated with vertebral body malformations and occasionally with a visible connection between the subarachnoid space and the enteric tract. Patients with neurenteric cysts are usually young adults. They may present with clinical signs and symptoms related to spinal cord compression. Other clinical manifestations include atypical respiratory symptoms, thoracic and/or abdominal pain, and meningitis [14].

On CT scan, neurenteric cysts are a mixture of isodense, hypodense, and hyperdense areas that sometimes have a widened spinal canal and congenital vertebral abnormalities. On the CT myelogram, the cysts are often intradural, extramedullary, and multilobulated. They can be similar to intraspinal ACs although most of them are iso- or slightly hyperintense compared to CSF on T1-weighted and typically hyperintense on T2-weighted MR imaging sequences. In truth, the image appearances may vary depending on the protein content [14, 18]. Peripheral rim enhancement is rare following contrast injection.

6.3 Ependymal Cysts

Intraspinal ependymal cysts, also known as neuroepithelial cysts, are rare benign congenital cysts lined by cuboidal ependymal cells that produce a clear serous liquid. Cyst expansion may be secondary to active fluid secretion [46]. They occur less frequently than ACs. The cysts are most commonly located within the spinal cord, anterior to the cervical cord or in the conus medullaris region, especially in the pediatric population. Associated spinal malformations are unusual. Ependymal cysts may be seen in all age groups. Usually, patients present with nonspecific clinical symptoms similar to those of any other intradural spinal lesion. However, pain is the most frequent symptom [71]. Symptomatic cases are usually correlated with large sizes.

On imaging, the margins of the cysts are smooth, well-defined, and distinct from the spinal cord parenchyma. Ependymal cysts are difficult to differentiate from spinal ACs. However, ACs are rarely seen intramedullary. Neuroepithelial cysts are isodense and isointense with CSF on CT scan and MR imaging respectively, without peripheral wall enhancement [46, 54, 71]. Sometimes, the cyst content may be hyperintense to CSF on T1-weighted MRI if there is a high protein concentration.

6.4 Bronchogenic Cysts

Spinal bronchogenic cysts (SBCs) are rare congenital lesions derived from the endodermal tract. They are considered the second most common foregut duplication cysts following neurenteric cysts [28]. Bronchogenic cysts are rarely seen within the spinal canal. They can occur anywhere in the spinal canal, but they are most often found in the cervical segment. The majority of cysts are intradural and extramedullary [49, 84]. They may enlarge slowly and cause an indolent course of spinal cord compression. Radiographs show imaging characteristics similar to CSF on all MRI sequences without contrast enhancement. Sometimes, the liquid content may have varying signal intensity on MR images due to the mixture of protein, water, and mucus. Spinal bronchogenic cysts are rarely diagnosed prior to surgery and the final diagnosis depends on the anatomopathological examination [49, 84].

7 Ventriculus Terminalis

The ventriculus terminalis (also known as persistent terminal ventricle, or fifth ventricle) is an ependymal lined cavity within the conus medullaris [42]. This entity differs from a "filar cyst" which is a rare small cyst located within the filum terminalis [21]. The ventriculus terminalis is in continuity with the central ependymal canal of the spinal cord and usually regresses during the first weeks after birth. This rare cystic anatomic variation may persist in adulthood causing neurologic and/or sphincter disturbances. Women in their 50s seem to be the most affected group [86].

On MRI, the ventriculus terminalis is usually described as a rounded or oval, non-enhancing lesion that appears hypointense on T1-weighted images and hyperintense on T2-weighted images with no perilesional edema. With regard to the cyst extension, no more than one or two vertebral segments are usually involved. According to a recent literature review, only 54 cases of surgically treated patients with a ventriculus terminalis have been reported [27, 68]. Distinguishing between a ventriculus terminalis and an intramedullary AC is difficult on neuroimaging. The final diagnosis can only be determined by histological examination.

8 Dural Ectasia

Dural ectasia, also known as an enlarged dural sac, refers to the ballooning or widening of the dural sac and/or spinal nerve root sleeves. This dural enlargement generally develops in the lumbosacral region where the CSF pressure is high. Dural ectasia can result in bony erosion especially as posterior vertebral scalloping. Pathogenesis of this rare entity is unknown; however, some cases were associated with generally weakened connective tissue as seen in Marfan syndrome, Ehlers-Danlos syndrome, Loeys-Dietz syndrome, or type 1 neurofibromatosis [23, 48]. Clinically, patients with an enlarged dural sac may present with low back pain, sciatica-like symptoms, lower limb weakness, sphincter disturbances, headache, or scoliosis [43]. But many patients will remain asymptomatic [23]. On lateral radiography and bony CT scan, posterior vertebral scalloping may be seen in the lumbosacral region. On MRI, there is an increase in the anteroposterior diameter of the dural sac with a lack of epidural fat. Signal content of the fluid inside the thecal sac is similar to that of CSF [23, 48].

9 Infectious Lesions

9.1 Hydatid Cysts

Hydatidosis is a rare parasitic disease principally caused by the larval cysts of the tapeworm *Echinococcus granulosus* less commonly *E. alveolaris* or *E. multilocularis.* The disease is endemic in those regions of the world where cattle and dogs live together and include the Mediterranean basin, the Middle East, Australia, and Latin America. The liver and lungs are the most common sites of infestation, unlike the skeleton. The spine is affected in less than 1% of all patients. The destruction of the vertebra causes spinal instability and secondary neurologic damage [2, 51].

In the spine, the cysts are usually microvesicular, multiple, and invasive. Typically, spinal hydatidosis is classified into five types [13]:

1. Intramedullary.
2. Intradural extramedullary.
3. Extradural intraspinal.
4. Vertebral.
5. Paravertebral.

Vertebral body lesions with extradural extension are the most frequent variation. In contrast, intradural hydatidosis is rare. The most common spinal sites involved are the lower thoracic and lumbar segments. Adult men are more commonly affected than women. The most frequent presenting symptoms are nonspecific and include back pain, radiculopathy, lower limb weakness, urinary/bowel disorder, and spinal deformity. Other signs and symptoms may be related to hepatic and pulmonary involvement. A previous history of hydatid disease will be evocative.

Plain X-ray and the CT scan reveal multiple, well-defined, osteolytic extensive cavitary vertebral areas without periosteal reaction or sclerosis. On CT scan, the occurrence of "classic" spherical lesions with several daughter cysts is frequent in the paravertebral soft tissues. Contrast enhance-

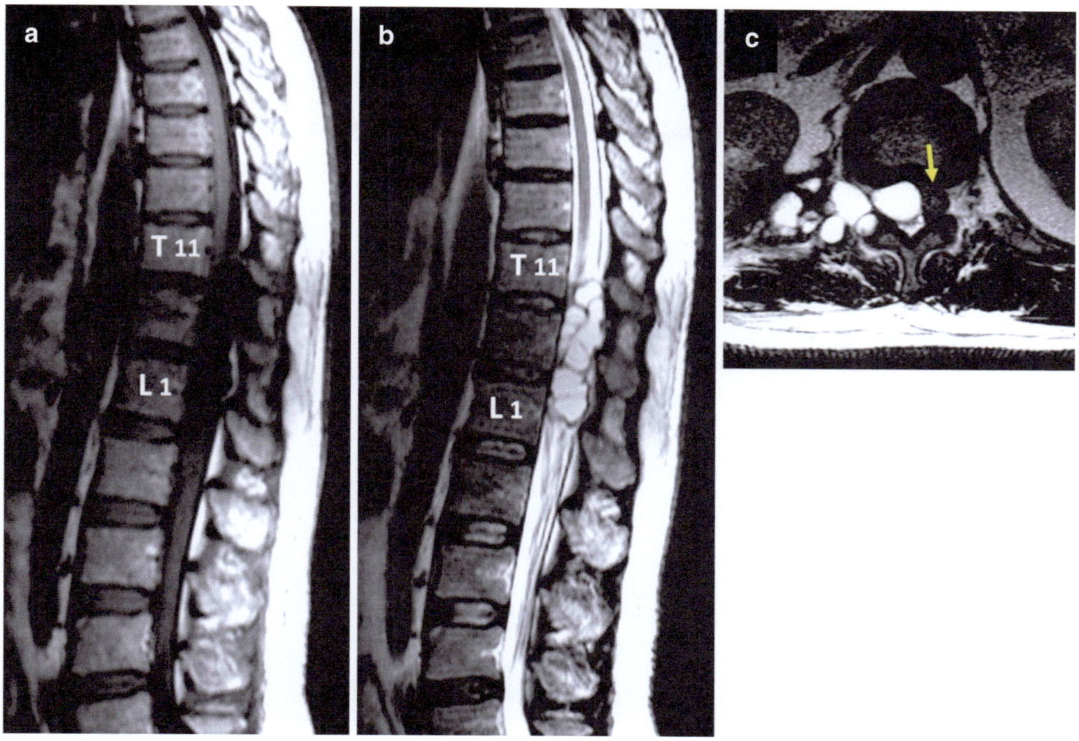

Fig. 4 Sagittal T1- (**a**) and sagittal (**b**) and axial (**c**) T2-weighted MR images revealing multiple epidural hydatid cysts from T11 to L1 without vertebral or paravertebral involvement. However, there is a right foraminal extension with spinal cord compression (arrow). The cyst contents are isointense to CSF

ment is rare and often related to bacterial co-infection. Whenever possible, it will be necessary to look for concomitant pulmonary and hepatic cysts. However, the majority of spinal ACs can be confused with type 2 and type 3 (Fig. 4) spinal hydatidosis, without vertebral or paravertebral involvement. In such cases, these parasitic cysts appear oblong like a "sausage" with thin uniform walls on MRI. These fluid-filled lesions demonstrate similar signal characteristics to CSF in all pulse sequences: low signal intensity on T1-weighted images and high intensity on T2-weighted images [2, 36, 51]. A modification in the signal intensity may suggest inactivation of the cyst viability. Classically, no walls enhance following gadolinium administration. Also, diffusion-weighted images can help differentiate hydatid cysts from spinal ACs and other suppurative collections. The degree and extent of the spinal cord compression will be better studied on sagittal T2-weighted images [70].

9.2 Suppurations

Most intraspinal canal infections are extradural. They are known as spinal epidural abscess (Figs. 5 and 6) and are less often seen within the spinal cord as an intramedullary abscess (Fig. 7) but they can also be intradural extramedullary in location. Abscesses contained in the intradural-extramedullary space are also called *spinal subdural abscess* or *spinal subdural empyema*. All spinal canal infections have the potential to cause permanent damage to the spinal cord and even sepsis and death [2, 22, 69].

Some epidural abscesses may be associated with a concomitant infection in the vertebral body (spinal osteomyelitis), disk space (discitis), or both (spondylodiscitis). In contrast, simultaneous vertebral and paraspinal infections are rare with other types of intradural suppuration.

Development of these different infectious disease types mainly occurs through hematogenous

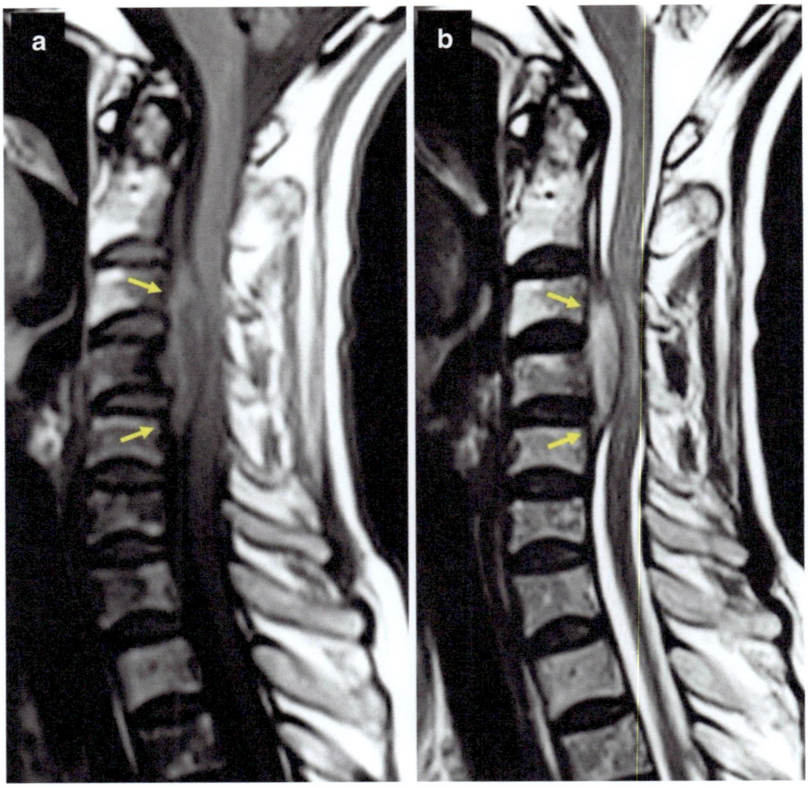

Fig. 5 Case 1. Sagittal T1- (**a**) and T2-weighted (**b**) MR images showing a C3–C5 anterior epidural abscess (arrows) causing spinal cord compression

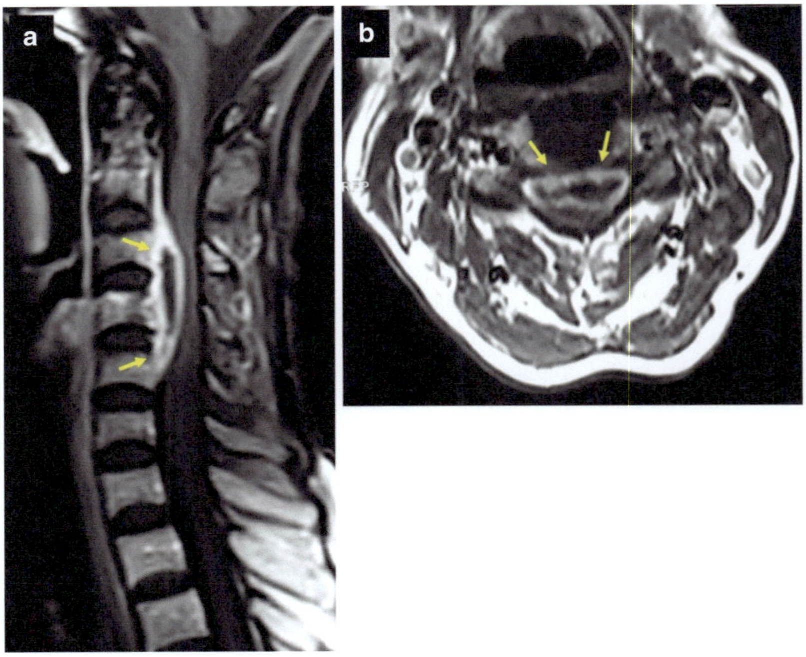

Fig. 6 Case 1. The epidural abscess (arrows) enhance peripherally around a central area of hypointensity on post-gadolinium sagittal (**a**) and axial (**b**) T1-weighted MR images

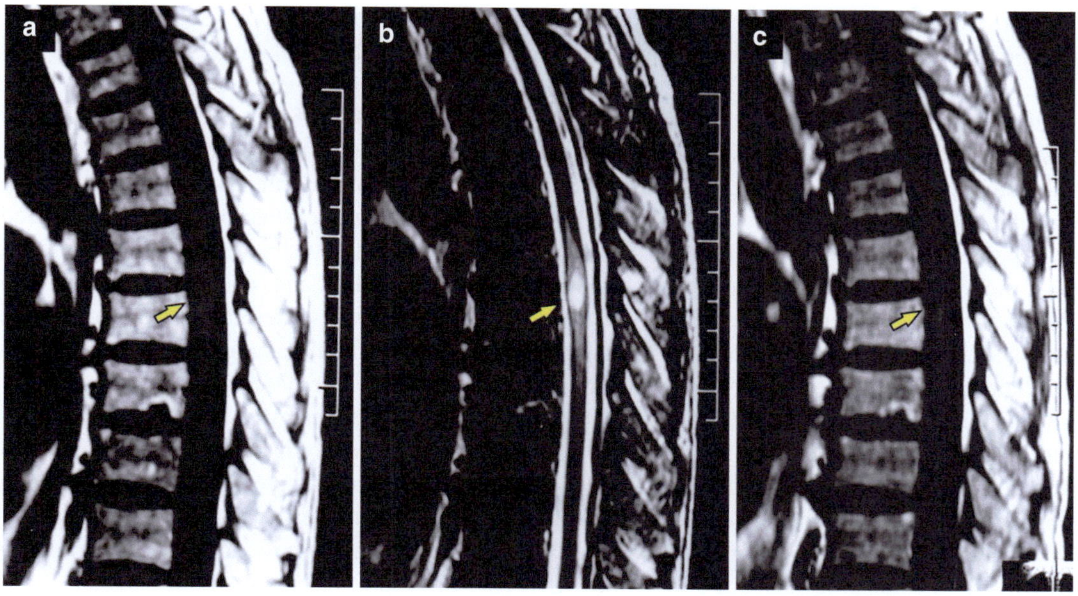

Fig. 7 Sagittal T1-weighted MRI after gadolinium administration (**a**) and on T2-weighted sequence (**b**). This midthoracic intraparenchymatous spinal cord ring-like lesion was proved to be an abscess (arrow). The patient was treated with antibiotic therapy and corticosteroids with a good recovery. The complete resolution of the abscess is seen on postcontrast sagittal T1-weighted images performed 12 weeks later. There is a moderate spinal atrophy without gadolinium enhancement (**c**) (arrow). (Reproduced from Akhaddar A. (2017) Spinal Cord Abscesses. In: Atlas of Infections in Neurosurgery and Spinal Surgery. Springer, Cham. https://doi.org/10.1007/978-3-319-60086-4_20; with permission)

spread from a remote source of infection, contiguous expansion from an adjacent infection, and direct inoculation. However, some cases remain cryptogenic. A number of underlying diseases and some predisposing factors can be identified in patients with intraspinal infectious collections and include intravenous drug abuse, HIV infection, diabetes mellitus, chronic renal failure, hepatic cirrhosis, alcoholism, underlying malignancy, morbid obesity, rheumatic heart valve disease, and tuberculosis. Furthermore, any immunosuppressive treatment can predispose to support spinal canal infections [2].

Thoracic and lumbar vertebral columns are the sites for infectious predilection. Because the extradural space has no smooth anatomic border like those found in the subdural space, epidural empyemas are often more focal and limited than subdural ones. Moreover, extradural suppurations are more common in the aging population with multiple comorbidities and are relatively unusual among children. Conversely, SCA are more frequent in male children, due to the increased potential for congenital midline defects [69].

Signs and symptoms of intraspinal canal infections are often nonspecific. Initially, clinical findings may be subtle and confusing due to other underlying medical issues. Acute forms present as an acute spinal cord syndrome mimicking "acute transverse myelitis," especially in intradural forms. Fever and back and/or root pain constitute typical presenting symptoms in addition to progressive neurological deficit below the level of the lesion. Initially, there is no spinal tenderness (except with spinal epidural abscess). Meningismus is a common symptom in intradural forms. Indeed, systemic signs of infection (fever, malaise, irritability, night sweats, and headache) are common but inconsistent [22, 69].

Chronic varieties tend to have a less specific symptomatology mimicking spinal cord tumors with a progressive neurological deficit and low back pain without fever. Nevertheless, signs and symptoms depend on the location of the lesion, the volume and number of collections/abscesses, and their chronicity.

Apparent etiologies, recent history of sepsis or an invasive procedure, or an anatomical spinal defect such as a congenital anomaly should constantly be taken into consideration.

Plain radiographies are normal unless there is an associated spondylodiscitis. CT scan may better define the destructive bony changes and intraspinal gas (bubbles of air) may be seen. A combination of spinal osteomyelitis and discitis on radiographic images is uncommon [22].

MRI is the imaging technique of choice to confirm the presence of a suppurative collection and to determine its exact location within the spinal canal. Typical suppurations appear as hypo or isointense collections on T1-weighted images and hyperintense collections on T2-weighted images with gadolinium enhancement. Collections that are fluid-filled and thus easily drained tend to be hyperintense on T2-weighted images and will enhance peripherally around a central core of hypointensity on T1-weighted images (Figs. 5 and 6). Fat suppression sequences may help in making the diagnosis by removing the increased signals of extradural fat and bone marrow [2].

Also, the purulent fluid demonstrates a high signal intensity on DWI and low ADC values reflecting decreased diffusion properties unlike those for ACs. Spinal subdural and intramedullary abscesses appear poorly defined compared to epidural collections. Screening for a congenital spine anomaly can help determine the diagnosis, especially in children.

9.3 Cysticercosis

Cysticercosis is the most common parasitic infection of the CNS worldwide, commonly affecting the brain. The disease is caused by the larva of the tapeworm Taenia solium. This parasitic disease is endemic in most parts of Asia, Latin America, and Sub-Saharan African countries. Intraspinal involvement is rare and is usually associated with intracranial cysticercosis [2, 17]. Classically, neurocysticercosis is categorized into four forms: vesicular, colloidal vesicular, granular nodular, and calcified nodular. Two types of cysts tend to develop in the spinal canal, primarily intradurally and may be confused with intraspinal ACs: simple cysts (Cysticercus cellulosae) and multiples cysts (Cysticercus racemosus). Both cystic forms may involve spinal cord parenchyma and subarachnoid spaces. Among these, leptomeningeal cysts are the most common. Spinal cysticercosis may cause arachnoiditis, meningitis, myelitis, or spinal cord compression. The most common clinical signs associated with intramedullary lesions are myelopathy and progressive motor weakness secondary to spinal cord compression. While back pain and radicular pain are the most frequent symptoms found with extramedullary cysts [17, 56].

Most spinal cysticercosis cysts are similar in appearance to a spinal AC with a signal intensity similar to that of the CSF on both T1- and T2-weighted images without restricted diffusion. Contiguous edema and post-gadolinium rim enhancement can be seen with parasitic cysts [64]. It is well known that the individual scolex is difficult to detect on MR imaging. The scolex can be seen within the cyst as a "mural nodule": a high intensity focus on T1-weighted images that is low intensity on T2-weighted images. The cystic lesions can be solitary or multiple, simple or multiloculated [51, 56, 64]. In addition, there are other findings suggesting the existence of this parasitic disease that complement the MRI results: medical history and by immunology workup that includes enzyme-linked immunosorbent assay and electroimmuno-transfer blot assay [17]. Conversely, these cystic lesions may be associated with concomitant intracranial cysts [39].

10 Meningoceles and Pseudomeningoceles

A spinal pseudomeningocele is an abnormal collection of CSF that communicates with the subarachnoid space surrounding the spinal cord, nerve roots, and cauda equina. These collections are mainly seen as a result of a traumatic injury or a surgical procedure [10, 31]. The CSF collection has no surrounding membrane, but it is contained in a cavity within the soft tissues. In contrast, in a "real meningocele" the CSF is contained within an extension of the meningeal layers. Meningoceles are typically classified as "congenital." They result from herniation of the meninges through a defect in the vertebral column (e.g. spina bifida) usually involving the soft tissues under the skin surface. Conversely, the majority of spinal pseudomeningoceles are "iatrogenic" and mainly occur in the posterior lumbosacral region following spinal surgery (Figs. 8 and 9). In brachial plexus injury, the key finding is that the nerve root avulsion pseudomeningocele does not contain any neural structures [24]. Pseudomeningoceles are frequently asymptomatic, but some patients may present with recurrent low back pain, lower extremity radiculopathy, nerve root entrapment, subcutaneous swelling, or symptoms of intracranial hypotension [4, 31]. CSF leakage from the wound may be the cause of severe subarachnoid and CNS infections. On CT scan, a pseudomeningocele appears as a low-density collection that extends to the dura with little or no peripheral contrast enhancement. Both on MRI and CT scan, the cyst content has similar features to CSF. Although MRI is the neurodiagnostic procedure of choice, CT-myelography and a radionuclide myelographic study may be useful tools in some situations [31]. Suspected fluid can be examined for detecting Beta2 transferrin which is a sensitive and specific method for diagnosing a CSF leak. Unlike the majority of intraspinal ACs, pseudomeningoceles are extradural and the diagnosis will be highly evocative when there is a previous history of spinal surgery or traumatic injury. Also, congenital meningoceles are defects of the neural tube, most are associated with neuroimaging with an anterior or posterior bony defect in the vertebral column [10, 24, 31].

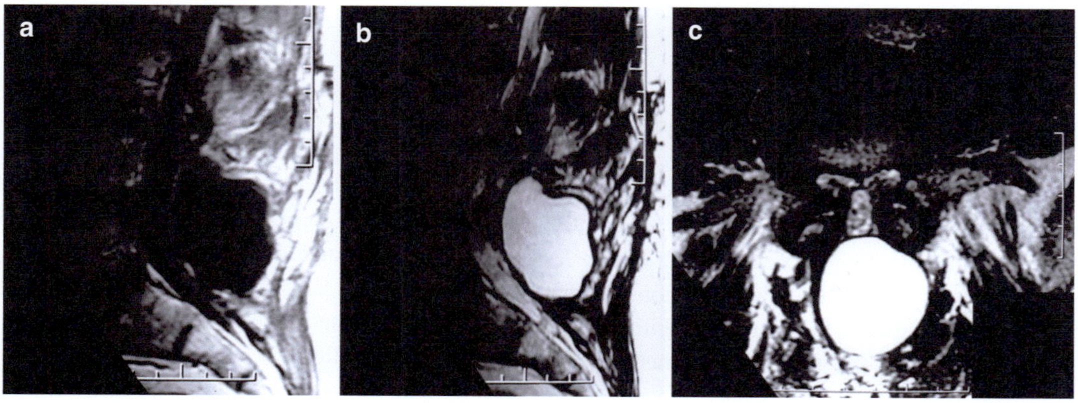

Fig. 8 Posterior lumbo-sacral pseudomeningoceles following L4–L5 laminectomy in a patient operated on 6 months previously for a lumbar spinal stenosis in another institution. Sagittal T1- (**a**) and sagittal (**b**) and axial (**c**) T2-weighted MR images

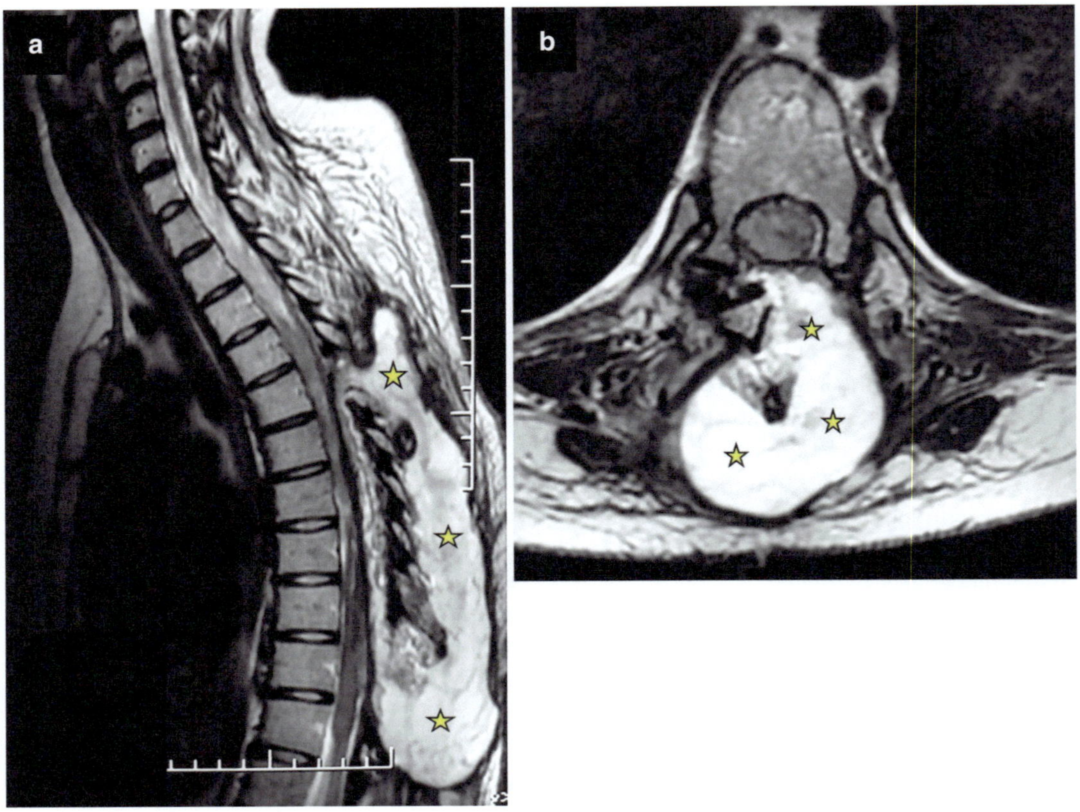

Fig. 9 Posterior mid-thoracic pseudomeningoceles (stars) following T6–T10 laminotomy in a young patient operated on 4 months previously for a thoracic spinal cord tumor in another neurosurgical center. Sagittal (**a**) and axial (**b**) T2-weighted MR images

11 Spinal Degenerative Cysts

Spinal degenerative cysts include a heterogeneous group of cystic lesions that potentially share a common etiology supporting a theory of degeneration. At least, increased motion and the role of trauma seem to have a responsibility in the formation of many cysts. This group includes the following types [7, 8, 12, 58, 74]:

- Juxtafacet cysts which include synovial cysts and ganglion cysts.
- Ligamentum flavum cysts also known as flaval cysts.
- Discal cysts.
- Posterior longitudinal ligament cysts.
- Cysts associated with Baastrup disease.

These cystic collections have been categorized using various combinations of topographic and pathological characteristics and by their attachment to or communication with a specific spinal structure such as a facet joint, intervertebral disc, and/or various spinal ligaments. Cyst walls are composed of fibrous tissue of varying thickness and cellularity without signs of infection or inflammation. The cyst composition is variable: serous, proteinaceous, hemorrhagic, or a mixture of all of them. Sometimes, the cyst walls are calcified or the cyst fluid may contain gas. Finally, distinction between these 6 types of cysts may sometimes be difficult and is clinically unimportant for many authors [29, 38, 52]. Most cysts are epidural, small, benign, and often occur in the lumbar spine. Synovial cysts develop more commonly in the lateral epidural space in the proximity of a lumbar facet joint (Fig. 10). Ligamentum flavum cysts are attached to the LF laterally. Discal cysts, ganglion cysts, and posterior longitudinal ligament cysts (Fig. 11) occur in the antero-lateral epidural space [8]. However, cysts of Baastrup disease are found in the posterior median epidural region. With the increasing usage of neuroimaging techniques, many incidental asymptomatic cysts are being discovered on CT scan and MR imaging in middle aged and elderly patients. Nevertheless, other cysts may produce acute or chronic symptoms. These symptoms are highly variable and depend principally on the anatomic location, cyst dimension, and chronological evolution. Generally, most patients have low back pain and/or radicular symptoms mimicking a lumbar disc herniation or lumbar spinal stenosis.

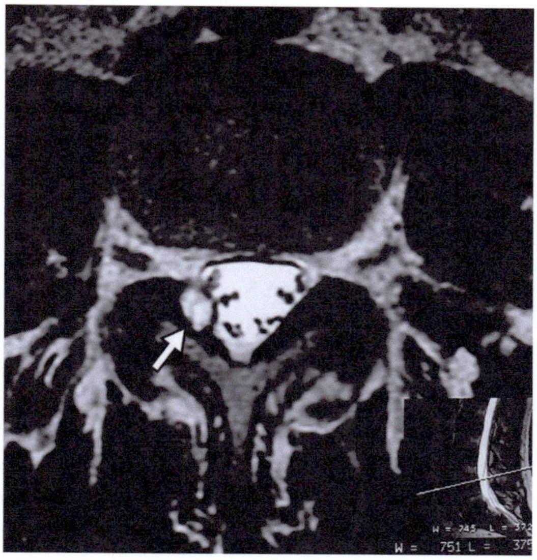

Fig. 10 Right extradural L4–L5 synovial cyst (arrow) mimicking a Tarlov cyst. Axial T2-weighted MR image

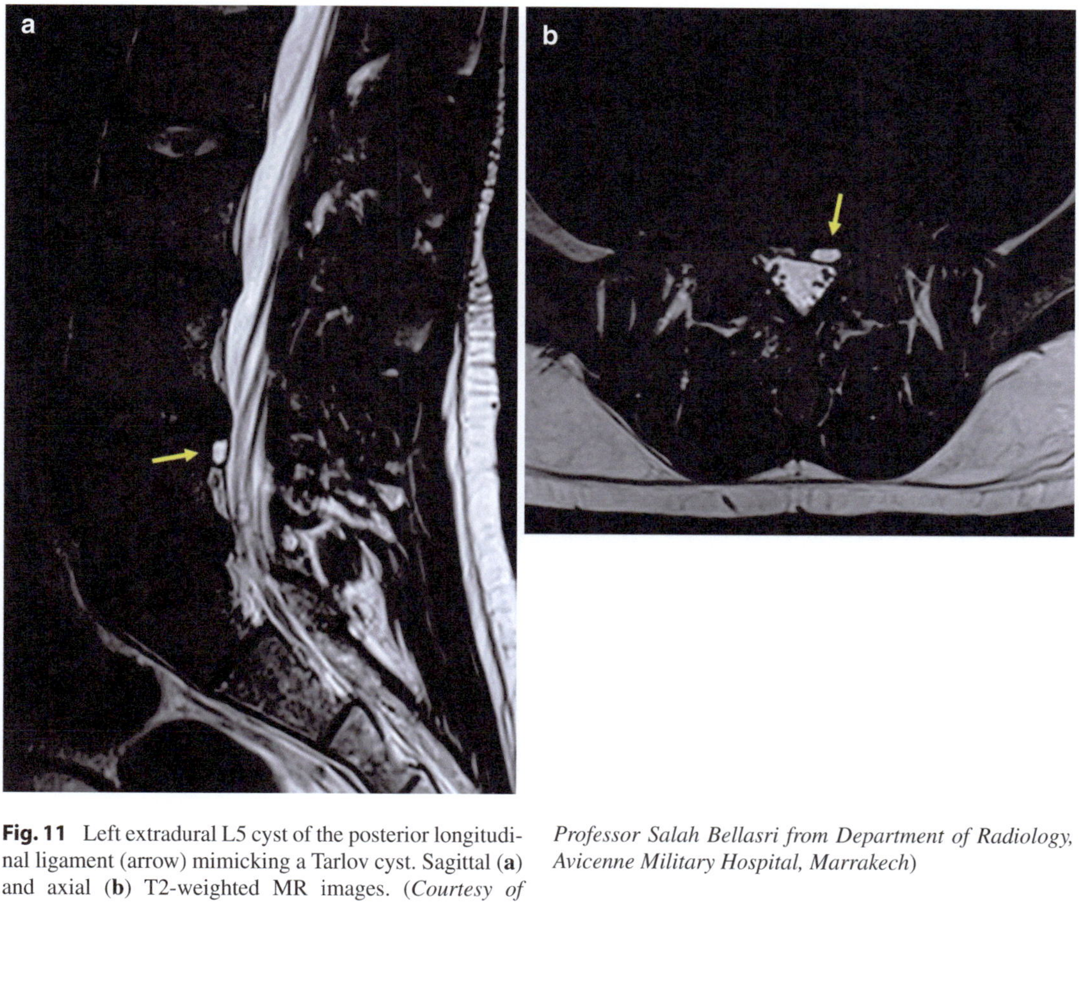

Fig. 11 Left extradural L5 cyst of the posterior longitudinal ligament (arrow) mimicking a Tarlov cyst. Sagittal (**a**) and axial (**b**) T2-weighted MR images. (*Courtesy of Professor Salah Bellasri from Department of Radiology, Avicenne Military Hospital, Marrakech*)

Spinal degenerative cysts are rarely confused with spinal ACs. However, some degenerative cysts have unenhanced signal features very similar to those of CSF. On MRI, most degenerative cysts are well-defined thin-walled lesions usually centered on their originating structures and the contents display the signal intensity of water on all sequences. Mural enhancement may be seen following contrast injection. However, gadolinium administration is rarely required. Very rarely secondary acute bleeding or infection may occur within the cyst, changing its signal characteristics, and it may present with high signal on T1 and heterogeneous low signal on T2-weighted images. Possible bone remodeling/erosion and a calcified rim are better seen on CT scan. Intracystic contrast injection can be useful in differentiating between synovial cysts, discal cysts, and the other degenerative cysts [8].

12 Spinal Cord Herniation

A spinal cord herniation is an unusual pathologic entity caused by a defect in the arachnoid layer, with tethering of the spinal cord in close contact with the subdural space [73]. Although post-surgical or post-traumatic cases were previously reported, most cases are considered "idiopathic" or spontaneous spinal cord herniations because no obvious secondary cause is identified. Generally, most patients presented with focal myelopathy such as Brown-Séquard syndrome or spastic paraparesis. Idiopathic herniation of the spinal cord classically occurs in the kyphotic mid-thoracic spine area. More spinal cords herniate through a small anterior or a far *lateral* arachnoid defect. On sagittal MR images, a focal anterior displacement/angulation of the spinal cord is observed, generally limited to 1 or 2 vertebral segments with or without spinal cord atrophy. Also, a high T2 signal intensity may be seen within the spinal cord parenchyma. Interestingly, there was no CSF seen between the spinal cord parenchyma and the subarachnoid space but there was an enlargement of the subarachnoid space on the opposite side, which should be differentiated from subdural intraspinal ACs [11, 59]. Myelography combined with CT myelography is helpful for the diagnosis; however, MRI remains the gold standard for differentiating the majority of other cystic lesions [9]. For some authors, phase-contrast pulse cine MRI can easily exclude an associated posterior ACs [15].

13 Other Cyst-Like Entities

More intricate intraspinal fluid collections may be confused with a spinal ACs and can also be included in the present list such as vascular malformations (dural fistula, arteriovenous malformation, or other vascular anomalies), hematomas (spontaneous or secondary), varices, gas/pneumatic pseudocysts [6], or arachnoiditis (infectious, inflammatory, or iatrogenic).

14 Conclusion

Although intraspinal ACs have been considered uncommon for a very long time, these cysts are more and more often seen in our regular spinal imaging studies. Among asymptomatic and symptomatic cases, the practitioner should consider other spinal and intraspinal cystic lesions or normal anatomic variants that can occasionally be confused with "real" spinal ACs. In the case of a diagnostic uncertainty or unusual neuroimaging features, additional improved MR imaging should be requested whenever possible. This additional imaging may indicate the exact topography of the cysts and their inner structures, defining the exact margins of the collections, and determining the relationship of the cysts with contiguous anatomic structures as well as any communication between the cyst and adjacent subarachnoid spaces. Such information, in addition to the clinical presentation and occasionally biological data, will be essential to improve our capacity to determine the best therapeutic decision for each case.

References

1. Aithala GR, Sztriha L, Amirlak I, Devadas K, Ohlsson I. Spinal arachnoid cyst with weakness in the limbs and abdominal pain. Pediatr Neurol. 1999;20:155–6. https://doi.org/10.1016/s0887-8994(98)00131-3.
2. Akhaddar A, editor. Atlas of infections in neurosurgery and spinal surgery. Cham: Springer International; 2017. https://doi.org/10.1007/978-3-319-60086-4.
3. Akhaddar A, Ajja A, Albouzidi A, Elmostarchid B, Boucetta M. Cystic schwannoma of the cauda equina mimicking hemangioblastoma. Neurochirurgie. 2008;54:101–3. https://doi.org/10.1016/j.neuchi.2008.01.007.
4. Akhaddar A, Boulahroud O, Boucetta M. Nerve root herniation into a calcified pseudomeningocele after lumbar laminectomy. Spine J. 2012;12:273. https://doi.org/10.1016/j.spinee.2012.02.008.
5. Akhaddar A, el Hassani MY, Ghadouane M, Hommadi A, Chakir N, Jiddane M, et al. Dermoid cyst of the conus medullaris revealed by chronic urinary retention. Contribution of imaging. J Neuroradiol. 1999;26:132–6.
6. Akhaddar A, Eljebbouri B, Naama O, Boucetta M. Sciatica due to lumbar intraspinal gas pseudocyst. Intern Med. 2010;49:2647. https://doi.org/10.2169/internalmedicine.49.4474.
7. Akhaddar A, Qamouss O, Belhachmi A, Elasri A, Okacha N, Boucetta M. Cervico-thoracic juxtafacet cyst causing spinal foraminal widening. Joint Bone Spine. 2008;75:747–9. https://doi.org/10.1016/j.jbspin.2008.04.009.
8. Aljuboori Z, Altstadt T. Symptomatic lumbar discal cyst: a rare entity that can mimic other lumbar cystic lesions. Cureus. 2019;11:e5453. https://doi.org/10.7759/cureus.5453.
9. Bartanusz V, Savage JG, Belayev A. Spinal cord herniation or intradural arachnoid cyst? Spine J. 2014;14:385. https://doi.org/10.1016/j.spinee.2013.05.045.
10. Beretta F, Bernucci C, D'Aliberti G. Anterior spinal pseudomeningocele after C0-C2 traumatic injuries: role of the "dural transitional zone" in the etiopathogenesis. Eur Spine J. 2013;22(Suppl 6):S889–93. https://doi.org/10.1007/s00586-013-3029-5.
11. Berg-Johnsen J, Ilstad E, Kolstad F, Züchner M, Sundseth J. Idiopathic ventral spinal cord herniation: an increasingly recognized cause of thoracic myelopathy. J Cent Nerv Syst Dis. 2014;6:85–91. https://doi.org/10.4137/JCNSD.S16180.
12. Biji B, Moorthy RK, Rajshekhar V. Posterior longitudinal ligament cyst as a rare cause of lumbosacral radiculopathy with positive straight leg raising test. Neurol India. 2008;56:96–7. https://doi.org/10.4103/0028-3886.39330.
13. Braithwaite PA, Lees RF. Vertebral hydatid disease: radiological assessment. Radiology. 1981;140:763–6. https://doi.org/10.1148/radiology.140.3.7280247.
14. Brooks BS, Duvall ER, el Gammal T, Garcia JH, Gupta KL, Kapila A. Neuroimaging features of neurenteric cysts: analysis of nine cases and review of the literature. AJNR Am J Neuroradiol. 1993;14:735–46.
15. Brugières P, Malapert D, Adle-Biassette H, Fuerxer F, Djindjian M, Gaston A. Idiopathic spinal cord herniation: value of MR phase-contrast imaging. AJNR Am J Neuroradiol. 1999;20:935–9.
16. Burtis MT, Ulmer JL, Miller GA, Barboli AC, Koss SA, Brown WD. Intradural spinal vein enlargement in craniospinal hypotension. AJNR Am J Neuroradiol. 2005;26:34–8.
17. Carpio A. Neurocysticercosis: an update. Lancet Infect Dis. 2002;2:751–62. https://doi.org/10.1016/s1473-3099(02)00454-1.
18. Chakraborty S, Priamo F, Loven T, Li J, Insinga S, Schulder M. Supratentorial neurenteric cysts: case series and review of pathology, imaging, and clinical management. World Neurosurg. 2016;85:143–52. https://doi.org/10.1016/j.wneu.2015.08.057.
19. Chatzidakis EM, Volikas Z, Condilis N, Lypiridis S, Fratzoglou M, Simopoulos K. Spinal cystic meningioma presenting as a ring enhancing lesion on MRI. Ann Ital Chir. 2008;79:197–8.
20. Cho DY, Hur JW, Shim JH, Kim JS. Cystic giant sacral schwannoma mimicking aneurysmal bone cyst: a case report and review of literatures. J Korean Neurosurg Soc. 2013;54:350–4. https://doi.org/10.3340/jkns.2013.54.4.350.
21. Choi JH, Lee T, Kwon HH, You SK, Kang JW. Outcome of ultrasonographic imaging in infants with sacral dimple. Korean J Pediatr. 2018;61:194–9. https://doi.org/10.3345/kjp.2018.61.6.194.
22. Darouiche RO, Hamill RJ, Greenberg SB, Weathers SW, Musher DM. Bacterial spinal epidural abscess. Review of 43 cases and literature survey. Medicine (Baltimore). 1992;71:369–85.
23. de Kleuver M, van Jonbergen JP, Langeloo DD. Asymptomatic massive dural ectasia associated with neurofibromatosis type 1 threatening spinal column support: treatment by anterior vascularized fibula graft. J Spinal Disord Tech. 2004;17:539–42. https://doi.org/10.1097/01.bsd.0000117544.88865.f0.
24. Drzymalski DM, Tuli J, Lin N, Tuli S. Cervicothoracic intraspinal pseudomeningocele with cord compression after a traumatic brachial plexus injury. Spine J. 2010;10:e1–5. https://doi.org/10.1016/j.spinee.2010.08.002.
25. Elder BD, Ishida W, Goodwin RC, Bydon A. Iatrogenic spinal subdural extra-arachnoid hygroma following uncomplicated lumbar decompression. Cureus. 2017;9:e1171. https://doi.org/10.7759/cureus.1171.
26. Fattahi A, Taheri M, Majdi M. Lymphangioma of the thoracic spine with epidural compression: a case report. Iran J Med Sci. 2019;44:172–5.
27. Fletcher-Sandersjöö A, Edström E, Bartek J Jr, Elmi-Terander A. Surgical treatment for symptomatic ventriculus terminalis: case series and a literature

review. Acta Neurochir. 2019;161:1901–8. https://doi.org/10.1007/s00701-019-03996-0.
28. Fortuna A, Mercuri S. Intradural spinal cysts. Acta Neurochir. 1983;68:289–314. https://doi.org/10.1007/BF01401186.
29. Freidberg SR, Fellows T, Thomas CB, Mancall AC. Experience with symptomatic spinal epidural cysts. Neurosurgery. 1994;34:989–93. https://doi.org/10.1227/00006123-199406000-00006.
30. French H, Somasundaram A, Biggs M, Parkinson J, Allan R, Ball J, et al. Idiopathic intradural dorsal thoracic arachnoid cysts: a case series and review of the literature. J Clin Neurosci. 2017;40:147–52. https://doi.org/10.1016/j.jocn.2017.02.051.
31. Hawk MW, Kim KD. Review of spinal pseudomeningoceles and cerebrospinal fluid fistulas. Neurosurg Focus. 2000;9:e5. https://doi.org/10.3171/foc.2000.9.1.5.
32. Holly LT, Batzdorf U. Syringomyelia associated with intradural arachnoid cysts. J Neurosurg Spine. 2006;5:111–6. https://doi.org/10.3171/spi.2006.5.2.111.
33. Hsieh JK, Colby S, Nichols D, Kondylis E, Liu JKC. Delayed development of spinal subdural hematoma following cranial trauma: a case report and review of the literature. World Neurosurg. 2020;141:44–51. https://doi.org/10.1016/j.wneu.2020.05.158.
34. Hughes G, Ugokwe K, Benzel EC. A review of spinal arachnoid cysts. Cleve Clin J Med. 2008;75:311–5. https://doi.org/10.3949/ccjm.75.4.311.
35. Jiang G, Sun LL, Ye YJ, Yang ZT, Ji QL, Pang J, et al. Giant cell tumors of the mobile spine with invasion of adjacent vertebrae: an unusual imaging finding. BMC Musculoskelet Disord. 2021;22:726. https://doi.org/10.1186/s12891-021-04610-0.
36. Kafaji A, Al-Zain T, Lemcke J, Al-Zain F. Spinal manifestation of hydatid disease: a case series of 36 patients. World Neurosurg. 2013;80:620–6. https://doi.org/10.1016/j.wneu.2013.06.013.
37. Kasliwal MK, Kale SS, Sharma BS, Suri V. Totally cystic intradural extramedullary schwannoma. Turk Neurosurg. 2008;18:404–6.
38. Khalatbari K, Ansari H. MRI of degenerative cysts of the lumbar spine. Clin Radiol. 2008;63:322–8. https://doi.org/10.1016/j.crad.2007.05.020.
39. Kimura-Hayama ET, Higuera JA, Corona-Cedillo R, Chávez-Macías L, Perochena A, Quiroz-Rojas LY, et al. Neurocysticercosis: radiologic-pathologic correlation. Radiographics. 2010;30:1705–19. https://doi.org/10.1148/rg.306105522.
40. Kobayashi K, Imagama S, Ando K, Nishida Y, Ishiguro N. Acute non-traumatic idiopathic spinal subdural hematoma: radiographic findings and surgical results with a literature review. Eur Spine J. 2017;26:2739–43. https://doi.org/10.1007/s00586-017-5013-y.
41. Kobayashi K, Ando K, Kato F, Sato K, Kamiya M, Tsushima M, et al. Variety of preoperative MRI changes in spinal cord ependymoma of WHO grade II: a case series. Eur Spine J. 2019;28:426–33. https://doi.org/10.1007/s00586-018-5760-4.
42. Koehler PJ. Isaäc Van Deen and benedikt stilling: a controversy on the function of the spinal cord in the 19th century. J Hist Neurosci. 1992;1:189–200. https://doi.org/10.1080/09647049209525532.
43. Kow CY, Tee JW, Jithoo R. Incidental dural ectasia associated with scoliosis. Spine J. 2016;16:e25–6. https://doi.org/10.1016/j.spinee.2015.08.043.
44. Kranz PG, Luetmer PH, Diehn FE, Amrhein TJ, Tanpitukpongse TP, Gray L. Myelographic techniques for the detection of spinal CSF leaks in spontaneous intracranial hypotension. AJR Am J Roentgenol. 2016;206:8–19. https://doi.org/10.2214/AJR.15.14884.
45. Krishnan P, Banerjee TK. Classical imaging findings in spinal subdural hematoma—"Mercedes-Benz" and "Cap" signs. Br J Neurosurg. 2016;30:99–100. https://doi.org/10.3109/02688697.2015.1071319.
46. Lalitha AV, Rout P, Souza FD, Shailesh, Rao S. Spinal intramedullary neuroepithelial (ependymal) cyst. A rare cause of treatable acute para paresis. Indian J Pediatr. 2006;73:945–6. https://doi.org/10.1007/BF02859294.
47. Lehman RA, Fieger HG Jr. Arachnoid cyst producing recurrent neurological disturbances. Surg Neurol. 1978;10:134–6.
48. Lundby R, Rand-Hendriksen S, Hald JK, Lilleås FG, Pripp AH, Skaar S, et al. Dural ectasia in Marfan syndrome: a case control study. AJNR Am J Neuroradiol. 2009;30:1534–40. https://doi.org/10.3174/ajnr.A1620.
49. Ma X, Li W, Niu C, Liang F, Guo L, Shakir TM, Zhang M. Intraspinal bronchogenic cyst: series of case reports and literature review. J Spinal Cord Med. 2017;40:141–6. https://doi.org/10.1080/10790268.2017.1279816.
50. Mack J, Squier W, Eastman JT. Anatomy and development of the meninges: implications for subdural collections and CSF circulation. Pediatr Radiol. 2009;39:200–10. https://doi.org/10.1007/s00247-008-1084-6.
51. Majmundar N, Patel PD, Dodson V, Tran A, Goldstein I, Assina R. Parasitic infections of the spine: case series and review of the literature. Neurosurg Focus. 2019;46:E12. https://doi.org/10.3171/2018.10.FOCUS18472.
52. Marshman LA, Benjamin JC, David KM, King A, Chawda SJ. "Disc cysts" and "posterior longitudinal ligament ganglion cysts": synonymous entities? Report of three cases and literature review. Neurosurgery. 2005;57:E818. https://doi.org/10.1093/neurosurgery/57.4.e818.
53. Matsumoto H, Matsumoto S, Yoshida Y. Concomitant intracranial chronic subdural hematoma and spinal subdural hematoma: a case report and literature review. World Neurosurg. 2016;90:706.e1–9. https://doi.org/10.1016/j.wneu.2016.03.020.
54. McNutt SE, Mrowczynski OD, Lane J, Jafrani R, Rohatgi P, Specht C, et al. Congenital spinal cysts: an update and review of the literature. World Neurosurg.

2021;145:480–91.e9. https://doi.org/10.1016/j.wneu.2020.08.092.
55. Milhorat TH, Capocelli AL Jr, Anzil AP, Kotzen RM, Milhorat RH. Pathological basis of spinal cord cavitation in syringomyelia: analysis of 105 autopsy cases. J Neurosurg. 1995;82:802–12. https://doi.org/10.3171/jns.1995.82.5.0802.
56. Pant I, Chaturvedi S, Singh G, Gupta S, Kumari R. Spinal cysticercosis: a report of two cases with review of literature. J Craniovertebr Junction Spine. 2016;7:285–8. https://doi.org/10.4103/0974-8237.193261.
57. Parisi G, Tropea R, Giuffrida S, Lombardo M, Giuffrè F. Cystic meningiomas. Report of seven cases. J Neurosurg. 1986;64:35–8. https://doi.org/10.3171/jns.1986.64.1.0035.
58. Park JW, Lee BJ, Jeon SR, Rhim SC, Park JH, Roh SW. Surgical treatment of lumbar spinal discal cyst: Is it enough to remove the cyst only without following discectomy? Neurol Med Chir (Tokyo). 2019;59:204–12. https://doi.org/10.2176/nmc.oa.2018-0219.
59. Parmar H, Park P, Brahma B, Gandhi D. Imaging of idiopathic spinal cord herniation. Radiographics. 2008;28:511–8. https://doi.org/10.1148/rg.282075030.
60. Pierce JL, Donahue JH, Nacey NC, Quirk CR, Perry MT, Faulconer N, et al. Spinal hematomas: what a radiologist needs to know. Radiographics. 2018;38:1516–35. https://doi.org/10.1148/rg.2018180099.
61. Prevo RL, Hageman G, Bruyn RP, Broere G, van de Stadt J. Extended extradural spinal arachnoid cyst: an unusual cause of progressive spastic paraparesis. Clin Neurol Neurosurg. 1999;101:260–3. https://doi.org/10.1016/s0303-8467(99)00050-5.
62. Raco A, Piccirilli M, Landi A, Lenzi J, Delfini R, Cantore G. High-grade intramedullary astrocytomas: 30 years' experience at the neurosurgery department of the university of Rome "Sapienza". J Neurosurg Spine. 2010;12:144–53. https://doi.org/10.3171/2009.6.SPINE08910.
63. Radmanesh F, Nejat F, El Khashab M. Dermal sinus tract of the spine. Childs Nerv Syst. 2010;26:349–57. https://doi.org/10.1007/s00381-009-0962-z.
64. Rajbhandari S, Gurung P, Yadav J, Rajbhandari P, Acharya S, Pant B. A case report of multiple isolated intradural neurocysticercosis of the lumbo-sacral spine. Int J Surg Case Rep. 2021;87:106434. https://doi.org/10.1016/j.ijscr.2021.106434.
65. Raz E, Zagzag D, Saba L, Mannelli L, Di Paolo PL, D'Ambrosio F, et al. Cyst with a mural nodule tumor of the brain. Cancer Imaging. 2012;12:237–44. https://doi.org/10.1102/1470-7330.2012.0028.
66. Rico-Santos M, Villafani J, Sáiz A, Oliva NP. Progressive back pain due to epidural hygroma: an infrequent complication of lumbar puncture in adults. BMJ Case Rep. 2015;2015:bcr2015211379. https://doi.org/10.1136/bcr-2015-211379.
67. Russo S, Belli A, Eynon A, Nader-Sepahi A. Post-traumatic spinal hygroma causing cord compression in type III odontoid fracture with vertical atlantoaxial instability. Spine (Phila Pa 1976). 2017;42:E1092–4. https://doi.org/10.1097/BRS.0000000000002081.
68. Sandersjöö A, Edström E, Bartek J Jr, Elmi-Terander A. Surgical treatment for symptomatic ventriculus terminalis: case series and a literature review. Acta Neurochir. 2019;161:1901–8. https://doi.org/10.1007/s00701-019-03996-0.
69. Sandler AL, Thompson D, Goodrich JT, van Aalst J, Kolatch E, El Khashab M, et al. Infections of the spinal subdural space in children: a series of 11 contemporary cases and review of all published reports. A multinational collaborative effort. Childs Nerv Syst. 2013;29:105–17. https://doi.org/10.1007/s00381-012-1916-4.
70. Secer HI, Anik I, Celik E, Daneyemez MK, Gonul E. Spinal hydatid cyst mimicking arachnoid cyst on magnetic resonance imaging. J Spinal Cord Med. 2008;31:106–8. https://doi.org/10.1080/10790268.2008.11753990.
71. Sharma A, Sayal P, Badhe P, Pandey A, Diyora B, Ingale H. Spinal intramedullary arachnoid cyst. Indian J Pediatr. 2004;71:e65–7.
72. She DJ, Lu YP, Xiong J, Geng DY, Yin B. MR imaging features of spinal pilocytic astrocytoma. BMC Med Imaging. 2019;19:5. https://doi.org/10.1186/s12880-018-0296-y.
73. Shimizu S, Kobayashi Y, Oka H, Kumabe T. Idiopathic spinal cord herniation: consideration of its pathogenesis based on the histopathology of the dura mater. Eur Spine J. 2019;28:298–305. https://doi.org/10.1007/s00586-017-5147-y.
74. Singh V, Rustagi T, Mahajan R, Priyadarshini M, Das K. Ligamentum flavum cyst: rare presentation report and literature review. Neurol India. 2020;68:1207–10. https://doi.org/10.4103/0028-3886.299172.
75. Sneyers B, Ramboer K. Spinal subdural hygroma. Acta Neurol Belg. 2021;121:311–9. https://doi.org/10.1007/s13760-020-01558-1.
76. Srinivasan VM, Fridley JS, Thomas JG, Omeis I. Nuances in localization and surgical treatment of syringomyelia associated with fenestrated and webbed Intradural spinal arachnoid cyst: a retrospective analysis. World Neurosurg. 2016;87:176–86. https://doi.org/10.1016/j.wneu.2015.11.004.
77. Tang L, Cianfoni A, Imbesi SG. Diffusion-weighted imaging distinguishes recurrent epidermoid neoplasm from postoperative arachnoid cyst in the lumbosacral spine. J Comput Assist Tomogr. 2006;30:507–9. https://doi.org/10.1097/00004728-200605000-00026.
78. Ursini T, Rodari P, Badona Monteiro G, Barresi V, Cicciò C, Moscolo F, et al. Large multicystic spinal lesion in a young African migrant: a problem of differential diagnosis. BMJ Case Rep. 2021;14:e242690. https://doi.org/10.1136/bcr-2021-242690.
79. van Aalst J, Hoekstra F, Beuls EA, Cornips EM, Weber JW, Sival DA, et al. Intraspinal dermoid and epidermoid tumors: report of 18 cases and reappraisal of the literature. Pediatr Neurosurg. 2009;45:281–90. https://doi.org/10.1159/000235602.

80. Vassilouthis J, Ambrose J. Computerized tomography scanning appearances of intracranial meningiomas. An attempt to predict the histological features. J Neurosurg. 1979;50:320–7. https://doi.org/10.3171/jns.1979.50.3.0320.
81. Wang DD, Martin KW, Auguste KI, Sun PP. Fast dynamic imaging technique to identify obstructive lesions in the CSF space: report of 2 cases. J Neurosurg Pediatr. 2015;15:519–23. https://doi.org/10.3171/2014.11.PEDS13620.
82. Wang Q, Cheng J, Zhang S, Ju Y, Liu W, Hui X. Central nervous system hemangioblastomas in the elderly (over 65 years): clinical characteristics and outcome analysis. Clin Neurol Neurosurg. 2020;189:105622. https://doi.org/10.1016/j.clineuro.2019.105622.
83. Weindling SM, Kotsenas AL. Spontaneous craniospinal hypotension. J Magn Reson Imaging. 2005;22:804–9. https://doi.org/10.1002/jmri.20441.
84. Weng JC, Ma JP, Hao SY, Wang L, Xu YL, Yang J, et al. Intradural extramedullary bronchogenic cyst: clinical and radiologic characteristics, surgical outcomes, and literature review. World Neurosurg. 2018;109:e571–80. https://doi.org/10.1016/j.wneu.2017.10.023.
85. Zhang J, Chen ZH, Wang ZF, Sun P, Jin JT, Zhang XH, et al. Epidural cystic spinal meningioma: a case report. Medicine (Baltimore). 2016;95:e3030. https://doi.org/10.1097/MD.0000000000003030.
86. Zhang L, Zhang Z, Yang W, Jia W, Xu Y, Yang J. Cystic dilation of the ventriculus terminalis: report of 6 surgical cases treated with cyst-subarachnoid shunting using a T-catheter. World Neurosurg. 2017;104:522–7. https://doi.org/10.1016/j.wneu.2017.05.017.
87. Zileli M, Isik HS, Ogut FE, Is M, Cagli S, Calli C. Aneurysmal bone cysts of the spine. Eur Spine J. 2013;22:593–601. https://doi.org/10.1007/s00586-012-2510-x.

Part V

Options in Operative Management of Arachnoid Cysts

Editor's Summary

In this "Part V: Options in Operative Management of Arachnoid Cysts," there are a total of seven chapters describing the options for the operative management of arachnoid cysts (ACs). Once the presumed diagnosis of the presence of an AC that is potentially causing symptoms has been made, a number of different surgical techniques can be considered and employed for the successful treatment of symptomatic ACs. Beginning with simply aspirating and draining the AC as proposed in 24 to the much more refined microsurgical approach to the removal of ACs as presented in the following chapter. Diversion of the fluid within the cyst can be accomplished through the placement of a conventional shunting device or by stereotactic internal diversion as described in Chapters 26 and 27, respectively. With endoscopy becoming an increasingly useful technique for performing numerous neurosurgical procedures both cranial and spinal in nature, the utility for successfully treating ACs is featured in 28. Spinal ACs can require surgical management because of the profound symptomatology that they can cause when left untreated or with a delay in their diagnosis. As with all surgical procedures involving the central nervous system, some form of complication is always possible as discussed in the concluding 30 for this part.

Aspiration and Drainage of Arachnoid Cysts

Ahmad Pour-Rashidi and Sara Hanaei

1 Introduction

Arachnoid cyst (ACs), an extra-axial cerebrospinal fluid (CSF) collection inside the arachnoid layer, is a congenital benign non-neoplastic abnormality made by arachnoid-related serous tissues. It accounts for about 1% of intracranial and 1–3% of spinal space-occupying lesions (SOL) with an approximate male/female ratio of 2:1. This cystic lesion may be present in various forms. In some cases, the cyst is linked to the adjacent cisterns freely, while it makes a limited SOL without any connection to the intracranial CSF in others. Additionally, it can have different contents including bloody fluid, high protein content, or xanthochromic fluid [1, 2].

ACs may be seen solely or as part of a syndrome or association. These CSF collections should be considered in genetic disorders such as Marfan syndrome, neurofibromatosis type 1, glutaric aciduria, acro-callosal syndrome, and autosomal dominant polycystic kidney disease (ADPKD). They show various behaviors during the patient's lifetime, from a rare spontaneous disappearance to slowly growing cysts. The latter occurs when a unidirectional valve allows the CSF to enter with no exit point, leading to progressive cyst enlargement. Despite these features, most cysts have a stable size during the patient's entire life. Accordingly, there are some other probable factors determining the surgical necessity including superimposed infection and intracystic bleeding [29].

Patients with these abnormal cysts may present with a wide variety of symptoms depending on their location. Although asymptomatic at the time of diagnosis, and detected as an incidental finding in many cases, a group of patients may become symptomatic. Headache, neurodevelopmental delay, intractable seizure, focal neurological deficits, and macrocephaly are some of the symptoms associated with ACs as a result of cyst mass effect. However, sometimes finding a relationship between the symptoms and the cyst will become more complicated [8, 29].

Many patients may have ACs with no symptoms, whose cyst may become symptomatic at one point of their life. The exact risk factors to make these cysts symptomatic might be unidentifiable or unclear. In some situations, such as bleeding inside the cyst or by cyst contamination with bacteria, we are able to determine why the patient is symptomatic pre- or intraoperatively, while in other conditions, finding a definite mechanism is not possible, and patient's symptoms may not be explainable.

A. Pour-Rashidi
Department of Neurosurgery, Sina Hospital, Tehran University of Medical Sciences (TUMS), Tehran, Iran

S. Hanaei (✉)
Department of Neurosurgery, Imam Khomeini Hospital Complex, Tehran University of Medical Sciences (TUMS), Tehran, Iran

Universal Scientific Education and Research Network (USERN), Tehran, Iran

M. Turgut et al. (eds.), *Arachnoid Cysts*, https://doi.org/10.1007/978-3-031-22701-1_24

2 Treatment Options for Arachnoid Cysts

To recommend the best treatment modality for ACs, different factors should be considered including the patient's signs and symptoms, cyst size, cyst location, cyst type, and previous treatments. Owing to the varied presentation and different forms of ACs, as well as their unclear natural course, deciding on the optimal method for treatment is still controversial. Therefore, different therapeutic approaches with different outcomes have been discussed in the literature that may not be straightforward in all patients with ACs [6].

Headache is the most common presentation of these cysts occurring because of cyst mass effect, increased intracranial pressure (ICP), and consequently hydrocephalus. Importantly, in some patients the headache might be unrelated to the AC; therefore, in these cases, a watchful waiting approach along with regular visits could be an option. There are no definite intervals for follow-up visits and neuroimaging, but the location of AC has a significant role to introduce an appropriate interval for follow-up. For instance, short intervals may be recommended to follow quadrigeminal ACs. Invasive ICP monitoring can be applied as well, although it remains a challenging method [29].

In patients whose headache is unrelated to the cyst or in asymptomatic cases, some authors suggested a preventive surgery to reduce the cyst complications during different situations that may cause unpredictable consequences. For instance, they believed that high altitude could cause cyst rupture due to atmospheric pressure alterations. Also, they reported that head trauma could lead to cyst rupture, then a subdural hygroma/hematoma, or an intracystic hematoma leading to acute neurologic deficits. However, the cumulative risk for such horrible complications was less than 3%, where the risk of those adverse consequences has been reported as 5% or more after cyst surgery. On the other hand, there is some evidence of cyst disappearance following spontaneous or traumatic rupture. Given that, preventive surgery has no beneficial role in AC treatment [21, 26, 27].

In other symptomatic patients, a multitude of surgical techniques is available. Surgical excision of the cyst concomitant with marsupialization is a method to treat AC; however, it should be considered that complete cyst resection may not be achieved because of the cyst wall adhesion to the underlying cerebral structures. According to the literature, craniotomy and cyst fenestration were the most favorable choices of treatment for ACs [27]. Cyst fenestration through a microsurgical keyhole approach or endoscopic approach in order to connect the cyst to normal intracranial CSF flow is another option [23]. Although this method became a popular trend after the rapidly increasing neuroendoscopy utilization for treating many intracranial lesions, including ACs, there was no significant difference between open and endoscopic approaches regarding some complications such as subdural hygroma/hematoma [26]. Furthermore, the endoscopic approach limits the surgeon in terms of intraoperative bleeding control compared to open craniotomy, even though it may be more effective in suprasellar and quadrigeminal cistern ACs in addition to a shorter hospitalization period [9, 10].

Cyst aspiration and drainage by a needle via burr hole craniotomy and cyst shunting are considered the other approaches that will be helpful in selected patients, which will be discussed in the following sections [8, 23, 31].

3 Cystoperitoneal (CP) Shunting as Primary Treatment

As discussed earlier, open craniotomy and maximal safe cyst wall excision were considered as the treatment of choice since the 1980s [24]. In this way, the surgeons were able to achieve two goals simultaneously: first to eliminate the cyst mass effect and second to obtain a histopathologic sample to rule out the neoplastic characteristics of the cyst [24]. Nevertheless, both early and late complications of this type of surgery included subdural hygroma/hematoma, cyst recurrence (approximately, 25%), and associated hydrocephalus needing a shunt placement (approximately, 30–100%). Moreover, another important limitation was a mortality rate of approximately 20% after open craniotomy, particularly in pediatrics. Therefore, this led to considering cystoperitoneal (CP) shunt implantation as the primary treatment [13].

Some surgeons recommended the CP shunting as the primary treatment of ACs in select patients. They considered different factors to estimate the rate of postoperative events leading them to insert a shunt and then introduced this method as the first therapeutic option. The most important factor to determine the efficacy of primary shunt placement was the communication of the cysts with other cisterns and subarachnoid spaces. Hence, utilizing precise preoperative investigations is a requirement for optimal decision-making. Despite the existence of several imaging modalities including computed tomography (CT) cisternography and cine magnetic resonance imaging (MRI), it is not always very straightforward to confirm the presence of a connection between the cyst and free CSF [24]. Importantly, connection of the AC to the free CSF circulation and concurrent hydrocephalus were both considered as determining factors, since primary shunt implantation was more beneficial in such cases [24]. Therefore, in these two groups of patients, craniotomy and cyst wall excision could be considered as second-line therapy in case of shunt failure.

Generally, two forms of shunting could be considered for ACs: (1) CP shunt and (2) CP concomitant with ventriculoperitoneal (VP) shunt (Fig. 1). The latter should be used in cases of concurrent hydrocephalus with AC. On the other hand, there are two protocols for CP shunting:

1. In the first one, a small craniotomy is performed, and the cyst wall is removed as much as possible, allowing the cyst to collapse. Then, a shunt tube is placed in the cyst cavity, followed by both cyst and dura matter stitching that is thought to prevent a subdural hygroma/hematoma.
2. The second technique is similar to VP shunting; it means that after craniotomy, the cyst will only be punctured to introduce the shunt tube [25].

Similar to all therapeutic modalities, shunting has complications which are similar to other types of shunt devices. One of these complications is shunt infection. Despite a sterile operation along with perioperative intravenous antibiotics, CP shunt infection was reported between 1.3% and 8.7% in studies with more than 5 years of follow-up compared to 1–15% following VP shunt placement [22, 25]. Shunt malfunction is predictable due to a list of reasons comprising shunt fracture, occlusion, distraction,

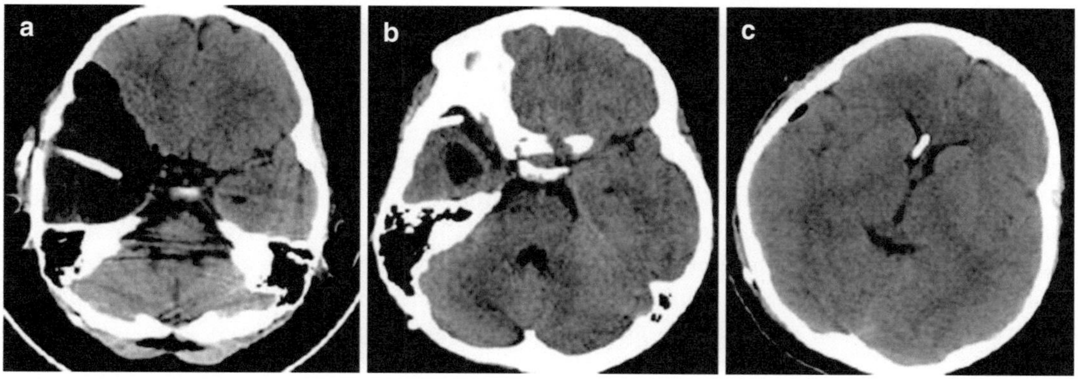

Fig. 1 Brain computed tomography (CT) scans of a 5-year-old boy. (**a**) Shunt insertion in a right temporal arachnoid cyst (ACs). (**b**) A CT scan shows obliterated cyst, but typical symptoms of pseudotumor cerebri were presented after 6 years. (**c**) A ventriculoperitoneal (VP) shunt was inserted that resulted in symptom disappearance

over-drainage, and under-drainage, as it occurs after VP shunting as well. This adverse event with an incidence rate as high as 50% is more frequent in CP shunting than VP shunt placement which may be due to the different underlying pathology of this disease [25]. Rarely, patients who underwent shunt insertion present with walking difficulties displaying cervical myelopathy. This condition was reported after VP shunting as called "over-shunting-associated myelopathy" or "Miyazaki syndrome." A total number of 14 patients with VP shunting and 2 patients with CP shunting were reported in the literature so far to have this complication [28].

Shunt dependency is another concern after shunting the AC with a rate of 0.9–37% [17]. When a shunt stays in the brain for a long time, the absorptive mechanism of cerebral tissues will be impaired, and the replaced fibrosis makes the brain less elastic with low compliance, which results in the brain tendency to keep the shunt in place [25]. The diagnostic triad of shunt dependency is [7, 16]:

1. Symptoms of intermittent and unexplainable raised ICP.
2. Symptom improvement by lowering the ICP through injection of osmotic agents such as mannitol or confirming increased ICP by utilizing an ICP monitoring system.
3. Delayed filling of the shunt reservoir.

In some patients, acquired Chiari malformation type 1 was reported after CP shunting because of craniocerebral disproportion leading to hindbrain herniation [17]. This complication was serious enough for some neurosurgeons to ignore CP shunting as the first-line method while the others tried to overcome it [12, 25]. The factor that has a crucial role in dependency is shunt duration, as a longer shunt duration may lead to a higher rate of dependency. Therefore, there were some investigations to determine the optimal time for shunt removal. Accordingly, in a large series by Arai et al., it was revealed that the average interval between shunt insertion and the occurrence of shunt dependency was approximately 6.2 years (range, 0.6–10 years). Therefore, the authors recommended shunt removal as early as cyst obliteration [3].

Moreover, there are some methods to avoid or treat shunt dependency such as replacing the shunt with another catheter, using a programmable shunt to increase the shunt valve resistance [11], and replacing the shunt system with a lumboperitoneal shunt. Sometimes replacing the shunt with another catheter may be difficult due to the small size of the ventricles. In this situation, lumboperitoneal shunt or intracranial shunt using a navigation system could be helpful [15, 25]. In addition, Dong et al. presented an approach in which they resected the collapsed cyst wall as much as possible via microscopic keyhole surgery. They reported two cases operated via this approach in whom the results were promising and they could treat shunt dependency [7].

4 Needle Aspiration or Burr Hole Drainage for the Arachnoid Cysts

Occasionally, some ACs may disappear due to an unclear mechanism. While trivial trauma and infection were reported so far to explain this mechanism, the other relevant factors are still unknown. It is noteworthy that AC resolution may occur completely without any presentation, which could be considered as a part of the cyst natural course. Nonetheless, the actual natural history of an AC is not yet clear [19].

Subdural hygroma/hematoma is a complication of AC rupture following head injury. Furthermore, there are several reports of vanishing ACs during a patients' follow-up period. It is believed that head injury may cause tearing in the cyst membrane and open its cavity into the subdural space, which leads to the cyst fading away. According to this hypothesis, neurosur-

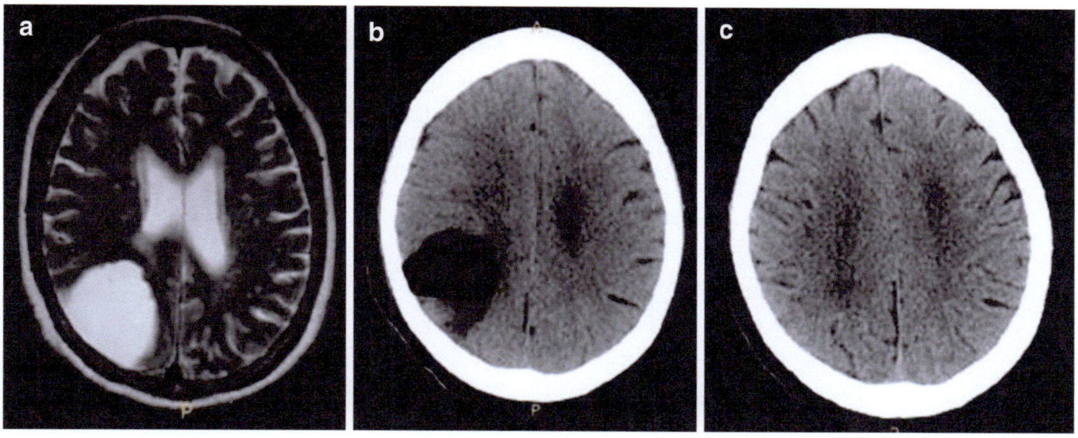

Fig. 2 (**a**) A brain magnetic resonance imaging (MRI) showed a right parietal convexity AC. (**b**) A brain CT scan after burr hole drainage. (**c**) A postoperative 3-month CT scan showed complete disappearance of the AC

geons designed a trauma-like approach to treat ACs. They performed trephination (artificial trauma) localized on the cyst location to simulate a head trauma leading to cyst rupture and then slowly and progressively cause cyst regression by burr hole drainage [14]. Indeed, the surgeon first changes an AC to a subdural collection and then treats it as a subdural hygroma/hematoma (Fig. 2).

Another approach to the ACs is the cyst aspiration using CT scan, MRI, or stereotactically. In this approach, only a few patients may fulfill the selection criteria, and CT-guided, MR-guided, or stereotactic aspiration of the cyst could be carried out [4, 5, 20]. The advantages of the MR-guided approach are a more targeted aspiration while showing around neural structures in greater detail accompanied by displaying probable immediate complications such as epidural bleeding [4]. Rarely, an Ommaya reservoir may be implanted in super-selective patients for periodic cyst aspiration that prevents shunt necessity and its complications [30].

Based on the available data about the AC aspiration and burr hole drainage, the first method is not acceptable and is not adequate enough as the first-line therapy, even though it was used in some cases with spinal cord ACs. The only indication of AC aspiration is the small cysts without apparent subarachnoid communication [18]. Besides, burr hole drainage is recommended in limited situations such as when a subdural hygroma/hematoma occurred after opening the cyst to subdural space [14].

Figure 3 has summarized the treatment options for AC.

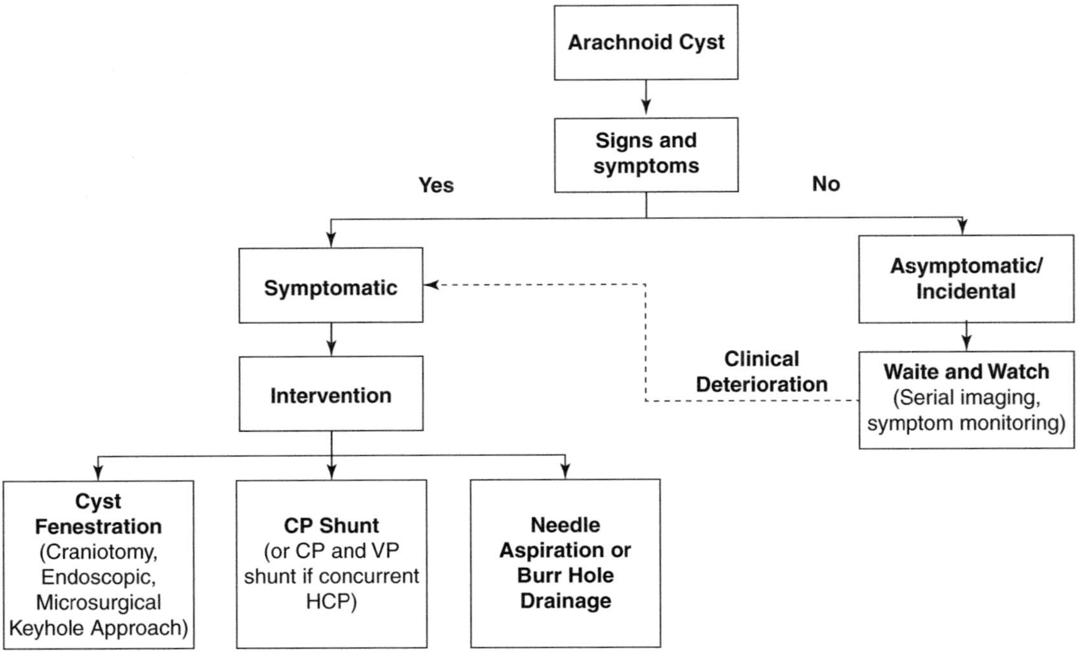

Fig. 3 Therapeutic algorithm for ACs

5 Conclusion

Despite the extensive research concerning different aspects of ACs, the underlying pathology is not clarified yet. Also, the scant data in terms of definite treatment has resulted in a multitude of therapeutic approaches without level I of evidence. Accordingly, and concerning all of the therapeutic approaches, precise patient selection would be a critical step in the management of ACs. CP shunting as the primary treatment for ACs is controversial, although some authors recommended it only for selected patients according to indications. The cyst aspiration and burr hole drainage are not well studied yet, but they are not as popular as the other therapeutic modalities and are associated with limited indications. As the current knowledge about the treatment of ACs are mainly based on case reports and case series (evidence level—IV), further research with a higher level of evidence is required to determine the optimal therapeutic approach for this disease.

References

1. Abdelhameed E, Morsy AA. Surgical outcome of primary intradural spinal arachnoid cysts: a series of 10 cases. Egypt J Neurol Psychiatry Neurosurg. 2021;57(1):1–6.
2. Alexiou GA, et al. Shunting for the treatment of arachnoid cysts in children. Neurosurgery. 2010;67(6):1632–6; discussion 1636.
3. Arai H, et al. Arachnoid cysts of the middle cranial fossa: experience with 77 patients who were treated with cystoperitoneal shunting. Neurosurgery. 1996;39(6):1108–13.
4. Bellavia R, et al. Percutaneous aspiration of an intradural/extradural thoracic arachnoid cyst: use of MR imaging guidance. J Vasc Interv Radiol. 2000;11(3):369–72.
5. Bond AE, et al. Spinal arachnoid cysts in the pediatric population: report of 31 cases and a review of the literature. J Neurosurg Pediatr. 2012;9(4):432–41.
6. Boutarbouch M, et al. Management of intracranial arachnoid cysts: institutional experience with initial 32 cases and review of the literature. Clin Neurol Neurosurg. 2008;110(1):1–7.
7. Dong F, et al. Shunt dependency syndrome after cyst-peritoneal shunt resolved by keyhole microsurgical cyst resection: two case reports and literature review. Neuropediatrics. 2018;49(05):310–3.

8. Elhammady MS, Bhatia S, Ragheb J. Endoscopic fenestration of middle fossa arachnoid cysts: a technical description and case series. Pediatr Neurosurg. 2007;43(3):209–15.
9. Gangemi M, et al. Endoscopy versus microsurgical cyst excision and shunting for treating intracranial arachnoid cysts. J Neurosurg Pediatr. 2011;8(2):158–64.
10. Hall S, et al. Clinical and radiological outcomes following surgical treatment for intra-cranial arachnoid cysts. Clin Neurol Neurosurg. 2019;177:42–6.
11. Hamid NA, Sgouros S. The use of an adjustable valve to treat over-drainage of a cyst-peritoneal shunt in a child with a large sylvian fissure arachnoid cyst. Childs Nerv Syst. 2005;21(11):991–4.
12. Kang JK, et al. Shunt-independent surgical treatment of middle cranial fossa arachnoid cysts in children. Childs Nerv Syst. 2000;16(2):111–6.
13. Kaplan BJ, Mickle JP, Parkhurst R. Cystoperitoneal shunting for congenital arachnoid cysts. Childs Brain. 1984;11(5):304–11.
14. Kim DU, et al. Disappearance of arachnoid cyst after burrhole trephination: case series. Korean J Neurotrauma. 2019;15(2):170–5.
15. Kim SK, et al. Shunt dependency in shunted arachnoid cyst: a reason to avoid shunting. Pediatr Neurosurg. 2002;37(4):178–85.
16. Li C, et al. Shunt dependency syndrome after cystoperitoneal shunting of arachnoid cysts. Childs Nerv Syst. 2014;30(3):471–6.
17. Martínez-Lage JF, et al. CSF overdrainage in shunted intracranial arachnoid cysts: a series and review. Childs Nerv Syst. 2009;25(9):1061.
18. Moses ZB, Chi JH, Chavali R. Direct puncture for diagnosis of intradural spinal arachnoid cyst and fenestration using 3D rotational fluoroscopy: technical note and the "jellyfish sign". J Neurosurg Spine. 2018;29(6):720–4.
19. Nadi M, et al. Resolution of middle fossa arachnoid cyst after minor head trauma-stages of resolution on MRI: case report and literature review. Pediatr Neurosurg. 2017;52(5):346–50.
20. Pell MF, Thomas DG. The management of infratentorial arachnoid cyst by CT-directed stereotactic aspiration. Br J Neurosurg. 1991;5(4):399–403.
21. Prokopienko M, Kunert P, Marchel A. Unusual volume reduction of Galassi grade III arachnoid cyst following head trauma. J Neurol Surg A Cent Eur Neurosurg. 2013;74(Suppl 1):e198–202.
22. Raygor KP, et al. Ventriculoperitoneal shunt infection rates using a standard surgical technique, including topical and intraventricular vancomycin: the Children's Hospital Oakland experience. J Neurosurg Pediatr. 2020;26:1–9.
23. Shim KW, et al. Treatment option for arachnoid cysts. Childs Nerv Syst. 2009;25(11):1459–66.
24. Stein SCJN. Intracranial developmental cysts in children: treatment by cystoperitoneal shunting. Neurosurgery. 1981;8(6):647–50.
25. Takaoki K, et al. Chapter 12—Shunt techniques—cystoperitoneal shunt; 2018. p. 165–72.
26. Tamburrini G. Controversies in the management of intracranial arachnoid cysts. In: Arachnoid cysts. Amsterdam: Elsevier; 2018. p. 93–104.
27. Tamburrini G, Dal Fabbro M, Di Rocco C. Sylvian fissure arachnoid cysts: a survey on their diagnostic workout and practical management. Childs Nerv Syst. 2008;24(5):593–604.
28. Tomonori I, et al. A case of miyazaki syndrome caused by arachnoid cyst-peritoneal shunt. World Neurosurg. 2021;146:85–9.
29. Westermaier T, Schweitzer T, Ernestus R-I. Arachnoid cysts. Adv Exp Med Biol. 2012;724:37–50.
30. Yang S, et al. Intracerebral arachnoid cyst treated with ommaya reservoir implantation in a patient younger than two years. J Craniofac Surg. 2014;25(4):e378–80.
31. Zhang B, Zhang Y, Ma Z. Long-term results of cystoperitoneal shunt placement for the treatment of arachnoid cysts in children. J Neurosurg Pediatr. 2012;10(4):302–5.

Microsurgical Approach to Arachnoid Cysts

Michelle E. De Witt and Walter A. Hall

1 Introduction

Intracranial arachnoid cysts (ACs) are extraparenchymal, intra-arachnoidal collections filled with a fluid similar in composition to cerebrospinal fluid (CSF). They are generally believed to be due to congenital splitting or duplication of the arachnoid membrane [8, 65, 76], although case reports of de novo AC cyst development do exist [8, 61, 66, 78].

1.1 Incidence

In adults, estimates of AC incidence based on either computed tomography (CT) or magnetic resonance imaging (MRI) range from as low as 0.3% up to 1.8% [3, 22, 39, 83, 84]. Of these, larger studies using MRI imaging to diagnose an AC suggest an incidence of at least 1% [3, 83, 84]. The reported incidence of pediatric ACs in the literature ranges from 0.5% to 2.6% [4, 34, 36, 41]. Increasing incidence is quoted in the literature over time, likely reflective of choice of CT versus MRI and advances in imaging techniques [39, 41, 83, 84, 91].

M. E. De Witt · Walter A. Hall (✉)
Department of Neurosurgery, SUNY Upstate University Hospital, Syracuse, NY, USA
e-mail: Dewittm@upstate.edu; Hallw@upstate.edu

1.2 Natural History

The natural history of most ACs is benign and they remain asymptomatic over time. ACs are not static entities however. Fluctuation in size may occur and indeed has been well described [3, 4, 12, 44, 45, 55, 66, 67]. Enlarging ACs may ultimately require treatment [3, 4, 44, 45, 55, 66]. Conversely, ACs may decrease in size over time, although this is thought to be uncommon [3, 12, 45, 67]. There are additionally case reports of spontaneous resolution of ACs [1, 47, 55, 63, 70, 81, 85].

1.3 Location

ACs may be located in any arachnoid space; however, the vast majority of ACs are supratentorial [3, 4, 73]. Of these, middle fossa ACs represent the most common supratentorial location, comprising anywhere from 34 to 60% of ACs [3, 4, 9, 24, 29, 37, 59, 84, 86]. Other locations include the suprasellar cistern, interhemispheric fissure, hemispheric convexity, and retrocerebellar and quadrigeminal cisterns [3, 4, 10, 30, 35, 40, 75, 77]. Intraventricular cysts are thought to be quite rare [15].

M. Turgut et al. (eds.), *Arachnoid Cysts*, https://doi.org/10.1007/978-3-031-22701-1_25

2 Presentation

Many ACs are asymptomatic and found incidentally on imaging studies performed for other indications [3, 4, 65] including routine prenatal imaging [26, 28, 73].

Symptomatic ACs may present with a variety of complaints. ACs are often associated with non-specific symptoms [14, 25, 74, 87], with headache being the most common complaint described in many studies [5, 17, 82]. Other symptoms associated with high intracranial pressure (ICP) such as seizures, vomiting, and lethargy have been reported [17, 82]. Cognitive issues ranging from vague cognitive complaints [2, 32, 87, 89] to short-term memory deficits [5] and delayed developmental milestones in children have all been reported [17]. Focal motor deficits, gait abnormalities, visual changes, and cranial neuropathies have all been described [17, 82]. In children, macrocephaly, increasing head circumference, and temporal bone bowing have all been seen [17, 73, 82]. Endocrinopathies ranging from growth hormone deficiency to precocious puberty to panhypopituitarism have also been described [56, 69, 77].

Initial presentation with subdural hygroma or subdural hematoma (SDH) or intracystic hemorrhage from AC rupture is a well-described occurrence [11, 16, 21, 27, 57, 62, 88]. Larger cyst size at presentation and a history of recent head trauma have been found to be risk factors for presentation with a hemorrhage in these patients [16].

Expectedly, AC symptomatology can often be location dependent as a result of direct mass effect of the AC on adjacent neurological structures. Thus, patients with suprasellar ACs may present with visual problems, endocrinopathies [77], or hydrocephalus [3]. Patients with ambient cistern, quadrigeminal cistern, or retrocerebellar ACs often present with hydrocephalus [3, 4, 73] although the latter is suggested to have a more insidious onset [73]. A cerebellopontine angle location may be associated with vertigo, tinnitus, ipsilateral sensorineural hearing loss, or facial palsy [3, 33]. ACs located in the temporal fossa may be associated with bowing of the temporal bone [82].

In Al-Holou et al.'s natural history study, ACs in the suprasellar location, the cerebellopontine angle, the ambient cistern, and the quadrigeminal cistern had a higher likelihood of being symptomatic compared to ACs located in the middle fossa or retrocerebellar space. They also found that, in adults, a younger age and larger cyst size were more likely to be symptomatic [3]. Similarly, Ali et al., in their pediatric case series, found that cyst size and younger age at diagnosis were significant predictive factors for undergoing surgery [9].

3 Indications for Surgical Intervention

In general, there is a consensus in the literature that intervention is indicated for symptomatic ACs [23, 25, 37, 51, 59, 82]. Symptoms such as refractory epilepsy, focal neurological deficits, and hydrocephalus are clear indications for therapeutic treatment [30, 33, 90]. For these patients, the debate mainly focuses on the choice of intervention. The clinical challenge that arises lies in determining if other signs and symptoms that a patient presents with are indeed caused by the AC.

Headaches, the most common presenting sign of an AC, may be significantly improved after surgical intervention [46]; however, they may also persist despite AC treatment and radiographic improvement [18]. In a 2008 survey of the neurosurgical management of ACs, chronic headache was a major indication for offering surgical intervention in 35.5% of those surveyed [80].

In those patients with a subdural hematoma (SDH) or hygroma, treatment of the SDH via evacuation may be indicated; studies assessing SDHs report good outcomes without a surgical intervention directly addressing the AC [21, 27, 49, 57, 62]. An intracystic hemorrhage may be an indication for treatment [27]; however, Domenicucci et al. argue that in the setting of a concurrent chronic SDH, the blood products seen in the AC are from the movement of the blood breakdown products from the SDH into the AC through the cyst membrane, thus addressing the cyst may not be warranted [21].

Other diagnostic tests may be deemed necessary prior to proceeding with intervention. Those patients presenting with seizures may benefit from electroencephalogram (EEG) monitoring to localize the seizure to the parenchyma adjacent to the AC prior to offering surgical intervention [80, 90]. Some studies have looked at neuropsychological testing with positive performance gains on these tests after postoperative cyst reduction or elimination. These authors advocate for a role, currently undefined, for neuropsychological testing in AC patients and suggest having a lower threshold at which to offer surgical intervention [32, 87, 89]. Di Rocco et al. described intraparenchymal ICP monitoring for patients with middle fossa ACs and used the documented presence of intracranial hypertension to guide intervention [19]. Martinez-Lage et al. suggested the use of cerebral 99 mTc-HMPAO single photon emission computed tomography (SPECT) to assess for a decrease in regional cerebral blood flow (rCBF) in the brain parenchymal zone around the AC [53].

The role of surgery in the asymptomatic patient has also been debated in the literature with advocates for prophylactic treatment of ACs. Proponents of interventional treatment in these patients cite concern for future hemorrhage [80]. However, while the true hemorrhage risk is unknown, it does appear to be quite low [3, 4, 16]. Increasing radiographic size [9, 43] is also sometimes considered an indication for treatment, but, given the generally benign natural history and the documented, though uncommon, occurrence of spontaneous regression, this indication is also debated [3, 45]. A patient with an unclear association of symptomatology with his AC would likely benefit from interval follow-up to elucidate if there is a true correlation between the two.

4 Treatment Options

Treatment options may include both observational follow-up and surgical interventions. Conservative management may be the preferred treatment course in the cases of asymptomatic ACs with interval follow-up with imaging studies and clinical exam. Interventions broadly fall into one of three categories: CSF diversion procedures, endoscopic fenestration of the AC, and microsurgical excision or fenestration of the AC.

4.1 Conservative Management

Taken together, the relatively stable natural history of ACs with the often non-specific complaints at the time of diagnosis shows a distinct role for clinical observation. An incidentally discovered AC should be watched and followed clinically in the event of symptom development or cyst growth. The patient in whom there is clinical uncertainty as to whether the AC is symptomatic would likely benefit from observational follow-up to further elucidate the correlation of the symptoms with the AC.

4.2 Microsurgery

Microsurgical intervention can comprise of a craniotomy followed by either cyst fenestration into a CSF cistern (subarachnoid space, ventricle, or basal cistern) or may be excisional with resection of the cyst wall. There are no comparative studies assessing differences in recurrence rates or other clinical outcomes between cyst excision and cyst fenestration. Some authors favor cyst excision [17]; however cyst fenestration seems to be the more common choice of technique [73, 80]. In a 2008 survey of international neurosurgical practices for a symptomatic middle fossa AC, microsurgical fenestration was the practicing neurosurgeon's treatment modality of choice among all treatment options [80], although there is a current trend in the literature toward the use of neuroendoscopy.

Microsurgery has been found to be safe and effective in the treatment of ACs in many studies with improved clinical and radiological outcomes in 79–100% in large case series [31, 37, 46, 68, 71]. The possibility of shunt independence in successfully treated patients is a significant consideration when choosing microsurgical intervention [9, 82]. Compared to endoscopy, microsurgical intervention may be favored for small ACs or those located over the hemispheric cortex [25, 71].

There may be a significant technical advantage in using a microsurgical technique over the endoscopic approach. The ability to perform bimanual instrument manipulation within the working field without compromising the visual fields, greater depth perception, and a wider visual field are some of the advantages of using the operative microscope. There is additionally a superior ability to obtain hemostasis [46, 72, 80, 82]. With the microsurgical technique, the operator lifts the cyst wall away from the surrounding structures before sharply dissecting the wall. Thus, there may be an additional value in this technique when working in areas where sensitive structures are immediately adjacent to the AC [9, 82], as with the endoscopic technique there is blunt dissection of the cyst wall without the ability to lift the cyst wall up and away from other structures when performing the dissection. Indeed, Turhan et al., in their retrospective comparison study between neuroendoscopy and microsurgery for Galassi type II or III Sylvian fissure ACs [24], found similar outcomes between the two techniques, but based on these technical differences, they favored the microsurgical approach as the more likely safer methodology [82]. Furthermore, the practicing neurosurgeon may have greater familiarity and comfort with using the operative microscope.

Surgical complications which may be seen postoperatively include CSF leak, pseudomeningocele formation [46, 64], meningitis [46], wound dehiscence, hemiparesis [64], cranial nerve palsies [29, 37, 46], seizures [46], and persistent hydrocephalus [64]. Subdural hygromas may occur in 2%–40% of cases [30, 46, 50, 64, 71] which may be managed with external drainage or require subdural-peritoneal shunt placement [79]. Subdural hematomas may also be seen [37, 50]. Cyst recurrence and the need for revision surgery are some major complications [23, 25, 29, 37, 46, 50, 64, 71, 90]. In a large review, the revision rate after craniotomy for pediatric supratentorial ACs was 29%; this was not statistically significant but showed a trend toward a lower revision rate versus other surgical techniques [9]. The subsequent need for CSF diversion after microsurgical fenestration has been reported in anywhere from 4 to 24.1% of patients [43, 46, 65]. A pediatric series of 26 patients with middle fossa ACs treated with microsurgical cyst fenestration found younger age, progressive cyst expansion before fenestration, and macrocephaly to be significantly associated with the need for shunt placement following fenestration [43]. Other studies have shown an association with an increased need for secondary CSF diversion with hydrocephalus at presentation [23] or macrocephaly in infants [91]. Silva et al., in a case series of 16 pediatric patients with middle fossa ACs, suggested concurrent shunt placement due to complications with CSF leak, citing a trend toward decreased rates of revision surgery; however, in those treated concurrently with combined microsurgical fenestration and cystoperitoneal (CP) shunt placement, 18.75% still needed shunt revision [72], which is comparable to the reported rates of the need for CSF diversion after microsurgery alone.

Other authors have suggested there is a higher failure rate in infants [19, 73, 90], and some have suggested initial or concurrent CP shunt placement [73]. However, while the risk of needing CSF diversion is not insignificant, the comparative effectiveness of the timing of the interventions – concurrent CSF diversion and microsurgical cyst elimination, initial microsurgical cyst elimination followed by CSF diversion, or CSF diversion followed by microsurgery—has not been well defined.

4.3 Neuroendoscopy

In the recent decades, neuroendoscopic cyst fenestration has emerged as an interventional modality which can offer the possibility for definitive treatment of an AC and subsequent shunt independence [9]. There have been some studies that have suggested that endoscopic cyst fenestration may result in lower rates of radiographic improvement in cyst size, yet studies on clinical outcomes have not shown either method to be superior [9, 82]. Success rates for neuroendoscopy as a primary intervention range from 81 to 91% [20, 25, 38, 60]. For suprasellar ACs, neuroendoscopy is favored [9, 25] due to the ease of access and lower rates of injury to the surrounding neural structures. Indeed, in a recent meta-analysis by Kelly et al., endoscopic ventriculocystocisternostomy was found to have the lowest revision rates and best rates of clinical resolution of symptoms [40]. Copley et al. also showed good results in his case series of intraventricular ACs treated using an endoscopic technique [15]. Studies additionally have shown that endoscopic cyst fenestration is associated with a shorter hospital stay [9].

There are similar morbidity risks compared to microsurgery. Some report morbidity rates may be lower than that for microsurgery [58, 60], yet other authors have found no significant difference [9, 71]. As a surgical technique, neuroendoscopy has a significant learning curve [46, 72, 80]. Technical limitations of this technique may contribute to morbidity risk in these patients. Small or hemispheric ACs may pose a challenge for neuroendoscopic techniques, and microsurgery may be the preferred technique. As with both primary CPS and microsurgery, there is a high rate of revision surgery with reported revision rates ranging from 14.6 to 43% [8, 58].

4.4 CSF Diversion

CSF diversion procedures used in the treatment of patients with ACs include direct diversion of the cyst with a CP shunt or less commonly a cystoventricular shunt [48, 54]. A ventriculoperitoneal (VP) shunt may be placed, or an endoscopic third ventriculostomy may be performed for the treatment of hydrocephalus associated with the AC. Subdural peritoneal (SDP) shunts may be second-line interventions as treatment for postoperative subdural hygromas [19, 79]. SDP shunt placement as initial treatment for presentation with subdural hygromas is controversial [6, 33, 49].

Drawbacks of CP shunts include life-long shunt dependence [42]. Shunt overdrainage [13, 52], infection, and shunt failure all contribute to a high rate of revision surgery [7, 9, 72, 73]. Some patients may develop slit-cyst syndrome [72]. Reoperation rates for CP shunt when used as the index intervention were reported as high as 50% in a large meta-analysis; these rates were significantly higher than those for either endoscopic intervention or microsurgery, although there was determined to be no difference in quality of life among all techniques at 5 years [9].

Direct diversion of the cyst into the peritoneal cavity is sometimes used as a first-line intervention and can be associated with cyst size reduction and symptomatic improvement [7, 14, 17]. Some authors have proposed a combined initial approach of microsurgical cyst fenestration and CP shunt placement [65, 72]. Due to these above complications, other authors argue that CP shunt placement should be the last recourse treatment [42, 82]. Additionally, certain cyst locations may not be amenable to shunt placement due to difficulty of access and risk of injury to the surrounding neural structures during CP shunt placement [8].

4.5 Choice of Treatment Modality

For the AC patient who is deemed a surgical candidate, a number of factors may influence the neurosurgeon's choice of surgical intervention. These include patient age, cyst size and location, risks associated with intervention, and surgeon preference or comfort with technique [73]. A summary comparing the advantages and disadvantages of various surgical interventions for ACs is listed in Table 1.

The optimal treatment algorithm for the patient with a symptomatic AC has yet to be defined. Creating one is limited by the quality of the available data as most of the literature is based on small retrospective studies. Larger case series have not shown significant differences in reoperation rates, morbidity rates, or rates of symptomatic improvement [9, 82].

Table 1 Comparison of surgical interventions

Intervention	Advantages	Disadvantages
CSF diversion	Technically less demanding	Shunt dependent High revision rate
Endoscopic fenestration	Shunt independent Decreased hospital stay Better for suprasellar ACs	Difficult to access small hemispheric or temporal cysts Learning curve
Microsurgery	Shunt independent Can access structures not amenable to endoscopy	Longer hospital stay

5 Conclusion

ACs are clinical entities that are seen not infrequently by practicing neuroradiologists, neurologists, neurosurgeons, primary care providers, and emergency medicine providers. Conservative management may be the preferred treatment course in the cases of asymptomatic ACs with interval follow-up with imaging studies and clinical exams.

Correlation of patient symptoms with ACs can be a diagnostic challenge in many circumstances. Symptomatic ACs may benefit from an appropriately selected surgical intervention. To date, no clear treatment modality is clearly superior to other methods. Patient age, cyst location, and surgical morbidities may all play a role in dictating the choice of treatment. In the appropriate patient, microsurgical cyst excision or marsupialization is an effective surgical option with good clinical and radiographic outcomes. Where there is clinical equipoise in the choice of technique, a detailed discussion of therapeutic options with the attendant benefits and risks of each should be undertaken with the patient. Additionally, there is a clear need for future prospective studies to better delineate both the indications for therapeutic intervention and to further investigate which subset of patients may respond best to microsurgical treatment or another therapeutic modality.

References

1. Adilay U, Guclu B, Tiryaki M, Hicdonmez T. Spontaneous resolution of a sylvian arachnoid cyst in a child: a case report. Pediatr Neurosurg. 2017;52:343–5.
2. Agopian-Dahlenmark L, Mathiesen T, Bergendal Å. Cognitive dysfunction and subjective symptoms in patients with arachnoid cyst before and after surgery. Acta Neurochir. 2020;162:1041–50.
3. Al-Holou WN, Terman S, Kilburg C, Garton HJ, Muraszko KM, Maher CO. Prevalence and natural history of arachnoid cysts in adults. J Neurosurg. 2013;118:222–31.
4. Al-Holou WN, Yew AY, Boomsaad ZE, Garton HJ, Muraszko KM, Maher CO. Prevalence and natural history of arachnoid cysts in children. J Neurosurg Pediatr. 2010;5:578–85.
5. Albakr A, Sader N, Lama S, Sutherland GR. Interhemispheric arachnoid cyst. Surg Neurol Int. 2021;12:125.
6. Albuquerque FC, Giannotta SL. Arachnoid cyst rupture producing subdural hygroma and intracranial hypertension: case reports. Neurosurgery. 1997;41:951–5; discussion 955–6.
7. Alexiou GA, Varela M, Sfakianos G, Prodromou N. Shunting for the treatment of arachnoid cysts in children. Neurosurgery. 2010;67:1632–6; discussion 1636.
8. Ali M, Bennardo M, Almenawer SA, Zagzoog N, Smith AA, Dao D, Ajani O, Farrokhyar F, Singh SK. Exploring predictors of surgery and comparing operative treatment approaches for pediatric intracranial arachnoid cysts: a case series of 83 patients. J Neurosurg Pediatr. 2015;16:275–82.
9. Ali ZS, Lang SS, Bakar D, Storm PB, Stein SC. Pediatric intracranial arachnoid cysts: comparative effectiveness of surgical treatment options. Childs Nerv Syst. 2014;30:461–9.
10. André A, Zérah M, Roujeau T, Brunelle F, Blauwblomme T, Puget S, Bourgeois M, Sainte-Rose C, Ville Y, Di Rocco F. Suprasellar arachnoid cysts: toward a new simple classification based on prognosis and treatment modality. Neurosurgery. 2016;78:370–9; discussion 379–80.
11. Bilginer B, Onal MB, Oguz KK, Akalan N. Arachnoid cyst associated with subdural hematoma: report of three cases and review of the literature. Childs Nerv Syst. 2009;25:119–24.
12. Boutarbouch M, El Ouahabi A, Rifi L, Arkha Y, Derraz S, El Khamlichi A. Management of intracranial arachnoid cysts: institutional experience with initial 32 cases and review of the literature. Clin Neurol Neurosurg. 2008;110:1–7.
13. Caldarelli M, Novegno F, Di Rocco C. A late complication of CSF shunting: acquired Chiari I malformation. Childs Nerv Syst. 2009;25:443–52.

14. Ciricillo SF, Cogen PH, Harsh GR, Edwards MS. Intracranial arachnoid cysts in children. A comparison of the effects of fenestration and shunting. J Neurosurg. 1991;74:230–5.
15. Copley P, Kirkman MA, Thompson D, James G, Aquilina K. Endoscopic surgery for intraventricular arachnoid cysts in children: clinical presentation, radiological features, management, and outcomes over a 12-year period. Childs Nerv Syst. 2018;34:257–66.
16. Cress M, Kestle JR, Holubkov R, Riva-Cambrin J. Risk factors for pediatric arachnoid cyst rupture/hemorrhage: a case-control study. Neurosurgery. 2013;72:716–22; discussion 722.
17. Deopujari CE, Shaikh ST, Karmarkar VS, Sudke AY, Mohanty CB, Biyani NK. Experience with management of intracranial arachnoid cysts. J Neurol Surg A Cent Eur Neurosurg. 2021;82:43–52.
18. Di Rocco C. Sylvian fissure arachnoid cysts: we do operate on them but should it be done? Childs Nerv Syst. 2010;26:173–5.
19. Di Rocco C, Tamburrini G, Caldarelli M, Velardi F, Santini P. Prolonged ICP monitoring in sylvian arachnoid cysts. Surg Neurol. 2003;60:211–8.
20. Di Rocco F, Syril RJ, Roujeau T, Puget S, Sainte-Rose C, Zerah M. Limits of endoscopic treatment of sylvian arachnoid cysts in children. Childs Nerv Syst. 2010;26:155–62.
21. Domenicucci M, Russo N, Giugni E, Pierallini A. Relationship between supratentorial arachnoid cyst and chronic subdural hematoma: neuroradiological evidence and surgical treatment. J Neurosurg. 2009;110:1250–5.
22. Eskandary H, Sabba M, Khajehpour F, Eskandari M. Incidental findings in brain computed tomography scans of 3000 head trauma patients. Surg Neurol. 2005;63:550–3; discussion 553.
23. Fewel ME, Levy ML, McComb JG. Surgical treatment of 95 children with 102 intracranial arachnoid cysts. Pediatr Neurosurg. 1996;25:165–73.
24. Galassi E, Tognetti F, Gaist G, Fagioli L, Frank F, Frank G. CT scan and metrizamide CT cisternography in arachnoid cysts of the middle cranial fossa: classification and pathophysiological aspects. Surg Neurol. 1982;17:363–9.
25. Gangemi M, Seneca V, Colella G, Cioffi V, Imperato A, Maiuri F. Endoscopy versus microsurgical cyst excision and shunting for treating intracranial arachnoid cysts. J Neurosurg Pediatr. 2011;8:158–64.
26. Gedikbasi A, Palabiyik F, Oztarhan A, Yildirim G, Eren C, Ozyurt SS, Ceylan Y. Prenatal diagnosis of a suprasellar arachnoid cyst with 2- and 3-dimensional sonography and fetal magnetic resonance imaging: difficulties in management and review of the literature. J Ultrasound Med. 2010;29:1487–93.
27. Gregori F, Colistra D, Mancarella C, Chiarella V, Marotta N, Domenicucci M. Arachnoid cyst in young soccer players complicated by chronic subdural hematoma: personal experience and review of the literature. Acta Neurol Belg. 2020;120:235–46.
28. Grossman TB, Uribe-Cardenas R, Radwanski RE, Souweidane MM, Hoffman CE. Arachnoid cysts: using prenatal imaging and need for pediatric neurosurgical intervention to better understand their natural history and prognosis. J Matern Fetal Neonatal Med. 2021;35:1–8.
29. Helland CA, Lund-Johansen M, Wester K. Location, sidedness, and sex distribution of intracranial arachnoid cysts in a population-based sample. J Neurosurg. 2010;113:934–9.
30. Hoffman HJ, Hendrick EB, Humphreys RP, Armstrong EA. Investigation and management of suprasellar arachnoid cysts. J Neurosurg. 1982;57:597–602.
31. Holst AV, Danielsen PL, Juhler M. Treatment options for intracranial arachnoid cysts: a retrospective study of 69 patients. Acta Neurochir Suppl. 2012;114:267–70.
32. Isaksen E, Leet TH, Helland CA, Wester K. Maze learning in patients with intracranial arachnoid cysts. Acta Neurochir. 2013;155:841–8; discussion 848.
33. Jafrani R, Raskin JS, Kaufman A, Lam S. Intracranial arachnoid cysts: pediatric neurosurgery update. Surg Neurol Int. 2019;10:15.
34. Jansen PR, Dremmen M, van den Berg A, Dekkers IA, Blanken LME, Muetzel RL, Bolhuis K, Mulder RM, Kocevska D, Jansen TA, de Wit MY, Neuteboom RF, Polderman TJC, Posthuma D, Jaddoe VWV, Verhulst FC, Tiemeier H, van der Lugt A, White TJH. Incidental findings on brain imaging in the general pediatric population. N Engl J Med. 2017;377:1593–5.
35. Jones RF, Warnock TH, Nayanar V, Gupta JM. Suprasellar arachnoid cysts: management by cyst wall resection. Neurosurgery. 1989;25:554–61.
36. Jordan LC, McKinstry RC 3rd, Kraut MA, Ball WS, Vendt BA, Casella JF, DeBaun MR, Strouse JJ. Incidental findings on brain magnetic resonance imaging of children with sickle cell disease. Pediatrics. 2010;126:53–61.
37. Kang JK, Lee KS, Lee IW, Jeun SS, Son BC, Jung CK, Park YS, Lee SW. Shunt-independent surgical treatment of middle cranial fossa arachnoid cysts in children. Childs Nerv Syst. 2000;16:111–6.
38. Karabatsou K, Hayhurst C, Buxton N, O'Brien DF, Mallucci CL. Endoscopic management of arachnoid cysts: an advancing technique. J Neurosurg. 2007;106:455–62.
39. Katzman GL, Dagher AP, Patronas NJ. Incidental findings on brain magnetic resonance imaging from 1000 asymptomatic volunteers. JAMA. 1999;282:36–9.
40. Kelly KA, Sherburn MM, Sellyn GE, Ahluwalia R, Foster J, Shannon CN, Bonfield CM. Management of suprasellar arachnoid cysts in children: a systematic literature review highlighting modern endoscopic approaches. World Neurosurg. 2020;141:e316–23.

41. Kim BS, Illes J, Kaplan RT, Reiss A, Atlas SW. Incidental findings on pediatric MR images of the brain. AJNR Am J Neuroradiol. 2002;23:1674–7.
42. Kim SK, Cho BK, Chung YN, Kim HS, Wang KC. Shunt dependency in shunted arachnoid cyst: a reason to avoid shunting. Pediatr Neurosurg. 2002;37:178–85.
43. Kimiwada T, Hayashi T, Narisawa A, Shirane R, Tominaga T. Shunt placement after cyst fenestration for middle cranial fossa arachnoid cysts in children. J Neurosurg Pediatr. 2015;16:533–9.
44. Kurabe S, Sasaki O, Mitsuhashi D, Koike T. Growing posterior fossa arachnoid cyst causing tonsillar herniation and hydrocephalus. Arch Neurol. 2011;68:1606–7.
45. Lee JY, Kim JW, Phi JH, Kim SK, Cho BK, Wang KC. Enlarging arachnoid cyst: a false alarm for infants. Childs Nerv Syst. 2012;28:1203–11.
46. Levy ML, Wang M, Aryan HE, Yoo K, Meltzer H. Microsurgical keyhole approach for middle fossa arachnoid cyst fenestration. Neurosurgery. 2003;53:1138–44; discussion 1144-5.
47. Lim JW, Choi SW, Song SH, Kwon HJ, Koh HS, Youm JY. Is arachnoid cyst a static disease? A case report and literature review. Childs Nerv Syst. 2019;35:385–8.
48. Magnéli S, Cesarini KG, Grabowska A, Rostami E. Cystoventricular drainage of intracranial arachnoid cysts in adults. World Neurosurg. 2021;152:e297–301.
49. Maher CO, Garton HJ, Al-Holou WN, Trobe JD, Muraszko KM, Jackson EM. Management of subdural hygromas associated with arachnoid cysts. J Neurosurg Pediatr. 2013;12:434–43.
50. Marin-Sanabria EA, Yamamoto H, Nagashima T, Kohmura E. Evaluation of the management of arachnoid cyst of the posterior fossa in pediatric population: experience over 27 years. Childs Nerv Syst. 2007;23:535–42.
51. Martínez-Lage JF, Pérez-Espejo MA, Almagro MJ, López-Guerrero AL. Hydrocephalus and arachnoid cysts. Childs Nerv Syst. 2011;27:1643–52.
52. Martínez-Lage JF, Ruíz-Espejo AM, Almagro MJ, Alfaro R, Felipe-Murcia M, López-Guerrero AL. CSF overdrainage in shunted intracranial arachnoid cysts: a series and review. Childs Nerv Syst. 2009;25:1061–9.
53. Martínez-Lage JF, Valentí JA, Piqueras C, Ruiz-Espejo AM, Román F, Nuño de la Rosa JA. Functional assessment of intracranial arachnoid cysts with TC99 m-HMPAO SPECT: a preliminary report. Childs Nerv Syst. 2006;22:1091–7.
54. McBride LA, Winston KR, Freeman JE. Cystoventricular shunting of intracranial arachnoid cysts. Pediatr Neurosurg. 2003;39:323–9.
55. McDonald PJ, Rutka JT. Middle cranial fossa arachnoid cysts that come and go. Report of two cases and review of the literature. Pediatr Neurosurg. 1997;26:48–52.
56. Mohn A, Schoof E, Fahlbusch R, Wenzel D, Dörr HG. The endocrine spectrum of arachnoid cysts in childhood. Pediatr Neurosurg. 1999;31:316–21.
57. Müslüman AM, Özöner B, Kirçelli A, Can SM, Yilmaz A, Kaldirimoğlu A, Şahin B. Chronic subdural hematoma associated with arachnoid cyst of the middle fossa: surgical treatment and mid-term results in fifteen patients. Turk Neurosurg. 2017;32(6):1.
58. Nowosławska E, Polis L, Kaniewska D, Mikołajczyk W, Krawczyk J, Szymański W, Zakrzewski K, Podciechowska J, Polis B. Neuroendoscopic techniques in the treatment of arachnoid cysts in children and comparison with other operative methods. Childs Nerv Syst. 2006;22:599–604.
59. Oberbauer RW, Haase J, Pucher R. Arachnoid cysts in children: a European co-operative study. Childs Nerv Syst. 1992;8:281–6.
60. Oertel JM, Baldauf J, Schroeder HW, Gaab MR. Endoscopic cystoventriculostomy for treatment of paraxial arachnoid cysts. J Neurosurg. 2009;110:792–9.
61. Okumura Y, Sakaki T, Hirabayashi H. Middle cranial fossa arachnoid cyst developing in infancy. Case report. J Neurosurg. 1995;82:1075–7.
62. Parsch CS, Krauss J, Hofmann E, Meixensberger J, Roosen K. Arachnoid cysts associated with subdural hematomas and hygromas: analysis of 16 cases, long-term follow-up, and review of the literature. Neurosurgery. 1997;40:483–90.
63. Peterson C, Lawless M, Sood S. Spontaneous resolution of asymptomatic pediatric suprasellar arachnoid cysts: report of 2 cases and review of the literature. Pediatr Neurosurg. 2020;55:62–6.
64. Pradilla G, Jallo G. Arachnoid cysts: case series and review of the literature. Neurosurg Focus. 2007;22:E7.
65. Raffel C, McComb JG. To shunt or to fenestrate: which is the best surgical treatment for arachnoid cysts in pediatric patients? Neurosurgery. 1988;23:338–42.
66. Rao G, Anderson RC, Feldstein NA, Brockmeyer DL. Expansion of arachnoid cysts in children: report of two cases and review of the literature. J Neurosurg. 2005;102:314–7.
67. Russo N, Domenicucci M, Beccaglia MR, Santoro A. Spontaneous reduction of intracranial arachnoid cysts: a complete review. Br J Neurosurg. 2008;22:626–9.
68. Sato H, Sato N, Katayama S, Tamaki N, Matsumoto S. Effective shunt-independent treatment for primary middle fossa arachnoid cyst. Childs Nerv Syst. 1991;7:375–81.
69. Savas Erdeve S, Ocal G, Berberoglu M, Siklar Z, Hacihamdioglu B, Evliyaoglu O, Fitoz S. The endocrine spectrum of intracranial cysts in childhood and review of the literature. J Pediatr Endocrinol Metab. 2011;24:867–75.
70. Seizeur R, Forlodou P, Coustans M, Dam-Hieu P. Spontaneous resolution of arachnoid cysts: review and features of an unusual case. Acta Neurochir. 2007;149:75–8; discussion 78.
71. Shim KW, Lee YH, Park EK, Park YS, Choi JU, Kim DS. Treatment option for arachnoid cysts. Childs Nerv Syst. 2009;25:1459–66.

72. Silav G, Sarı R, Bölükbaşı FH, Altaş M, Işık N, Elmacı İ. Microsurgical fenestration and cystoperitoneal shunt through preauricular subtemporal keyhole craniotomy for the treatment of symptomatic middle fossa arachnoid cysts in children. Childs Nerv Syst. 2015;31:87–93.
73. Soleman J, Kozyrev DA, Constantini S, Roth J. Surgical treatment and outcome of posterior fossa arachnoid cysts in infants. J Neurosurg Pediatr. 2021;28:544–52.
74. Spacca B, Kandasamy J, Mallucci CL, Genitori L. Endoscopic treatment of middle fossa arachnoid cysts: a series of 40 patients treated endoscopically in two centres. Childs Nerv Syst. 2010;26:163–72.
75. Spennato P, Ruggiero C, Aliberti F, Buonocore MC, Trischitta V, Cinalli G. Interhemispheric and quadrigeminal cysts. World Neurosurg. 2013;79:S20.e1–7.
76. Starkman SP, Brown TC, Linell EA. Cerebral arachnoid cysts. J Neuropathol Exp Neurol. 1958;17:484–500.
77. Starzyk J, Kwiatkowski S, Urbanowicz W, Starzyk B, Harasiewicz M, Kalicka-Kasperczyk A, Tylek-Lemańska D, Dziatkowiak H. Suprasellar arachnoidal cyst as a cause of precocious puberty—report of three patients and literature overview. J Pediatr Endocrinol Metab. 2003;16:447–55.
78. Struck AF, Murphy MJ, Iskandar BJ. Spontaneous development of a de novo suprasellar arachnoid cyst. Case report. J Neurosurg. 2006;104:426–8.
79. Tamburrini G, Caldarelli M, Massimi L, Santini P, Di Rocco C. Subdural hygroma: an unwanted result of sylvian arachnoid cyst marsupialization. Childs Nerv Syst. 2003;19:159–65.
80. Tamburrini G, Dal Fabbro M, Di Rocco C. Sylvian fissure arachnoid cysts: a survey on their diagnostic workout and practical management. Childs Nerv Syst. 2008;24:593–604.
81. Thomas BP, Pearson MM, Wushensky CA. Active spontaneous decompression of a suprasellar-prepontine arachnoid cyst detected with routine magnetic resonance imaging. Case report. J Neurosurg Pediatr. 2009;3:70–2.
82. Turhan T, Erşahin Y, Akıntürk N, Mutluer S. Fenestration methods for sylvian arachnoid cysts—endoscopy or microsurgery. Childs Nerv Syst. 2012;28:229–35.
83. Vernooij MW, Ikram MA, Tanghe HL, Vincent AJ, Hofman A, Krestin GP, Niessen WJ, Breteler MM, van der Lugt A. Incidental findings on brain MRI in the general population. N Engl J Med. 2007;357:1821–8.
84. Weber F, Knopf H. Incidental findings in magnetic resonance imaging of the brains of healthy young men. J Neurol Sci. 2006;240:81–4.
85. Weber R, Voit T, Lumenta C, Lenard HG. Spontaneous regression of a temporal arachnoid cyst. Childs Nerv Syst. 1991;7:414–5.
86. Wester K. Peculiarities of intracranial arachnoid cysts: location, sidedness, and sex distribution in 126 consecutive patients. Neurosurgery. 1999;45:775–9.
87. Wester K. Intracranial arachnoid cysts—do they impair mental functions? J Neurol. 2008;255:1113–20.
88. Wester K, Helland CA. How often do chronic extra-cerebral haematomas occur in patients with intracranial arachnoid cysts? J Neurol Neurosurg Psychiatry. 2008;79:72–5.
89. Wester K, Hugdahl K. Arachnoid cysts of the left temporal fossa: impaired preoperative cognition and postoperative improvement. J Neurol Neurosurg Psychiatry. 1995;59:293–8.
90. Yang SH, Lee KS, Sung JH, Son BC, Jeun SS, Kang JK. Surgical decompression of supratentorial arachnoid cysts in pediatric patients younger than one year. Pediatr Neurosurg. 2008;44:465–70.
91. Zada G, Krieger MD, McNatt SA, Bowen I, McComb JG. Pathogenesis and treatment of intracranial arachnoid cysts in pediatric patients younger than 2 years of age. Neurosurg Focus. 2007;22:E1.

Shunt Placement for Arachnoid Cysts

Kemal Ertilav and Ali Serdar Oğuzoğlu

1 Introduction

Arachnoid cysts (ACs) are benign, congenital, non-neoplastic, extra-axial, fluid-filled intra-arachnoidal lesions similar to cerebrospinal fluid (CSF). These are the most common intracranial cysts and constitute 1% of intracranial space-occupying lesions [19, 12]. Primary ACs are congenitally formed by the collection of CSF between the arachnoid layers [24, 18, 13]. Although ACs can be seen at any age, 75% of them are seen in children. The male/female ratio is 3:1 [33]. In secondary ACs, CSF is trapped within the arachnoid scar tissue after trauma, bleeding, chemical irritation, tumor, or inflammatory events. Thus, the fluid within the cyst may be stained with hemosiderin and contain inflammatory cells [18, 26]. Histopathologically, it consists of a simple single layer of arachnoid cells in a vascular collagenous membrane continuous with the arachnoid layer. The cyst, which is filled with a clear fluid resembling CSF, can sometimes be xanthochromic, proteinous, or hemorrhagic. Secondary ACs may show histopathologically prior inflammatory changes such as gliosis and hemosiderin in the wall. In addition, they may carry loculated and/or protein content depending on the underlying pathological processes [14]. Apart from this, ACs may be associated with some congenital anomalies such as corpus callosum agenesis, and sometimes they can be seen bilaterally in siblings or the same child [1].

Ninety percent of ACs are located in the supratentorial compartment of the brain, and the rest are located infratentorially. Forty-nine percent of the supratentorial cysts are located in the middle cranial fossa and the Sylvian fissure. Some ACs completely fill the temporal fossa and extend to the frontal cortex. Other localization areas include the convexity, interhemispheric area, and sellar, suprasellar, and intraventricular region. Those located in the posterior fossa are found in the ponto-cerebellar corner, vermis, supra- and intra-cerebellar hemispheres, and clival and interpeduncular areas [11, 28, 29]. Most ACs, especially those with supratentorial localization, are asymptomatic. Symptomatic lesions, on the other hand, may show various symptoms depending on the location, size, and effect on CSF circulation [21]. Approximately 75% of intracranial ACs occur before the age of 3 years. Some are asymptomatic for life. Those with Sylvian fissures usually present with an intracranial pressure syndrome accompanied by nausea, vomiting and papilledema, and headache symptoms. The most common symptom is an epileptic seizure. The seizure may be focal, partial, or generalized. In many cases, the etiology of the seizure is unknown. Massive midline shift can lead to chronic herniation, midbrain compression, and hemiparesis [15, 18, 33]. Midline posterior fossa

K. Ertilav (✉) · A. S. Oğuzoğlu
Department of Neurosurgery, Süleyman Demirel University School of Medicine, Isparta, Turkey

M. Turgut et al. (eds.), *Arachnoid Cysts*, https://doi.org/10.1007/978-3-031-22701-1_26

cysts most often present with obstructive hydrocephalus findings. Ataxia and cranial nerve pathologies are among the rare findings [22, 31]. Suprasellar cysts usually cause hydrocephalus by extending into the third ventricle or by obstructing the aqueductus sylvii [17]. Bobble-head doll syndrome is seen in suprasellar ACs [10, 32]. In this syndrome, rhythmic, non-voluntary, forward, and backward rocking head movements are observed two or three times per second. Suprasellar cysts may also cause bitemporal hemianopsia or visual acuity abnormalities [17]. In intrasellar ACs, endocrinopathy findings such as precocious puberty, hypopituitarism, and growth retardation may be observed. This condition should be differentiated from Rathke's cleft cysts [22]. In interhemispheric cysts, signs of increased intracranial pressure can be observed in varying degrees. In addition, growth retardation, hyper- or hypotonia, hemiparesis, ocular changes, and epilepsy may occur. Convexity ACs usually present with headache and epileptic seizures. Cranial asymmetry may be detected, and transillumination testing may reveal the cyst [22].

2 Diagnosis

Recently, an increasing number of diagnoses of intracranial ACs have been made by prenatal ultrasonography. This method is a noninvasive, inexpensive diagnostic method and an effective screening tool, especially for cerebral malformations [27].

Computed tomography (CT) has become the standard neuroimaging technique for the detection and characterization of AC over time. The cyst is seen as a hypodense lesion with attenuation values similar to the CSF on CT. Contrast-enhanced series can be obtained to differentiate ACs from cystic tumors. The cyst wall is distinguished by a lack of contrast enhancement [3, 31].

Recently, magnetic resonance imaging (MRI) has become the standard neuroimaging technique for the detection and characterization of all ACs, particularly posterior fossa cysts [8, 30]. MRI is the preferred imaging modality because it provides information in three planes, eliminates bone artifact, and helps in planning surgery. In addition, it may show anomalies such as agenesis of the corpus callosum or aqueductal stenosis. The differential diagnosis of ACs, including epidermoid tumor, which is most frequently confused with diffusion MRI, can be made [3, 31]. Galassi et al. made a classification according to the appearance of ACs in the Sylvian fissure. Type I cysts are small lenticular cysts in the Sylvian fissure, anterior pole of the middle fossa, and posterior to the sphenoid wing; they do not cause mass effect and midline shift. Type II cysts appear rectangular and involve the middle and proximal aspect of the fissure outside the insular cortex. There is minimal midline shift [3]. Type III cysts are large lenticular-shaped lesions and usually cause shift in the midline. Type III includes the entire Sylvian fissure. These cysts almost completely cover the temporal fossa and have a large cerebral hemisphere area separating the Sylvian fissure opercle. The temporal lobe is severely atrophic, and both the frontal and parietal lobes are greatly compressed so that most of one side of the cranial cavity can be occupied. A striking mass effect is the rule. The ventricles and midline structures are markedly and sometimes extremely distorted and pushed to the opposite side. Cranial deformities and angiographic pathological changes are consistently present and very prominent [3].

3 Conservative Treatment

Although there is no consensus in the literature, there are studies showing that ACs in different localizations go into spontaneous resolution or regression with a conservative approach [23]. A conservative approach is generally recommended in asymptomatic patients. If an asymptomatic AC patient is to be followed up conservatively, the patient should be followed at regular intervals (every 6 months for the first 2 years) with cranial CT and/or MRI. If the cyst is stable after 2 years, follow-up should be continued at 1-year intervals [7]. Especially, middle cranial fossa cysts may show an increase in intracystic hemorrhage and mass effect as a result of spontaneous hemorrhage or trauma. Since the widespread opinion exists that intracystic hemorrhage and increased mass effect require surgery, it would be appropriate to inform the relatives of the patients about the possible symptoms [20].

4 Surgical Treatment

The most important factor affecting the success of the surgical treatment of ACs is to choose the correct indication. Clinical and radiological findings, cyst location, age, and cyst size should be evaluated in detail. Clinical findings include headache that cannot be explained by other causes accompanied by a large radiologically detected cyst, hydrocephalus due to cyst obstruction of the ventricles, endocrinological and visual disturbances due to cyst compression, and epileptic seizure due to compression. Radiologically, effacement of the subarachnoid spaces due to the mass effect of the cyst can be observed. Cyst location is extremely important in terms of surgical decision-making.

Cysts located in the sellar-suprasellar area and quadrigeminal cistern can be treated early, especially in the developmental period, in order to prevent endocrine and visual symptoms.

In cysts located in the posterior fossa, close follow-up may be required as it may cause obstructive hydrocephalus. It should be kept in mind that temporally located cysts may cause seizure formation and interhemispheric and cortical located cysts may cause seizure formation and clinical findings due to corpus callosum compression [6]. In patients who do not show increased intracranial pressure and focal neurological signs, follow-up with CT or MRI is a valid management plan [16].

The main purpose of the surgical treatment of ACs can be summarized as connecting the cyst content with the CSF pathways or evacuation of the cyst content into other body cavities.

The main methods that serve this purpose are as follows: In addition to cystoperitoneal (CP) and ventriculoperitoneal (VP) shunt placement, fenestration is provided between the cyst and the cisterns or ventricles by craniotomy or endoscopic intervention. In this section, we will talk about CP shunt placement in the surgical treatment of ACs. Cyst location is important in determining the surgical technique. In the company of current technological developments, endoscopic fenestration and microsurgical fenestration have become more widely and successfully used compared to placing shunt systems.

Especially in suprasellar cysts, the endoscopic technique is more advantageous than microsurgical fenestration and shunt placement with a high success rate (92.5%) [4, 11]. Similarly, the endoscopic technique is more widely used in the treatment of deeply located cysts such as in the quadrigeminal cistern. In the treatment of ACs of Sylvian origin, it was emphasized in a study that the most common clinical remission method was CP shunt placement (96.8%) [2] (Figs. 1, 2 and 3). The success rate of shunt surgery in convexity and interhemispheric ACs has been reported to be 100% [5].

Approximately 90% of ACs are detected in the supratentorial area, and if there is no ventricular enlargement in supratentorial ACs, a CP shunt alone is an extremely effective treatment method. However, if supratentorial ACs are accompanied by hydrocephalus, it is more appropriate to con-

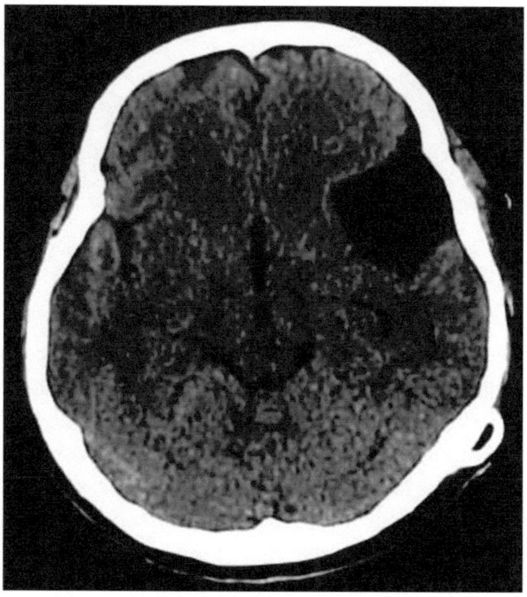

Fig. 1 Preoperative axial computed tomography (CT) image of galassi type 2 AC patient

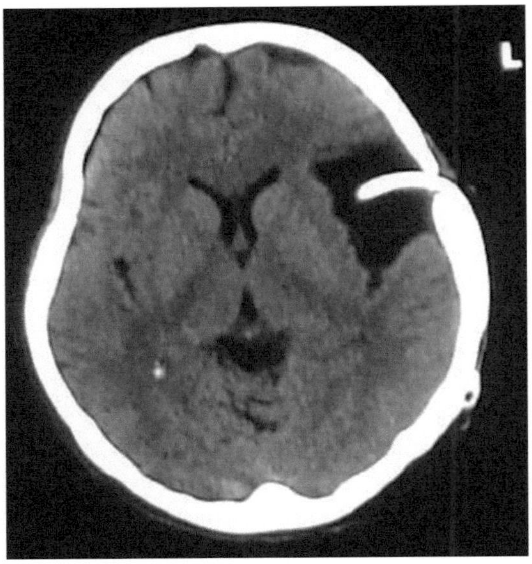

Fig. 2 Early postoperative axial CT image of galassi type 2 AC patient

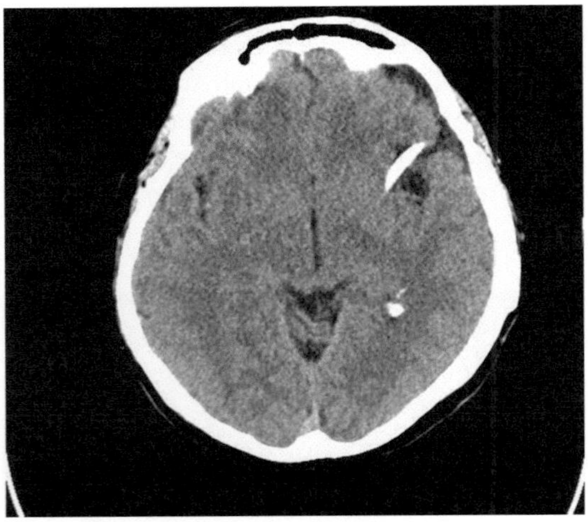

Fig. 3 Postoperative late axial CT image of galassi type 2 AC patient

nect the cyst and the ventricles with a "Y" connector and insert a VP shunt. In cases where shunt surgery will be performed, the option of evacuation of cyst and ventricular contents together via "Y" connector should not be forgotten, as well as VP shunt or CP shunt options. It should also be noted that shunt surgery options have disadvantages such as making the patient shunt dependent, infection, shunt dysfunction, excessive drainage, and repeat surgery. Shunt occlusion and the need for repetitive operation, slit ventricular condition due to excessive drainage, shunt dependence syndrome, and subdural hemorrhage are rare but serious complications of shunt placement for ACs.

Recently, a high-pressure valve or a flow-controlled shunt has been used, especially to prevent excessive drainage problems. Achieving a shunt-free state should be the ultimate goal for all shunted patients [9, 25].

5 Conclusion

Optimal treatment of ACs is a frequently discussed and renewed issue depending on current technological developments and especially the continuous development of endoscopic systems. However, a CP shunt combined with a VP shunt remains currently a safe and effective method, especially for the treatment of supratentorial cysts accompanied by hydrocephalus.

References

1. Albright AL. Treatment of bobble-head doll syndrome by transcallosal cystectomy. Neurosurgery. 1981;8:593–5.
2. Bahk WM, Pae CU, Chae JH, Jun TY, Kim KS. A case of brief psychosis associated with an arachnoid cyst. Psychiatry Clin Neurosci. 2002;56:203–5.
3. Beltramello A, Mazza C. Spontaneous disappearance of a large middle fossa arachnoid cyst. Surg Neurol. 1985;24:181–3.
4. Benton JW, Hellhaus G, Huttenlocher PR, Ojemann RG, et al. The bobble-head doll syndrome. Neurology. 1996;16:725–9.
5. Cagnoni G, Fonda C, Pancani S, Pampaloni A, Mugnaini L. Intracranial arachnoid cysts in pediatric age. Pediatr Med Chir. 1996;18:85–90.
6. Chunde L, Yin L, Jiang T, Ma Z, Jia G. Shunt dependency syndrome after cystoperitoneal shunting of arachnoid cysts. Childs Nerv Syst. 2014;30(3):471–6.
7. Cincu R, Agrawal A, Eiras J. Intracranial arachnoid cysts: current concepts and treatmentalternatives. Clin Neurol Neurosurg. 2007;109:837–43.
8. Ciricillo SF, Cogen PH, Harsh GR, Edwards MS. İntracranial arachnoid cysts in children. A comparison of the effects of fenestrastion and shunting. J Neurosurg. 1991;74:230–5.
9. Clemenceau S, Carpenter A. Intracranial arachnoid cysts. A review. Rev Neurol (Paris). 1999;155:604–8.

10. Cokluk C, Senel A, Celik F, Ergur H. Spontaneous disappearance of two asymptomatic arachnoid cysts in two different locations. Minim Invasive Neurosurg. 2003;46(2):110–2.
11. Crimmins DW, Pierre-Kahn A, Sainte-Rose C, Zerah M. Treatment of suprasellar cysts and patient outcome. J Neurosurg. 2006;105:107–14.
12. Decq P, Brugieres P, Le Guerinel C, Djindjian M, Keravel Y, Nguyen JP. Percutaneous endoscopic treatment of suprasellar arachnoid cysts: ventriculocystostomy or ventriculocystocisternostomy? Technical note. J Neurosurg. 1996;84:696–701.
13. Dyck P, Gruskin P. Supratentorial arachnoid cysts in adults: a discussion of two cases from a pathophysiologic and surgical perspective. Arch Neurol. 1977;34:276.
14. Galassi E, Tognetti F, Gaist G, et al. CT scan and metrizamide CT cisternography in arachnoid cysts of the middle fossa: classification and pathophysiological aspects. Surg Neurol. 1982;17(5):363–9. https://doi.org/10.1016/0090-3019(82)90315-9.
15. Gangemi M, Seneca V, Colella G, Cioffi V, Imperato A, Maiuri F. Endoscopy versus microsurgical cyst excision and shunting for treating intracranial arachnoid cysts. J Neurosurg Pediatr. 2011;8(2):158–64.
16. Go KG. The diagnosis and treatment of intracranial arachnoid cysts. Neurosurg Quart. 1995;5(3):187204.
17. Hoffman HJ, Hendrick EB, Humphreys RP, Armstrong EA. Investigation and management of suprasellar arachnoid cysts. J Neurosurg. 1982;57:597–602.
18. Hornig GW, Zervas NT. Slit defect of the diaphragma sellae with valve effect: observation of a "slit valve". Neurosurgery. 1992;30:265–7.
19. Karnazes AC, Kei J, Le MV. Image diagnosis: arachnoid cysts. Perm J. 2015;19:110–1.
20. Kemerdere R, Kafadar AM, Erdinçler P. Treatment options of arachnoid cysts. Türk Nöroşirurji Dergisi. 2013;23(2):220–5.
21. Krawchenko J, Collins GH. Pathology of an aracnoid cysts. Case report. J Neurosurg. 1979;50:224–8.
22. McLone DG. The subarachnoid space: a review. Childs Brain. 1980;6:113–30.
23. Mottolese C, Szathmari A, Simon E, Ginguene C, Ricci-Franchi AC, Hermier M. The parallel use of endoscopic fenestration and a cystoperitoneal shunt with programmable valve to treat arachnoid cysts: experience and hypothesis. J Neurosurg Pediatr. 2010;5(4):408–14.
24. Pascual-Castroviejo I, Roche MC, Bermejo AM, Arcas J, et al. Primary intracranial arachnoid cysts. A study of 67 childhood cases. Childs Nerv Syst. 1991;7:257–63.
25. Patel TR, Bannister CM, Thorne J. A study of prenatal ultrasound and postnatal magnetic imaging in the diagnosis of central nervous system abnormalities. Eur J Pediatr Surg. 2003;13(Suppl 1):S18–22.
26. Pilu G, De Palma L, Romero R. The fetal subarachnoid sisterns: an ultrasound study with report of a case of congenital communicating hydrocephalus. J Ultrasound Med. 1986;5:365–72.
27. Raffel C, McComb JG. Arachnoid cysts. In: Cheek W, editor. Pediatric neurosurgery. Philadelphia: WB Saunders; 1994. p. 104–10.
28. Rengachary SS, Kennedy JD. Intracranial arachnoid and ependymal cysts. In: Wilkins R, Rengachary S, editors. Neurosurgery. New York: McGraw-Hill; 1996. p. 3709–28.
29. Rengachary SS, Watanabe I, Brackett CE. Pathogenesiz intracranial aracnoid cysts. Surg Neurol. 1981;40:61–83.
30. Robinson RG. Congenital cysts of the brain: arachnoid malformations. Neurol Surg. 1971;4:133–73.
31. Starkman SP, Brawn TC, Linelli EA. Cerebral aracnoid cysts. J Neurooncol. 1958;17:484–500.
32. Sommer IEC, Smit LME. Congenital supratentorial arachnoidal and giant cysts in children: a clinical study with arguments for a conservative approach. Childs Nerv Syst. 1997;13:8–12.
33. Swett HA, Nixon GW. Agenesis of the corpus callosum with interhemispheric cyst. Radiology. 1975;114:641–5.

Stereotactic Internal Diversion of Arachnoid Cysts

Elias Rizk

1 Introduction

Arachnoid cysts (ACs) are non-traumatic, cerebral spinal fluid masses in the arachnoid membranes (Fig. 1). These masses are the most commonly found intracranial cysts and account for about 1.5% of all intracranial lesions [9, 12]. The cytology of the ACs has been an unclear and controversial issue. However, in several reports, ACs are demonstrated as liquid masses surrounded by the arachnoid membrane [1]. The fluid usually is present within the margins of cerebral spinal fluid, such as in the Sylvian fissures, suprasellar, quadrigeminal, posterior-infratentorial cisterns, and cerebellopontine angle [20]. It has been proposed that these cysts primarily formed from the splitting and duplication of the arachnoid endomenix. Commonly the arachnoid endomenix develops into pia and forms the arachnoid and subarachnoid space [23]. The ACs are distinguished from the pia and cortex within the subarachnoid space. This space is a transparent and thin region containing blood-containing vessels spread around the whole brain. The expansion of cysts, especially during the stages of development, can be due to multiple reasons [48]. Yamanouchi et al. proposed that the cyst's growth is linked to the difference in cerebrospinal fluid pressure or may be due to the one-directional ball-valve process [28]. Kusaka et al. postulate that the expansion results from the oncotic gradient that is caused due to the increased concentration of protein inside the cysts. However, Yamanouchi et al. [48] discussed the secretory ability of membrane proteins, which can potentially be the cause of cyst expansion.

ACs can be classified as congenital, also called true ACs. The congenital ACs occur due to embryonic abnormalities [10]. The second class is the secondary ACs, also known as acquired cysts. Secondary ACs usually result from the sequestration of cerebral spinal fluid due to several processes such as inflammation, trauma, tumors, and hemorrhage [1]. Most ACs are asymptomatic, benign, and found incidentally on brain images for various conditions [4]. Many theories proposed the genesis and agenesis of the ACs in the brain [10, 22]. The smaller ACs usually exhibit no symptoms, but larger cysts such as supratentorial, posterior fossa, and suprasellar cysts can present with headaches, neurologic dysfunction, and seizures [19, 24, 27]. As a matter of fact, more than two-thirds of symptomatic patients with AC(s) show a common headache symptom [24].

E. Rizk (✉)
Department of Neurosurgery, College of Medicine, The Pennsylvania State University, Hershey, PA, USA

Department of Neurosurgery, Penn State Health Milton S. Hershey Medical Center, Hershey, PA, USA
e-mail: ebr10@psu.edu; erizk@pennstatehealth.psu.edu

M. Turgut et al. (eds.), *Arachnoid Cysts*, https://doi.org/10.1007/978-3-031-22701-1_27

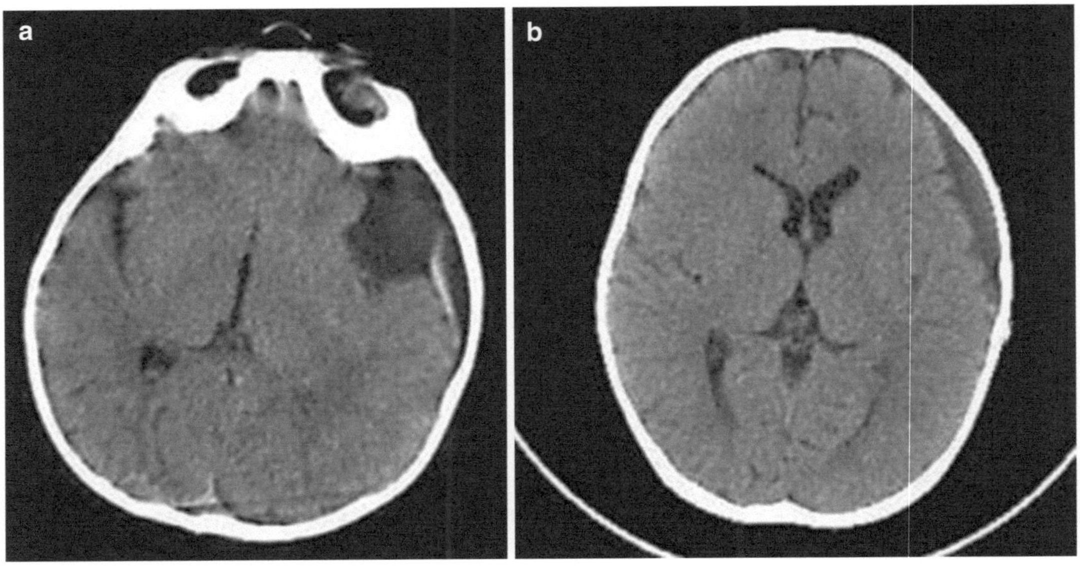

Fig. 1 A computed tomography (CT) image of a patient suffering from an arachnoid cyst (ACs). (**a**) shows the preoperative condition indicating an AC located in the middle fossa. (**b**) shows the CT scan after 18 months of surgery-based removal of an AC

2 Prevalence of Arachnoid Cysts

With the increased use of imaging techniques such as magnetic resonance imaging (MRI) and CT, diagnosing ACs has become prevalent [47, 50]. ACs are more prevalent in males than females and are reported more often in the middle fossa [25]. ACs in the intracranial region may lead to cranial abnormalities or increased head size, seizures, cognitive disorders, hydrocephalus, headaches, and other neurological disorders like visual and cerebellar abnormalities [4]. An accurate understanding of the nature and prevalence of ACs can lead to better identification and patient selection for surgical purposes. Several clinical case series proposed that ACs can be treated surgically with fenestrations based on endoscopy techniques [41, 49], craniotomy [29, 41], or placement of shunts [38]. Each of these operative techniques is linked with a morbidity and/or mortality potential [14, 37, 43]. Around 30–60% of the patients suffering from symptomatic ACs exhibit signs and symptoms of hydrocephalus [34]. Patients younger than 2 years of age are more prone to macrocephaly than other symptoms [46]. Sommer et al. report that the cause and effect linkage with ACs is weaker with the signs such as aphasia, headaches, and attention deficiency disorder [42]. Sometimes, when the ACs rupture, they may develop intracranial hypertension and subdural hygromas [2]. A direct linkage between the ACs and the abnormal flow dynamics of cerebrospinal fluid has been observed. Several reports also describe other presentations including subdural hygroma [14], cerebral spinal fluid leakage [37], subdural hematoma and empyema [24], pseudomeningocele, meningitis [43], spasticity [37], hydrocephalus, seizures, and cranial nerve palsy [48]. Other reports describe the occurrence of impaired autoregulation secondary to ACs. This could be due to the cyst interfering with the normal flow of cerebral blood and its perfusion [40]. The cerebral perfusions are also responsible for the initiation of papilledema and headaches especially after the operation.

It is important to mention that some reports suggest the disappearance of ACs over time, especially those associated with head injury [33]. In addition, some reports showed the spontaneous disappearance of ACs without head injury. The proposed mechanism of this natural recovery is the breakage of the inner and outer arachnoid membranes that may facilitate the absorption of its content [48]. However, the spontaneous cyst resolution after the injury of the head and its relation with the direct absorption through the cyst's wall is still under debate.

3 Treatments of Intracranial Arachnoid Cysts

Treating ACs could be fraught with multiple needs for another surgery [24, 30, 41]. The preference for one surgical treatment over another is under debate. Despite the risk of complications, many authors suggest that the surgical treatment of ACs exhibits apparent symptoms [25]. Leon et al. report that the prevalence of headaches and seizures after the surgical removal of ACs remains increased [13, 29]. Some clinicians also propose monitoring intracranial pressure as a feasible tool to select the patient for surgical treatment [31]. Others demonstrated the feasibility of using the single-photon emission computed tomography (SPECT) imaging of cerebral blood flow to identify the need for surgical treatment [45].

A report by Tamburrini notes that 31.1% of the surgeons recommended surgery for patients with psychomotor delay, 13.3% recommended prophylactic treatment, 35.5% suggested surgery for patients showing signs of headaches, and the remaining 17.7% of surgeons considered surgery for the Galassi type 2 or more Sylvian cysts. In short, better knowledge of the nature and prevalence of ACs can lead to more accurate surgical decisions. Al-Holou conducted research on 11 patients for 3.5 years and emphasized the avoidance of surgical treatment until the ACs became symptomatic [4]. He further elaborated that an increase in the size of cysts despite symptoms also doesn't indicate the need for surgical treatment. The earlier clinical symptoms of the patient offer a direct link between the cysts and the choice of surgery. Zada et al. proposed that the extent of cyst development and its relation to the ventricular space exhibits another significant risk factor in predicting the need for shunt placement [50]. Other safe options are endoscopic and craniotomy fenestrations [17, 21].

4 Craniotomy Fenestration to Treat Arachnoid Cysts

A craniotomy exposes the AC for direct fenestration. Neurosurgeons open the cyst and fenestrate its contents into the subarachnoid space. Sixty percent of patients have a notable improvement following adequate fenestration [39]. Cyst fenestration offers an advantage regarding the independence of shunt placement needs [32]. Yang et al. conducted a retrospective study on patients less than 2 years of age [49]. A craniotomy was performed to fenestrate the cyst, and the results discussed the efficacy of surgical interventions depending on the symptoms. However, there are associated inherent risks with open craniotomy and cyst fenestration. Some authors [6] reported the prevalence of intraparenchymal hemorrhage as a rare complication occurring while treating ACs through open fenestration. Others reported that cyst excision has also been associated with intracranial hemorrhage. It has been proposed that reperfusion injury is due to the dysfunction of cerebrovascular autoregulation. Seemingly slow but continuous cyst decompression may reduce complications [36]. Cerebral infarction is also a notable complication following craniotomy and cyst fenestration [5]. Figures 2 and 3 show an ipsilateral hemorrhagic in an 18-year-old female patient who underwent craniotomy fenestration to remove ACs. Other complications include the development of subdural hygromas requiring further treatments [41, 44].

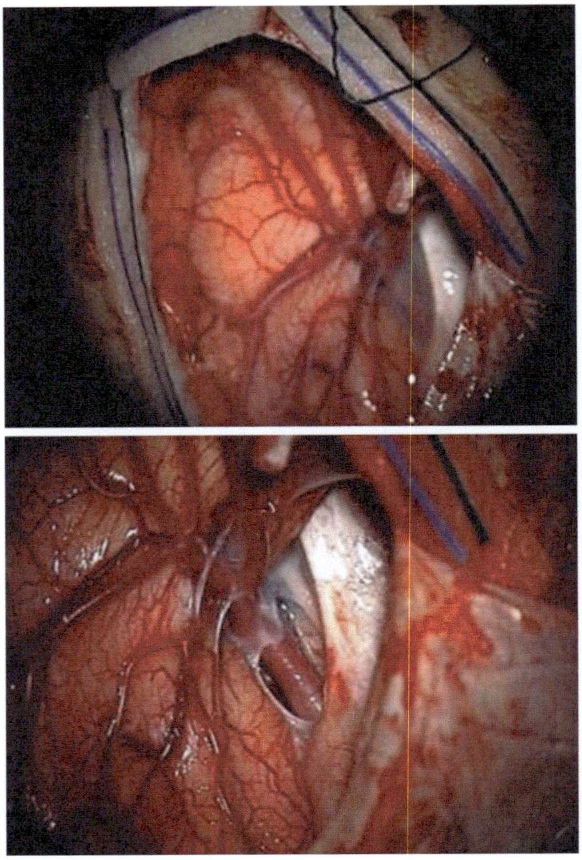

Fig. 2 Intraoperative photographs of ACs, a visual representation of opticocarotid cistern. The upper image shows condition before fenestration procedure, while the lower image represents condition after fenestration procedure [5]

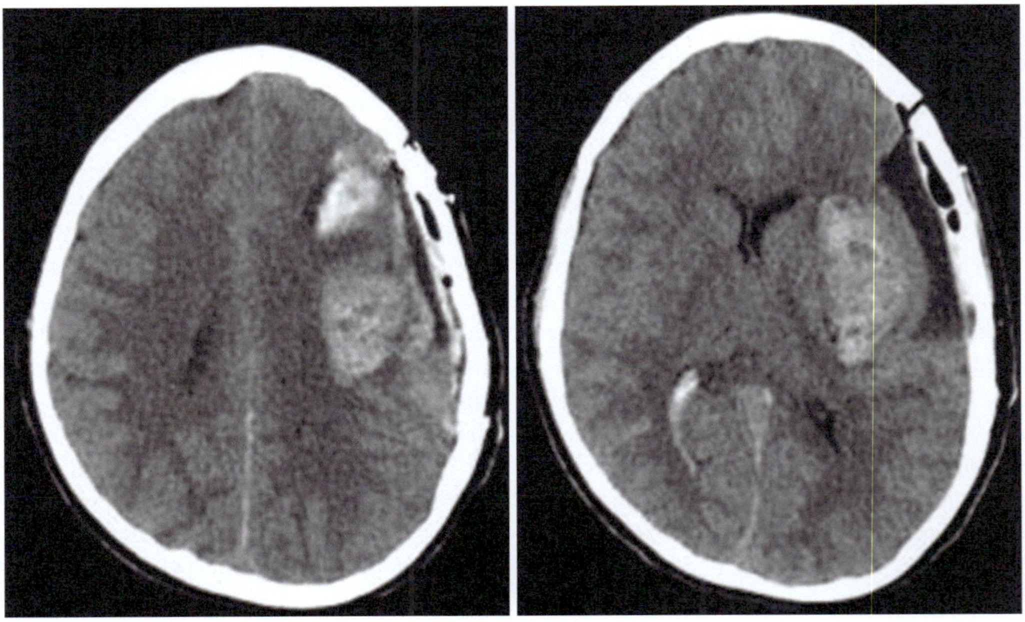

Fig. 3 Images from CT providing evidence for the various foci of intraparenchymal hemorrhage resulting after fenestration of cysts. The upper image is the representation of the axial region, while the lower image shows the coronal part after the operation [5]

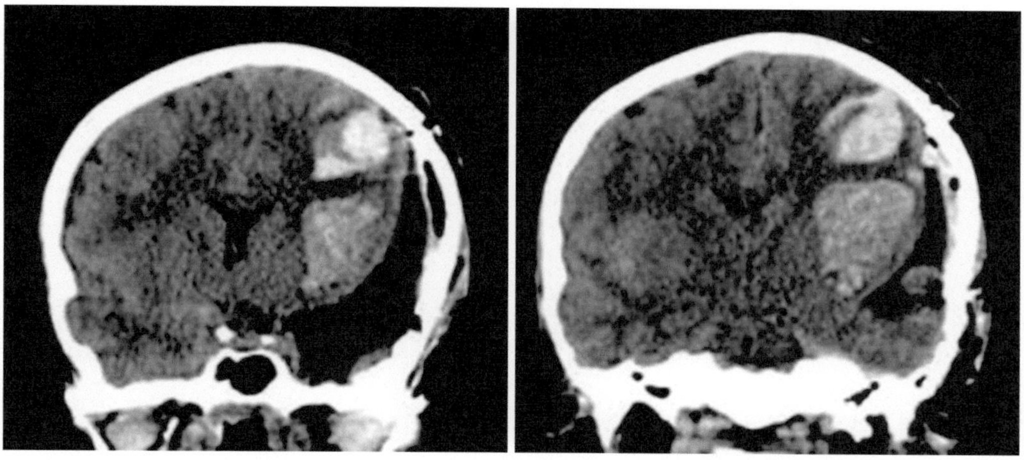

Fig. 3 (continued)

5 Endoscopic Fenestration for the Treatment of Arachnoid Cysts

Endoscopic fenestration is an effective and safe treatment to treat suprasellar ACs [43]. This has also been suggested as a surgical treatment for spinal ACs to decrease the risk of multiple laminectomies that can cause kyphotic deformity, requiring spinal fixation [18]. Endoscopic fenestration is a technique to reduce the risks of open cranial surgery [7]. Several reports favor endoscopic fenestration, suggesting it is an effective and safe procedure [15, 26]. Drawbacks of endoscopic fenestration include insufficient fenestration due to the vascularity of the membrane of the ACs and the shortcomings related to the rigidity of the endoscope. Papadimitiou reviewed the potential for endoscopic fenestration to treat spinal ACs [35]. The author proposed an opening at the caudal and cranial end of the spinal AC, followed by a minor dural opening to insert the endoscope and drain and divert the fluid (Fig. 4).

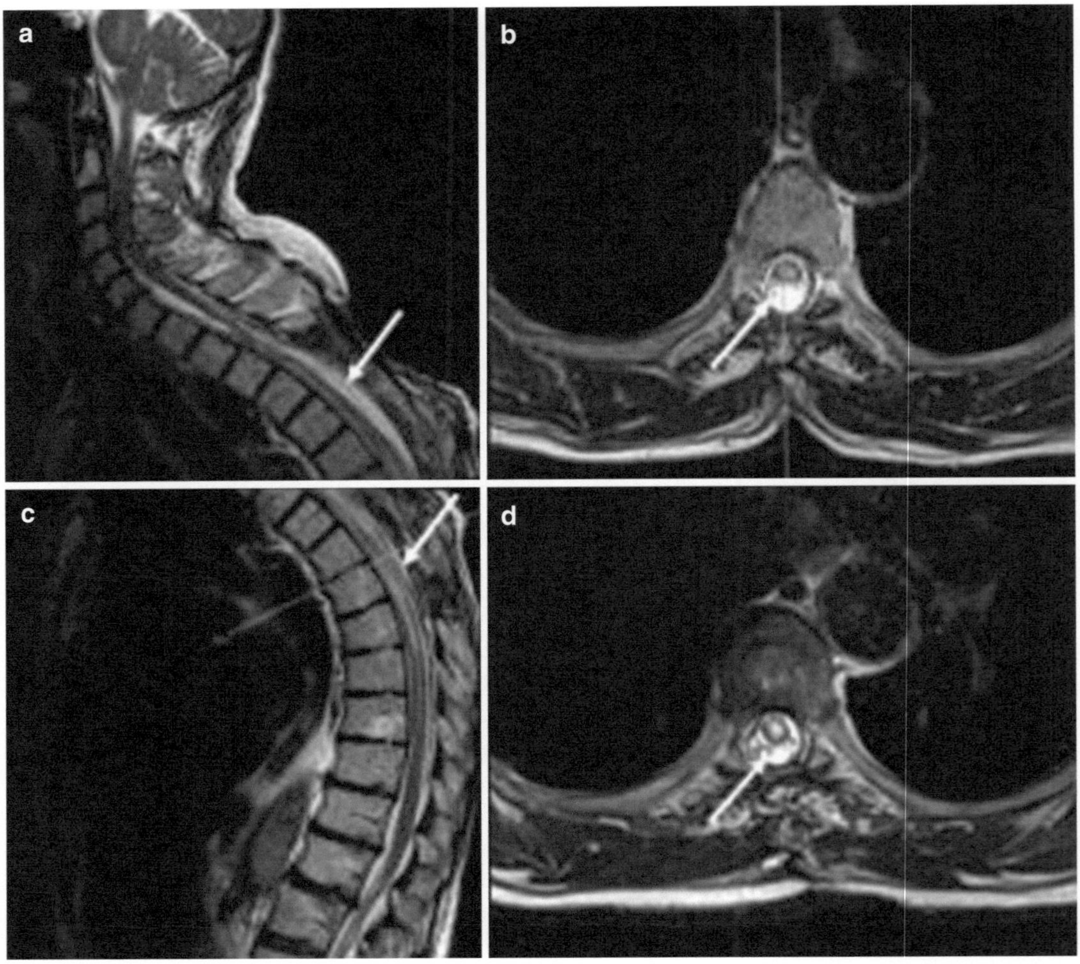

Fig. 4 Magnetic resonance imaging (MRI) micrographs of a patient undergoing endoscopic fenestration for the treatment of spinal ACs. (**a**) and (**c**) represent the sagittal MRI view, and (**b**) and (**d**) represents the MRI axial view. The patient experienced improvement after the treatment [35]

6 Shunt Placement for the Treatment of Arachnoid Cysts

Diverting shunts divert extra cerebrospinal fluid to alleviate increased intracranial pressure. Shunting procedures typically have a lower risk than cyst fenestration [25]. Drainage of the AC using a stereotactically placed burr hole is practical and straightforward. Shunt placement is proposed as a simple surgical treatment with reduced mortality, morbidity, and recurrence rates. Ciricillo compared the efficacy of fenestration treatment of children suffering from ACs with shunt placement [11]. In his cohort, fenestrated patients did not show clinical improvement. However, patients treated with shunt placement showed significant improvement. In another study by [38], the comparison between shunt placement and fenestration was compared. The authors reported 34 cases of ACs and found that 24% of the cases required shunt placement after being treated with cyst fenestration. However, a 41.7% revision rate was noted in patients treated through shunt placement. Stereotaxy is quickly becoming the gold standard with the adequate placement of catheter for the successful treatment of ACs.

Nevertheless, various researchers support shunt placement due to its outcomes despite the increased number of revisions [8, 16]. Alexiou et al. also demonstrated their confidence in shunt placement as an effective and safe surgical technique due to its significant outcomes, especially in children, such as rapid relief of the symptoms and reduction in the ACs size [3].

7 Conclusion

The literature review shows a need for further research reviewing various treatments of ACs. In addition, controversy remains regarding the adequate treatment of ACs effectively. Thus, further research and studies are required to determine which of these procedures are better for patient care.

References

1. Aicardi J, Bax M, Gillberg C, Ogier H. Diseases of the nervous system in childhood. London: Mac Keith Press; 1992.
2. Albuquerque FC, Giannotta SL. Arachnoid cyst rupture producing subdural hygroma and intracranial hypertension. Neurosurgery. 1997;41(4):951–6.
3. Alexiou GA, Varela M, Sfakianos G, Prodromou N. Shunting for the treatment of arachnoid cysts in children. Neurosurgery. 2010;67(6):1632–6.
4. Al-Holou WN, Terman S, Kilburg C, Garton HJ, Muraszko KM, Maher CO. Prevalence and natural history of arachnoid cysts in adults. J Neurosurg. 2013;118(2):222–31.
5. Auschwitz T, DeCuypere M, Khan N, Einhaus S. Hemorrhagic infarction following open fenestration of a large intracranial arachnoid cyst in a pediatric patient. J Neurosurg Pediatr. 2015;15(2):203–6.
6. Bahl A, Connolly DJ, Sinha S, Zaki H, McMullan J. Rapid brain shift, remote site hemorrhage, and a spinal hematoma after craniotomy for a large arachnoid cyst. J Pediatr Neurosci. 2012;7(2):106.
7. Basaran R, Kaksi M, Efendioglu M, Onoz M, Balkuv E, Kaner T. Spinal arachnoid cyst associated with arachnoiditis following subarachnoid haemorrhage in adult patients: a case report and literature review. Br J Neurosurg. 2015;29(2):285–9.
8. Boltshauser E, Martin F, Altermatt S. Outcome in children with space-occupying posterior fossa arachnoid cysts. Neuropediatrics. 2002;33(03):118–21.
9. Choi J-U, Kim D-S. Pathogenesis of arachnoid cyst: congenital or traumatic? Pediatr Neurosurg. 1998;29(5):260–6.
10. Cincu R, Agrawal A, Eiras J. Intracranial arachnoid cysts: current concepts and treatment alternatives. Clin Neurol Neurosurg. 2007;109(10):837–43.
11. Ciricillo SF, Cogen PH, Harsh GR, Edwards MS. Intracranial arachnoid cysts in children. A comparison of the effects of fenestration and shunting. J Neurosurg. 1991;74(2):230–5.
12. Di Rocco C, Caldarelli M. Suprasellar arachnoidal cysts. In: Intracranial cyst lesions. New York, NY: Springer; 1993. pp 113–128.
13. Di Rocco C, Tamburrini G, Caldarelli M, Velardi F, Santini P. Prolonged ICP monitoring in Sylvian arachnoid cysts. Surg Neurol. 2003;60(3):211–8.
14. Elhammady MSA, Bhatia S, Ragheb J. Endoscopic fenestration of middle fossa arachnoid cysts: a technical description and case series. Pediatr Neurosurg. 2007;43(3):209–15.
15. Eneling J, Boström S, Rossitti S. Subarachnoid hemorrhage-associated arachnoiditis and syringomyelia. Clin Neuroradiol. 2012;22(2):169–73.
16. Erdincler P, Kaynar MY, Bozkus H, Ciplak N. Posterior fossa arachnoid cysts. Br J Neurosurg. 1999;13(1):10–7.
17. Erşahin Y, Kesikçi H, Rüksen M, Aydın C, Mutluer S. Endoscopic treatment of suprasellar arachnoid cysts. Childs Nerv Syst. 2008;24(9):1013–20.
18. Fam MD, Woodroffe RW, Helland L, Noeller J, Dahdaleh NS, Menezes AH, Hitchon PW. Spinal arachnoid cysts in adults: diagnosis and management. A single-center experience. J Neurosurg Spine. 2018;29(6):711–9.
19. Galassi E, Gaist G. Dynamics of intracranial cyst formation and expansion. In: Intracranial cyst lesions. New York, NY: Springer; 1993. pp 53–77.
20. Gandy SE, Heier LA. Clinical and magnetic resonance features of primary intracranial arachnoid cysts. Ann Neurol. 1987;21(4):342–8.
21. Gangemi M, Colella G, Magro F, Maiuri F. Suprasellar arachnoid cysts: endoscopy versus microsurgical cyst excision and shunting. Br J Neurosurg. 2007;21(3):276–80.
22. Handa J, Okamoto K, Sato M. Arachnoid cyst of the middle cranial fossa: report of bilateral cysts in siblings. Surg Neurol. 1981;16(2):127–30.
23. Hassan J, Sepulveda W, Teixeira J, Cox PM. Glioependymal and arachnoid cysts: unusual causes of early ventriculomegaly in utero. Prenat Diagn. 1996;16(8):729–33.
24. Helland CA, Wester K. A population-based study of intracranial arachnoid cysts: clinical and neuroimaging outcomes following surgical cyst decompression in children. J Neurosurg Pediatr. 2006;105(5):385–90.
25. Kang J-K, Lee KS, Lee IW, Jeun SS, Son BC, Jung CK, Park YS, Lee SW. Shunt-independent surgical treatment of middle cranial fossa arachnoid cysts in children. Childs Nerv Syst. 2000;16(2):111–6.
26. Kashcheev AA, Arestov SO, Gushcha AO. Flexible endoscopy in surgical treatment of spinal adhesive arachnoiditis and arachnoid cysts. Zh Vopr Neirokhir Im N N Burdenko. 2013;77(5):44–54.

27. Koch CA, Voth D, Kraemer G, Schwarz M. Arachnoid cysts: does surgery improve epileptic seizures and headaches? Neurosurg Rev. 1995;18(3):173–81.
28. Kusaka Y, Luedemann W, Oi S, Shwardfegar R, Samii M. Fetal arachnoid cyst of the quadrigeminal cistern in MRI and ultrasound. Childs Nerv Syst. 2005;21(12):1065–6.
29. Leòn OH, Falero RAP, Rodrìguez IFA, Palacio CLC. Microsurgical keyhole approach for middle fossa arachnoid cyst fenestration. Neurosurgery. 2005;56(5):E1166.
30. Marin-Sanabria EA, Yamamoto H, Nagashima T, Kohmura E. Evaluation of the management of arachnoid cyst of the posterior fossa in pediatric population: experience over 27 years. Childs Nerv Syst. 2007;23(5):535–42.
31. Martínez-Lage JF, Valentí JA, Piqueras C, Ruiz-Espejo AM, Román F, de la Rosa JAN. Functional assessment of intracranial arachnoid cysts with TC99 m-HMPAO SPECT: a preliminary report. Childs Nerv Syst. 2006;22(9):1091–7.
32. McDonald PJ, Rutka JT. Middle cranial fossa arachnoid cysts that come and go. Pediatr Neurosurg. 1997;26(1):48–52.
33. Mori T, Fujimoto M, Sakae K, Sakakibara T, Shin H, Yamaki T, Ueda S. Disappearance of arachnoid cysts after head injury. Neurosurgery. 1995;36(5):938–42.
34. Naidich TP, McLone DG, Radkowski A. Intracranial arachnoid cysts. Pediatr Neurosurg. 1985;12(2):112–22.
35. Papadimitiou K, Cossu G, Maduri R, Valerio M, Vamadevan S, Daniel RT, Messerer M. Endoscopic treatment of spinal arachnoid cysts. Heliyon. 2021;7(4):e06736.
36. Pierangeli E, Gigante N, Pizzoni C. Tapping of a type II sylvian fissure arachnoid cyst. Neurol India. 2003;51(4):553.
37. Pradilla G, Jallo G. Arachnoid cysts: case series and review of the literature. Neurosurg Focus. 2007;22(2):1–4.
38. Raffel C, McComb JG. To shunt or to fenestrate: which is the best surgical treatment for arachnoid cysts in pediatric patients? Neurosurgery. 1988;23(3):338–42.
39. Rao G, Anderson RC, Feldstein NA, Brockmeyer DL. Expansion of arachnoid cysts in children: report of two cases and review of the literature. J Neurosurg Pediatr. 2005;102(3):314–7.
40. Sgouros S, Chapman S. Congenital middle fossa arachnoid cysts may cause global brain ischaemia: a study with 99Tc-hexamethylpropyleneamineoxime single photon emission computerised tomography scans. Pediatr Neurosurg. 2001;35(4):188–94.
41. Shim K-W, Lee Y-H, Park E-K, Park Y-S, Choi J-U, Kim D-S. Treatment option for arachnoid cysts. Childs Nerv Syst. 2009;25(11):1459–66.
42. Sommer IEC, Smit LME. Congenital supratentorial arachnoidal and giant cysts in children: a clinical study with arguments for a conservative approach. Childs Nerv Syst. 1997;13(1):8–12.
43. Spacca B, Kandasamy J, Mallucci CL, Genitori L. Endoscopic treatment of middle fossa arachnoid cysts: a series of 40 patients treated endoscopically in two centres. Childs Nerv Syst. 2010;26(2):163–72.
44. Tamburrini G, Caldarelli M, Massimi L, Santini P, Di Rocco C. Subdural hygroma: an unwanted result of sylvian arachnoid cyst marsupialization. Childs Nerv Syst. 2003;19(3):159–65.
45. Tamburrini G, Del Fabbro M, Di Rocco C. Sylvian fissure arachnoid cysts: a survey on their diagnostic workout and practical management. Childs Nerv Syst. 2008;24(5):593–604.
46. Terao T, Sawauchi S, Hashimoto T, Miyazaki Y, Akiba Y, Abe T. A case of spontaneous rupture of a suprasellar cystic mass. No Shinkei Geka. 2001;29(8):755–8.
47. Weber F, Knopf H. Incidental findings in magnetic resonance imaging of the brains of healthy young men. J Neurol Sci. 2006;240(1–2):81–4.
48. Yamanouchi Y, Someda K, Oka N. Spontaneous disappearance of middle fossa arachnoid cyst after head injury. Childs Nerv Syst. 1986;2(1):40–3.
49. Yang S-H, Lee K-S, Sung JH, Son BC, Jeun S-S, Kang J-K. Surgical decompression of supratentorial arachnoid cysts in pediatric patients younger than one year. Pediatr Neurosurg. 2008;44(6):465–70.
50. Zada G, Krieger MD, McNatt SA, Bowen I, McComb JG. Pathogenesis and treatment of intracranial arachnoid cysts in pediatric patients younger than 2 years of age. Neurosurg Focus. 2007;22(2):1–5.

Endoscopic Approach to Arachnoid Cysts

George W. Koutsouras, Maham Ahmed, and Zulma Tovar-Spinoza

1 Introduction

Arachnoid cysts (ACs) are confined collections contained within a capsule of arachnoid mater that lack communication with the cerebral ventricular system. Patients are generally asymptomatic from these lesions that are discovered incidentally on brain imaging. The prevalence of ACs has increased with the increasing use of neuroimaging such as MRI and CT, with a reported prevalence of 1.4% comprising 1% of all intracranial masses [3]. The prevalence is reportedly higher in children at 2.6% and has a female preponderance in the adult population [23]. Of those reported, 5% are symptomatic, and of those up to 75% are pediatric cases. When symptomatic, surgical options for their management include open fenestration and endoscopic fenestration. We discuss the indications, considerations, and technique of the endoscopic intervention for ACs.

2 Pathophysiology

While most ACs are congenital, as they formed by the in utero division of the arachnoid layer, creating a space for the fluid to collect, secondary ACs may also occur. These are typically associated with trauma, infection, surgical intervention, and bleeding. Histopathological analysis dictates the derivation of the cyst walls from splitting of the arachnoid membrane with the presence of an inner and outer leaflet but the absence of an epithelial lining and a lack of vasculature along the cyst wall [13, 26].

Most ACs are asymptomatic and discovered incidentally on brain imaging. Symptomatology is dependent on the size and location of the cyst (Table 1). Larger-sized cysts are more likely to be symptomatic due to local mass effect on neurovascular structures and the brain parenchyma and alterations in CSF flow. In contrast, smaller cysts are typically clinically silent. Most cysts remain stable in size, while a minority may shrink or enlarge in size over time during observation. While the exact mechanism for size alterations is unknown, several plausible theories have been proposed. These include (a) the continued CSF production by cells lining the cyst wall, (b) diffusion of fluid down the electrochemical gradient from surrounding vasculature to the cyst interior, and (c) the ball-valve mechanism allowing for fluid entrapment within the cyst [10, 14].

While they may occur anywhere there is arachnoid mater, the location of ACs is organized into anterior cranial fossa, middle cranial fossa, cerebral convexity, interhemispheric, supracerebellar, retrocerebellar, cerebellopontine angle (CPA), ambient cistern, quadrigeminal cistern, brain stem, craniospinal junction, and along the spine (Fig. 1) [23, 29]. Most cysts are in the mid-

G. W. Koutsouras (✉) · M. Ahmed
Z. Tovar-Spinoza
Department of Neurosurgery, Upstate University Hospital, Syracuse, NY, USA
e-mail: koutsoug@upstate.edu;
ahmedmah@upstate.edu; tovarspz@upstate.edu

M. Turgut et al. (eds.), *Arachnoid Cysts*, https://doi.org/10.1007/978-3-031-22701-1_28

Table 1 Cyst location, symptomatology, and surgical considerations

Cyst location	Common symptoms	Considerations
Middle cranial fossa	Epilepsy	Sylvian fissure vessels Opticocarotid recess
Suprasellar (prepontine)	Hydrocephalus Panhypopituitarism Ocular disturbance Head bobbing	No diathermy; cranial nerves, rain stem, pituitary gland, basilar artery VCC or VC
CPA/posterior fossa	Vertigo Sensorineural hearing loss Nausea	Lower cranial nerves Brain stem; CC
Quadrigeminal	Hydrocephalus	VC; transient diabetes insipidus
Intraventricular	Hydrocephalus	VC with cisternostomy or VC alone
Para-axial/interhemispheric supratentorial		CV
Spinal	Backache Fluctuating leg weakness	Thoracic (most commonly); open

ICA interval carotid artery, *VCC* ventriculocystocisternostomy, *VC* ventriculocystostomy, *CC* cystocisternostomy, *CV* cystoventriculostomy

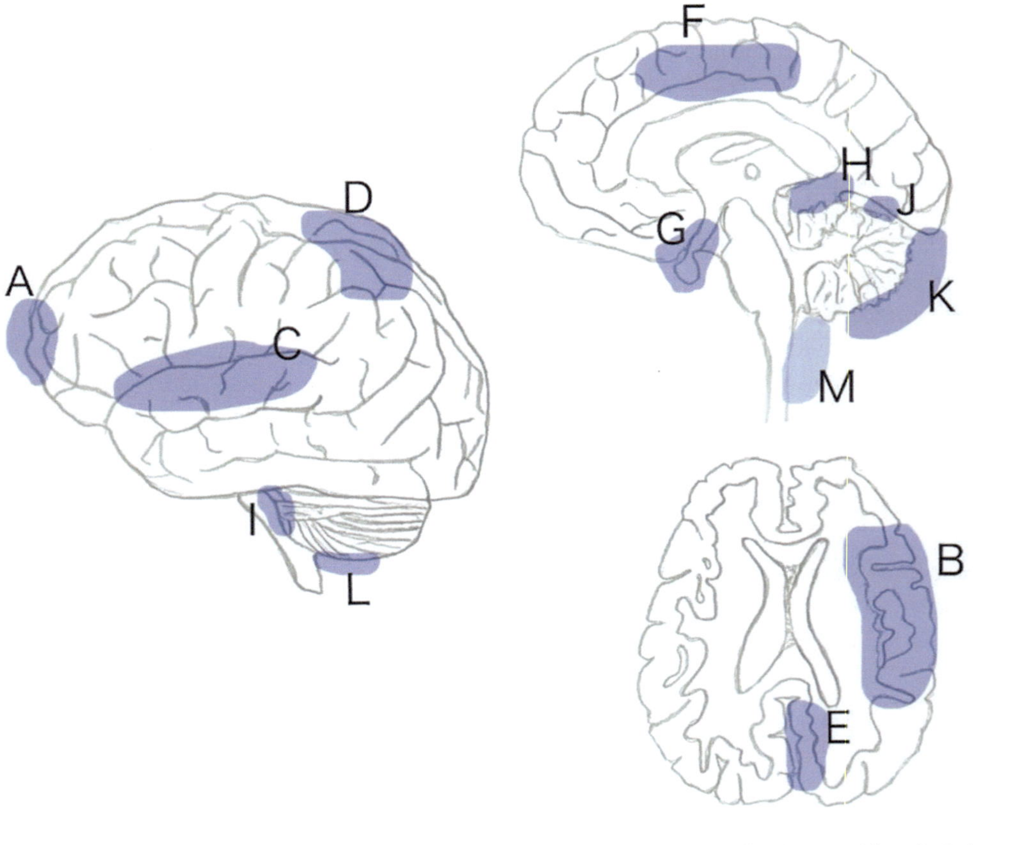

Fig. 1 Common locations of ACs. Common locations of ACs are depicted (violet): A = anterior cranial fossa, B = middle cranial fossa, C = Sylvian fissure (middle cranial fossa), D = convexity, E = parafalcine, F = interhemispheric, G = sellar/suprasellar, H = quadrigeminal cistern, I = skull base, J = supracerebellar, K = retrocerebellar, L = cisterna magna, M = cerebrospinal junction

dle cranial fossa, followed by retrocerebellar, cerebral convexity, and CPA regions. Most commonly symptomatic cysts are those located in the suprasellar region, presenting with endocrine abnormalities due to disruption of the hypothalamic-pituitary axis or symptoms due to impingement of the optic pathway in the near vicinity. The initial clinical presentation is typically not associated with cyst location-specific symptoms but rather non-specific ones, including nausea, vomiting, macrocrania, visual disturbances, and unsteadiness; this may delay considering a CNS abnormality until imaging studies are obtained. Nevertheless, the most commonly reported symptoms are headache and seizures, while some specific localization symptoms may also present, as reported in Table 1 [24].

Brain imaging is the ideal method for diagnosing an AC. MRI is the imaging modality of choice because it allows for the determination of size, location, and involvement of structures located near the cyst. An MRI may also allow for a broad differential diagnosis refinement, including epidermoid cyst, dermoid cyst, abscess, metastasis, and other cysts. In each sequence, the AC follows CSF signals, with a characteristic thin wall and lack of enhancement from inflammation allowing for differentiation from other pathologies [27, 30, 31].

3 History of Neuroendoscopy

Figure 2 describes the historical timeline of neuroendoscopy. Maximilian Nitz is accredited with the creation of the first endoscope in 1879, a device for enhanced illumination with a relatively larger visual field due to a light source at the tip of the scope and telescoping optics technology [1]. Endoscope technology was utilized in neurological surgery for the first time in 1910. Prior to this, it had been advanced through various fields of medicine, including gastroenterology, urology, pulmonology, and obstetrics and gynecology. In fact, its first application in neurosurgery was by Victor Lespinasse, a urologist at the Wesley Hospital in Chicago, USA, in 1910 [1, 2]. He used the cystoscope to perform a bilateral fulguration of the choroid plexus to treat hydrocephalus in an infant duo.

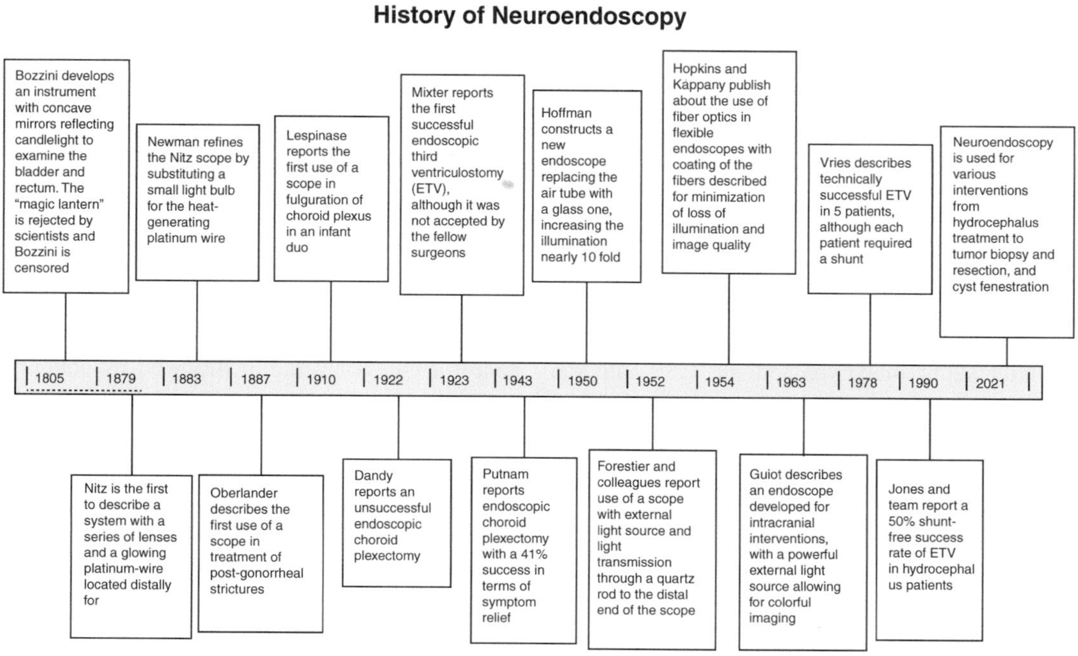

Fig. 2 Evolution of neuroendoscopy

While Lespinasse merely presented his work in a local gathering and did not publish it formally, in 1918, Walter Dandy published his technique of ventriculostomy and choroid plexus extirpation following his understanding of CSF dynamics from his work with Kenneth Blackfan. Although his original technique was unpolished, it required the drainage of the entire volume of CSF before ligation and removal of the choroid plexus. Dandy published an update on the technique in 1922, where he described it as choroid plexectomy via cystoscopy through the lateral ventricles. Following that, in 1923 W. Jason Mixter published the first report of an endoscopic third ventriculostomy (ETV) with the use of a urethroscope in an infant with non-communicating hydrocephalus, although his contemporary colleagues did not highly regard his work and the limitations of his equipment did not abet his claims. Over a decade later, John Scarff at Columbia University performed the same procedure utilizing an improved endoscope with an opening tip, built-in electrocautery, and an irrigation system that maintained the patency of the ventricular system. He achieved significant symptom reduction in the patient initially until their rapid decline, and the autopsy exposed the necessity for a larger incision rather than a minor puncture at the floor of the third ventricle for a successful procedure.

The fifth and sixth decades of the twentieth century brought about a period of pause in neuroendoscopy, as shunting and microsurgery gained popularity for the same procedures with a significant procedure success rate and a low mortality rate [1]. In 1949, Frank Nulsen and Eugene Spitz successfully treated hydrocephalus via a rubber tubbing shunt that bypassed the CSF into the venous system. Following that, the advent of microsurgery in 1960 further pushed neuroendoscopy into the background. Microsurgery was equipped with the two factors absent in endoscopy, namely, the ability to work in deep brain structures without the concern for significant damage to brain tissue and having high magnification and ample illumination. Publications on neuroendoscopy were sparse during this time due to the prevalence of other more efficient techniques. Meanwhile, pioneering scientists worked on the development of components of the novel endoscope that would soon revive neuroendoscopy without the limitations of its predecessors. Holter Hopkins, a British optical physicist, invented variable refractive lenses, deducing that a glass rod with interspersed air lenses may allow for a greater field of vision and illumination (up to ten times that of its predecessor) as compared to the air rod with glass lenses of previous endoscopes. This rod-lens system forms the basis of the present-day rigid endoscope. In 1969, George Smith and Willian Boyle invented the charged-couple device as a component of the novel endoscope, which converted optical stimuli to electrical impulses allowing for image capturing with improved quality and further miniaturization of the technology. The device was perfect for use in low-illumination environments with high sensitivity to light. Finally, from the initial advent of fiber optics in the 1950s until their improvements in the 1970s, it allowed for the use of powerful light sources placed distally in the scope and transmitted efficiently to locations of interest without a loss of luminescence. With the components of enhanced resolution video capturing and significantly improved illumination and visual field magnitude via advanced optical systems, interest in neuroendoscopy was revived anew.

The first report of neuroendoscopy for AC fenestration was reported by Pierre-Kahn and his team in 1990 [21, 22]. The French Hospital Necker group of surgeons analyzed 20 cases of ACs treated in their institution between 1972 and 1988. The earlier cases utilized stereotactic guidance for cyst fenestration followed by shunting but later evolved to ventriculoscopy for the last four cases. The surgeons concluded that the procedure was a feasible alternative and advantageous in its ease of perforation with the coagulator and avoidance of requiring radiological equipment [21]. An increasing use of neuroendoscopic fenestration for AC was reported since then and onward to the 2010s.

4 Surgical Indications

Asymptomatic ACs are typically monitored for the development of symptoms and with serial imaging. Most long-term follow-up cases describe the lesion's stability, while a minority may show the development of new symptoms based on mass effect or hydrocephalus. Rarely, cyst rupture may occur spontaneously or due to trauma, resulting in a subdural hygroma or hemorrhage [15]. These new entities may be monitored over time without the need for immediate intervention.

Specific guidelines for surgical intervention for AC do not currently exist, although literature recommendations consider symptomatology and cyst location indicators for possible intervention. This practice is supported by the persistence of symptoms such as headache and seizures in many reported cases despite surgical intervention [3, 7]. ACs leading to hydrocephalus or intracranial hypertension are shown to derive the most significant benefit from intervention. At the same time, those with non-specific symptoms such as nausea, vomiting, headache, seizures, vertigo, developmental delay, and visual changes are reported to obtain minimal to no benefit from treatment. Therefore, current recommendations for surgical intervention in ACs are passive observation of asymptomatic cases and intervention only in the case of known intracranial hypertension or hydrocephalus, because radiological and clinical improvement shows no correlation in the other symptom instances [7, 13].

Gallasi criteria for middle cranial fossa ACs, described in Table 2, are used by many neurosurgeons to determine the need for surgical intervention for the largest category of ACs [11, 16]. Gallasi type II and III ACs are often selected for surgical intervention, whether symptomatic or not, due to the prophylactic measures against the risk for hemorrhage or hygroma formation in the event of cyst rupture [3]. Also, larger cysts are generally surgically managed due to the potential for mass effect on cerebrovascular structures should passive observation be selected.

Surgical options for ACs include microsurgical fenestration via craniotomy, shunting, and neuroendoscopy. While there is no current consensus on the ideal surgical method, increasing the use of neuroendoscopy is reported due to a high procedural success rate, less severe associated complications, and a lower complication and cyst recurrence rate. In contrast to a report of 240 cases in France in the pediatric population, microneurosurgical intervention showed longer event-free survival and fewer complications compared to neuroendoscopy. However, this was a single-center study with twice as many open procedures versus endoscopic interventions [4].

Cyst location is an essential factor in choosing surgical technique, where suprasellar, quadrigeminal, and posterior fossa cysts are reported to have significantly higher successful treatment rates via neuroendoscopy than those located over the cortical convexities and in the interhemispheric region [12]. While it has been reported that any of the three surgical techniques is efficacious in treating middle cranial fossa cysts, the endoscopic approach is recommended as the primary approach due to safety considerations, with the use of the other two being recommended only if symptoms persist [6]. Shunting is usually avoided due to the associated serious complications that include infection, CSF over-drainage, and shunt dependency [7].

Table 2 The Gallasi criteria for the middle cranial fossa AC

Type	Description
I	– Typically clinically silent – Localized to the anterior middle cranial fossa
II	– Symptomatic or asymptomatic – Extends towards the Sylvian fissure, displacing the temporal lobe
III	– Typically symptomatic – Occupying the entire middle cranial fossa, displacing temporal lobe and impinging on frontal and parietal structures

5 Surgical Technique

AC surgery intends to decompress the cyst by fenestration of the cyst into the normal cerebrospinal fluid spaces, removing the cyst wall, aspiration of the cyst, or via shunting. Open or endoscopic approaches can accomplish fenestration or cyst excision. Fenestration into normal CSF spaces, such as subarachnoid cisterns, ventricles, or both, is possible. Endoscopic treatment alone confers a minimally invasive approach [18, 20].

All procedures are performed under general anesthesia, along with preoperative antibiotic prophylaxis. Rigid head fixation is usually performed, and frameless stereotaxy assists in planning the craniotomy location [13]. Prior to incision, the trajectory for endoscope insertion is often determined to minimize cortical or intraventricular damage and to allow for the most direct and linear access to the cyst-cisternal interface of interest. Keeping these two goals in mind, a small incision with a small craniotomy, commonly a burr-hole craniotomy, can be accomplished [20]. After durotomy/corticectomy, a Cottonoid or fibrin glue can be used to limit the loss of CSF or cyst fluid.

Generally, a multichannel rigid or flexible endoscope is utilized. Commonly, Gaab 5.4 mm or Aesculap 6.4 mm, four-channel neuroendoscopes [17], or the Oi-Handi 4.4 mm three-lumen endoscope are used. Navigation may assist with the insertion of the working endoscopic sheath that can be registered to the frameless system. A standard digital camera is used. An endoscopic holder can also be used. Continuous irrigation allows for clear visualization of the cyst membrane and brain surfaces through the camera, as well as hemostasis. A continuous purge of this irrigation fluid prevents over-insufflation of the intracranial and cystic compartments and the inadvertent elevation in intracranial pressure. Figure 2a demonstrates a preoperative MRI of a complex intraventricular AC treated with endoscopic fenestration. Visualization of the AC lining can be seen in Fig. 2b, where fenestration through the lining of the septum pellucidum was performed once the AC was fenestrated.

Fenestration of a cyst first begins after the proper inspection of all surrounding structures and careful inspection of the cyst surface. The cyst can be opened using bipolar coagulation, forceps, and micro scissors. Figures 3 and 4 demonstrate the use of forceps to allow fenestration of a pontine AC and blunt fenestration for a precerebellar AC. Following cyst fenestration, the opening is typically further enlarged using a number of techniques, such as balloon dilation, forceps separation, or division with the scissors. Irrigation is discontinued, and visualization of the anticipated flow of CSF pulsations can be seen with each cardiac cycle. The perforation was inspected for incidental damage, and hemostasis can be achieved via an embolectomy catheter, bipolar cauterization, or irrigation.

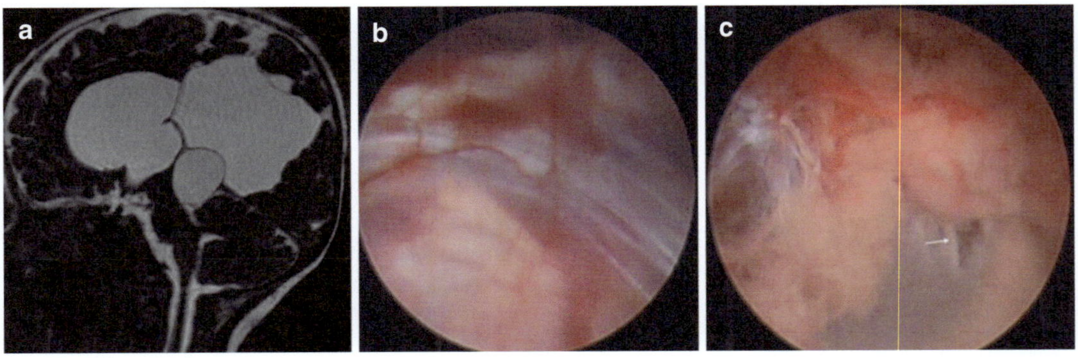

Fig. 3 Pineal region AC. (**a**) Sagittal T2 steady-state magnetic resonance imaging sequence demonstrating enlargement of the ventricular system, with pineal region cyst present. (**b**) AC lining seen via endoscope. (**c**) AC lining perforation after the use of forceps instrumentation

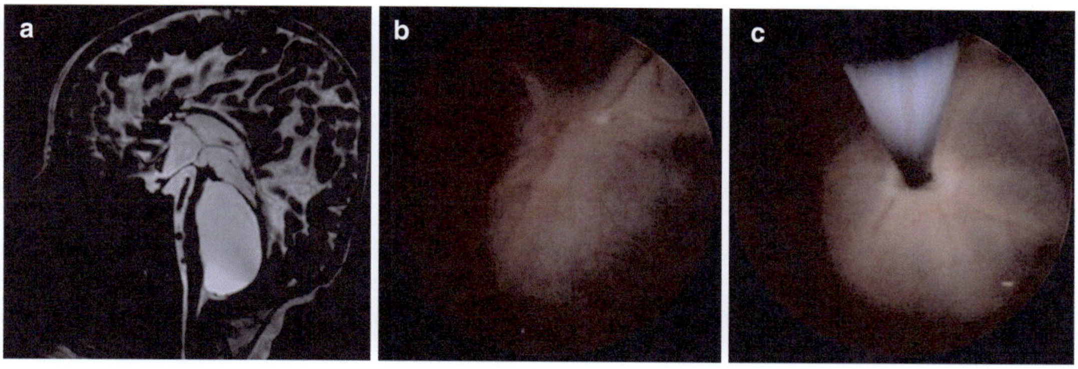

Fig. 4 Posterior fossa precerebellar cyst. (**a**) Sagittal T2 steady-state magnetic resonance imaging sequence demonstrating large precerebellar cyst with bowing and thinning of the brain stem, mass effect on the cerebellum. (**b**) AC lining visualized through endoscope. (**c**) AC lining fenestration being performed with blunt instrumentation

The four most frequent endoscopic surgical procedures are described [20]. In the cystocisternostomy technique, the AC is first entered beneath the burr hole, and the basal cisterns are approached through the body of the cyst. The thickened arachnoid membranes must be reliably opened around key structures, such as the optic nerve, carotid artery, and third nerve. The second most often described case is ventriculocystostomy, in which the cyst is approached through the ventricle. The key component of this procedure is to penetrate the thick and resistant cystic arachnoid membrane from the ventricular side. Suprasellar, quadrigeminal, and Sylvian cysts have all been approached via this technique.

In the cystoventriculostomy approach, attention must be directed to reduce AC fluid in order to avoid brain shift that can affect the stoma that must be created through the brain tissue into the ventricular side. Suprasellar, quadrigeminal, Sylvian, and even interhemispheric cysts have all been approached via this technique. Ventriculocystocisternostomy is like ventriculocystostomy, but in addition to creating a stoma in the arachnoid membrane on the ventricular side, an opening into the basal cisterns is made. This technique is commonly applied to suprasellar-located cysts. Copley et al. described their success rates over their 12-year cohort. They saw an improved result in their cohort in which a ventriculocystocisternostomy was performed in addition to cisternostomy alone [8].

Care must be taken when removing the cyst because adherence to the surrounding neurovascular structures is common. Removal of the cyst wall or fenestration into the cyst will direct the surgeon into normal subarachnoid spaces, where critical neurovascular structures are located. For example, the cisternal opening of the middle cranial fossa or temporobasal ACs will be located near the optic-carotid recess. In suprasellar cysts, the prepontine recess, the basilar artery, or abducens nerves will be close by, and the pituitary gland and stalk are also at risk [30].

The location of cysts will result in different neurovascular structure considerations (Table 1). For example, temporobasal ACs will prompt the surgeon to monitor for third or fourth nerve palsies or even the development of diabetes insipidus. Proximity of the lower cranial nerves to the posterior circulation must be recognized when surgically managing posterior fossa cysts [18, 19].

6 Strengths and Limitations of Neuroendoscopy in Arachnoid Cyst

Neuroendoscopy is recommended as the primary method for surgical fenestration of ACs in the recent neurosurgical literature [18, 28]. The surgical technique is advantageous in its single burr-hole approach, minimally invasive nature, and direct access to the space-occupying lesions [16, 25, 32]. The convenience of the technique also allows for simultaneous cyst fenestration along with treatment of co-existing hydrocephalus, thus minimizing the need for additional invasive procedures. Neuroendoscopy is associated with a smaller volume of blood loss, decreased operative time length, and lower rate of cyst recurrence when compared to non-endoscopic methods. Also, a greater total resection rate of cysts has been reported, possibly due to better and more precise visualization through endoscopy of closed spaces and the various membranes that must be opened to allow for proper CSF flow and cyst drainage [9]. Clinical improvement has been reported in up to 60–100% of patients, with improved radiographic outcomes ranging from 50 to 100% [5, 6, 18]. Neuroendoscopic surgical treatment of ACs is also associated with less post-operative hydrocephalus, lower neurologic morbidity rates, shorter length of hospital stay, and earlier return to the workforce [32].

The risk of damage to neurovascular structures and brain parenchyma with alterations in instruments and optical equipment is also decreased once the endoscope is positioned. An especially appealing prospect of this technique is the less severe and more treatable nature of the associated complications, with the most common of which being meningitis, post-operative fever, subdural effusion or hematoma, and CSF leak (Table 3).

Table 3 Strengths and limitations of endoscopic approaches

Strengths	Limitations
Minimally invasive—smaller volume blood loss	Single-instrument space through working channel
Higher total cyst resection rate	Challenging visualization of large cysts due to significant distortion of the anatomy
Lower recurrence rate	Rapid reduction in visualization in the setting of a bleed
Simultaneous treatment of hydrocephalus, biopsy, excision, fenestration	Limited scope length (20 mm)
Greater illumination	Fish-eye distortion of the visual field

Post-operative fever and subdural fluid accumulation are the most commonly reported complications of AC neuroendoscopy. The fever is typically non-infectious, as determined from CSF analysis and culture, and likely results from intracerebroventricular rinsing during the surgery. Subdural fluid is monitored and is usually absorbed within 3 months without intervention [25]. Complication rates vary across studies, age ranges, and properties of the cyst in terms of size and location. However, they are reported to be lower in magnitude than those from non-endoscopic methods [16].

Technical limitations of neuroendoscopy in AC fenestration stem from the use of instruments only through the working channel, limiting the ways of manipulating the arachnoid membrane for opening. While microsurgical fenestration through craniotomy can utilize two instruments to pull the membrane with one hand and open it with the other, a single endoscopic instrument can achieve both tasks by the forceps pulling and opening the membrane simultaneously. To overcome this, a larger-diameter bone window can be created, and the use of a wider endoscope can allow for the passage of two instruments. However, both instruments are in the same axis of the working passage regardless, and the increased exposure eliminates the minimally invasive advantage of neuroendoscopy. Importantly, accurate positioning of the endoscope is difficult due to continuous cyst fluid release and resulting repositioning of brain tissue, despite the presence of neuronavigation. A minor limitation is the maximum 20 mm length of the endoscope, preventing access to deeper located cysts [25]. The use of a flexible endoscope and combined microsurgical techniques is alternative options to assist in managing these cysts.

Visibility is a significant issue associated with the endoscopic technique, and understanding the spatial orientation and accounting for the fish-eye point of view may be challenging. Large cysts may cause substantial distortion of the anatomy, and the light through the initial insertion of the endoscope can be insufficient to localize in the absence of a navigation system. While the cystic space may initially appear dark, deeper insertion can overcome this limitation sufficiently for surgical intervention. Also, using anatomical markers such as arteries, veins, cranial nerves, cisterns, and the Sylvian fissure can allow for timely localization. One significant and characteristic limitation of neuroendoscopy is a bleeding-associated rapid reduction in visualization, to the extent that the procedure may be abandoned for an alternative method [9]. To deal with such an issue in the case of bleeding, copious and patient irrigation with body temperature crystalloid solution is required to stop the bleeding and clear the cavity of residual hematomas.

7 Conclusion

The use of endoscopy for treating ACs is a dependable option in AC surgical management. Location and expertise are crucial factors, and the surgeon should be ready to convert the surgery into an open procedure if the endoscopic option is not anatomically or technically feasible.

References

1. Abbott R. History of neuroendoscopy. Neurosurg Clin N Am. 2004;15(1):1–7.
2. Abd-El-Barr MM, Cohen AR. The origin and evolution of neuroendoscopy. Childs Nerv Syst. 2013;29(5):727–37.
3. Al-Holou WN, Terman S, Kilburg C, Garton HJ, Muraszko KM, Maher CO. Prevalence and natural history of arachnoid cysts in adults. J Neurosurg. 2013;118(2):222–31.
4. Amelot A, Beccaria K, Blauwblomme T, Bourgeois M, Paternoster G, Cuny ML, et al. Microsurgical, endoscopic, and shunt management of pediatric temporosylvian arachnoid cysts: a comparative study. J Neurosurg Pediatr. 2019;23(6):749–57.
5. Azab WA, Almanabri M, Yosef W. Endoscopic treatment of middle fossa arachnoid cysts. Acta Neurochir. 2017;159(12):2313–7.
6. Chen Y, Fang HJ, Li ZF, Yu SY, Li CZ, Wu ZB, et al. Treatment of middle cranial fossa arachnoid cysts: a systematic review and meta-analysis. World Neurosurg. 2016;92:480–90.
7. Choi JW, Lee JY, Phi JH, Kim SK, Wang KC. Stricter indications are recommended for fenestration surgery in intracranial arachnoid cysts of children. Childs Nerv Syst. 2015;31(1):77–86.
8. Copley P, Kirkman MA, Thompson D, James G, Aquilina K. Endoscopic surgery for intraventricular arachnoid cysts in children: clinical presentation, radiological features, management, and outcomes over a 12-year period. Childs Nerv Syst. 2018;34(2):257–66.
9. Di Rocco F, Roujeau T, Puget S, Sainte-Rose C, Zerah M. Limits of endoscopic treatment of sylvian arachnoid cysts in children. Childs Nerv Syst. 2010;26(2):155–62.
10. Dyck P, Gruskin P. Supratentorial arachnoid cysts in adults. A discussion of two cases from a pathophysiologic and surgical perspective. Arch Neurol. 1977;34(5):276–9.
11. Galassi E, Tognetti F, Gaist G, Fagioli L, Frank F, Frank G. CT scan and metrizamide CT cisternography in arachnoid cysts of the middle cranial fossa: classification and pathophysiological aspects. Surg Neurol. 1982;17(5):363–9.
12. Gangemi M, Maiuri F, Donati P, Sigona L, Iaconetta G, De Divitiis E, Neuroendoscopy. Personal experience, indications and limits. J Neurosurg Sci. 1998;42(1):1–10.
13. Greenfield JP, Souweidane MM. Endoscopic management of intracranial cysts. Neurosurg Focus. 2005;19(6):E7.
14. Halani SH, Safain MG, Heilman CB. Arachnoid cyst slit valves: the mechanism for arachnoid cyst enlargement. J Neurosurg Pediatr. 2013;12(1):62–6.
15. Hall S, Smedley A, Sparrow O, Mathad N, Waters R, Chakraborty A, et al. Natural history of intracranial arachnoid cysts. World Neurosurg. 2019;126:e1315–20.
16. Mustansir F, Bashir S, Darbar A. Management of arachnoid cysts: a comprehensive review. Cureus. 2018;10(4):e2458.
17. Nowoslawska E, Polis L, Kaniewska D, Mikolajczyk W, Krawczyk J, Szymanski W, et al. Neuroendoscopic techniques in the treatment of arachnoid cysts in children and comparison with other operative methods. Childs Nerv Syst. 2006;22(6):599–604.
18. Oertel J, Linsler S, Wagner W, Gaab M, Schroeder H, Rediker J. Endoscopic treatment of intracranial arachnoid cysts: a retrospective analysis of a 25-year experience. Oper Neurosurg. 2020;20(1):32–44.
19. Oertel JM, Baldauf J, Schroeder HW, Gaab MR. Endoscopic cystoventriculostomy for treatment of paraxial arachnoid cysts. J Neurosurg. 2009;110(4):792–9.
20. Oertel JM, Wagner W, Mondorf Y, Baldauf J, Schroeder HW, Gaab MR. Endoscopic treatment of arachnoid cysts: a detailed account of surgical techniques and results. Neurosurgery. 2010;67(3):824–36.
21. Pierre-Kahn A, Capelle L, Brauner R, Sainte-Rose C, Renier D, Rappaport R, et al. Presentation and management of suprasellar arachnoid cysts. Review of 20 cases. J Neurosurg. 1990;73(3):355–9.

22. Pierre-Kahn A, Capelle L, Sainte-Rose C, Renier D, Hoppe-Hirsch E, Hirsch JF. Treatment of suprasellar arachnoid cysts by percutaneous transfrontal ventriculocystostomy. Apropos of a series of 17 cases. Neurochirurgie. 1990;36(6):370–7.
23. Pradilla G, Jallo G. Arachnoid cysts: case series and review of the literature. Neurosurg Focus. 2007;22(2):E7.
24. Proimos E, Chimona T, Memtsas Z, Papadakis C. Middle fossa arachnoid cysts and inner ear symptoms: are they related? Hippokratia. 2014;18(2):168–71.
25. Qin B, Gao L, Hu J, Wang L, Chen G. Intracerebral hematoma after endoscopic fenestration of an arachnoid cyst: a case report. Medicine. 2018;97(44):e13106.
26. Rengachary SS, Watanabe I. Ultrastructure and pathogenesis of intracranial arachnoid cysts. J Neuropathol Exp Neurol. 1981;40(1):61–83.
27. Santamarta D, Aguas J, Ferrer E. The natural history of arachnoid cysts: endoscopic and cine-mode MRI evidence of a slit-valve mechanism. Minim Invasive Neurosurg. 1995;38(4):133–7.
28. Schulz M, Oezkan Y, Schaumann A, Sieg M, Tietze A, Thomale UW. Surgical management of intracranial arachnoid cysts in pediatric patients: radiological and clinical outcome. J Neurosurg Pediatr. 2021;2021:1–11.
29. Valluru B, Raj R. Images in clinical medicine. Arachnoid cyst. N Engl J Med. 2015;373(11):e13.
30. Wang JC, Heier L, Souweidane MM. Advances in the endoscopic management of suprasellar arachnoid cysts in children. J Neurosurg. 2004;100(5):418–26.
31. Wang X, Chen JX, You C, Jiang S. CT cisternography in intracranial symptomatic arachnoid cysts: classification and treatment. J Neurol Sci. 2012;318(1-2):125–30.
32. Zhao P, Wang X, Li C, Gui S, Zong X, Zhang Y. The effectiveness of neuroendoscopic versus non-neuroendoscopic procedures in the treatment of lateral ventricular cysts: a retrospective medical record review study. BMC Neurol. 2013;13:59.

Surgical Management of Spinal Arachnoid Cysts

Ali Akhaddar and Mohamed Boucetta

1 Introduction

The occurrence of spinal arachnoid cysts (ACs) is much lower than that of intracranial ACs. In the spine, ACs can be extradural (Figs. 1 and 2), intradural extramedullary (Fig. 3), perineural (Figs. 4 and 5), or more rarely within the spinal cord. The most common site is in the middle/lower thoracic spine with limited vertebral segments being involved [3, 12, 18, 47]. Spinal ACs are extra-axial and surrounded by arachnoid membranes that may or may not communicate with the subarachnoid space. These cysts are benign, and most are congenital in origin, although a small group may arise following inflammation, infection, bleeding, trauma, or even surgery. Less common locations of intraspinal ACs are in the lumbar and lumbosacral, thoracolumbar, and sacral spine. The cervical spine is rarely involved [47, 49–51]. The vast majority of cysts are typically limited to three or four vertebral body levels craniocaudally and therefore restricted to a single spinal segment or the junction between two spinal segments [5, 18]. However, extensive cysts involving multiple segments of the spinal axis have also been reported [17, 25, 53]. Clinical presentations are highly variable and depend primarily on the anatomic location, cyst volume, duration of symptoms, and the patient's age. Some patients manifest simple rachialgia, while others present with complete paraplegia/quadriplegia [46, 52, 55, 68]. With the extensive usage of spinal magnetic resonance imaging (MRI) techniques, many incidental asymptomatic cysts are being discovered in all age groups. Although many authors recommend no treatment for small or asymptomatic cysts, there is still some debate regarding the best treatment strategy for symptomatic lesions.

Once the surgical indication is determined, the management of intraspinal ACs consists of surgical exploration and decompression via total/partial cyst excision, marsupialization, fenestration, ligation of the communication site, shunting, or a combination of these techniques [3, 10, 35, 51].

The indications for and performance of surgery for the various forms of intraspinal ACs are presented in this chapter that deals primarily with the current techniques applied in the surgical management of intraspinal cystic lesions. At the end of this chapter, there is a section addressing postoperative complications.

A. Akhaddar (✉)
Department of Neurosurgery, Avicenne Military Hospital of Marrakech, Mohammed V University in Rabat, Rabat, Morocco

M. Boucetta
Department of Neurosurgery, Avicenne Military Hospital of Marrakech, Mohammed V University in Rabat, Rabat, Morocco

Department of Neurosurgery, Mohammed V University in Rabat, Rabat, Morocco

M. Turgut et al. (eds.), *Arachnoid Cysts*, https://doi.org/10.1007/978-3-031-22701-1_29

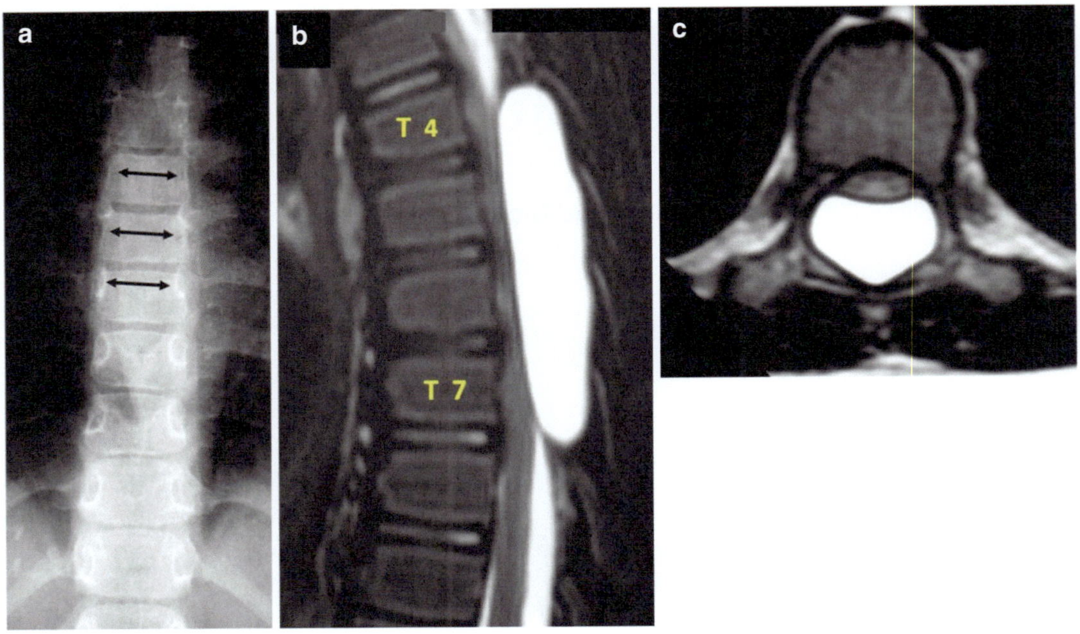

Fig. 1 T4–T7 spinal extradural AC with posterior spinal cord compression in an 8-year-old boy. Enlarged spinal canal (double arrows) on anteroposterior spinal thoracic radiogram (**a**). Sagittal (**b**) and axial T2-weighted magnetic resonance imaging (MRI) (**c**)

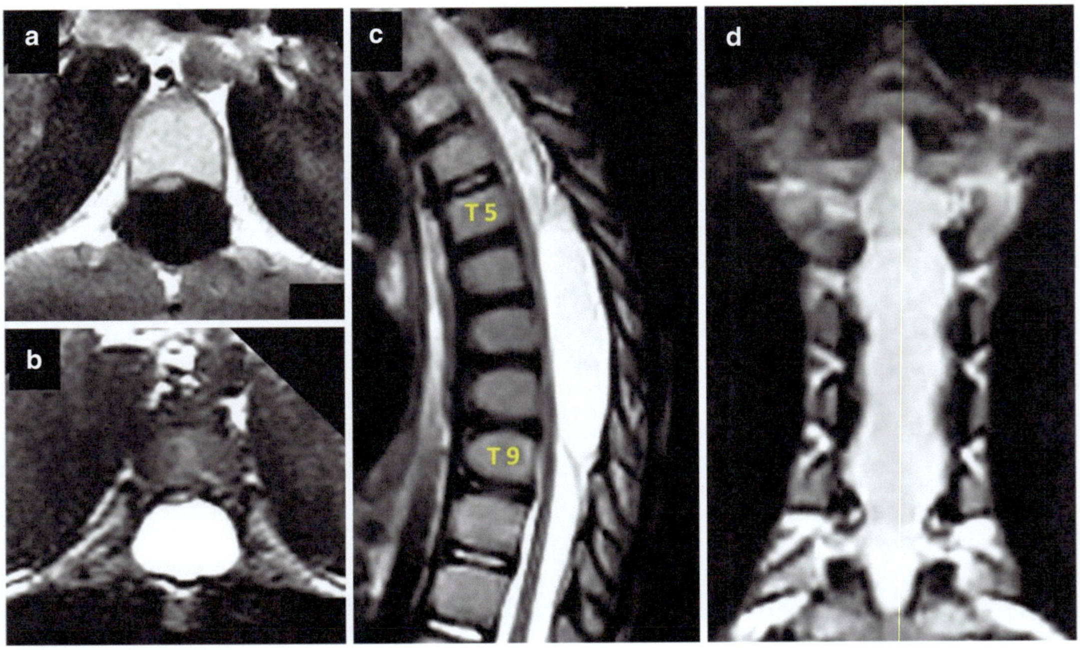

Fig. 2 T5–T9 spinal extradural AC located posterior to the spinal cord in an 11-year-old girl. Axial T1-weighted (**a**) and T2-weighted (**b**) MRI, sagittal (**c**) and coronal T2-weighted images (**d**)

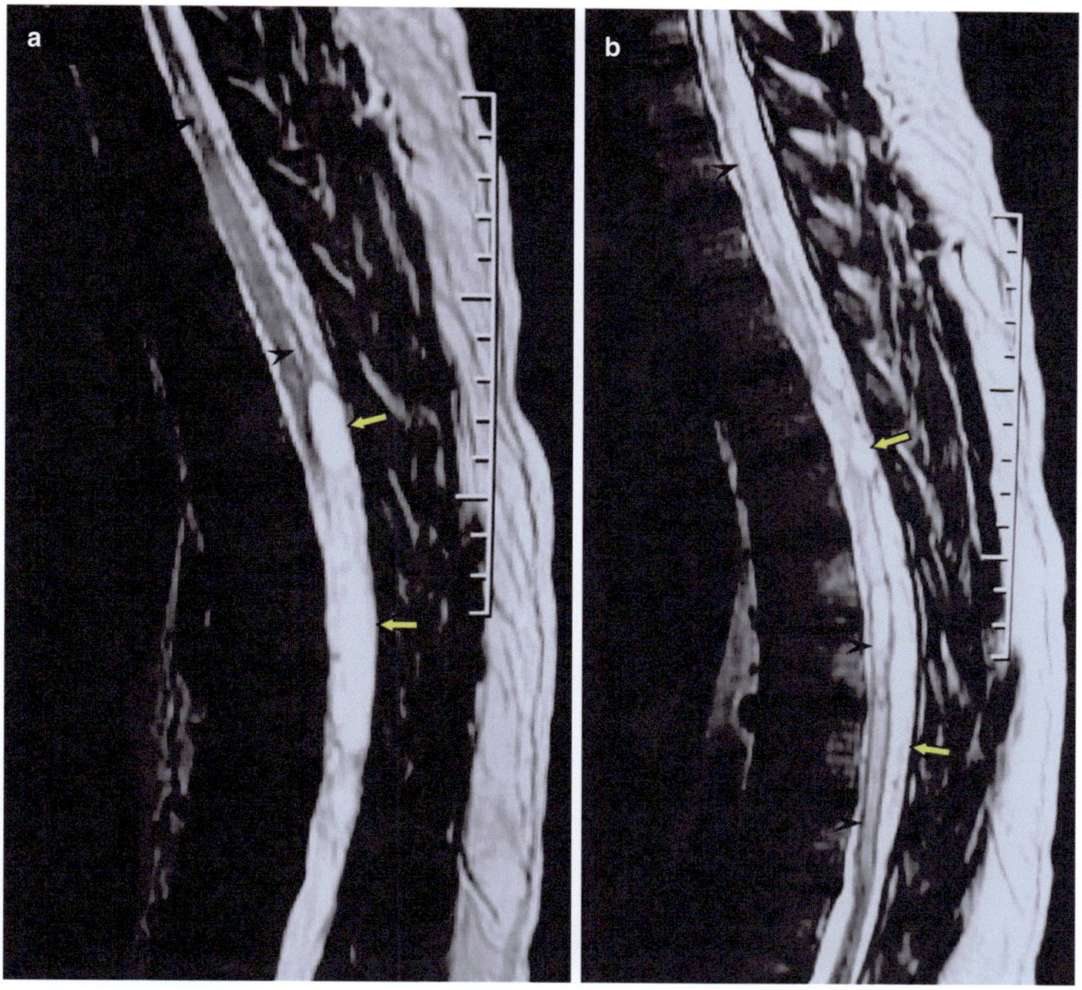

Fig. 3 Spinal tuberculous arachnoiditis in a 38-year-old man with a history of tuberculous meningitis 2 years previously. Sagittal T2-weighted MRI (**a**, **b**) showing multiloculated cystic lesions surrounding the thoracic spinal cord (arrows). Note the high signal within the spinal cord (head arrows). Changes of arachnoiditis may be focal, multifocal, or diffuse (Reproduced from Akhaddar A. (2017) Spinal Tuberculosis. In: Atlas of Infections in Neurosurgery and Spinal Surgery. Springer, Cham. https://doi.org/10.1007/978-3-319-60086-4_24; with permission)

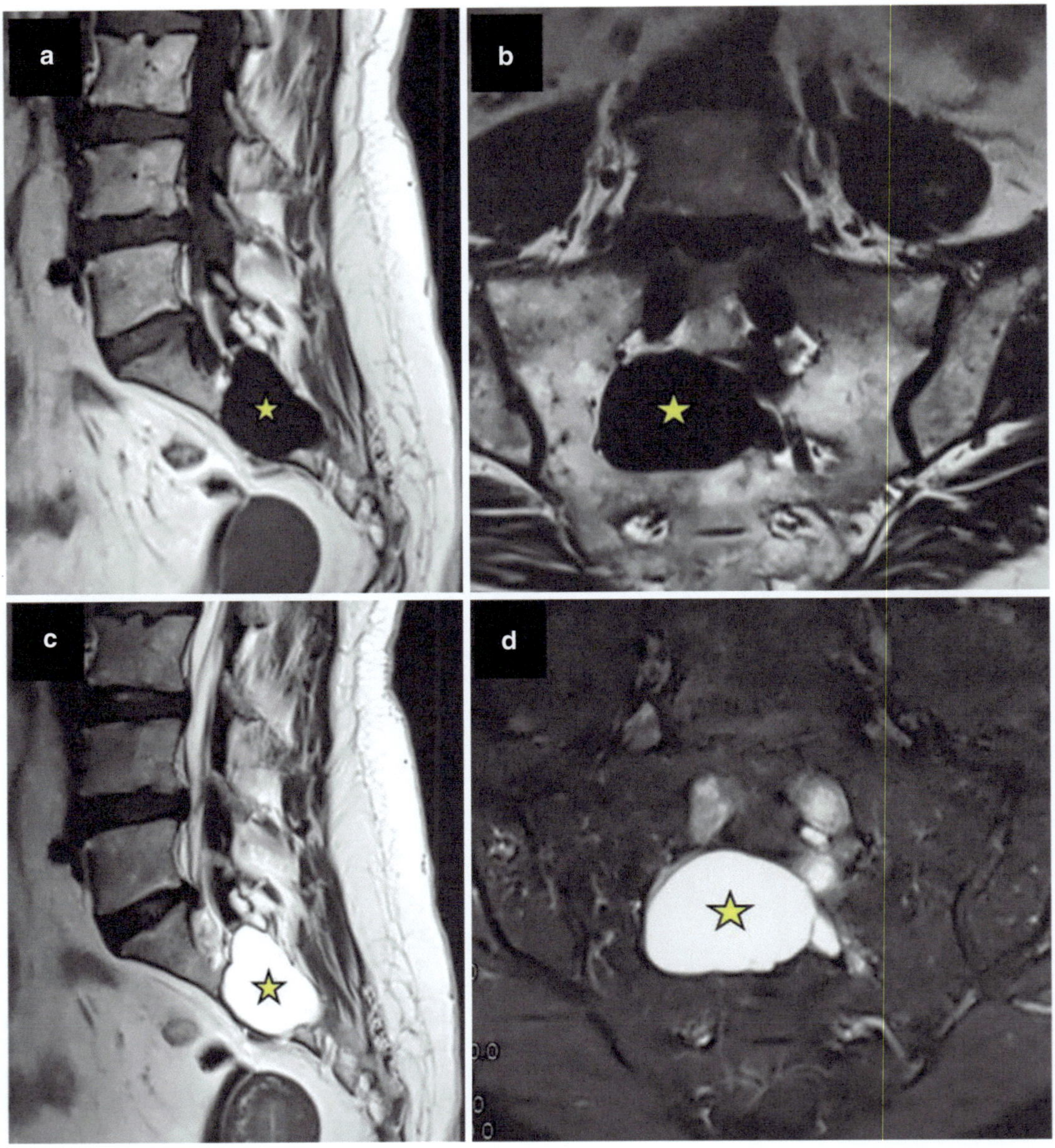

Fig. 4 S2 Tarlov cyst in an adult (stars). Sagittal (**a**) and coronal (**b**) T1-weighted MRI. Sagittal T2-weighted image (**c**) and coronal MRI on FLAIR sequence (**d**)

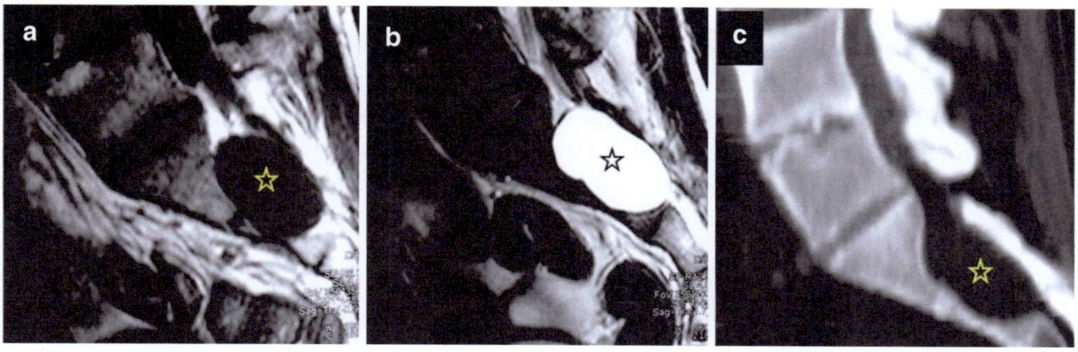

Fig. 5 S1–S2 Tarlov cyst in an adult (stars). Sagittal T1-weighted (**a**) and T2-weighted (**b**) MRI. Sagittal spinal computed tomography (CT) scan on bone window (**c**)

2 Patient Selection and Preoperative Evaluation

Prior to any successful treatment, the initial diagnosis of spinal ACs should be suspected and confirmed promptly. The clinical presentation and neuroimaging evaluation are essential factors that enhance our ability to determine the best therapeutic plan for each case. Furthermore, various cystic spinal lesions may mimic ACs. Chapter "Differential Diagnosis of Intraspinal Arachnoid Cysts" of the current book provides a review of the main differential diagnosis of intraspinal ACs. MRI is now the primary imaging modality of choice that may indicate the exact topography of the cysts and their inner structures, define the exact margins of the collections, and determine the relationship of the cysts with contiguous anatomic structures as well as any communication between the cyst and adjacent subarachnoid spaces (Figs. 1, 2, 3, and 4).

Many authors recommend not treating asymptomatic ACs that cause no pain or neurological symptoms/signs that are without mass effect, regardless of their size and spinal location. However, no clear association exists between the volume of an AC and the need for surgical excision. Consequently, "asymptomatic" patients may require an MRI each year to detect any cystic progression or new anomaly. However, if they become "symptomatic," patients should be reevaluated, without delay, clinically, and by MRI.

Surgery is the treatment of choice for symptomatic patients, especially those with intractable pain, if neurological signs/symptoms progress secondary to nerve root or spinal cord compression or if the patient presents with spinal instability or cyst extension [51].

3 Surgical Principles

ACs are rare pockets of the arachnoid membrane that were first described intracranially by Bright in 1842 [6]. One decade later, the French physician and physiologist François Magendie (1783–1855) published the earliest observation of an intraspinal AC in 1842 [31]. The initial record of spinal intradural cysts compressing the spinal cord and being successfully treated by surgery was reported by Spiller in 1903 [58] followed by Skoog in 1915 [56].

The key aim of the surgery for spinal ACs should be neurologic decompression and prevention of cyst recurrence. These goals will be achieved by total resection of the cyst wall and closure of the communication between the cyst and the subarachnoid space. In surgical practice, however, this is not always possible primarily because some cyst walls adhere to varying degrees to neurologic structures and secondly because other ACs are situated anteriorly or antero-laterally to the spinal cord. In addition, some cysts may be multiple, very extensive, and/or have multiple septations [3, 5, 12, 14, 18].

For the traditional posterior approach, the operation is performed under general anesthesia with the patient in the prone position. A bladder catheter is placed, and good venous access is ensured. Some authors believe that the use of electrophysiologic monitoring for somatosensory/motor-evoked potentials and anal electromyography may improve the safety of the procedure by alerting the surgeon to unintentional excessive traction/dissection/manipulation that may occur during surgery [12, 14, 36, 60, 66]. Preoperative radiological localization or intraoperative fluoroscopy is used to identify the correct vertebral level for surgery [16, 36]. After a posterior midline skin incision is made, the muscle and ligaments are separated from the spinous processes, lamina, and facet complexes. The laminectomy/laminotomy is carried out that includes one vertebral level above and below the position of the cyst. In most cases, a total bilateral laminectomy was performed. However, this relatively invasive surgery may result in postoperative subluxation or kyphosis, especially in the cervical or thoracic spinal areas. To prevent these postoperative problems, the length of laminectomy should be kept to a minimum (less than five segments) [44]. For Lee et al., a minimal skipped hemilaminectomy was a feasible technique for the treatment of large intraspinal ACs [27]. In recent years, many surgeons have favored the laminoplasty technique in order to decrease the chance of postoperative kyphosis [12, 18, 36].

More anterior ventral ACs may require extension of the surgical approach by drilling the inner part of the adjacent facet joints [14]. When the stability of the spine is lessened, surgical stabilization with osteosynthesis/fusion is required. Some ventrally situated cervical ACs may be excised through a conventional anterior cervical approach with corpectomy and spinal reconstruction [10, 37, 54, 59].

The surgeon should attempt to remove ACs completely but without causing additional injury. Furthermore, in cases with many adhesions and multiple septations, especially in those spinal AC secondary to trauma, inflammation, infection, or bleeding, partial resection as widely as possible is sometimes indicated [9]. In some anterior or extensive intraspinal ACs, other alternative surgical techniques can be used such as stenting, cystic shunting, or simple percutaneous needle aspiration [35, 40, 44, 57, 62].

For intradural spinal ACs, some authors suggest placing a small silastic shunt into the cyst cavity to drain into the subarachnoid CSF space [66]. The distal end of this catheter was then sutured to the pia mater and positioned in a site far removed from the nerve roots.

Sometimes, additional shunting may be required if the cyst fails to resolve after marsupialization/fenestration or even partial resection. These cystic diversions were previously reported into the peritoneal cavity, pleural cavity, or the atrium of the heart [2, 24, 32, 40, 42]. In addition, Rabb et al. recommended using a dural patch graft consolidated by fibrin glue before considering permanent shunt insertion, especially in patients with a large dural defect [48].

At the end of the surgery, the dura is closed in a continuous manner, and the suture line is reinforced with fibrin glue or a tissue dural patch. A Valsalva maneuver should be performed to verify the integrity of the impermeable dural closure. The wound is then closed in layers. All of these precautions were undertaken in order to avoid a postoperative CSF fistula and pseudomeningocele.

In child and adolescents, a hyperextension brace is recommended for several weeks if an extensive conventional laminectomy was required.

4 Surgical Therapy for Extradural Arachnoid Cysts

Extradural ACs will be apparent as soon as the posterior vertebral elements are removed via laminectomy or laminotomy (Figs. 2 and 6). Using the operative microscope, the cyst wall can be carefully dissected from the thecal sac until a small pedicle through a dural defect is identified, usually on the dorsal aspect of the junction with a nerve root (Fig. 7). The pedicle (also known as the cervix or ostium through which the cyst com-

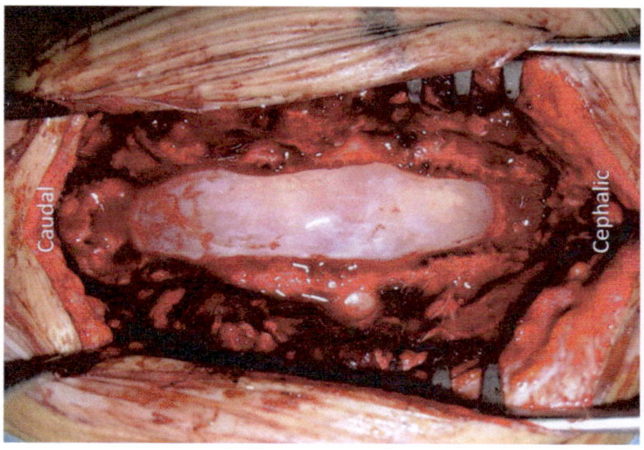

Fig. 6 Operative view following laminectomy showing the T5–T9 extradural ACs located posterior to the thecal sac

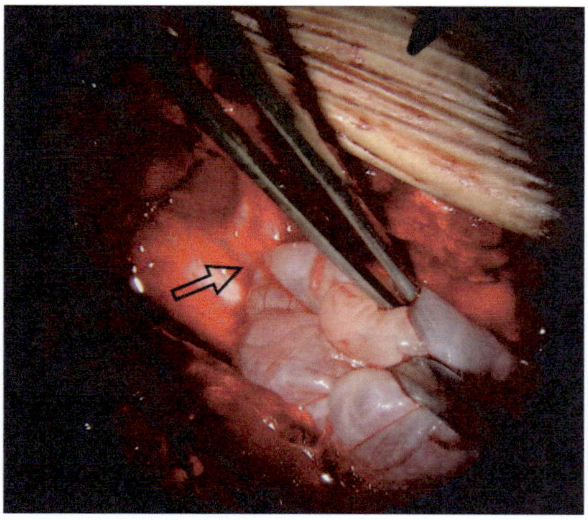

Fig. 7 Operative view under the operative microscope showing a small pedicle through a dural defect (arrow) on the dorsal aspect of the junction with a nerve root

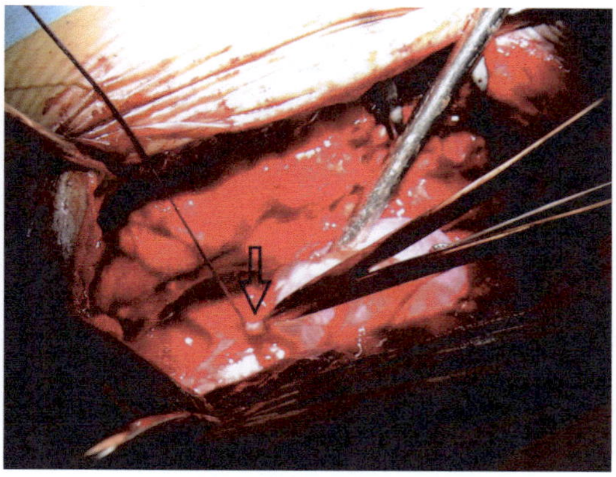

Fig. 8 Operative view under the operative microscope: the small pedicle (cervix or ostium through which the cyst communicates with the intradural space) was ligated (arrow)

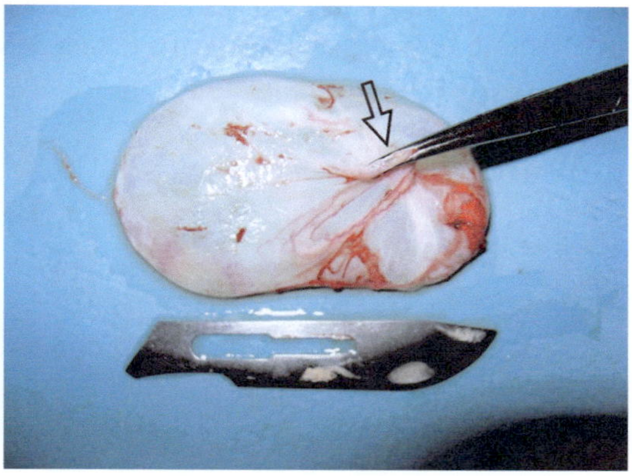

Fig. 9 The extradural AC was completely removed after cutting the small communicating pedicle (arrow)

municates with the intradural space) will be ligated, transected, and the cyst removed (Figs. 8 and 9). Then, the dural defect can usually be sutured closed and reinforced with fibrin glue to prevent CSF leakage [29]. If the AC does not communicate with the subarachnoid space, a complete excision can be performed without a subsequent repair or the obliteration of the dural communicating pedicle [30].

Sometimes, the nervous tissue may be found within the cysts. In this situation, the cyst could be removed, but the nerve roots should be preserved. Consequently, a duraplasty will be necessary [26].

For lumbar lateralized extradural ACs, Ido et al. recommended using a trans-foraminal approach that seems to be more useful and effective than a traditional laminectomy/laminotomy because it can offer a more adequate visual field with better visualization with less risk of spine destabilization [22].

In cases of extradural spinal ACs that have both intraspinal and extraspinal components, the cyst should be removed through the enlarged intervertebral foramina. Extraspinal components are relatively easy to remove. Also, the resection of the intraspinal component is similar to the technique used for isolated extradural cysts [9]. In the event of spine instability, surgical stabilization with osteosynthesis may be needed.

5 Surgical Therapy for Intradural Extramedullary Arachnoid Cysts

Intradural ACs are generally apparent on opening the dura mater via posterior midline durotomy (Figs. 3 and 10). Intraoperative ultrasonography may assist with the localization of intradural cysts, assessing their morphology and evaluating the cyst dimensions [14, 36]. Using the surgical microscope, the complete or partial drainage of large cysts may help facilitate resection of the thick cyst wall. Also, some authors stress the need to perform a cystic fenestration into the subarachnoid space before cystic wall excision [66]. A combination of sharp and blunt microsurgical dissection should be used to carefully separate the cyst wall from the adjacent neural tissues and blood vessels. Also, the arachnoid wall that is adherent to the dura may need a more aggressive resection to prevent any recurrence (Fig. 10). For Wang et al., gentle dissection of any arachnoid adhesions around the spinal cord parenchyma should also be performed in order to release the spinal cord [66].

In cases with monocompartimental spinal intradural cysts without intracystic septations (especially for idiopathic cysts), Schmutzer et al. recommend performing only a unilateral monosegmental approach followed by an excision of the upper pole of the cyst wall in order to create a stoma into the subarachnoid space [51]. When a bilateral approach is needed, laminoplasty seems to be an alternative to laminectomy, particularly for patients with multisegmental cervicothoracic cysts. Multiple laminectomies can compromise spinal alignment and stability [43, 69].

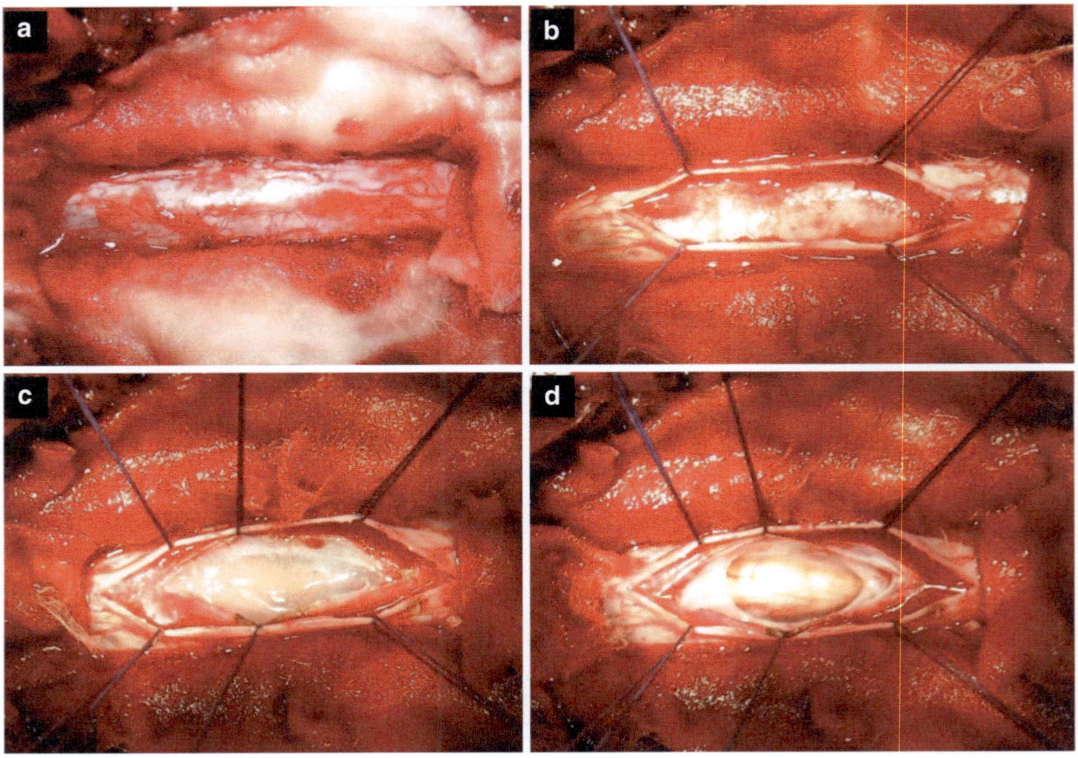

Fig. 10 Intraoperative views after limited posterior thoracic laminectomy (**a**–**d**). The dura mater was opened (**b**). Note the important adhesive and arachnoid thickening with fibrosis (a web-like appearance) (**c**). Spinal cord appearance following gentle arachnoid dissection (**d**) (Reproduced from Akhaddar A. (2017) Spinal Tuberculosis. In: Atlas of Infections in Neurosurgery and Spinal Surgery. Springer, Cham. https://doi.org/10.1007/978-3-319-60086-4_24; with permission)

In order to avoid neurological damage from excision of an adherent cyst wall, the surgeon should consider alternative options. When cysts cannot be completely resected, wide fenestration or marsupialization of the cyst wall should be performed. In this same situation, some authors suggest using additional cyst diversion or shunting (see below). Simple aspiration of the cyst contents provides only a temporary solution.

Occasionally, a dural patch was used to repair the dura defect and/or to allow more space for the spinal cord [16]. Indeed, duraplasty increases the dimensions of the intradural space to avoid spinal cord tethering [36].

Concerning an associated syringomyelia, Schmutzer et al. noticed a total disappearance of the intramedullary syrinx in 7 of 14 thoracic cases after surgical resection or fenestration of the intradural spinal ACs [51].

6 Surgical Therapy for Intramedullary Arachnoid Cysts

Intramedullary spinal ACs are rare; only 18 cases have been reported previously and surgically treated [1, 21, 34, 39, 64]. Marsupialization of the cyst was achieved in 11 cases and removal of the cyst wall in 7 patients. The cyst wall was entirely excised in only 1 patient out of 18 [19]. The majority of cases underwent a classic dorsomedial myelotomy. A DREZ (dorsal root entry zone) myelotomy was performed in only two patients [20]. This last procedure would allow for better circulation of CSF between the residual cystic cavity and the subarachnoid space in addition to reducing the chance of spinal cord injury and scar fibrosis [39]. None of the 18 patients required a shunting procedure; however, recurrence was reported in one case [21]. In this 4-year-old boy, the cystic cavity increased in size, and the symptoms recurred 27 months after the first cystic fenestration. To prevent the recurrence of the cyst, Sun suggested that the residual cyst wall should be sutured to the pia mater to ensure adequate communication between the cyst cavity and the subarachnoid compartment [60]. On occasion, a wall biopsy may be necessary to exclude a secondary lesion.

7 Surgical Therapy for Tarlov Cysts

Sacral extradural spinal meningeal/perineural cysts, also known as Tarlov cysts [63], can be managed in the same manner (Figs. 4 and 5). However, if nerve root fibers are found within the cystic cavity, the cyst wall could be removed, but the nerve roots should be preserved. Consequently, a duraplasty will be required to reconstruct the nerve root sheath [15, 26]. Also, Neulen et al. considered that microsurgical fenestration between perineural cysts and the thecal sac at the level of the distal dural sleeve was a safe surgical approach for the treatment of symptomatic Tarlov cysts [38]. Other surgical techniques include cyst wall removal and filling of the remaining cavity with autologous muscle and fat in the lumbosacral canal [45, 61, 65] and titanium clipping [7]. Some small non-compressive epidural ACs could be treated simply by closing the pedicle between the cyst and the subarachnoid space without cyst resection [61]. More recently, authors report Tarlov cyst resection assisted with endoscopy (see below) [67].

8 Minimally Invasive Techniques

In order to reduce some surgical complications such as spinal cord injury, postoperative deficits, and kyphotic deformity, some authors promoted the use of the endoscope. Furthermore, this technique improves visualization of the cystic lesion.

Endo et al. advocated the use of endoscope in the management of six cases of intradural spinal ACs with the intention to reduce the size of the laminectomy. After restricted laminectomy/hemilaminectomy, the cyst wall was partially resected through the bone fenestration after which an endoscope was placed into the cyst cavity and moved in an up/down direction to fenestrate the cyst wall. This last maneuver allowed for the communication between the cyst fluid contents and the subarachnoid CSF space [11]. Also, using a flexible endoscope, Papadimitriou performed a cysto-peritoneal diversion of a T3–T10 spinal AC in a 79-year-old man [42].

Recently, Wang et al. reported their useful experience of endoscopic-assisted fenestration of a series of 15 patients with sacral Tarlov cysts [67]. After making a bone window in the lamina, the endoscope was advanced into the spinal canal to provide visibility. The excellent visualization allowed for easy distinction between the cyst wall and the nerve roots. The cyst wall was incompletely resected under endoscopic guidance, and the site of communication between the cyst cavity and the subarachnoid space was carefully identified.

CT scan-guided percutaneous aspiration is a well-known minimally invasive method used for perineural/Tarlov cysts in the lumbosacral region [15]. It is also considered an important prognostic procedure to help select cases where surgical treatment might be favorable [28]. In contrast, many authors believe that percutaneous needle aspiration is an inadequate procedure for treating intraspinal ACs because of the high rate of cyst recurrence [40, 44, 57]. However, this simple and quick method may be reserved for patients in poor general health status who are unable to endure a major spinal surgical procedure [4, 10]. For Takahashi et al., percutaneous drainage under MRI guidance was considered prior to a more invasive surgical approach [62].

9 Postoperative Complications

Despite the low rate of postoperative complications following surgery for spinal ACs [12, 13, 16, 18, 67], surgeons should know about these possible problems and clearly describe them to the patients and/or their family before surgery. Many alternatives exist for the management of these complications, but none of them can be thought of as a standard of care. When a repeat surgical procedure is contemplated, it should be considered in select patients based on a benefit-risk evaluation.

Postoperative wound infection (three cases reported) [14, 41, 51], poor wound healing [36], CSF leakage [25, 33], postoperative epidural hematoma (two cases) [36, 51], pseudomeningocele (two cases) [16, 36], and postoperative kyphosis [43, 69] are some important nonspecific complications of surgical treatment of intraspinal ACs.

There is no reported case of death except for Palmer's patient. This 3-year-old boy was operated on three times for an anterior intradural upper cervical AC. Postoperatively, the patient developed a wound infection with progressive tetraparesis and respiratory failure. He died 2 weeks following the third operation [41].

Recurrence and insufficient shrinkage of the cyst are important complications of the surgery for intraspinal ACs. Globally, the recurrence rate was less than 12.5% realizing that the highest incidence was seen in intradural forms. However, we must distinguish the relative low recurrence rate for intradural idiopathic cysts (12%) from that of post-hemorrhagic cysts (66%) [13, 36, 49, 51]. Indeed, a correlation analysis finds an important risk factor for revision involving post-hemorrhagic intradural ACs [51]. Consequently, cysts with multiple septations and those that evolved following bleeding must undergo whenever possible an extended cyst wall resection to decrease the risk of cyst recurrence.

Recurrent intraspinal ACs that cannot be completely resected following the first surgical procedure have subsequently been treated by cyst shunting [5, 8, 23].

10 Conclusion

Intraspinal ACs represent an unusual heterogeneous pathologic entity with various clinical presentations and neuroimaging appearances. Consequently, surgical management is more complex than previously thought. For symptomatic patients, complete surgical excision of the cyst is the treatment of choice. However, specific surgical goals are determined by the cyst subtype and its relationship with adjacent neural structures. In standard practice, extradural ACs are typically resected with closure of the dural defect, whereas intradural or anterior cysts are usually fenestrated. Cysts with associated nerve fibers should be managed carefully in order to preserve the neurologic function. Despite the fact that endoscopic techniques are less invasive and are correlated with less risk of complications, endoscopic procedures for spinal disorders require a significant learning phase before obtaining satisfactory results.

Finally, there is no standard protocol for the management of intraspinal ACs. However, when surgery is discussed, the surgeon should always consider his experience and institutional practice, the cyst's underlying etiology, clinical signs and symptoms, the patient's age and comorbid conditions, the cyst appearance and its exact location, the relationship between the cyst and contiguous anatomic structures as well as the communication between the cyst and adjacent subarachnoid spaces, and any congenital lesions that could be associated. Additionally, care and prudence must be taken perioperatively and during the surgical intervention to diminish postoperative adverse events that increase morbidity.

References

1. Alugolu R, Arradi V, Sahu BP. Intramedullary arachnoid cyst in an adult: case report and review. Asian J Neurosurg. 2016;11:70. https://doi.org/10.4103/1793-5482.145054.
2. Andrews BT, Weinstein PR, Rosenblum ML, Barbaro NM. Intradural arachnoid cysts of the spinal canal associated with intramedullary cysts. J Neurosurg. 1988;68:544–9. https://doi.org/10.3171/jns.1988.68.4.0544.
3. Baig Mirza A, Bartram J, Sinha S, Gebreyohanes A, Boardman T, Vastani A, et al. Surgical management and outcomes in spinal intradural arachnoid cysts: the experience from two tertiary neurosurgical centres. Acta Neurochir. 2021. https://doi.org/10.1007/s00701-021-05027-3.
4. Bellavia R, King JT Jr, Naheedy MH, Lewin JS. Percutaneous aspiration of an intradural/extradural thoracic arachnoid cyst: use of MR imaging guidance. J Vasc Interv Radiol. 2000;11:369–72. https://doi.org/10.1016/s1051-0443(07)61432-8.
5. Bond AE, Zada G, Bowen I, McComb JG, Krieger MD. Spinal arachnoid cysts in the pediatric population: report of 31 cases and a review of the literature. J Neurosurg Pediatr. 2012;9:432–41. https://doi.org/10.3171/2012.1.PEDS11391.
6. Bright R. Serous cysts in the arachnoid diseases of the brain and nervous system. In: Reports of medical cases selected with a view of illustrating the symptoms and cure of diseases by a reference to morbid anatomy. Part I, vol. 2. London: Longman; 1831. p. 437–9.
7. Cantore G, Bistazzoni S, Esposito V, Tola S, Lenzi J, Passacantilli E, et al. Sacral Tarlov cyst: surgical treatment by clipping. World Neurosurg. 2013;79:381–9. https://doi.org/10.1016/j.wneu.2012.06.015.
8. Carrillo R. Lumbar cerebrospinal fluid drainage for symptomatic sacral nerve root cysts: an adjuvant diagnostic procedure and/or alternative treatment? Technical case report. Neurosurgery. 1998;42:952–3. https://doi.org/10.1097/00006123-199804000-00162.
9. Chen Z, Sun XL, Zhao Y, Wang K, Jian FZ. Dural dissection cyst: a more accurate term for extradural meningeal cyst. CNS Neurosci Ther. 2014;20:515–20. https://doi.org/10.1111/cns.12246.
10. Cloward RB. Congenital spinal extradural cysts: case report with review of literature. Ann Surg. 1968;168:851–64. https://doi.org/10.1097/00000658-196811000-00011.
11. Endo T, Takahashi T, Jokura H, Tominaga T. Surgical treatment of spinal intradural arachnoid cysts using endoscopy. J Neurosurg Spine. 2010;12:641–6. https://doi.org/10.3171/2009.12.SPINE09577.
12. Eroglu U, Bozkurt M, Kahilogullari G, Dogan I, Ozgural O, Shah KJ, et al. Surgical management of spinal arachnoid cysts in adults. World Neurosurg. 2019;122:e1146–52. https://doi.org/10.1016/j.wneu.2018.11.005.
13. Evangelou P, Meixensberger J, Bernhard M, Hirsch W, Kiess W, Merkenschlager A, et al. Operative management of idiopathic spinal intradural arachnoid cysts in children: a systematic review. Childs Nerv Syst. 2013;29:657–64. https://doi.org/10.1007/s00381-012-1990-7.
14. Fam MD, Woodroffe RW, Helland L, Noeller J, Dahdaleh NS, Menezes AH, et al. Spinal arachnoid cysts in adults: diagnosis and management. A single-center experience. J Neurosurg Spine. 2018;29:711–9. https://doi.org/10.3171/2018.5.SPINE1820.
15. Fletcher-Sandersjöö A, Mirza S, Burström G, Pedersen K, Kuntze Söderqvist Å, Grane P, et al. Management of perineural (Tarlov) cysts: a population-based cohort study and algorithm for the selection of surgical candidates. Acta Neurochir.

2019;161:1909–15. https://doi.org/10.1007/s00701-019-04000-5.
16. French H, Somasundaram A, Biggs M, Parkinson J, Allan R, Ball J, et al. Idiopathic intradural dorsal thoracic arachnoid cysts: a case series and review of the literature. J Clin Neurosci. 2017;40:147–52. https://doi.org/10.1016/j.jocn.2017.02.051.
17. Fukumoto H, Samura K, Katsuta T, Miki K, Fukuda K, Inoue T. Extensive multilocular spinal extradural meningeal cyst that developed 16 years after traumatic brachial plexus injury: a case report. World Neurosurg. 2016;86:510. https://doi.org/10.1016/j.wneu.2015.10.027.
18. Garg K, Borkar SA, Kale SS, Sharma BS. Spinal arachnoid cysts - our experience and review of literature. Br J Neurosurg. 2017;31:172–8. https://doi.org/10.1080/02688697.2016.1229747.
19. Gelabert-González M, Cutrín-Prieto JM, García-Allut A. Spinal arachnoid cyst without neural tube defect. Childs Nerv Syst. 2001;17:179–81. https://doi.org/10.1007/s003810000367.
20. Gezici AR, Ergün R. Intramedullary arachnoid cyst: 3-year follow up after bilateral dorsal root entry zone myelotomy. Acta Neurochir. 2008;150:595–7. https://doi.org/10.1007/s00701-007-1501-x.
21. Ichinose T, Miyashita K, Tanaka S, Oikawa N, Oishi M, Nambu I, et al. Recurrent spinal intramedullary arachnoid cyst: case report and literature review. World Neurosurg. 2020;138:68–72. https://doi.org/10.1016/j.wneu.2020.02.106.
22. Ido K, Matsuoka H, Urushidani H. Effectiveness of a transforaminal surgical procedure for spinal extradural arachnoid cyst in the upper lumbar spine. J Clin Neurosci. 2002;9:694–6. https://doi.org/10.1054/jocn.2002.1138.
23. James HE, Postlethwait R. Spinal peritoneal shunts for conditions other than hydrocephalus and pseudotumor cerebri: a clinical report. Pediatr Neurosurg. 2007;43:456–60. https://doi.org/10.1159/000108787.
24. Jensen F, Knudsen V, Troelsen S. Recurrent intraspinal arachnoid cyst treated with a shunt procedure. Acta Neurochir. 1977;39:127–9. https://doi.org/10.1007/BF01405250.
25. Kahraman S, Anik I, Gocmen S, Sirin S. Extradural giant multiloculated arachnoid cyst causing spinal cord compression in a child. J Spinal Cord Med. 2008;31:306–8. https://doi.org/10.1080/10790268.2008.11760728.
26. Kleib AS, Salihy SM, Hamdi H, Carron R, Soumaré O. A rare cause of thoracic spinal cord compression by multiple large tarlov cysts. Korean J Neurotrauma. 2018;14:35–8. https://doi.org/10.13004/kjnt.2018.14.1.35.
27. Lee HJ, Cho WH, Han IH, Choi BK. Large thoracolumbar extradural arachnoid cyst excised by minimal skipped hemilaminectomy: a case report. Korean J Spine. 2013;10:28–31. https://doi.org/10.14245/kjs.2013.10.1.28.
28. Lee JY, Impekoven P, Stenzel W, Löhr M, Ernestus RI, Klug N. CT-guided percutaneous aspiration of Tarlov cyst as a useful diagnostic procedure prior to operative intervention. Acta Neurochir. 2004;146:667–70. https://doi.org/10.1007/s00701-004-0274-8.
29. Lee SH, Shim HK, Eun SS. Twist technique for removal of spinal extradural arachnoid cyst: technical note. Eur Spine J. 2014;23:1755–60. https://doi.org/10.1007/s00586-014-3393-9.
30. Liu JK, Cole CD, Kan P, Schmidt MH. Spinal extradural arachnoid cysts: clinical, radiological, and surgical features. Neurosurg Focus. 2007;22:E6. https://doi.org/10.3171/foc.2007.22.2.6.
31. Magendie F. Recherches physiologiques et cliniques sur le liquide céphalorachidien ou cérébrospinal. Paris: Méquignon-Marvis fils; 1842. http://catalogue.bnf.fr/ark:/12148/cb308573129.
32. Maiuri F, Iaconetta G, Esposito M, Neurological picture. Recurrent episodes of sudden tetraplegia caused by an anterior cervical arachnoid cyst. J Neurol Neurosurg Psychiatry. 2006;77:1185–6. https://doi.org/10.1136/jnnp.2006.092312.
33. Matsumoto H, Matsumoto S, Miki T, Miyaji Y, Minami H, Masuda A, et al. Surgical treatment of sacral perineural cyst–case report. Neurol Med Chir. 2011;51:867–71. https://doi.org/10.2176/nmc.51.867.
34. Medved F, Seiz M, Baur MO, Neumaier-Probst E, Tuettenberg J. Thoracic intramedullary arachnoid cyst in an infant. J Neurosurg Pediatr. 2009;3:132–6. https://doi.org/10.3171/2008.10.PEDS08202.
35. Morio Y, Nanjo Y, Nagashima H, Minamizaki T, Teshima R. Sacral cyst managed with cyst-subarachnoid shunt: a technical case report. Spine. 2001;26:451–3. https://doi.org/10.1097/00007632-200102150-00025.
36. Moses ZB, Friedman GN, Penn DL, Solomon IH, Chi JH. Intradural spinal arachnoid cyst resection: implications of duraplasty in a large case series. J Neurosurg Spine. 2018;28:548–54. https://doi.org/10.3171/2017.8.SPINE17605.
37. Muhammedrezai S, Ulu MO, Tanriöver N, Moghaddam AM, Akar Z. Cervical intradural ventral arachnoid cyst resected via anterior corpectomy with reconstruction: a case report. Turk Neurosurg. 2008;18:241–4.
38. Neulen A, Kantelhardt SR, Pilgram-Pastor SM, Metz I, Rohde V, Giese A. Microsurgical fenestration of perineural cysts to the thecal sac at the level of the distal dural sleeve. Acta Neurochir. 2011;153:1427–34. https://doi.org/10.1007/s00701-011-1043-0.
39. Novegno F, Umana G, Di Muro L, Fraioli B, Fraioli MF. Spinal intramedullary arachnoid cyst: case report and literature review. Spine J. 2014;14:e9–e15. https://doi.org/10.1016/j.spinee.2013.10.051.
40. Osenbach RK, Godersky JC, Traynelis VC, Schelper RD. Intradural extramedullary cysts of the spinal canal: clinical presentation, radiographic diagnosis, and sur-

gical management. Neurosurgery. 1992;30:35–42. https://doi.org/10.1227/00006123-199201000-00007.
41. Palmer JJ. Cervical intradural arachnoid cyst in a 3-year-old child. Report of a case. Arch Neurol. 1974;31:214–5. https://doi.org/10.1001/archneur.1974.00490390096014.
42. Papadimitriou K, Cossu G, Maduri R, Valerio M, Vamadevan S, Daniel RT, Messerer M. Endoscopic treatment of spinal arachnoid cysts. Heliyon. 2021;7:e06736. https://doi.org/10.1016/j.heliyon.2021.e06736.
43. Papagelopoulos PJ, Peterson HA, Ebersold MJ, Emmanuel PR, Choudhury SN, Quast LM. Spinal column deformity and instability after lumbar or thoracolumbar laminectomy for intraspinal tumors in children and young adults. Spine. 1997;22:442–51. https://doi.org/10.1097/00007632-199702150-00019.
44. Petridis AK, Doukas A, Barth H, Mehdorn HM. Spinal cord compression caused by idiopathic intradural arachnoid cysts of the spine: review of the literature and illustrated case. Eur Spine J. 2010;19(Suppl 2):S124–9. https://doi.org/10.1007/s00586-009-1156-9.
45. Potts MB, McGrath MH, Chin CT, Garcia RM, Weinstein PR. Microsurgical fenestration and paraspinal muscle pedicle flaps for the treatment of symptomatic sacral tarlov cysts. World Neurosurg. 2016;86:233–42. https://doi.org/10.1016/j.wneu.2015.09.055.
46. Prevo RL, Hageman G, Bruyn RP, Broere G, van de Stadt J. Extended extradural spinal arachnoid cyst: an unusual cause of progressive spastic paraparesis. Clin Neurol Neurosurg. 1999;101:260–3. https://doi.org/10.1016/s0303-8467(99)00050-5.
47. Qi J, Yang J, Wang G. A novel five-category multimodal T1-weighted and T2-weighted magnetic resonance imaging-based stratification system for the selection of spinal arachnoid cyst treatment: a 15-year experience of 81 cases. Neuropsychiatr Dis Treat. 2014;10:499–506. https://doi.org/10.2147/NDT.S52517.
48. Rabb CH, McComb JG, Raffel C, Kennedy JG. Spinal arachnoid cysts in the pediatric age group: an association with neural tube defects. J Neurosurg. 1992;77:369–72. https://doi.org/10.3171/jns.1992.77.3.0369.
49. Sadek AR, Nader-Sepahi A. Spinal arachnoid cysts: presentation, management and pathophysiology. Clin Neurol Neurosurg. 2019;180:87–96. https://doi.org/10.1016/j.clineuro.2019.03.014.
50. Samura K, Morioka T, Miyagi Y, Nagata S, Mizoguchi M, Mihara F, et al. Surgical strategy for multiple huge spinal extradural meningeal cysts. Case report. J Neurosurg. 2007;107(4 Suppl):297–302. https://doi.org/10.3171/PED-07/10/297.
51. Schmutzer M, Tonn JC, Zausinger S. Spinal intradural extramedullary arachnoid cysts in adults-operative therapy and clinical outcome. Acta Neurochir. 2020;162:691–702. https://doi.org/10.1007/s00701-019-04156-0.
52. Shaaban A, Abdelrahman A, Jarir RA, Al-Bozom I, Raza A. Thoracic spinal intramedullary arachnoid cyst presented with myelopathy with marked post-operative improvement: a case report and review of literature. Asian J Neurosurg. 2019;14:981–4. https://doi.org/10.4103/ajns.AJNS_72_19.
53. Sharma A, Karande S, Sayal P, Ranadive N, Dwivedi N. Spinal intramedullary arachnoid cyst in a 4-year-old girl: a rare cause of treatable acute quadriparesis: case report. J Neurosurg. 2005;102(4 Suppl):403–6. https://doi.org/10.3171/ped.2005.102.4.0403.
54. Shrestha P, Shrestha P, Devkota UP. Excision of an anterior intradural arachnoid cyst of the cervical spine through central corpectomy approach. Eur Spine J. 2017;26(Suppl 1):154–7. https://doi.org/10.1007/s00586-017-4973-2.
55. Singh S, Bhaisora KS, Sardhara J, Das KK, Attri G, Mehrotra A, et al. Symptomatic extradural spinal arachnoid cyst: more than a simple herniated sac. J Craniovertebr Junct Spine. 2019;10:64–71. https://doi.org/10.4103/jcvjs.JCVJS_12_19.
56. Skoog A. Spinal cord compression from leptomeningeal cysts. With a report of two cases. JAMA. 1915;65:394–8.
57. Spiegelmann R, Rappaport ZH, Sahar A. Spinal arachnoid cyst with unusual presentation. Case report. J Neurosurg. 1984;60:613–6. https://doi.org/10.3171/jns.1984.60.3.0613.
58. Spiller WG. A case of intradural arachnoid cyst with operation and recovery. Trans Coll Physicians. 1913;25:1–18.
59. Srinivasan US, Bangaari A, Senthilkumar G. Partial median corpectomy for C2-C3 intradural arachnoid cyst: case report and review of the literature. Neurology. 2009;57:803–5. https://doi.org/10.4103/0028-3886.59484.
60. Sun J. Classification, mechanism and surgical treatments for spinal canal cysts. Chin Neurosurg J. 2016;2:7. https://doi.org/10.1186/s41016-016-0022-y.
61. Sun JJ, Wang ZY, Teo M, Li ZD, Wu HB, Yen RY, et al. Comparative outcomes of the two types of sacral extradural spinal meningeal cysts using different operation methods: a prospective clinical study. PLoS One. 2013;8:e83964. https://doi.org/10.1371/journal.pone.0083964.
62. Takahashi S, Morikawa S, Egawa M, Saruhashi Y, Matsusue Y. Magnetic resonance imaging-guided percutaneous fenestration of a cervical intradural cyst. Case report. J Neurosurg. 2003;99(3 Suppl):313–5. https://doi.org/10.3171/spi.2003.99.3.0313.
63. Tarlov IM. Spinal perineurial and meningeal cysts. J Neurol Neurosurg Psychiatry. 1970;33:833–43. https://doi.org/10.1136/jnnp.33.6.833.

64. Thakur VV, Rangnekar RD, Aroor S, Kesavapisharady K, Abraham M. Conus medullaris intramedullary arachnoid cyst- case report and review of the literature. Surg Neurol Int. 2021;12:370. https://doi.org/10.25259/SNI_525_2021.
65. Tsitsopoulos PP, Marklund N, Salci K, Holtz A, Mani M. Management of symptomatic sacral perineural cysts with microsurgery and a vascularized fasciocutaneous flap. J Spine Surg. 2018;4:602–9. https://doi.org/10.21037/jss.2018.07.02.
66. Wang MY, Levi AD, Green BA. Intradural spinal arachnoid cysts in adults. Surg Neurol. 2003;60:49–55. https://doi.org/10.1016/s0090-3019(03)00149-6.
67. Wang Z, Jian F, Chen Z, Wu H, Wang X, Duan W, et al. Percutaneous spinal endoscopic treatment of symptomatic sacral Tarlov cysts. World Neurosurg. 2021;158:e598–604. https://doi.org/10.1016/j.wneu.2021.11.019.
68. Wenger M, Zobor N, Markwalder R, Vogt E, Markwalder TM. Intradural extramedullary arachnoid cyst of the thoracic spine associated with cord compression. J Clin Neurosci. 2007;14:693–6. https://doi.org/10.1016/j.jocn.2006.02.011.
69. Yasuoka S, Peterson HA, MacCarty CS. Incidence of spinal column deformity after multilevel laminectomy in children and adults. J Neurosurg. 1982;57:441–5. https://doi.org/10.3171/jns.1982.57.4.0441.

Postoperative Complications Associated with Arachnoid Cysts

Gıyas Ayberk and Atilla Kazancı

1 Introduction

Arachnoid cyst (ACs) is a congenital lesion characterized by the accumulation of a cerebrospinal fluid (CSF) between the arachnoid leaves. Bright [8] was the first to describe AC as an entity in 1831. Although the first theories about the origin of ACs were attributed to anomalies during the formation of the subarachnoid space in the early embryonic period, these theories have not been validated today [10, 38, 53]. The fact that ACs are more frequently observed around the Sylvian fissure suggests that they are formed during the folding of the subarachnoid cistern and encephalon [26, 27, 56, 63]. ACs may occur secondary to trauma in infants [53]. Familial ACs are rare and show genetic heterogeneity rather than a specific gene mutation [69].

Although many theories have been proposed regarding the growth of ACs, such as the ball-valve mechanism, the osmotic pressure difference between the intra- and extracystic media, fluid accumulation due to lobar agenesis, and secretion from the cells on the luminal side, none of them can explain why the growth of cysts occurs [7, 13].

ACs constitute 1% of the intracranial space-occupying lesions and 1–3% of all mass lesions in the spinal canal [23, 34]. The autopsy and magnetic resonance imaging (MRI) series incidence is 0.75–1% and 0.75%, respectively [53]. Prevalence is around 2% [2]. The pediatric age group constitutes 60–90% of the mixed adult and pediatric AC series [30]. They are located supratentorially (70–90%), infratentorially (5–10%), or near the spinal cord (1–3%) [4, 19, 53, 58]. Although ACs are more common in the temporal fossa (72.5%) of adults, they constitute one-third of ACs in pediatric age group [3, 4, 31]. Other areas where ACs are common in adults are in the frontal region (15.4%) and the posterior fossa (8.3%) [31].

2 Treatment Methods for Arachnoid Cysts

Surgical operations are not necessary for all ACs. The patient should be treated in the case where an AC causes clinical symptoms such as headache, focal neurological findings, seizures, and cognitive changes due to increased intracranial pressure [25, 54, 68]. The primary goal of surgical treatment is to prevent reaccumulation of the cysts and the recurrence of symptoms by avoiding complications. There are various factors which affect the results of an AC surgery; however, these factors have not been determined completely [69]. There is no consensus on which AC should be treated, which symptoms will improve after the operation, and whether prophylactic treatment is required [18].

G. Ayberk · A. Kazancı (✉)
Department of Neurosurgery, Ankara Yıldırım Beyazıt University School of Medicine, Ankara, Turkey

M. Turgut et al. (eds.), *Arachnoid Cysts*, https://doi.org/10.1007/978-3-031-22701-1_30

Treatment options include stereotactic aspiration, open surgical techniques such as craniotomy and fenestration (CF), craniotomy and fenestration with cyst excision (CFE), external cystoperitoneal (CP) shunting, internal shunting (cystosubdural (CS) or cystoventricular CV), and endoscopic cystocisternostomy (ECC) [15, 19]. Stereotactic aspiration failed due to reaccumulation and is not used today [30]. The issue of which treatment method is the best is still controversial today. Advances in endoscopic techniques have brought ECC to be the primary surgical method for the treatment of AC.

3 Complications of Arachnoid Cyst Surgery

3.1 Anesthetic Consideration

Endoscopic AC surgery must not be performed under local anesthesia since continuous saline infusion may cause vomiting during surgery [11, 12, 14]. Pneumocephalus becomes a critical problem after neuroendoscopic interventions. In order to prevent this development, it is necessary to place a burr hole at the top of the skull. Therefore, the air inside the skull is removed with saline irrigation [11, 12, 14]. Additionally, restoring the end-tidal carbon dioxide level and maintaining adequate hydration will allow the brain to regain its original shape [47]. In cases where postoperative pneumocephalus is severe, giving pure oxygen through a face mask facilitates air resorption.

3.2 Surgical Complications

AC surgery is not the simple excision or puncture of a thin membrane of the cyst. The primary goal in AC surgery is to ensure communication between the cyst and the subarachnoid space without any complications. All of the general complications observed in neurosurgical operations may also occur in all types of AC surgery. Therefore, regardless of the technique used for AC treatment, the surgeon must follow basic neurosurgical principles to prevent complications.

Open craniotomy techniques (CF, CFE), external (CP) or internal shunting (CS, CV), and ECC are the surgical procedures currently used in the treatment of ACs. With the development of neuroendoscopic techniques following the 1990s, the use of endoscopy in the treatment of ACs has become widespread [45, 46, 61, 67].

Endoscopic surgery causes minimal damage to the surrounding tissues, shortens the patient's length of stay in the operating room and hospital, and prevents the patient from being dependent on a shunt [11, 47, 49, 50, 55, 60, 61, 65]. Endoscopic surgical techniques are not uncomplicated procedures. The complication rate was reported as 13.8% in patients who underwent intracranial endoscopic surgery [14]. Preventing complications begins with appropriate preoperative planning, such as determining the trajectory for the endoscope and whether to use a single or multiple trajectories [1]. For example, if a burr hole is placed too anteriorly, the endoscope may enter the foramen of Monro by mistake [1]. Using two endoscopes in different directions helps prevent complications by providing a better view for the surgeon [1]. An inexperienced surgeon may lose their orientation quickly due to obscure anatomy. In the absence of anatomic landmarks inside the cyst or the ventricle, neuronavigation may help identify the best trajectory [1]. A tiny amount of blood will prevent the endoscopist from performing the procedure. Adequate hemostasis must be achieved before opening the dura. All of these described general principles are important in the prevention of complications in neuroendoscopic surgery.

The rate of subdural effusion has been reported to be 2–40% in microsurgical or endoscopic treatment of temporal ACs and requires treatment with a subduroperitoneal shunt if it fails to resolve spontaneously [14, 33, 36, 37, 59, 62]. The cause of subdural effusion may be related to the size of the cyst or the size of the fenestration [65].

Bleeding during the operation, especially in the endoscopic treatment of ACs, is one of the most critical intraoperative complications, which causes vision loss. In order to avoid bleeding, the cyst wall must be well coagulated before the insertion of the endoscope. In the literature, intraoperative bleeding occurs in between 3% and 14% of cases [50, 64]. If bleeding occurs, switching from endoscopic surgery to a microsurgical craniotomy may be necessary. However, most bleeding stops with irrigation or bipolar coagulation. Good hemostasis is also critical in keeping the fenestration open [12].

The suprasellar ACs originate from defects in the diencephalic membrane and present surgical challenges due to their proximity to the optic chiasm, hypothalamus, and critical vascular structures [44]. VC or VCC is the endoscopic method used to treat suprasellar ACs and requires the crossing of many arachnoid membranes [44]. Accessibility of the endoscope from a small corridor to a deep region in suprasellar ACs is easy, and endoscopic fenestration is being used for all ages, more frequently and safely [9, 28, 40, 57]. Erşahin et al. [24] reported bleeding in three patients (17.6%) during endoscopic treatment in a suprasellar AC series and how it was controlled with irrigation or bipolar coagulation. In 25 patients with suprasellar ACs, intraoperative bleeding occurred in one patient (4%) and was stopped with irrigation [21]. In suprasellar ACs, the visible part of the cyst from the foramen of Monro is the ceiling of the third ventricle. Therefore, coagulation should be used to a minimum in order to avoid diencephalic complications [51]. If the cyst collapses after perforation of the diencephalic membrane, the inside of the cyst should be seen with flash irrigation [51]. Memory loss may occur due to excessive manipulation of the cyst or during perforation of the upper wall of the suprasellar cysts [17]. The diencephalic membrane of the suprasellar AC wall is thick in 40% of the patients, and fenestration is complex where perforation must be accomplished with a sharp tool to prevent bleeding or excessive manipulation of the cyst [20, 21]. The lateral part of the diencephalic membrane attaches to the pia of the mesial temporal lobe [43]. The posterior communicating artery penetrates the diencephalic membrane, and particular attention should be given to this structure during perforation [43]. It is necessary to perforate the mesencephalic membrane to perform VCC. This membrane emerges from the anterior part of the tentorium on both sides and attaches to the posterior infundibulum and pituitary stalk [43]. Perforation of the thick mesencephalic membrane may stretch the infundibulum or pituitary stalk and may cause diabetes insipidus or syndrome of inappropriate ADH secretion (SIADH). Care should be taken when perforating the diencephalic and mesencephalic membranes during VCC because the chiasm is displaced downward and the mammillary bodies upward [68]. Shim et al. [61] performed VCC in six-case intrasellar cyst series. Two patients developed SIADH that recovered after 4–6 weeks [61]. Sharp tools must be used to fenestrate the thick mesencephalic membrane to avoid bleeding of the vascular structures on the cyst wall and SIADH [21]. Distinguishing communicating or non-communicating suprasellar AC is vital to prevent vascular complications [46]. In communicating-type suprasellar AC, the basilar artery is located inside the cyst; however, in the non-communicating type, the basilar artery is located behind a transparent membrane [46].

During temporal AC treatment, a third nerve palsy is common after an open craniotomy or endoscopic techniques [15, 43]. Arachnoid membranes are thicker and stiffer when arteries or cranial nerves pass through a cistern [73]. Arachnoid membranes in these regions cannot be opened simply by spreading via the forceps or by puncturing with blunt-ended instruments. The percentage of occurrence of a third nerve palsy is between 1.5% and 11.8% in endoscopic techniques, and fenestration should be performed between the ICA and the third nerve in order to prevent its occurrence [16, 29, 50, 51, 72]. In the case of a thickened arachnoid membrane, the surgeon should switch from the endoscope to the open craniotomy technique to avoid complications.

In endoscopic or open craniotomy techniques, sudden drainage of cyst fluid may cause intracerebral or intracystic bleeding [12, 13, 60]. The reason for this unfortunate complication is hyperperfusion injury which may occur after cyst evacuation due to failed cerebral blood flow autoregulation. The way to prevent this complication is to avoid loss of CSF by opening the dura to the entire sheath diameter in endoscopic techniques [72]. Bleeding from the Sylvian bridging veins may occur after cyst evacuation due to the collapse of the supporting brain [71]. In case of hemorrhagic complications, external ventricular drainage or craniotomy may be performed.

In the International Sylvian AC survey conducted in 2008 to treat temporal ACs, CF was still the most often performed surgery among neurosurgeons, although 28.8% preferred pure endoscopic or endoscope-assisted cyst fenestration and the least commonly used technique was cyst shunting [66]. The advantages of open surgical techniques include direct inspection inside the cyst, excision of the cyst wall, treatment of multilocular cysts, stereoscopic vision, using both hands with standard instruments, and prevention of shunt dependency [30, 53]. However, postoperative complications are common in open surgical techniques, such as subdural hematoma (SDH), subdural hygroma, CSF fistula, third nerve palsy, and infection. In 33 pediatric temporal fossa ACs out of 44, CFE and cyst excision were performed without fenestration in two patients [36]. Postoperative SDH developed in five patients. The cause of SDH was thought to be a rupture of the anastomotic vessels between the arachnoid and the dura mater, and the cyst wall should be excised as minimally as possible to prevent SDH formation [5]. In another pediatric series, CF was performed in 8 patients out of 16 with ACs in different locations [30]. Fifty percent of patients recurred in the CF group. The reason for the high recurrence rate and unsuccessful results was the incomplete excision of the cyst wall [30]. Although it is recommended to perform the cyst wall excision as little as possible to prevent SDH, it is still recognized as one of the reasons for surgical failure in this series [30]. The incidence of CSF fistula and meningocele has been reported as 6% and 2.7%, respectively [35, 42]. Postoperative CSF fistula usually resolves with lumbar drainage.

After endoscopic or open craniotomy techniques and due to poor subdural absorption of the CSF, a subdural hygroma can occur [22, 48]. In a pediatric series of 40 patients with temporal AC, all patients were treated endoscopically, and subdural hygroma requiring subdural peritoneal shunt was observed in five (12.5%) patients [62]. Transcortical intervention prevents hygroma formation; however it is inevitable in cases when subdural absorption is poor [22, 48]. In addition, the transcortical approach may cause complications such as epilepsy [41]. In addition to cyst wall excision, cisternal fenestration is necessary to prevent the development of hygroma [28, 48].

Internal shunts are alternative shunting techniques used for the prevention of SDH or hygroma. They allow the achievement of physiological intracranial pressure by connecting the cyst with subdural space [55]. Inserting the distal shunt end into the subdural space prevents the complete collapse of the cyst and SDH or subdural hygroma [70]. Wester et al. [70] treated 12 ACs in adult patients (9 temporal, 3 frontal convexities) by inserting a CS shunt. An angled Holter ventricular catheter was inserted through the parietal cyst wall and the distal edge into the subdural space. SDH or hygroma occurred in two patients with Galassi type II or III temporal AC. Helland et al. [32] performed CS shunt in 31 adult patients with AC, 21 of which were located in the temporal fossa and 10 over the frontal convexity. There were seven complications observed in this series, and all had Galassi type II or III temporal AC. CSH and hygroma developed in five and two patients, respectively. Shunt failure was observed in three patients due to the membrane's occlusion of the intracystic catheter. The development of SDH or hygroma is more common in Galassi type II or III temporal ACs [32, 70]. This result may be due to the separation of dural border cells and arachnoid barrier cells or the tearing of anastomotic vessels between the cyst wall and the dura mater.

CP shunts have been used in the treatment of AC for a long time. Shunting of a cyst is a minor operation with a lower risk and fewer complications. However, despite the improvements in shunt and valve systems, shunt dysfunction and infection still pose a serious problem [52]. Overdrainage causing subdural hematoma or effusion may lead to shunt malfunction. An excessively large durotomy should be avoided to prevent a subdural effusion from forming [30]. The most crucial cause of shunt dysfunction is shunt infection, with a frequency of 8–15% [52]. Arai et al. [6] treated 77 temporal fossa ACs with CP shunting in adult and pediatric-aged groups. Postoperatively, one epidural hematoma, one shunt infection, and eight shunt malfunctions occurred. The outer cyst wall excision and the low-pressure valve CP shunt without an anti-siphon device should be inserted to prevent shunt dysfunction [6]. In 44 pediatric temporal fossa ACs, CP or VP shunt was performed in 7 patients, and cyst excision with CP shunt in 2 patients [36]. Shunt infection developed in one of three patients with a VP shunt. The use of a no-touch technique, minimal operating room traffic, and expedient surgery are essential to minimize shunt infection.

Shunt dependence has been known for a long time in hydrocephalic patients. However, shunt dependence after CP shunting has not attracted attention since Arai et al. [6]. Four of eight patients with shunt failure had increased intracranial pressure, although there was no change in their cyst size. The cause of increased intracranial pressure in four patients was found to be shunt dependency [6]. The shunt should be removed when the cyst becomes obliterated to prevent shunt dependence [6]. Kim et al. [39] reported eight patients with shunt dependency. Shunt dependency is not related to the age of the patient at the time of the first shunt insertion, the location and size of the cyst, the characteristics of the valve system of the shunt, or the number of previous shunting procedures [39]. After CP shunt insertion, shunt dependence develops in 42 months (ranges between 17 and 80 months) [39]. To prevent shunt dependence in symptomatic or asymptomatic patients, the first option should be craniotomy and fenestration [39].

4 Conclusion

The size of ACs remains stable or increases over time. While the treatment is necessary for ACs causing mass effect, the treatment of asymptomatic cysts is controversial. Fenestration of ACs is performed by endoscopic surgery or craniotomy. If these methods are unsuccessful, the patient should be treated with external or internal shunts. Each technique that is used in the treatment has its own complications. In order to minimize complications, the patient should be evaluated appropriately in the preoperative period. The size and location of the cyst and the duration of the symptoms should be taken into consideration. To prevent complications and recurrence, cyst fenestration should be performed in two areas: the entrance of the cisterns and the deep subarachnoid portion adjacent to them. Appropriate techniques should be used to prevent vascular and cranial nerve complications in the fenestration of the cyst.

References

1. Abbott R. The endoscopic management of arachnoidal cysts. Neurosurg Clin N Am. 2004;15:9–17.
2. Al-Holou WN, Terman S, Kilburg C, Garton HJL, Muraszko KM, Maher CO. Prevalence, and natural history of arachnoid cysts in adults. J Neurosurg. 2013;118:222–31.
3. Albuquerque FC, Giannotta SL. Arachnoid cyst rupture producing subdural hygroma and intracranial hypertension: case reports. Neurosurgery. 1997;41(4):951–6.
4. Ali ZS, Lang SS, Bakar D, Storm PB, Stein SC. Pediatric intracranial arachnoid cysts: comparative effectiveness of surgical treatment options. Childs Nerv Syst. 2014;30:461–9.
5. Aoki N, Sakai T. Intraoperative subdural hematoma in a patient with arachnoid cyst in the middle cranial fossa. Childs Nerv Syst. 1990;6:44–6.
6. Arai H, Sato K, Wachi A, Okuda O, Taked N. Arachnoid cysts of the middle cranial fossa: experience with 77 patients who were treated with cystoperitoneal shunting. Neurosurgery. 1996;39:1108–13.
7. Basaldella L, Orvieto E, Dei Tos AP, Della Barbera M, Valente M, Longatti P. Causes of arachnoid cyst development and expansion. Neurosurg Focus. 2007;15:22.

8. Bright R. Serous cysts in the arachnoid. In: Rees O, Brown G, editors. Diseases of the brain and nervous system. Part I. London: Longman Group Ltd; 1831. p. 437–9.
9. Buxton N, Vloeberghs M, Punt J. Flexible neuroendoscopic treatment of suprasellar arachnoid cysts. Br J Neurosurg. 1999;13:316–8.
10. Catala M, Poirier J. Arachnoid cysts: a histologic, embryologic and physiopathologic review. Rev Neurol. 1998;154(6-7):489–501.
11. Chernov MF, Kamikawa S, Yamane F, Hori T. Double-endoscopic approach for management of convexity arachnoid cyst: case report. Surg Neurol. 2004;61:483–7.
12. Choi JU, Kim DS, Huh R. Endoscopic approach to arachnoid cyst. Childs Nerv Syst. 1999;15:285–91.
13. Choi JU, Kim DS. Pathogenesis of arachnoid cyst: congenital or traumatic? Pediatr Neurosurg. 1998;29:260–6.
14. Cinalli G, Spennato P, Ruggiero C, Aliberti F, Trischitta V, Buonocore MC, Cianciulli E, Maggi G. Complications following endoscopic intracranial procedures in children. Childs Nerv Syst. 2007;23:633–44.
15. Cincu R, Agrawal A, Eiras J. Intracranial arachnoid cysts: current concepts and treatment alternatives. Clin Neurol Neurosurg. 2007;109:837–43.
16. Couvreur T, Hallaert G, Heggen TVD, Baert E, Dewaele F, Kalala Okito J-P, Vanhauwaert D, Deruytter M, Roost DV, Caemaert J. Endoscopic treatment of temporal arachnoid cysts in 34 patients. World Neurosurg. 2015;84:734–40.
17. Decq P, Brugieres P, Le Guerinel C, Djindjian M, keravel Y, Nguyen JP. Percutaneous endoscopic treatment of suprasellar arachnoid cysts: ventriculocystostomy or ventriculocystocisternostomy? J Neurosurg. 1996;84:696–701.
18. Di Rocco F, James R, Roujeau T, Puget S, Sainte-Rose C, Zerah MR, James S, Roujeau T, Puget S, Sainte-Rose C, Zerah M. Limits of endoscopic treatment of sylvian arachnoid cysts in children. Childs Nerv Syst. 2010;26:155–62.
19. Duz B, Kaya S, Daneyemez M, Gonul E. Surgical management strategies of intracranial arachnoid cysts: a single institution experience of 75 cases. Turk Neurosurg. 2012;22(5):591–8.
20. El-Ghandour NMF. Endoscopic treatment of intraparenchymal arachnoid cysts in children. J Neurosurg Pediatr. 2014;14:501–7.
21. El-Ghandour NMF. Endoscopic treatment of suprasellar arachnoid cysts in children. Neurosurg Pediatr. 2011;8:6–14.
22. Elhammady MSA, Bhatia S, Ragheb J. Endoscopic fenestration of middle fossa arachnoid cysts: a technical description and case series. Pediatr Neurosurg. 2007;43:209–15.
23. Eroglu U, Bozkurt M, Kahilogullari G, Dogan I, Ozgural O, Shah KJ, Zaimoglu M, Al-Beyati ESM, Ugur HÇ, Aaron A, Cohen-Gadol AA. Surgical management of spinal arachnoid cysts in adults. World Neurosurg. 2018;122:e1146–52.
24. Erşahin Y, Kesikçi H, Rüksen M, Aydın C, Mutluer S. Endoscopic treatment of suprasellar arachnoid cysts. Childs Nerv Syst. 2008;24:1013–20.
25. Esmaeeli B, Eftekhar B. Intraparenchymal hemorrhage after surgical decompression of a Sylvian fissure arachnoid cyst. Neurology. 2006;54:320–1.
26. Galassi E, Piazza G, Gaist G, Frank F. Arachnoid cysts of the middle cranial fossa: a clinical and radiological study of 25 cases treated surgically. Surg Neurol. 1980;14(3):211–9.
27. Galassi E, Tognetti F, Gaist G, Fagioli L, Frank F, Frank G. CT scan and metrizamide CT cisternography in arachnoid cysts of the middle cranial fossa: classification and pathophysiological aspects. Surg Neurol. 1982;17(5):363–9.
28. Gangemi M, Vincenzo S, Collela G, Cioffi V, Imperto A, Maiuri F. Endoscopy versus microsurgical cyst excision and shunting for treating intracranial arachnoid cysts. J Neurosurg Pediatr. 2011;8:158–64.
29. Gui SB, Wang XS, Zong XY, Li CZ, Li B, Zhang YZ. Assessment of endoscopic treatment for middle cranial fossa arachnoid cysts. Childs Nerv Syst. 2011;27:1121–8.
30. Harsh GR, Edwards MSB, Wilson CB. Intracranial arachnoid cyst in children. J Neurosurg. 1986;64:835–42.
31. Helland CA, Wester K. A population-based study of intracranial arachnoid cysts: clinical and neuroimaging outcomes following surgical cyst decompression in adults. J Neurol Neurosurg Psychiatry. 2007;78(10):1129–35.
32. Helland CA, Wester K. Arachnoid cysts in adults: long-term follow-up of patients treated with internal shunts to the subdural compartment. Surg Neurol. 2006;66:56–61.
33. Hopf NJ, Perneczky A. Endoscopic neurosurgery and endoscope-assisted microneurosurgery for the treatment of intracranial cyst. Neurosurgery. 1998;43:1330–6.
34. Hughes G, Ugokwe K, Benzel EC. Areview of spinal arachnoid cyst. Cleve Clin J Med. 2008;75(4):311–5.
35. Kandenwein JA, Richter HP, Börm W. Surgical therapy of symptomatic arachnoid cysts – an outcome analysis. Acta Neurochir. 2004;146:1317–22.
36. Kang JK, Lee KS, Lee IW, Jeun SS, Son BC, Jung CK, Park YS, Lee SW. Shunt-independent surgical treatment of middle cranial fossa arachnoid cysts in children. Childs Nerv Syst. 2000;16:111–6.
37. Karabatsau K, Hayhurst C, Buxton N, O'Brien DF, Malluci CL. Endoscopic management of arachnoid cysts: an advancing technique. J Neurosurg. 2007;106:455–62.
38. Kato M, Nakada Y, Ariga N, Kokubo Y, Makino H. Prognosis of four cases of primary middle fossa arachnoid cyst in children. Childs Brain. 1980;7(4):195–204.

39. Kim SK, Cho BK, Chung YN, Hee-Soo Kim S, Wang KC. Shunt dependency in shunted arachnoid cyst: a reason to avoid shunting. Pediatr Neurosurg. 2002;37:178–85.
40. Kirollos RW, Javadpour M, May P, Mallucci C. Endoscopic treatment of suprasellar and third ventricle-related arachnoid cysts. Childs Nerv Syst. 2001;17:713–8.
41. Kramer U, Kanner AA, Siomin V, Harela S, Constantini S. No evidence of epilepsy following endoscopic third ventriculostomy: a short-term follow-up. Pediatr Neurosurg. 2001;34:121–3.
42. Levy LM, Wang M, Aryan HE, Yoo K, Meltzer H. Microsurgical keyhole approach for middle Possa arachnoid cyst fenestration. Neurosurgery. 2003;53:1138–45.
43. Lu J, Zhu X. Microsurgical anatomy of the interpeduncular cistern and related arachnoid membranes. J Neurosurg. 2005;103:337–41.
44. Maher CO, Liliana GL. The effectiveness of ventriculocystocisternostomy for suprasellar arachnoid cysts. Neurosurg Pediatr. 2011;7:64–72.
45. McBride LA, Winston KR, Freeman JE. Cystoventricular shunting of intracranial aracchnoid cysts. Pediatr Neurosurg. 2003;39(6):323–9.
46. Miyajima M, Arai H, Okuda O, Hishii M, Nakanishi H, Sato K. Possible origin of suprasellar arachnoid cysts: neuroimaging and neurosurgical observations in nine cases. J Neurosurg. 2000;93:62–7.
47. Nowosławska E, Polis Kaniewska D, Mikołajczyk W, Krawczyk J, Szymański W, Zakrzewski K, Podciechowska J, Polis B. Neuroendoscopic techniques in the treatment of arachnoid cysts in children and comparison with other operative methods. Childs Nerv Syst. 2006;22:599–604.
48. Oberbauer RW, Haase J, Pucher R. Arachnoid cyst in children: a European co-operative study. Childs Nerv Syst. 1992;8:281–6.
49. Oertel J, Linsler S, Wagner W, Gaab M, Schroeder H, Rediker J. Endoscopic treatment of intracranial arachnoid systs: a retrospective analysis of a 25-year experience (case series). Oper Neurosurg. 2020;2020:1–13.
50. Oertel JMK, Wagner W, Mondorf Y, Baldauf J, Schroeder HWS, Gaab MR. Endoscopic treatment of arachnoid cysts: a detailed account of surgical techniques and results. Neurosurgery. 2010;67:824–36.
51. Özek MM, Urgun K. Neuroendoscopic management of suprasellar arachnoid cysts. World Neurosurg. 2013;79(2):S19.e13–S19.e18.
52. Paff M, Alexandru-Abrams D, Muhonen M, Loudon W. Ventriculoperitoneal shunt complications: a review. Interdiscip Neurosurg. 2018;13:66–70.
53. Pradilla G, Jallo G. Arachnoid cysts: case series and review of the literature. Neurosurg Focus. 2007;22(2):E7.
54. Qin B, Gao L, Hu J, Wang L, Chen G. Intracerebral hematoma after endoscopic fenestration of an arachnoid cyst A case report. Medicine. 2018;97(44):1–6.
55. Rappaport ZH. Suprasellar arachnoid cyst: options in operative management. Acta Neurochir. 1993;122:71–5.
56. Rengachary SS, Watanabe I. Ultrastructure and pathogenesis of intracranial arachnoid cysts. J Neuropathol Exp Neurol. 1981;40:61–83.
57. Rizk E, Chern JJ, Tagayun C, Tubbs RS, Hankinson T, Rozzelle C, Oakes WJ, Blount JP, Wellons JC. Institutional experience of endoscopic suprasellar arachnoid cyst fenestration. Childs Nerv Syst. 2013;29:1345–7.
58. Schmutzer M, Tonn JC, Zausinger S. Spinal intradural extramedullary arachnoid cysts in adults—operative therapy and clinical outcome. Acta Neurochir. 2020;163:691–702.
59. Schroeder HWS, Oertel J, Gaab MR. Incidence of complications in neuroendoscopic surgery. Childs Nerv Syst. 2004;20:878–83.
60. Shim KW, Lee YH, Park EK, Park YS, Choi JU, Kim DS. Treatment option for arachnoid cysts. Childs Nerv Syst. 2009;25:1459–66.
61. Shim KW, Park EK, Lee YH, Kim SH, Kim DS. Transventricular endoscopic fenestration of intrasellar arachnoid cyst. Neurosurgery. 2013;72:520–8.
62. Spacca B, Kandasamy J, Mallucci CL, Genitori L. Endoscopic treatment of middle fossa arachnoid cysts: a series of 40 patients treated endoscopically in two centres. Childs Nerv Syst. 2010;26:163–72.
63. Starkman SP, Brown TC, Linell EA. Cerebral arachnoid cysts. J Neuropathol Exp Neurol. 1958;17(3):484–500.
64. Talamonti G, D'Aliberti G, Picano M, Debernardi A, Collice M. Intracranial cysts containing cerebrospinal fluid-like fluid: results of endoscopic neurosurgery in a series of 64 consecutive cases. Neurosurgery. 2011;68:788–803.
65. Tamburrini G, Caldarelli M, Massimi L, Santini P, Di Rocco C. Subdural hygroma: an unwanted result of Sylvian arachnoid cyst marsupialization. Childs Nerv Syst. 2003;19:159–65.
66. Tamburrini G, D'Angelo L, Paternoster G, Massimi L, Caldarelli M, Di Rocco C. Endoscopic management of intra and paraventricular CSF cysts. Childs Nerv Syst. 2007;23:645–51.
67. Turhan T, Erşahin Y, Akıntürk N, Mutluer S. Fenestration methods for Sylvian arachnoid cysts-endoscopy or microsurgery. Childs Nerv Syst. 2012;28:229–35.
68. Wang XJ. Intraparenchymal hemorrhage after surgical decompression of an epencephalon arachnoid cyst: a case report. World J Clin Cases. 2021;9(1):274–7.
69. Wang Y, Cui J, Qin X, Hong X. Familial intracranial arachnoid cysts with a missense mutation (c.2576C>T) in RERE. A case report. Medicine. 2018;97:50.
70. Wester K. Arachnoid cysts in adults: experience with internal shunts to the subdural compartment. Surg Neurol. 1996;45:15–24.

71. Wester K, Helland CA. How often do chronic extra-cerebral hematomas occur in patients with intracranial arachnoid cysts? J Neurol Neurosurg Psychiatry. 2008;79:72–5.
72. Xu S, Wang Y, Luo Q, Jiang J, Zhong C. Endoscopic fenestration of twenty-six patients with middle fossa arachnoid cyst. J Craniofac Surg. 2016;27: 973–5.
73. Yaşargil MG, Kasdaglis K, Jain KK, Eber HP. Anatomical observations of the subarachnoid cisterns of the brain during surgery. J Neurosurg. 1976;44:298–302.

Part VI

Outcome and Prognosis of Arachnoid Cysts

Editor's Summary

In this "Part VI: Outcome and Prognosis of Arachnoid Cysts," there are a total of four chapters describing the outcomes associated with arachnoid cysts (ACs) and their prognosis. In general, the prognosis for these benign lesions is quite good with their prompt diagnosis and timely treatment if surgical intervention is deemed necessary. Despite intervention, there is a potential for recurrence with reparation of the cyst wall and with fluid reaccumulation as described in 31 of the last part of this book. With the slight chance for recurrence, there is a need for follow-up of ACs after their treatment which is discussed in 32. The evolution of the future management of ACs is presented in 33. It should be emphasized that ACs are intracranial and intraspinal space-occupying lesions that can cause neurological symptoms and morbidity with a delay in diagnosis and treatment. As exemplified through interesting case scenarios, this delay can lead to medicolegal consequences that are illustrated in several clinical cases described in the last chapter of this work.

Recurrence of Arachnoid Cysts

Brandon M. Wilkinson and Walter A. Hall

1 Introduction

Arachnoid cysts (ACs) are benign lesions which are frequently managed conservatively, although they may become symptomatic and a variety of surgical treatment options may be indicated in these cases. Unfortunately, recurrence of ACs may arise from inadequate fenestration into the surrounding cerebrospinal fluid (CSF) spaces, gradual closure of surgically created stomas, or shunt failure. Here a summary of the natural history and the various treatment options for ACs is provided in this chapter.

2 Natural History of Arachnoid Cysts

ACs are thought to develop from splitting and duplication of the developing endomeninx in embryogenesis [29, 30]. Secretory enzymes are contained within the cyst walls, with cyst enlargement resulting from accumulation of CSF. Additionally, a ball-valve mechanism may contribute to their enlargement [29]. A detailed discussion of their pathogenesis is provided elsewhere in this text. The clinical presentation of ACs varies, ranging from complications of cyst rupture including subdural hematoma/hygroma, to headache, focal neurological deficits based on cyst location, seizures, developmental delay, and behavioral changes [6, 31]. The most common site of origin is the middle cranial fossa, followed by the posterior fossa, frontal convexities, and the suprasellar region [1, 19]. Middle fossa ACs display a left-sided predominance and are more common in male patients [19]. A variety of surgical treatments have been described, including cyst wall fenestration with or without the use of endoscopy, microsurgical membrane resection, and cyst shunting.

Indications for surgery often include symptoms related to elevated intracranial pressure secondary to cyst mass effect and CSF flow obstruction, with resultant compression of surrounding neural structures [36]. In pediatric patients this often manifests as headache, nausea, vomiting, enlarging head circumference and full fontanelles in younger children, and papilledema in older children [2, 6]. Suprasellar cysts may also cause endocrine anomalies including precocious puberty as well as cranial nerve deficits [2, 6]. In adult patients, the incidence of ACs is approximately 1.4% [19]. They typically display a benign clinical course and similarly have a higher prevalence in men. Al-Holou et al. suggested sellar and suprasellar cysts are those most likely to be symptomatic in adults, with middle fossa cysts rarely manifesting with clinical symptoms. During a follow-up period of over 2 years,

B. M. Wilkinson (✉) · W. A. Hall
Department of Neurosurgery, SUNY Upstate Medical University, Syracuse, NY, USA
e-mail: wilkinsb@upstate.edu; hallw@upstate.edu

M. Turgut et al. (eds.), *Arachnoid Cysts*, https://doi.org/10.1007/978-3-031-22701-1_31

2% of cysts were found to enlarge and 1% were found to decrease in size. Only 24 of 661 patients identified required surgical treatment [1].

Spinal ACs may also occur less commonly than intracranial lesions. These patients may present with myelopathy or extremity numbness and weakness depending on the anatomic location. While typically intradural, the presence of a dural defect can give rise to extradural cysts as well [16].

A large number of cysts are discovered incidentally. In the absence of significant clinical symptoms, they are treated conservatively with imaging surveillance. Such cysts often remain stable in size and do not require surgery, unless complicated by rupture or subdural hematoma [1, 13]. Spontaneous resolution of ACs has also been described [26, 27]. In this chapter we focus on AC recurrence following surgical treatment.

3 Surgical Treatment of Arachnoid Cysts

A variety of surgical procedures for treatment of ACs may be performed, after careful consideration of the surrounding anatomic structures, degree of mass effect, and proximity to the ventricular system and surrounding cisterns. Treatments range from fenestration of the cyst wall into adjacent CSF spaces, resection of cyst walls, and cyst shunting. A detailed discussion of the various surgical approaches and associated technical nuances will be described elsewhere in this text.

In the case of cyst fenestration, open microsurgical fenestration began being largely described in the 1970s with moderate success. Fewel et al. reported a treatment success rate without subsequent intervention on the order of 50% in a case series of patients treated from 1976 to 1986. As surgical techniques improved, they reported an increased success rate of 60% in patients treated from 1987 to 1996. In patients without hydrocephalus, cyst fenestration had a significantly higher rate of success [14]. Subsequent studies have shown an improved rate of cyst resolution via microsurgical treatment [18]. In the case of middle fossa cyst, Levy et al. described a series of 50 patients treated via fenestration through a keyhole approach. Of all patients treated, 82% demonstrated decreased cyst size on serial imaging, with 18% demonstrating complete cyst effacement. Hemiparesis and cranial nerve palsies upon initial presentation were most likely to improve, whereas seizure disorders improved by 50% [23]. For suprasellar ACs, while ventriculocystostomy (VC) has been shown to be effective in many cases, some authors prefer to perform ventriculocystocisternotomy (VCC) to provide additional fluid outflow. Maher et al. suggested that while some studies lacking power have not validated the superiority of VCC, it may be associated with a decreased need for subsequent surgeries and can be considered the treatment of choice for patients with symptomatic supratentorial ACs [24].

The use of endoscopy has also been widely employed for cyst fenestration with similar rates of success [5, 8, 20, 33]. Advantages include a less invasive approach with smaller incision and burr hole craniotomy as opposed to a larger open craniotomy. Some authors have described however less ability to control bleeding, in some cases requiring conversion to open craniotomy [31]. Additionally, the absence of hydrocephalus makes fenestration into the ventricles impractical [9]. The rates of intraoperative bleeding complications overall appear similar when comparing endoscopy to microsurgical fenestration [5, 8, 20, 33]. Several case series have reported the success in reducing the radiographic size of ACs following endoscopic fenestration ranging from 70 to 90% [5, 8, 20, 31, 33]. Patients who did not achieve radiographic improvement often underwent subsequent surgical intervention via re-fenestration or cyst shunting. In considering the optimal technique, Gangemi et al. reported higher success rates using endoscopy for cysts located in the suprasellar and quadrigeminal regions and posterior fossa, whereas microsurgical fenestration or shunting may be favored for cortical cysts [15].

Cyst shunting has also been widely shown to be a valid method for achieving cyst decompression. Metabolic studies have demonstrated cortical metabolic improvement following cyst decompression resulting in improved language skills in patients with supratentorial cysts and pre-operative aphasia [12]. Multiple techniques have been described, including cyst-peritoneal, cyst-ventricular, cyst-subdural, and cyst-cisterno-ventricular shunting [25, 38]. Shunting into the ventricular system has been shown to help achieve normal physiologic intracranial pressure relationships. D'Angelo et al. demonstrated a progressive decrease in cyst volume in patients over the course of 1 year following cyst-ventricular shunting [10]. In some cases, reduction in cyst volume may be less apparent; however after improving communication between CSF compartments, symptomatic improvement has been shown in such patients where significant radiographic improvement did not occur [25].

While shunting does largely achieve good clinical and radiographic outcomes, shunt implantation does raise the possibility of permanent shunt dependence [3, 32]; thus many surgeons may opt for fenestration initially to avoid permanent hardware placement and the risks of future shunt failure. The most appropriate indication for shunt placement in AC patients is the presence of concomitant hydrocephalus, in some cases with placement of shunts both within the cyst and separately into the ventricular system [22].

Regardless of the shunting technique employed, surgical success rates appear similar when comparing cyst fenestration to shunting [25, 37, 38]. It should be noted that cyst or ventricular overdrainage may occur and can result in subdural hematoma or hygroma formation [38] requiring additional surgical intervention. This complication however does not appear to be isolated to shunted patients and has been reported following open and endoscopic fenestration [28, 35]. Both fixed-pressure and programmable valves may be used [17]; however careful consideration is required when deciding upon valve type to avoid post-operative complications.

4 Recurrence of Arachnoid Cysts Following Surgical Intervention

Given the overall success in alleviating symptoms and achieving good radiographic outcomes following surgical intervention, AC recurrence is relatively uncommon [21]. There appear to be two main reasons for cyst recurrence. First, the closure of fenestrated membranes may lead to cyst fluid reaccumulation and impaired communication with surrounding CSF spaces. Second, in patients treated with shunting, shunt failure also leads to cyst recurrence.

In the case of previously fenestrated membrane closure, several studies have proposed theories on why cyst wall closure occurs, raising into question whether cyst-ventricular or cyst-ventricular-cisternal fenestration should be performed. Crimmins et al. [9] studied 23 patients with suprasellar ACs requiring surgical intervention with a follow-up period of approximately 4 years. In their case series, VCC achieved a 100% success rate in radiographically reducing cyst size with clinical improvement in all patients, whereas VC was effective in 25% of cases with long-term follow-up. They observed a valve-like aperture in the cyst inferior membrane in several patients, hypothesizing that flow through the cyst may go in one direction, making it necessary to perforate both superior and inferior membranes in order to allow for communication, since perforation of the basal stoma allows flow into the basal cisterns. The upper stoma may close over time in such cases, leading to cyst recurrence. While failure rates did not achieve statistical significance due to the power of the study, failures were seen more often in VC alone and usually occurred within several months after surgery. Subsequent surgeries after recurrence may include repeat endoscopic fenestration; however this approach may often fail as well. While shunt implantation after initial failure is a valid option, many authors prefer repeat fenestration to avoid permanent hardware implantation in cases of late treatment failure.

Decq et al. described similar findings in a study comparing VC and VCC in two patients with suprasellar ACs [11]. Magnetic resonance CSF flow studies were performed pre- and post-operatively for both patients. In the patient treated initially with VCC, resolution of intracranial hypertension was achieved, and symptoms remained resolved after 2 years with no subsequent surgeries required. In the patient treated with VC however, symptoms returned after 18 months. CSF flow studies showed asynchronous flow between the cyst and the fourth ventricle, suggesting a closed stoma and impaired communication with the surrounding CSF spaces. A subsequent VCC was performed with good clinical outcome. In this patient, continued turbulent CSF flow around the cyst was noted after VC. The authors hypothesize that bowing of the third ventricle occurs and can cause direct obstruction of the apical stoma. In cases where the basal stoma is widely opened, this secondary obstruction does not occur. These findings are further supported in a case series of four patients by Caemaert et al. [4] treated with endoscopic fenestration, in which closures of the apical membrane were observed post-operatively.

Cases of recurrence after fenestration have also been described in convexity cysts [34]. Suzuki et al. described a case in which a 62-year-old woman with a right occipital convexity AC was treated with fenestration to the subarachnoid space. After a follow-up of 6 years, her initial visual symptoms and headache recurred, with MRI demonstrating cyst enlargement compared to post-operative imaging. She underwent subsequent membranectomy with a cyst Ommaya reservoir placed. A similar mechanism of membrane closure is suspected. While such cases are rare in the literature, reported delayed recurrence suggests long-term follow-up is appropriate for AC patients post-operatively.

In patients treated with shunting, AC recurrence due to shunt failure has been reported [7, 9, 37]. Ciricillo et al. reported 20 patients with ACs treated with a cyst-peritoneal shunt, many of which were subsequently placed following cyst fenestration. After a follow-up of 8 years, 30% of patients required shunt revision due to cyst recurrence [7]. While additional surgeries were required in these patients, a significant difference in the success rates was seen, with shunting appearing more efficacious than fenestration in achieving radiographic improvement. No predictors of shunt failure were determined; however no patients with middle fossa cysts required shunt revision, suggesting that this location may be more amenable to shunting compared to other locations.

Raffel et al. reported similar outcomes in a study analyzing 12 patients with ACs treated with cyst-peritoneal shunting [29]. Seven patients were treated with fenestration initially and underwent subsequent shunt placement, while five were treated with shunting upfront. Of the 12 total patients, 5 required one or more revision for cyst recurrence. They concluded that concomitant hydrocephalus should be treated with shunting, either with simultaneous cyst fenestration or by shunting alone, as 76% of patients without hydrocephalus remained shunt-free. The rates of shunt failure in AC patients appear similar to those associated with other pathologies [10, 17, 22].

5 Conclusion

ACs are benign lesions arising from duplication of arachnoid membranes in embryogenesis. When symptomatic, they can lead to headaches, macrocephaly, seizures, focal deficits, and elevated intracranial pressures. A variety of surgical treatment methods exist, including microsurgical or endoscopic cyst wall fenestration, membrane resection, and cyst shunting. Recurrence following surgical intervention may arise from impaired communication with surrounding CSF spaces with early or delayed stoma closure or in cases of shunt failure. While not shown to be statistically significant, cyst communication with surrounding cisterns in addition to the ventricular system may be favored over communication with the ventricular system alone in appropriate cases. Cyst fenestration is often preferred over shunt implantation as a first-line surgical treatment to avoid the potential for future shunt failure.

References

1. Al-Holou WN, Terman S, Kilburg C, Garton HJ, Muraszko KM, Maher CO. Prevalence and natural history of arachnoid cysts in adults. J Neurosurg. 2013;118(2):222–31.
2. Al-Holou WN, Yew AY, Boomsaad ZE, Garton HJ, Muraszko KM, Maher CO. Prevalence and natural history of arachnoid cysts in children. J Neurosurg Pediatr. 2010;5(6):578–85.
3. Arai H, Sato K, Wachi A, Okuda O, Takeda N. Arachnoid cysts of the middle cranial fossa: experience with 77 patients who were treated with cystoperitoneal shunting. Neurosurgery. 1996;39(6):1108–12; Discussion 1112-3.
4. Caemaert J, Abdullah J, Calliauw L, Carton D, Dhooge C, van Coster R. Endoscopic treatment of suprasellar arachnoid cysts. Acta Neurochir. 1992;119:68–73.
5. Choi JU, Kim DS, Huh R. Endoscopic approach to arachnoid cyst. Childs Nerv Syst. 1999;15:285–91.
6. Cilluffo JM, Onofrio BM, Miller RH. The diagnosis and surgical treatment of intracranial arachnoid cysts. Acta Neurochir. 1983;67(3-4):215–29.
7. Ciricillo SF, Cogen PH, Harsh GR, Edwards MS. Intracranial arachnoid cysts in children. A comparison of the effects of fenestration and shunting. J Neurosurg. 1991;74(2):230–5.
8. Couvreur T, Hallaert G, Van Der Heggen T, Baert E, Dewaele F, Okito JPK, Vanhauwaert D, Deruytter M, Roost DV, Caemaert J. Endoscopic treatment of temporal arachnoid cysts in 34 patients. World Neurosurg. 2015;84:734–40.
9. Crimmins DW, Pierre-Kahn A, Sainte-Rose C, Zerah M. Treatment of suprasellar cysts and patient outcome. J Neurosurg. 2006;105(2 Suppl):107–14.
10. D'Angelo V, Gorgoglione L, Catapano G. Treatment of symptomatic intracranial arachnoid cysts by stereotactic cyst-ventricular shunting. Stereotact Funct Neurosurg. 1999;72(1):62–9.
11. Decq P, Brugieres P, Le Guerinel C, Djindjian M, Keravel Y, Nguyen JP. Percutaneous endoscopic treatment of suprasellar arachnoid cysts: ventriculocystostomy or ventriculocystocisternostomy? Technical note. J Neurosurg. 1996;84:696–701.
12. De Volder AG, Michel C, Thauvoy C, Willems G, Ferrière G. Brain glucose utilisation in acquired childhood aphasia associated with a sylvian arachnoid cyst: recovery after shunting as demonstrated by PET. J Neurol Neurosurg Psychiatry. 1994;57:296–300.
13. Domenicucci M, Russo N, Giugni E, Pierallini A. Relationship between supratentorial arachnoid cyst and chronic subdural hematoma: neuroradiological evidence and surgical treatment. J Neurosurg. 2009;110(6):1250–5.
14. Fewel ME, Levy ML, McComb JG. Surgical treatment of 95 children with 102 intracranial arachnoid cysts. Pediatr Neurosurg. 1996;25(4):165–73.
15. Gangemi M, Seneca V, Colella G, Cioffi V, Imperato A, Maiuri F. Endoscopy versus microsurgical cyst excision and shunting for treating intracranial arachnoid cysts. J Neurosurg Pediatr. 2011;8(2):158–64.
16. Garg K, Borkar SA, Kale SS, Sharma BS. Spinal arachnoid cysts - our experience and review of literature. Br J Neurosurg. 2017;31(2):172–8.
17. Germano A, Caruso G, Caffo M, Baldari S, Calisto A, Meli F, Tomasello F. The treatment of large supratentorial arachnoid cysts in infants with cyst-peritoneal shunting and Hakim programmable valve. Childs Nerv Syst. 2003;19(3):166–73.
18. Gosalakkal JA. Intracranial arachnoid cysts in children: a review of pathogenesis, clinical features, and management. Pediatr Neurol. 2002;26(2):93–8.
19. Helland CA, Lund-Johansen M, Wester K. Location, sidedness, and sex distribution of intracranial arachnoid cysts in a population-based sample. J Neurosurg. 2010;113(5):934–9.
20. Hopf NJ, Perneczky A. Endoscopic neurosurgery and endoscope-assisted microneurosurgery for the treatment of intracranial cysts. Neurosurgery. 1998;43:1330–6.
21. Jallo GI, Woo HH, Meshki C, Epstein FJ, Wisoff JH. Arachnoid cysts of the cerebellopontine angle: diagnosis and surgery. Neurosurgery. 1997;40(1):31–7; Discussion 37-8.
22. Kaplan BJ, Mickle JP, Parkhurst R. Cystoperitoneal shunting for congenital arachnoid cysts. Childs Brain. 1984;11(5):304–11.
23. Levy ML, Wang M, Aryan HE, Yoo K, Meltzer H. Microsurgical keyhole approach for middle fossa arachnoid cyst fenestration. Neurosurgery. 2003;53(5):1138–44; discussion 1144–1145.
24. Maher CO, Goumnerova L. The effectiveness of ventriculocystocisternostomy for suprasellar arachnoid cysts. J Neurosurg Pediatr. 2011;7(1):64–72.
25. McBride LA, Winston KR, Freeman JE. Cystoventricular shunting of intracranial arachnoid cysts. Pediatr Neurosurg. 2003;39(6):323–9.
26. McDonald PJ, Rutka JT. Middle cranial fossa arachnoid cysts that come and go. Report of two cases and review of the literature. Pediatr Neurosurg. 1997;26(1):48–52.
27. Mokri B, Houser OW, Dinapoli RP. Spontaneous resolution of arachnoid cysts. J Neuroimaging. 1994;4(3):165–8.
28. Okano A, Ogiwara H. The effectiveness of microsurgical fenestration for middle fossa arachnoid cysts in children. Childs Nerv Syst. 2016;32(1):153–8. https://doi.org/10.1007/s00381-015-2908-y.
29. Raffel C, McComb JG. To shunt or to fenestrate: which is the best surgical treatment for arachnoid cysts in pediatric patients? Neurosurgery. 1988;23(3):338–42.
30. Rengachary SS, Watanabe I, Brackett CE. Pathogenesis of intracranial arachnoid cysts. Surg Neurol. 1978;9(2):139–44.
31. Schroeder HW, Gaab MR, Niendorf WR. Neuroendoscopic approach to arachnoid cysts. J Neurosurg. 1996;85:293–8.

32. Shim KW, Lee YH, Park EK, Park YS, Choi JU, Kim DS. Treatment option for arachnoid cysts. Childs Nerv Syst. 2009;25(11):1459–66.
33. Spacca B, Kandasamy J, Mallucci CL, Genitori L. Endoscopic treatment of middle fossa arachnoid cysts: a series of 40 patients treated endoscopically in two centres. Childs Nerv Syst. 2010;26(2):163–72.
34. Suzuki M, Tamaki T, Toda S, Tsuchiya M, Kogure K, Hosone M, Node Y, Teramoto A. Delayed recurrent arachnoid cyst of the occipital convexity in an elderly woman. Neurol Med Chir. 2009;49(3):134–7. https://doi.org/10.2176/nmc.49.134.
35. Tamburrini G, Caldarelli M, Massimi L, Santini P, Di Rocco C. Subdural hygroma: an unwanted result of Sylvian arachnoid cyst marsupialization. Childs Nerv Syst. 2003;19(3):159–65. https://doi.org/10.1007/s00381-003-0724-2.
36. Van der Meche FG, Braakman R. Arachnoid cysts in the middle cranial fossa: cause and treatment of progressive and non-progressive symptoms. J Neurol Neurosurg Psychiatry. 1983;46(12):1102–7.
37. Wang Y, Wang F, Yu M, Wang W. Clinical and radiological outcomes of surgical treatment for symptomatic arachnoid cysts in adults. J Clin Neurosci. 2015;22:1456–61.
38. Wester K. Arachnoid cysts in adults: experience with internal shunts to the subdural compartment. Surg Neurol. 1996;45(1):15–24.

Follow-Up of Arachnoid Cysts: Brain Plasticity Following Surgery for Arachnoid Cysts

Samuel Hall, Benjamin Gaastra, and Vassilios Tsitouras

1 Introduction

The majority of arachnoid cysts (ACs) are found incidentally and do not require surgical intervention. Surgical intervention is reserved for cysts which are causing symptoms due to mass effect or growing on surveillance imaging. It is expected that following surgical intervention the cyst will reduce in size and the brain expands to fill some, or all, of the space occupied by the AC. The change in the brain shape is referred to as brain plasticity. This chapter will explore how surgical intervention changes the cyst size, subsequent brain plasticity and what implications this has for patient outcomes.

2 Brain Compliance

Brain plasticity and the change in cyst volume are governed by the principles of compliance. Compliance is the tendency of a structure to change volume dependent on the change in pressure exerted against it. Elastance/stiffness is the inverse of compliance:

$$\text{Compliance} = \frac{\text{Change in volume}}{\text{Change in pressure}}$$

Although ACs are congenital, those that undergo surgery are likely symptomatic and thus growing. Growth occurs as intra-cystic pressure puts increased stress on the brain parenchyma, thus deforming it. When the intra-cystic pressure is reduced, following surgery, a new pressure gradient is generated across the cyst wall. The absolute value of pre-operative intra-cystic pressure does not relate to the degree of post-operative volume change [19]; thus variations in brain compliance likely determine the degree of post-operative brain expansion following the reduction of intra-cystic pressure.

Brain parenchyma is modelled as viscoelastic, and its stiffness is measured using the complex (dynamic) shear modulus. Complex shear modulus increases with age [34] and myelination [6] and varies within the brain. For example, the cerebellum is softer than the cerebrum [6]. Unlike elastic materials which do not lose energy when deformed (and thus demonstrate complete return to original size when stress is released), viscoelastic materials lose energy due to molecule reorganisation and thus display plastic deformation even if the stress is within the elastic limit (maximum degree of deformation before effect becomes permanent). These principles have been demonstrated based on short-term deformations, over seconds, and how they apply to the relaxation of the brain which has been deformed over

S. Hall (✉) · B. Gaastra
Department of Neurosurgery, University Hospital Southampton NHS Foundation Trust, Southampton, UK
e-mail: samuel.hall@doctors.org.uk

V. Tsitouras
Ippokratio General Hospital, Thessaloniki, Greece

M. Turgut et al. (eds.), *Arachnoid Cysts*, https://doi.org/10.1007/978-3-031-22701-1_32

weeks, months or even years is not known. The brain is far more complex than a simple polymer and exists in a dynamic environment; however, its viscoelastic nature may limit how much it will return to its original size.

3 How to Measure Cyst Volume

There are a number of techniques which can be used to measure AC volume depending on the imaging technology available. Techniques differ in their accuracy, skillset required to calculate and time requirement.

3.1 The MacDonald Method

The MacDonald method was initially described to measure tumour volumes using simple measures on cross-sectional imaging [10]. However, it is also translatable to measuring volumes of ACs [39, 40]. The modified MacDonald method uses linear measurements on cross-sectional imaging and takes the largest diameters of the cyst in cross section (named d1 and d2), the number of slices the cyst appears on (s) and the thickness of the slices (t). It is very similar to the better-known ABC/2 method with subtle differences generated by the incorporation of π. It does not require additional computational input beyond linear measurements on source images and is quick to calculate:

$$\text{Volume} = \frac{\pi \times d1 \times d2 \times s \times t}{6}$$

3.2 Volumetric Segmentation

Segmentation is the process of building a 3D model of a structure based on its boundaries as shown on radiological imaging such as CT or MRI. Many good descriptions on the science of volume segmentation have already been published [38], and further detail is beyond the scope of this chapter. There are a number of computer programmes available for clinicians which utilise DICOM data and simplify the process to produce a final volume. While previous work by the authors used the open-source 3D Slicer [16], there is no evidence that any one program is superior.

Choosing which imaging sequence to use for building a segmentation model will depend on the cyst anatomy. For example, large convexity cysts have boundaries that are easily visualised on any type of cross-sectional imaging and all MRI sequences. However small cysts in regions with multiple arachnoid layers (e.g. suprasellar cysts) require more sensitive MRI sequences such as a fine slice constructive interference in steady state (CISS) to best delineate the cyst margins. The slice thickness can influence model accuracy as the top and bottom boundaries of the cyst will lie between slices. The greater the slice thickness, the more cyst will be missed as the true boundary is further from the last slice on which the cyst is visible. This is illustrated in Fig. 1 with a theoretical spherical cyst with 50-mm diameter and assumes a slice thickness of 5 mm which demonstrates a potential 2% error for each end of the sphere. If the cyst is smaller and all other parameters are the same, then this error will be greater.

Defining volume boundaries is done either manually by tracing the outline on the imported imaging and repeating this for all the imaging slices for the object in question or automatically using the software's algorithms based on the contrast against surrounding structures. Once a 3D model has been built, the segmented volumes require surface smoothing and hole filling to generate a final volume.

3.3 Method Comparison

With the easy access of the necessary computer programmes, segmentation models are now the gold standard method for measuring cyst volume. Segmentation allows more accurate measurement, particularly of irregular shapes, than the MacDonald method. A study by Tamimi et al. [39] using a mixed cohort of locations and ages found that volumetric segmentation models generated a larger cyst volume than the modified

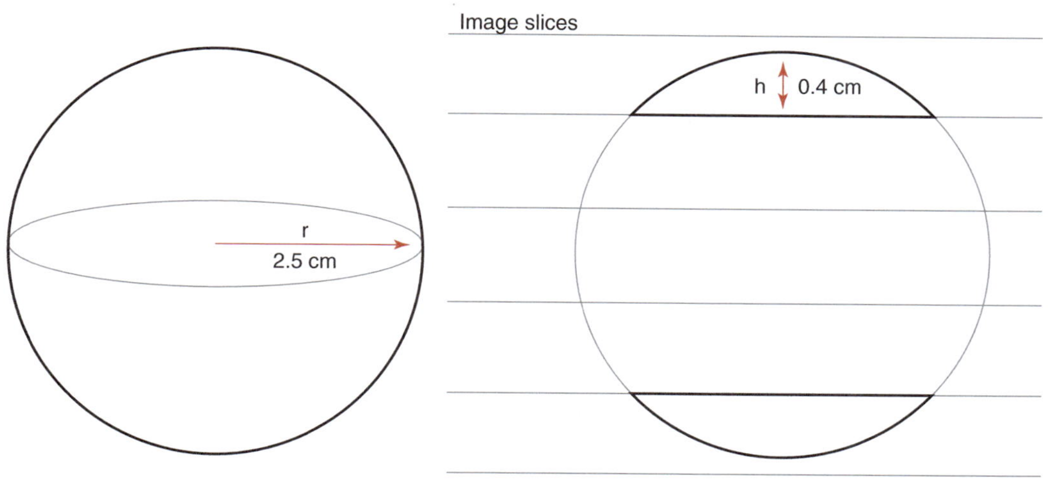

$$Volume = \frac{4}{3} x\pi \times r^3$$

$$65.45cm^3 = \frac{4}{3} x\pi \times 2.5^3$$

$$Volume\ a\ sphere\ part = \frac{1}{3} x\pi \times h^2 \times (3r - h)$$

$$1.19cm^3 = \frac{1}{3} x\pi \times 0.4^2 \times (3x\ 2.5 - 0.4)$$

Fig. 1 A schematic demonstrating total cyst volume (left) and the volume of cyst missed in imaging slices (right)

MacDonald method. However, the percentage volume change between pre- and post-operative scans was the same for both approaches. Neither method better correlated with symptom improvement. There is no consensus of whether automated or manual methods for defining the volume perimeter are more accurate, and it is likely that any differences are not clinically significant.

3.4 Classification of Post-Operative Radiological Outcomes

Once the cyst volume has been calculated pre- and post-operatively, it is possible to assign radiological outcomes based on the percentage of improvement. A volume reduction dichotomised to >50% or <50% is most commonly used in the literature to demonstrate surgical success. Helland et al. have expanded this to describe a simple 1–4 scoring system ranging from complete cyst disappearance (NOG1), >50% reduction (NOG2) and <50% reduction (NOG3) to no change (NOG4) [17]. How well these classifications actually relate to clinical outcome will be described below.

4 Influence of Surgical Modality on Brain Plasticity

As already well described, there are three broad categories for surgical intervention to treat an AC. These are endoscopic fenestration, microsurgical fenestration/marsupialisation and cysto-peritoneal shunting. Choosing between approaches is based on cyst location and surgeon preference and will not be discussed here nor will the clinical outcomes; however we will consider the effect of surgical approach on post-operative cyst volume change.

4.1 Endoscopic Series

4.1.1 Sylvian Fissure Cysts

The Sylvian fissure AC is the most common location, and its adjacence to the basal cisterns makes it ideal to be treated by fenestration. Over the last 30 years as endoscopic technology has improved, there has been a shift towards performing these fenestrations endoscopically.

Li et al. [25] used volumetric segmentation for their 28 patients and found average pre-operative volume of 135 cm^3 which reduced to 93 cm^3 at

4-month follow-up of which 21% of patients did not change their volume at all. The series from Couvreur et al. [8] reported that 91% of patients with a Sylvian cyst treated endoscopically saw at least a 10% cyst volume reduction afterwards. This was further itemised by Galassi classification with 100% of Galassi 1 and 88% of Galassi 3 cysts reaching the threshold of 10% reduction. Gui et al. [15] found that 16% of Sylvian cysts radiologically fully resolved, 60% showed partial reduction and 24% did not change in volume. Okano et al. [30] found similar results with 11% disappearing completely and the remainder showing partial resolution.

Notwithstanding the different reporting measures for radiological outcomes, all series of Sylvian cysts report up to 20% of patients showing no improvement with approximately 10–20% seeing full resolution.

4.1.2 Suprasellar Cysts

Suprasellar cysts are naturally much smaller than those in the Sylvian fissure, and thus the absolute volume reduction is not comparable. Given that they are less common, there are fewer series published on their radiological outcomes compared to the Sylvian location. A useful classification scheme from Paris combines an anatomical origin of these cysts with clinical and radiological features [5].

Gangemi et al. [13] published a series of five suprasellar cysts managed endoscopically using a mixture of ventriculo-cystostomy and ventriculo-cysto-cisternostomy (VCC). They found an average volume reduction of 34% including one patient whose cyst was unchanged. Ma et al. [26] presented a larger series of 23 patients treated predominantly with VCC and found a 68% average volume reduction, double that seen by Gangemi et al. The high pre-operative volume (mean 39 cm^3) in Ma et al. may have resulted in large volume changes. Rizk et al. [33] only had six patients but started with an even higher mean of 153 cm^3 and achieved a 75% volume reduction. Lastly, Maher and Goumnerova [27] treated 11 patients using VCC but did not use volumetrics for comparison although they did find that 73% of cysts fully resolved and only one did not change at all.

4.2 Open Series

Open microsurgical techniques depend on the cyst location and proximity to a CSF space, and the options include fenestration into a cistern or ventricle or marsupialisation (remove the parietal cyst membrane) or both.

The Helland and Wester group presented a series of 45 patients [21] treated with craniotomy, parietal cyst wall resection and cistern fenestration, all of which were Sylvian in location. Using their NOG outcome classification, 55% of their patients achieved a 50% reduction in cyst volume or better, and only 4% had no change in cyst volume.

The series of 20 patients by Tamimi et al. [39] contained an assortment of locations and patient ages treated with fenestration and cyst wall removal. Eighty-five percent of the series had a Sylvian/fronto-temporo-parietal cyst making it loosely comparable to Helland and Wester, and they achieved an overall reduction in cyst volume from 111 cm^3 to 34 cm^3 (70% reduction). Only two patients had a reduction of less than 10%. Unfortunately, because they report outcomes using different measures, it isn't possible to make further comparisons between these two purely open series.

4.3 Cysto-peritoneal Shunt Series

The large series by Zhang et al. [43] of primary cysto-peritoneal shunting in children reports that only 5% of cysts did not reduce in volume. This is comparable to the two open series described above. Unfortunately, Zhang et al. did not include further details on cyst volumes or percent (%) volume reduction which are required to further compare this series to volume reduction in other treatment methods [43].

4.4 Series Comparing Surgical Modalities

Our series contained 56 patients treated with any of the three modalities [16]. The overall cyst volume change ranged from 30 to 40% for each technique which is more modest than some of the open series described above. Even when we focused on the subgroup with Sylvian cysts, both the endoscopic and microsurgical groups only achieved 25–30% volume reduction which is much lower than the 70% reported by Tamimi et al. [39]. Our clinical outcomes were still comparable despite the lower volume reduction as will be discussed further below.

Amelot et al. [4] published a large series of patients with Sylvian ACs with an average pre-operative volume of 107 cm^3 which matches Tamimi et al. [39] above. However, they also found lower volume reduction than Tamimi et al. ranging from 45 to 60%. Amelot et al. confirmed our results that there is little difference in radiological outcome between endoscopic and microsurgical procedures. Amelot et al. were able to better compare CP shunts and demonstrated that cyst volume reduction was greater (60%) than the other techniques albeit not significantly so.

The trend of greater volume reduction following CP shunting has been repeated in several other studies comparing the three treatment modalities. Kandenwein et al. [22] compared open fenestration (+ cyst wall resection in one third) to cysto-peritoneal shunting and found a higher volume reduction in shunts than with open fenestration (74% vs. 58%). Shim et al. [36] measured how many patients achieved >50% cyst volume reduction and found this threshold was reached in 100% of CP shunt, 92% of open procedures and only 75% of endoscopic fenestrations. Lastly, a systematic review of AC treatment in patients over 60 years old [28] reported using the Helland and Wester classification found that 85–88% of patients treated with cysto-peritoneal shunting or cyst wall resection achieved at least >50% volume reduction, but this was only achieved by 68% of patients treated with fenestration (endoscopic or microsurgical). This last paper is slightly marred by the grouping of microsurgical and endoscopic fenestrations together but does raise the suggestion that cyst wall removal may provide superior radiological results compared to fenestration alone.

Chen et al. [7] published a meta-analysis of treatment methods for Sylvian ACs. They report on the rate of cyst reduction and found that 93% of cysts treated with CP shunts reduce in size compared to 87% managed with craniotomy and 76% managed with endoscopy.

Comparing the cyst volume reduction across surgical modalities is inherently limited due to the heterogeneity of the groups. The current evidence is limited to small-volume single-centre series and a single meta-analysis on Sylvian cysts. The mixture of ages and cyst locations as well as different measures for radiological success makes it difficult to make direct comparison between techniques. It also does not recognise that clinical success in different locations, e.g. suprasellar or posterior fossa, may be achieved with smaller cyst volume changes and the technique offering the highest change of cyst obliteration may not be necessary.

Similar measurements of the ventricular system after successful endoscopic third ventriculostomy [37] showed that the degree of volume reduction correlated with the initial size (larger ventricles showed smaller reduction) and the chronicity of the symptoms (longer duration had smaller reduction). In addition, the ventricular size even after some reduction and clinical improvement remained supernormal and stabilized between 3 and 6 months. In contrast, measurements in hydrocephalic patients treated with VP shunts showed more obvious volume reductions and a tendency to stabilise between 6 and 12 months [42].

5 Correlation of Symptomatology to Cyst Volume Reduction

The primary aim of surgical intervention for the large or growing AC is to improve the symptoms experienced by the patient. The symptoms vary by cyst location but can include headaches, focal neurology, seizures, papilledema and reduced level of consciousness. In order to manage surgical goals and patient expectations, it is important to understand how radiological outcomes relate to clinical outcomes and thus what degree of brain plasticity and cyst reduction constitute a surgical success.

In our own series of 56 patients [16] with symptomatic ACs treated by either endoscopic, microsurgical or shunting techniques, we dichotomised patients based on volume reduction of greater or less than 50%. We found that the percentage of patients with symptom improvement or resolution was approximately 90% in both groups. Galarza et al. [12] found similar results with 100% of patients symptom-free after surgery despite two thirds of patients having <50% reduction in cyst volume. This was true for both fenestration and shunting procedures. Other case series [3, 8, 14, 24] report no correlation between radiological and clinical outcomes without providing specific data.

Contrary to the above series, Kandenwein et al. found that the amount of cyst resolution weakly correlated with the degree of clinical improvement ($r = 0.34$, $p = 0.035$). Although when dichotomising cyst volume reduction >50% and <50% as the series above, despite a clear trend favouring more good outcomes in the >50% reduction group, there was no significant difference. Unlike the series above which group all degrees of partial improvement together, Kandenwein's assessment of clinical improvement divided partial improvement into *slight* and *significant*. Thus, patients with only slight improvement may be diluting the treatment effect of larger volume reductions in other series.

Tamimi et al. [39] analysed a cohort of mixed cyst location in adults and paediatric patients treated by microsurgical fenestration. They grouped patients in the opposite manner by either complete or partial resolution of symptoms and found no difference in the percentage reduction in cyst volume in either group (49 vs. 60%).

The work by Helland and Wester further confirms the lack of correlation between size reduction and clinical outcomes in adults [18]. They found that 85% of patients had symptom reduction/resolution in both the groups with >50% and <50% cyst volume reduction. However, in their series on paediatric ACs, they did find a significant association between clinical and radiological outcomes [17]. Whether or not a paediatric subgroup of patients demonstrate better correlation between brain re-expansion and cyst volume reduction than adults is difficult to confirm as other paediatric cohorts have found no correlation [32].

The above studies measured clinical outcome using change in symptoms; however Mørkve et al. [29] prospectively included quality-of-life metrics (SF-36 and Glasgow Benefit Inventory) in addition to clinical symptoms. While they confirmed that improvement of symptoms including headache and dizziness improved quality of life, the degree of reduction in cyst volume was not associated with improved quality of life. Using a maze learning test around the hospital corridors, the Wester group demonstrated that in a cohort of mixed ages and cyst locations, the post-operative group performed better in maze learning, compared to pre-operatively, which correlated with symptom improvement but not with the degree of cyst volume reduction [21].

Karabagli and Etus [23] found that despite a clinical success rate of 90% only 55% of patients showed a reduction in cyst volume. However more than three quarters of patients had radiological evidence of a patent fenestration which suggests that cyst communication and thus intracystic pressure reduction are more important than cyst volume.

In conclusion, the evidence on whether clinical symptom improvement correlates with the percentage of cyst size reduction is limited to single-centre case series. The majority of these series report improvement following surgery but do not show a relationship between symptom improvement and cyst volume change. However, these series are often a mixture of ages and locations and contain low numbers; thus it remains possible that in certain subgroups a correlation does exist.

6 Temporal Pattern of Cyst Volume Reduction

It is expected that cyst volumes will reduce following surgery, but over what time period does this occur? Understanding this will help with patient counselling and planning routine post-operative imaging. Most surgical series describe a single point of follow-up, usually at the latest time point available, which misses how the cyst changes over time.

The series by Rabiei et al. [32] on paediatric cysts provides good long-term follow-up. They imaged patients at 3 and 12 months and found a significant different between pre-operative and 3 months, but no significant difference in cyst volumes between 3 and 12 months.

Schulz et al. [35] followed a paediatric series with mixed locations and treatment types for a median of 26 months. The short-term post-operative radiological follow-up (2–4 months) showed significantly smaller cyst volumes compared to pre-operatively, but no further significant reduction was seen at long-term follow-up (16–34 months). Lastly, Pitsika and Sgouros [31] published a small cohort of four patients which further confirms this picture whereby most of the improvement occurs in the first 3–6 months and then no/minimal change up to 48 months.

The similar results of these series show that all significant post-operative changes occur within the first few months (up to 6 months). Unfortunately, both of these series include a mixture of open and endoscopic techniques, and thus any differences due to surgical approach are not seen. Furthermore, neither series included CP shunting which instinctively is likely to cause even more rapid drainage of the cyst contents.

7 Brain Plasticity in Adults Compared to Children

Children and adults have different brain compliance depending on their age. Older people are known to have decreased brain compliance [9] and thus a decreased change in volume per unit of pressure. This affects brain plasticity when the intra-cystic pressure is released and thus the final volume of the cyst following surgery.

Making comparisons of volume reduction based on age is challenging because the recent literature is heavily weighted towards reporting paediatric rather than adult series. Furthermore, different methods of reporting, i.e. absolute volumes versus classifications, make it difficult to directly compare outcomes across the series. In order to make some comparisons based on age, we will focus on discussing the Sylvian cyst, as the archetypical location, in order to remove cyst location as a confounder.

The series by Helland et al. [17] reported just over half of their paediatric temporal cysts were no longer visible on follow-up imaging and a further 21% were reduced to between 0 and 50% giving an overall rate of 75% experiencing at least 50% size reduction. By comparison their adult series [20] demonstrated lower extents of volume whereby only 28% were completely obliterated and a further 32% showed at least 50% reduction meaning only 60% of their patients achieved at least 50% reduction.

The results from the adult series by Wang et al. [41] do not split partial resolution into > or <50% and so are difficult to compare to Helland et al. [20]. However, their rate of complete cyst resolution (12%) is less than half that reported by Helland. Notably both of these adult series treated >80% of their Sylvian cysts via craniotomy and the remainder with shunts (cysto-subdural in Helland et al. or cysto-peritoneal in Wang et al.) so how comparable these findings are to modern practice which favours endoscopic fenestration and how much the differences in radiological outcome are due to the different shunt procedure are unknown.

Karabagli and Etus [23] reported only 50% of paediatric patients had any cyst volume reduction which is much lower than Helland et al. Among other paediatric series, the pre-operative volume of a Sylvian AC ranges from 65 to 230 cm^3 which reduced to 15–119 cm^3 following surgery with an average volume reduction of 45–61% [4, 31, 32, 35]. These figures include treatment through either endoscopic or microsurgical techniques.

Given that Karabagli and Etus [23] found 50% of paediatric cysts did not improve and Schulz et al. [35] found that 22% of patients had <10% improvement (akin to no improvement), the results from El-Ghandour [11] suggest that infant patients may be a distinct subgroup with regard to radiological outcomes. El-Ghandour found that only 6% of infants with middle fossa cysts did not show radiological improvement following endoscopic fenestration. Why infants show favourable radiological outcomes compared to other children has not been discussed, but potential mechanisms may include differing compliance of the unmyelinated brain or different CSF hydrodynamics that change with age.

The work by Tamimi et al. [39] comparing the modified MacDonald method to 3D segmentation for measuring volumes includes volume changes in adults and children for direct comparison. The series had a mixture of locations with 55% being Sylvian; however the spread of locations was comparable between age groups. Children exhibited approximately 20% greater reduction in cyst volume post-operatively compared to adults when measured with 3D volumetric models. Of note, the opposite results were found using the modified MacDonald method; however 3D segmentation is regarded as more accurate. This result is consistent with the work by Helland et al. above.

Li et al. [25] provide a further direct comparison between adults and children using 3D segmentation models in their series of Sylvian cysts. They found a statistically significant difference in the ages of patients whose cyst volumes reduced compared to those that remained unchanged (4.5 vs. 19 years).

8 Illustrative Cases

The following cases demonstrate some of the findings discussed above. All segmentation models have been generated by the authors using Brainlab (Munich, Germany).

8.1 Case 1: Sylvian Fissure

A 4-year-old female presented through the emergency department with a 10-day history of progressive headaches and vomiting following a minor head injury. She had not previously suffered with headaches nor any other neurological symptoms. She had no past medical history. On examination she was GCS 15/15 with no focal neurological deficit. She underwent CT scan in her local hospital which demonstrated a left Sylvian AC with hygroma and 5 mm of midline shift which was later confirmed with MRI. The pre-operative T2 MRI (Fig. 2a) demonstrates the membranous boundary between the AC and the subdural space which can be further identified by the vessels which run in the outer, parietal cyst membrane but do not transverse the subdural space (Fig. 2b). Segmentation models show that the cyst volume is 74 cm^3, and the ipsilateral hygroma is 202 cm^3 (Fig. 3).

The patient underwent endoscopic fenestration with a left temporal burr hole followed by fenestrations through the cyst wall into the optico-carotid and carotid oculo-motor triangle. Post-operatively the patient made a full recovery. Their post-operative MRI scan at 3 months (Fig. 2c) shows the cyst now measures 15 cm^3 (80% reduction) and the midline shift has resolved, but the subdural hygroma has not changed at 202 cm^3 (Fig. 3).

The patient likely started with a very large Galassi type 3 cyst which ruptured into the subdural space following trauma. The cyst itself is well decompressed as a result of a patent fenestration with some visible brain plasticity, notably the frontal operculum, and an objectively reduced cyst volume. Interestingly the hygroma remains unchanged as the severely deformed brain is unable to expand enough to fill the void likely due to the long-standing nature of the compression. The presence of a hygroma is clinically insignificant though the patient is asymptomatic, and over the following years, the brain may expand further.

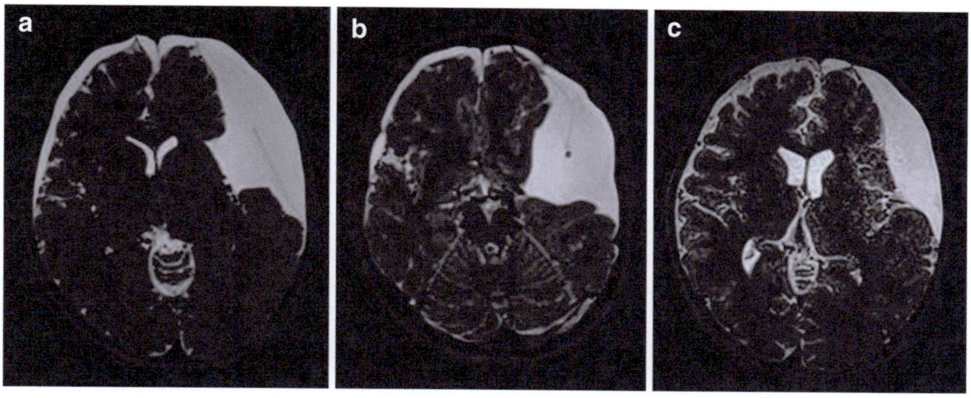

Fig. 2 Pre-operative MRI T2 sequence for case 1 (**a** + **b**) and post-operative MRI T2 (**c**)

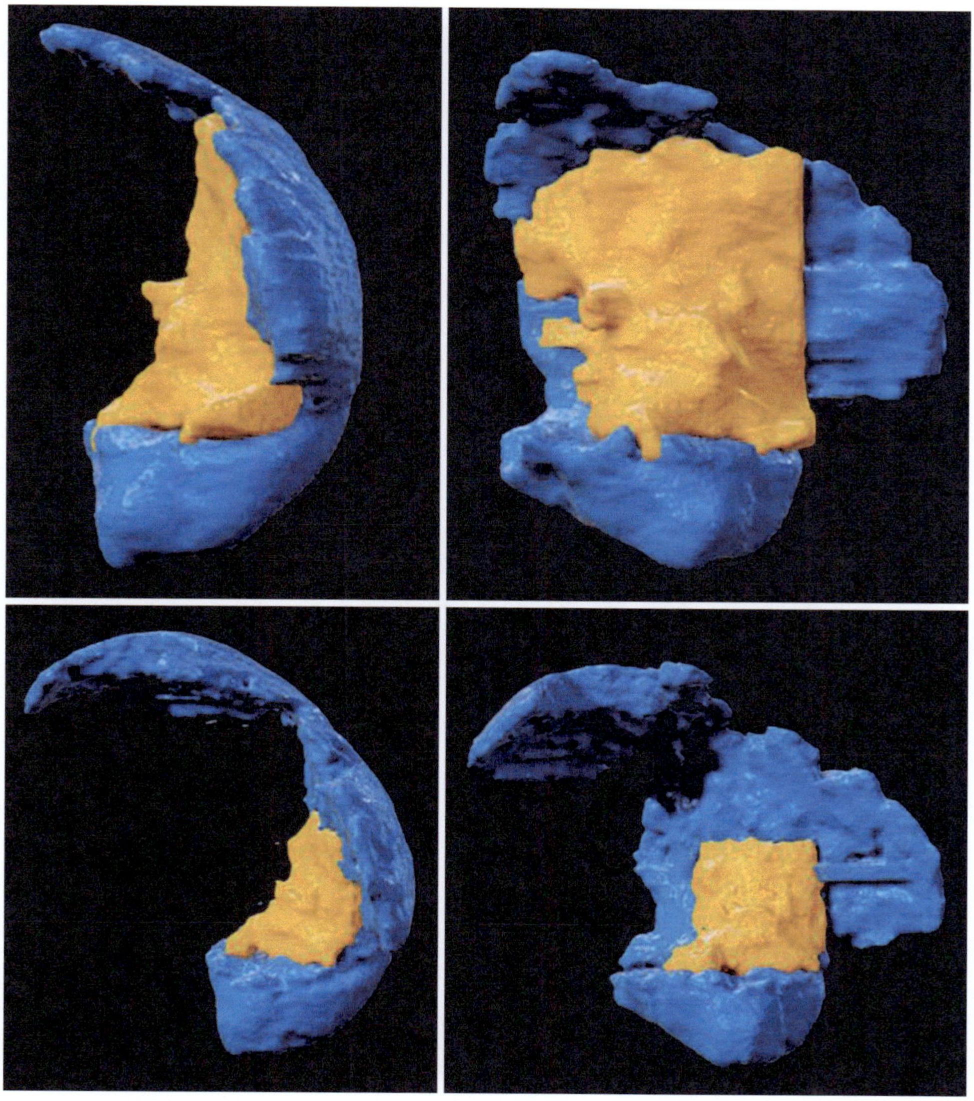

Fig. 3 Segmentation models demonstrating the cyst in yellow and subdural hygroma in blue (top, pre-operative; bottom, post-operative)

8.2 Case 2: Convexity AC

A male patient was born at term with an ante-natal diagnosis of a convexity AC. On examination he had macrocrania with a head circumference on the 99.6th centile but no other neurological deficit. He underwent MRI scan on day 2 of life (Fig. 4) which demonstrated a large convexity AC. Segmentation confirms the volume at 235 cm^3. Of note an ante-natal MRI scan 1 week prior to birth had a cyst volume of 201 cm^3.

The cyst wall extended to the quadrigeminal cistern which presents a potential site of fenestration. However, given the patient's young age and the high-risk anatomy in the quadrigeminal cistern, it was decided he should undergo a cysto-peritoneal shunt which was completed without incident on day 4. A post-operative MRI scan (Fig. 5) 1 month following surgery demonstrated complete obliteration of the cyst with a thin hygroma. He required no further surgical intervention and at 2 years of follow-up was developing normally, and his head circumference stabilised at the 91st centile.

This case demonstrates both the validity of minimally invasive approaches and the plasticity of the paediatric brain. While it is appealing to fenestrate the cyst because it is a definitive treatment option

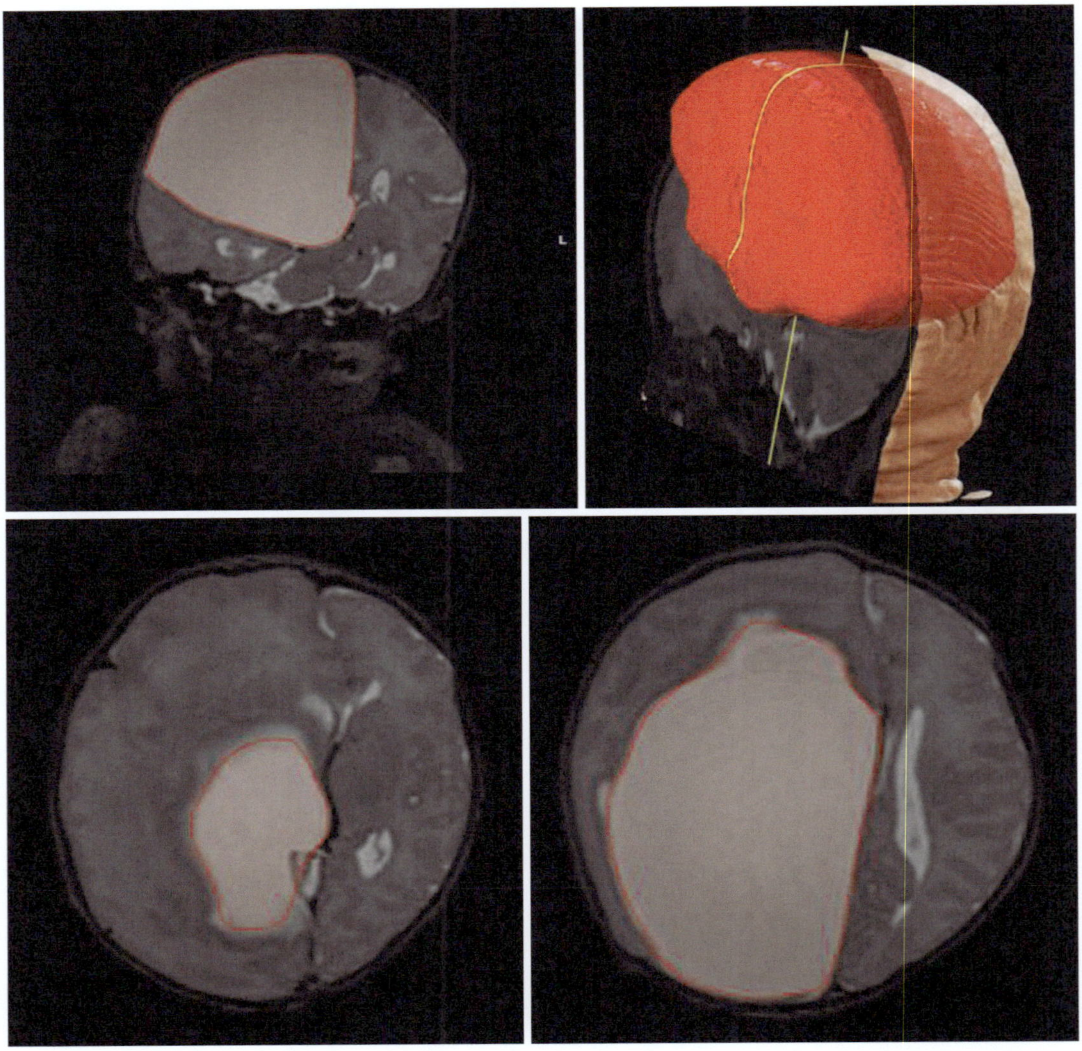

Fig. 4 Pre-operative MRI for case 2 including segmentation

and avoids the risk of shunt dependency, very good results are achievable with CP shunts. In this case the cyst rapidly emptied allowing full re-expansion of the brain. In the young, unmyelinated brain, there is little pressure differential across the stoma because the brain lacks stiffness to push against the cyst, whereas a shunt generates a much greater pressure differential between the intra-cystic and intra-abdominal compartments.

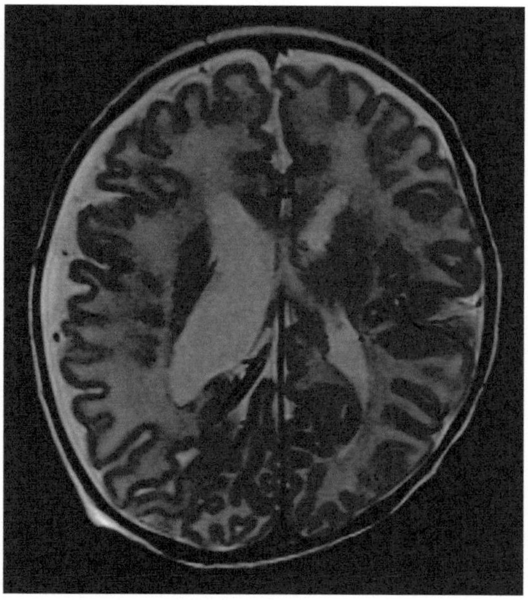

Fig. 5 Post-operative MRI for case 2

8.3 Case 3: Suprasellar AC

This 8-year-old girl is known to the neurosurgical department for undergoing a ventriculo-peritoneal shunt at 1 year of age to treat post-traumatic hydrocephalus. A routine MRI at 2 years of age demonstrated a suprasellar arachnoid cyst measuring 2.7 cm^3. This was managed conservatively with a repeat MRI at 8 years showing the cyst had grown to 3.7 cm^3 (Fig. 6a) and was now distorting the pituitary stalk and optic chiasm. Due to the concern of future endocrine and/or visual disturbance, she underwent an endoscopic ventriculo-cystostomy. Fenestration into the cistern was not possible due to thickened opaque arachnoid membranes which were not easily divided nor could vasculature be visualised. A post-operative MRI at 2 months (Fig. 6b) demonstrated the cyst volume had now reduced to 2.8 cm^3 (21% reduction) and the bowing of the pituitary stalk and optic tracts had reduced. Their post-operative course was uneventful, and they remain asymptomatic.

This case demonstrates the importance of the correct MRI sequences when dealing with small cysts in the suprasellar region. Being able to define the membranes is crucial in order to accurately measure the cyst volume especially when volumes are small and thus more suscep-

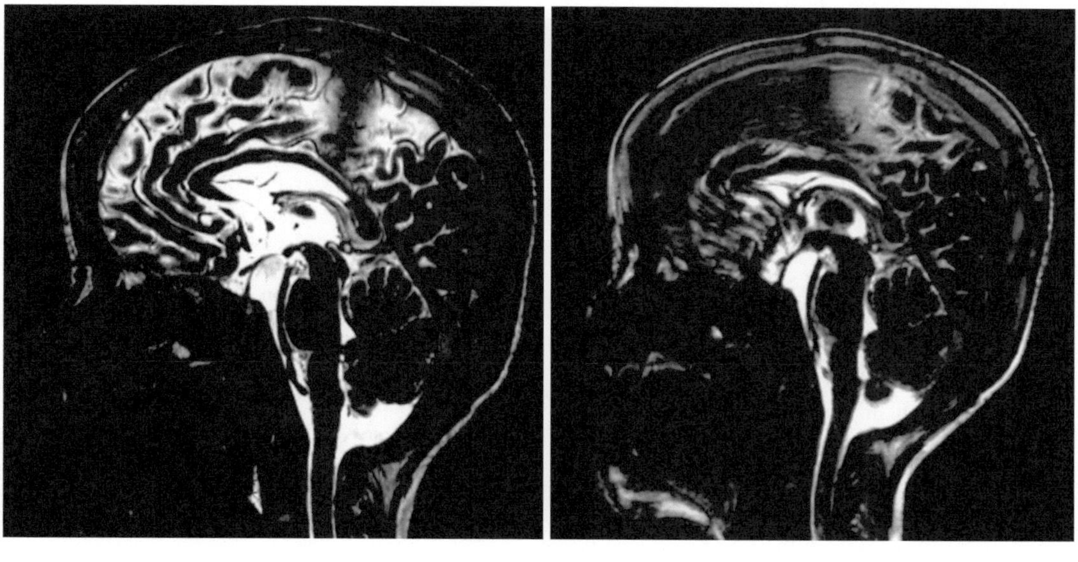

Fig. 6 Sagittal MRI for case 3 before (**a**) and after (**b**) surgery

tible to errors. It also demonstrates that cysts in some locations do not need a large volume change in order to achieve a clinically successful surgery.

9 Proposed Algorithm for the Follow-Up of Untreated Arachnoid Cysts

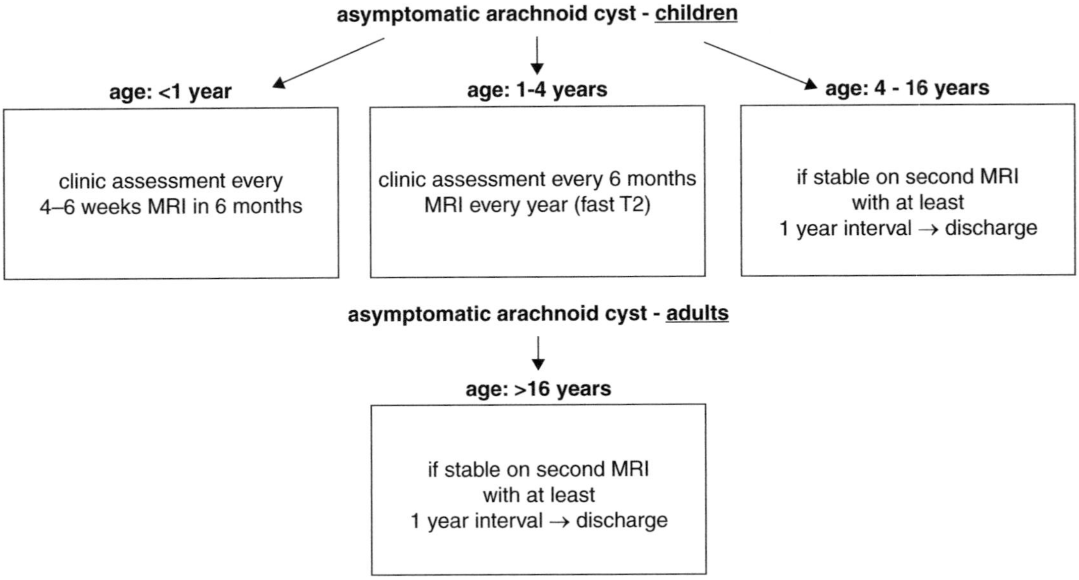

The above diagram shows an algorithm proposed by the senior author for the follow-up of asymptomatic ACs, based on the age of the patient at diagnosis. It is mostly applied for middle fossa ACs, and it's based on the seminal work of Al-Holou et al. [1, 2].

10 Conclusion

There is a significant literature reporting radiological outcomes after AC surgery. However, it is difficult to draw any conclusions on the cyst volume reduction following surgery due to the heterogeneity in outcome reporting. Ideally future series will present volumetric data in order to allow comparison between studies. A number of trends are noted in the studies discussed above. Firstly, cyst volume reduction following surgery does not correlate with clinical improvement. Secondly, the greatest change in cyst volume following surgery is seen in the first 6 months, with minimal reduction in volume seen beyond this time point. Finally, brain plasticity/cyst volume changes reduce as the patient ages. The primary role of post-operative imaging may therefore be to obtain a new baseline cyst volume to monitor for re-growth rather than as a marker of treatment success.

References

1. Al-Holou WN, Yew AY, Boomsaad ZE, Garton HJ, Muraszko KM, Maher CO. Prevalence and natural history of arachnoid cysts in children. J Neurosurg Pediatr. 2010;5(6):578–85.
2. Al-Holou WN, Terman S, Kilburg C, Garton HJ, Muraszko KM, Maher CO. Prevalence and natural history of arachnoid cysts in adults. J Neurosurg. 2013;118(2):222–31.
3. Ali M, Bennardo M, Almenawer SA, Zagzoog N, Smith AA, Dao D, et al. Exploring predictors of surgery and comparing operative treatment approaches for pediatric intracranial arachnoid cysts: a case series of 83 patients. J Neurosurg Pediatr. 2015;16(3):275–82.

4. Amelot A, Beccaria K, Blauwblomme T, Bourgeois M, Paternoster G, Cuny ML, et al. Microsurgical, endoscopic, and shunt management of pediatric temporosylvian arachnoid cysts: a comparative study. J Neurosurg Pediatr. 2019;23(6):749–57.
5. André A, Zérah M, Roujeau T, Brunelle F, Blauwblomme T, Puget S, et al. Suprasellar arachnoid cysts: toward a new simple classification based on prognosis and treatment modality. Neurosurgery. 2016;78(3):370–9; discussion 9-80.
6. Budday S, Ovaert TC, Holzapfel GA, Steinmann P, Kuhl E. Fifty shades of brain: a review on the mechanical testing and modeling of brain tissue. Arch Comput Methods Eng. 2020;27(4):1187–230.
7. Chen Y, Fang HJ, Li ZF, Yu SY, Li CZ, Wu ZB, et al. Treatment of middle cranial fossa arachnoid cysts: a systematic review and meta-analysis. World Neurosurg. 2016;92:480–90.e2.
8. Couvreur T, Hallaert G, Van Der Heggen T, Baert E, Dewaele F, Kalala Okito JP, et al. Endoscopic treatment of temporal arachnoid cysts in 34 patients. World Neurosurg. 2015;84(3):734–40.
9. Czosnyka M, Czosnyka ZH, Whitfield PC, Donovan T, Pickard JD. Age dependence of cerebrospinal pressure-volume compensation in patients with hydrocephalus. J Neurosurg. 2001;94(3):482–6.
10. Dang M, Modi J, Roberts M, Chan C, Mitchell JR. Validation study of a fast, accurate, and precise brain tumor volume measurement. Comput Methods Prog Biomed. 2013;111(2):480–7.
11. El-Ghandour NMF. Endoscopic treatment of intracranial cysts in infants: personal experience and review of literature. Childs Nerv Syst. 2021;37(11):3447–53.
12. Galarza M, Pomata HB, Pueyrredón F, Bartuluchi M, Zuccaro GN, Monges JA. Symptomatic supratentorial arachnoid cysts in children. Pediatr Neurol. 2002;27(3):180–5.
13. Gangemi M, Colella G, Magro F, Maiuri F. Suprasellar arachnoid cysts: endoscopy versus microsurgical cyst excision and shunting. Br J Neurosurg. 2007;21(3):276–80.
14. Gangemi M, Seneca V, Colella G, Cioffi V, Imperato A, Maiuri F. Endoscopy versus microsurgical cyst excision and shunting for treating intracranial arachnoid cysts. J Neurosurg Pediatr. 2011;8(2):158–64.
15. Gui S, Bai J, Wang X, Zong X, Li C, Cao L, et al. Assessment of endoscopic treatment for quadrigeminal cistern arachnoid cysts: a 7-year experience with 28 cases. Childs Nerv Syst. 2016;32(4):647–54.
16. Hall S, Smedley A, Rae S, Mathad N, Waters R, Chakraborty A, et al. Clinical and radiological outcomes following surgical treatment for intra-cranial arachnoid cysts. Clin Neurol Neurosurg. 2019;177:42–6.
17. Helland CA, Wester K. A population-based study of intracranial arachnoid cysts: clinical and neuroimaging outcomes following surgical cyst decompression in children. J Neurosurg. 2006;105(5 Suppl):385–90.
18. Helland CA, Wester K. Arachnoid cysts in adults: long-term follow-up of patients treated with internal shunts to the subdural compartment. Surg Neurol. 2006;66(1):56–61; discussion.
19. Helland CA, Wester K. Intracystic pressure in patients with temporal arachnoid cysts: a prospective study of preoperative complaints and postoperative outcome. J Neurol Neurosurg Psychiatry. 2007;78(6):620–3.
20. Helland CA, Wester K. A population based study of intracranial arachnoid cysts: clinical and neuroimaging outcomes following surgical cyst decompression in adults. J Neurol Neurosurg Psychiatry. 2007;78(10):1129–35.
21. Isaksen E, Leet TH, Helland CA, Wester K. Maze learning in patients with intracranial arachnoid cysts. Acta Neurochir. 2013;155(5):841–8. discussion 8.
22. Kandenwein JA, Richter HP, Börm W. Surgical therapy of symptomatic arachnoid cysts - an outcome analysis. Acta Neurochir. 2004;146(12):1317–22; discussion 22.
23. Karabagli H, Etus V. Success of pure neuroendoscopic technique in the treatment of Sylvian arachnoid cysts in children. Childs Nerv Syst. 2012;28(3):445–52.
24. Khan IS, Sonig A, Thakur JD, Nanda A. Surgical management of intracranial arachnoid cysts: clinical and radiological outcome. Turk Neurosurg. 2013;23(2):138–43.
25. Li Y, Chen X, Xu B. The efficacy of neuroendoscopic treatment for middle cranial fossa arachnoid cysts assessed by MRI 3D segmentation and modeling. Childs Nerv Syst. 2014;30(6):1037–44.
26. Ma G, Li X, Qiao N, Zhang B, Li C, Zhang Y, et al. Suprasellar arachnoid cysts in adults: clinical presentations, radiological features, and treatment outcomes. Neurosurg Rev. 2021;44(3):1645–53.
27. Maher CO, Goumnerova L. The effectiveness of ventriculocystocisternostomy for suprasellar arachnoid cysts. J Neurosurg Pediatr. 2011;7(1):64–72.
28. Merola J, Manivannan S, Ooi S, Chia WL, Makwana M, Lang J, et al. The efficacy of cystoperitoneal shunting for the surgical management of intracranial arachnoid cysts in the elderly: a systematic review of the literature. Surg Neurol Int. 2021;12:624.
29. Mørkve SH, Helland CA, Amus J, Lund-Johansen M, Wester KG. Surgical decompression of arachnoid cysts leads to improved quality of life: a prospective study. Neurosurgery. 2016;78(5):613–25.
30. Okano A, Ogiwara H. The effectiveness of microsurgical fenestration for middle fossa arachnoid cysts in children. Childs Nerv Syst. 2016;32(1):153–8.
31. Pitsika M, Sgouros S. Volume change of cranial arachnoid cysts after successful endoscopic fenestration in symptomatic children. Childs Nerv Syst. 2019;35(12):2313–8.
32. Rabiei K, Högfeldt MJ, Doria-Medina R, Tisell M. Surgery for intracranial arachnoid cysts in children-a prospective long-term study. Childs Nerv Syst. 2016;32(7):1257–63.
33. Rizk E, Chern JJ, Tagayun C, Tubbs RS, Hankinson T, Rozzelle C, et al. Institutional experience of endoscopic suprasellar arachnoid cyst fenestration. Childs Nerv Syst. 2013;29(8):1345–7.

34. Sack I, Streitberger KJ, Krefting D, Paul F, Braun J. The influence of physiological aging and atrophy on brain viscoelastic properties in humans. PLoS One. 2011;6(9):e23451.
35. Schulz M, Oezkan Y, Schaumann A, Sieg M, Tietze A, Thomale UW. Surgical management of intracranial arachnoid cysts in pediatric patients: radiological and clinical outcome. J Neurosurg Pediatr. 2021;2021:1–11.
36. Shim KW, Lee YH, Park EK, Park YS, Choi JU, Kim DS. Treatment option for arachnoid cysts. Childs Nerv Syst. 2009;25(11):1459–66.
37. St George E, Natarajan K, Sgouros S. Changes in ventricular volume in hydrocephalic children following successful endoscopic third ventriculostomy. Childs Nerv Syst. 2004;20(11-12):834–8.
38. Taha AA, Hanbury A. Metrics for evaluating 3D medical image segmentation: analysis, selection, and tool. BMC Med Imaging. 2015;15:29.
39. Tamimi AF, Al Ryalat NT, Al Qaisi AK, Juweid ME, Obeidat FN, Al Hyasat TG, et al. Microsurgical fenestration of intracranial arachnoid cysts: volumetric analysis and clinical outcome. Pediatr Neurosurg. 2021;56(1):35–44.
40. Tan Z, Li Y, Zhu F, Zang D, Zhao C, Li C, et al. Children with intracranial arachnoid cysts: classification and treatment. Medicine. 2015;94(44):e1749.
41. Wang Y, Wang F, Yu M, Wang W. Clinical and radiological outcomes of surgical treatment for symptomatic arachnoid cysts in adults. J Clin Neurosci. 2015;22(9):1456–61.
42. Xenos C, Sgouros S, Natarajan K, Walsh AR, Hockley A. Influence of shunt type on ventricular volume changes in children with hydrocephalus. J Neurosurg. 2003;98(2):277–83.
43. Zhang B, Zhang Y, Ma Z. Long-term results of cystoperitoneal shunt placement for the treatment of arachnoid cysts in children. J Neurosurg Pediatr. 2012;10(4):302–5.

Future Management of Arachnoid Cysts

Oreste de Divitiis, Vincenzo Meglio, Carmen Buchicchio, Elena d'Avella, and Giuseppe Cinalli

1 Introduction

Arachnoid cysts (ACs) are benign extra-axial fluid-filled neoformations, located within the layer of the arachnoid membrane, with an intensity of the contained liquid that resembles the cerebrospinal fluid (CSF) on magnetic resonance imaging (MRI) [17]. ACs are typically found in the pediatric population (75% of cases), even though they can be found among adults as well [1, 2, 22]. Since their first description by Richard Bright in 1831 [7], much progress has been made in their management, including the implementation of microscopic and endoscopic surgical approaches. However, nowadays a plateau seems to have been reached in this direction, with a slowing down in the developing of new treatment strategies.

In this chapter we attempt to provide a picture of what is the current scenario in AC treatment, trying to point out the main points of weakness, considering them as opportunities for harboring new research pathways to future implementation in the management of a such fascinating pathology.

O. de Divitiis (✉) · V. Meglio · C. Buchicchio
E. d'Avella
Division of Neurosurgery, Department of Neurosciences and Reproductive and Odontostomatological Sciences, Università degli Studi di Napoli Fedserico II, Naples, Italy

G. Cinalli
Department of Pediatric Neurosciences, Pediatric Neurosurgery Unit, Santobono-Pausilipon Children's Hospital, Naples, Italy

2 State of the Art

In order to approach the future, being aware of the present is mandatory. Currently, there are many possible therapeutic strategies available for the neurosurgeon that wants to treat a patient with ACs. According to the majority of the papers in the literature, observation via periodic imaging acquisitions is the main adopted strategy for the management of asymptomatic ACs that are the most common ones identified. However, there are some situations, namely, symptomatic or growing cysts, where adopting an active strategy turns out to be necessary. In these cases, surgery is the only possible choice since non-surgical options, such as acetazolamide, lead to poor results [31].

The principal aim of surgical treatment is to allow the trapped liquor to drain into other corridors, natural or artificial [15]. Moreover, another option is to obtain the complete excision of the cyst. In both cases, the final goals consist of reducing the pressure that the cysts exert on the surrounding structures or eliminating an eventual obstruction of CSF flow [27]. These objectives can be reached by adopting different strategies including cyst fenestration, aspiration of the cyst, shunting, and microscopic dissection, with cyst excision. These different conceptual possibilities translate into many different surgical techniques, namely, endoscopic fenestration, microsurgical open fenestration or excision, stereotactic intracavitary aspiration or irradiation, and cysto-

M. Turgut et al. (eds.), *Arachnoid Cysts*, https://doi.org/10.1007/978-3-031-22701-1_33

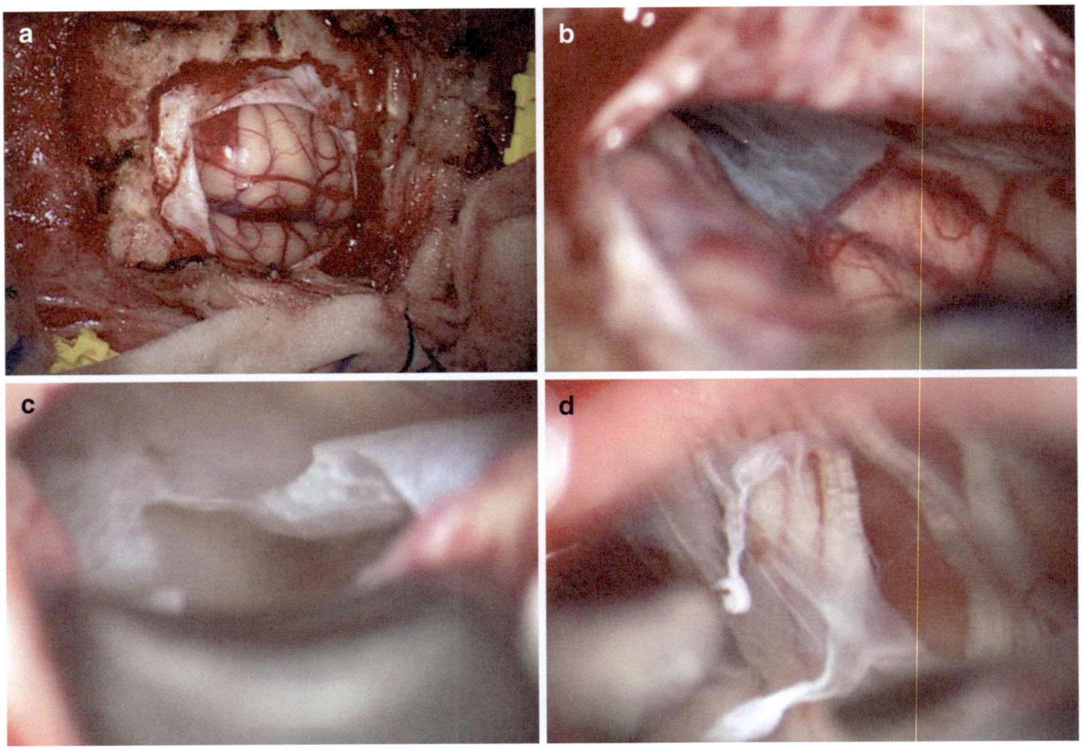

Fig. 1 Intraoperative images of a right cerebellopontine angle cyst, approached by a right retrosigmoid craniotomy. (**a**) After dural opening, the right cerebellum hemisphere is exposed. (**b**) Gentle retraction of the right cerebellar hemisphere and exposure of the cyst's wall. (**c**) Opening of the cyst's wall. (**d**) Visualization from the inside of the cyst. It's possible to recognize facial and stato-acoustic cranial nerves at the emergence in correspondence of the entry zone

peritoneal shunt, each one offering advantages and disadvantages (Fig. 1) [15, 27].

Neuroendoscopy has become more and more popular in the last decade, due to its minimally invasiveness; major safety; suitability in treating CSF-filled neoformations, like ACs; and the possibility of exploiting a natural road for CSF evacuation [13, 42, 51, 59, 67]. For all these reasons, it's being considered the method of choice in the surgical treatment of ACs, becoming the preferred approach of many neurosurgeons [51].

In addition, as meticulously reported by Oertel et al., the endoscopic approach comprises different application modalities, with specific indications, pros, and cons, namely, cisternostomy, cystoventriculostomy, ventriculocystostomy, and ventriculocysto-cisternostomy [52]. In actuating these different modalities, laser-assisted endoscopic fenestration is one of the most interesting applications in the field on neuroendoscopic AC management (Fig. 2) [8, 66].

Despite this multitude of options and the overall acceptable results obtained with them, there is no doubt that there are still margins for future improvements in giving the best possible long-term results to AC patients. Let's analyze these aspects more in depth.

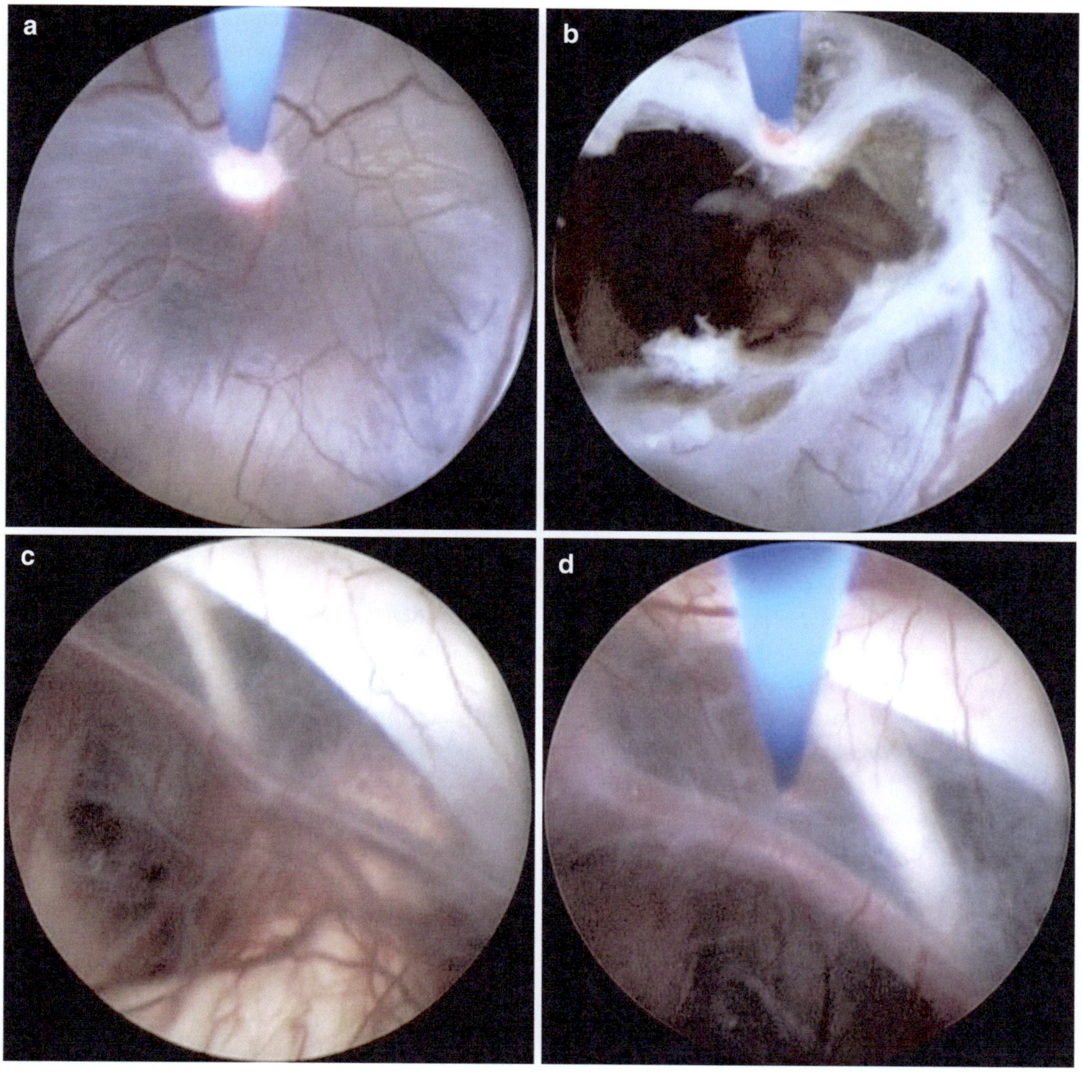

Fig. 2 Endoscopic trans-ventricular trans-foraminal endoscopic laser-assisted fenestration of a cyst of the choroidal fissure. (**a**, **b**) The cyst's wall laser fenestration. (**c**) Examination of the visceral layer of the AC's wall. It's possible to appreciate the tentorium, right third cranial nerve, right inner carotid artery with its bifurcation, and the optic chiasm. (**d**) Inner cyst's membrane fenestration. It's possible to recognize the basilar artery, the posterior cerebral artery, and the superior cerebellar artery

3 Future of AC Treatment

3.1 Indications: Signaling the Path

When planning the best treatment strategy for an AC patient, the first issue that immediately stands out is a lack of clear, solid, and unique guidelines or globally accepted criteria that are able to provide an unambiguous decisional base for neurosurgeons that approach this entity, especially for younger ones. This issue was already raised by other authors, like Juan F. Martínez-Lage et al., almost 10 years ago, but not much has changed since then [44, 59]. From an analysis of the literature, only a few defined guidelines are present, much regarding the management of obstructive hydrocephalus from suprasellar-prepontine ACs [46, 67]. These guidelines are derived from case reports and reported series, providing at most class II or III evidence. At the moment, to the best of our knowledge, treatment choices are taken mainly based on the surgeon's experience and preferences, representing, in our opinion, the first main issue in AC management, seeking for future improvements.

More specifically, in retracing all the decisional process to the best therapeutic strategy, two main criticisms stand out needing major attention from the neurosurgical society. The first main issue is the decision between adopting an active surgical approach and a conservative observation option. This topic, indeed, is still under debate among the scientific society mainly because of the lack of both randomized case-controlled class I studies and retrospective studies [45]. From an analysis of the literature over the last 30 years, it stands out that a certain grade of accordance is present in suggesting an observational approach for asymptomatic ACs, as surgery may be associated with morbidity [14, 36, 57]. In these cases, follow-up with neuroimaging modalities, namely, computed tomography (CT) and MRI, is the adopted treatment strategy. There are some authors, however, that are even in disagreement [56]. Mustansir et al., for example, recommend surgical treatment for all cysts that have large dimensions (Fig. 4), regardless of the presence of symptoms, and the observational approach is only for smaller asymptomatic ones. In this way, they focus more on cyst dimension rather than on the presence or not of symptoms [48]. Other authors also support this attitude [24, 38]. Masoudi et al., in a recent report of a series of 29 patients, suggest also treating asymptomatic patients with AC if they show macrocranium or increased head circumference. Interestingly, they also indicate observation as the first choice in symptomatic patients if headache is the only symptom. Thus, according to this group, the presence of symptoms is not enough to clearly indicate the necessity of a surgical approach [45]. According to Cincu et al., even in a frankly symptomatic AC patient, the relationship between the clinical manifestation and the cyst should be explored carefully, remarking on the necessity for objective criteria. Misjudging this correlation, indeed, may lead to a major risk of the procedure failing [15]. Tamburrini et al. also remarked on the uncertainty regarding the necessity or not of preventive surgery in asymptomatic patients, specifically regarding Sylvian fissure ACs. He concluded that most of the authors do not indicate this type of active approach, preferring a passive one. In conclusion, even today, choosing between an active surgical approach to ACs and a conservative one is still a matter of personal experience, and clear guidelines on the topic are lacking. Considering that this is a life-changing decision, this situation is no more acceptable in the age of the evidence-based medicine [67].

Secondly, which surgical approach to prefer is still a questioned issue, with a lot of controversies and variabilities among different centers and the final decision placed on the surgeon shoulders [14, 45, 57]. In our opinion, this represents a big issue that needs to be urgently clarified. Jung Won Choi et al., in 2015, advocated for "much clearer and stricter criteria for surgical treatment of ACs" and a set of guidelines, considering the undoubtable rising in prevalence that this pathology is showing in the modern neuroimaging era [14]. Interesting elements are already present in the literature. Oertel et al., in a paper presenting their experience of 95 endoscopic cyst fenestration procedures, suggest favoring the endoscopic technique when two anatomic elements are presents: a sufficient contiguity between the cyst and other CSF natural pathways and when the location of the cyst is particularly suitable to this approach. Regarding the latter, the suprasellar, quadrigeminal, and the posterior fossa are eligible locations for the endoscopic fenestration option [51]. Jung Won Choi et al., in a case series ranging over a 12-year period, also based their choice on the cyst's location. They opted, indeed, for the endoscopic approach in the case of deep-seated cysts and for the microsurgical one in the management of superficially located ACs. Interestingly, after having treated both locations with endoscopic approach for over 10 years, only after 2000 the authors moved to the microsurgical approach in case of superficial cysts. They justify this decision as an attempt in reducing the risk of post-operative CSF leakage. However, also for this group, the location is the main criteria for choosing the better approach. Finally, the authors suggest to prefer a cysto-peritoneal shunt as the approach of choice in infant patients, introducing the age of the patient as another criteria to consider [14]. As reported in a review of the literature, endoscopic fenestration is to be selected not only for suprasellar ACs but also in the case of multiloculated cysts, focusing in this way also on the composition of cyst and not just on its location. Always considering this aspect, craniotomy should be preferred instead for well-circumscribed ACs, if they are not associated with hydrocephalus or acute events, meaning that also clinical aspects play a role in determining the necessary type of surgery. Finally, the authors of the review indicate cyst shunting preferentially for middle cranial fossa cists (Fig. 3), with raised intracranial pressure [15]. Gustavo Pradilla et al. recommend cysto-peritoneal shunt not only for ACs associated with intracranial hypertension but also extend the indications of this technique to the cases of failed cyst fenestration [54].

In summary, there are many aspects that must be considered in choosing the best surgical technique for AC treatment, creating a difficult decision. Thus, in a future prospective, a more precise definition of the main criteria which can help the neurosurgeon in adopting one certain surgical approach over another, from our point of view, may bring a great improvement in the management of patients with ACs.

3.2 Future Improvements in Endoscopic Surgery: Cysto-E(Cho)Volution

Although for a long time the endoscopic approach for AC fenestration has been debated, the approach of choice in treating ACs in both infant and adult patients is further and further considered [14, 16, 21, 48, 57]. This diffusion is due to different reasons. One is, for example, the proximity of the cysts which are usually present near to the subarachnoid cisterns and the ventricular system. This aspect, indeed, offers the opportunity of fenestrating these cysts into the CSF spaces using a safe, minimally invasive, effective, and rapid technique, associated with a reduction in blood loss, in comparison to the open microsurgical approach. Moreover, this approach also avoids shunt-related complications [17], which is a considerable advantage especially for pediatric ACs.

Despite seeming to be so near to the perfect approach, there is no doubt that also the endoscopic approach presents some limits. Jung Won

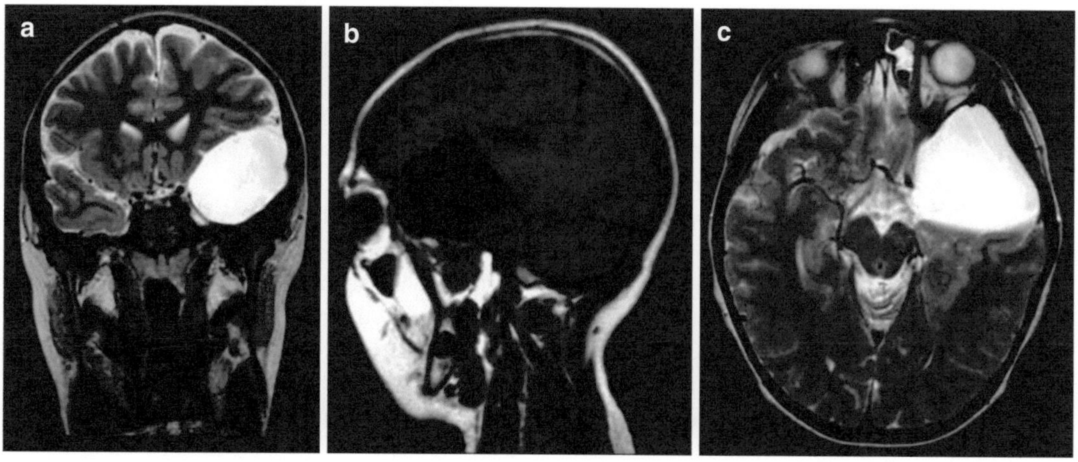

Fig. 3 Magnetic resonance imaging (MRI) sequences showing a middle cranial fossa cyst. From the coronal T2w (**a**), sagittal T1w (**b**), and axial T2w (**c**) MRI sequences, it's possible to appreciate the absence of cerebral parenchyma, filled by the cyst

Choi et al., in a study considering the surgical outcome from a series of patients endoscopically treated for intracranial ACs, reported that it carries more surgical complications than the open microscopic technique, especially in terms of CSF leakage rates and deficits in extraocular movement development, due to cranial nerve injury [14]. Other authors also remarked, instead, on the higher risk of reformation of membranes and the recurrence of the pathology, when the endoscopic approach is applied [23, 34, 48, 52]. Finally, also finding the right place to put the fenestration on the cyst's wall can be more difficult with the endoscopic visualization technique, instead of with the microsurgical approach [52].

Fortunately, we live in a high-tech phase of human evolution, where many intraoperative image-guidance systems have been implemented and are at the disposal of the neurosurgeon, leading to the so-called neuronavigation-supported surgery. The term neuronavigation indicates a well-accepted methodology of image-guided surgery which has proved to be useful in enhancing the safety and accuracy of many surgical procedures, minimizing the risks of injuring vital structures, also in neuroendoscopy. More precisely, neuronavigation is already used in the endoscopic treatment of ACs, chiefly in recent times, based on many different navigation methods, among which the preferred are intraoperative computed tomography, pre-operative or intraoperative MRI, stereotaxis, and even endoscopy itself [4, 66]. Despite being undoubtedly powerful and useful instruments for neuronavigation, there are some specific aspects that can undermine their surgical application [4]. The main aspect to focus on in considering the limits of these tools when applied to AC surgery is that these items are usually used based on pre-operative films. This is an issue, especially in considering that intraoperative landmarks change frequently their position during AC surgery, for technical reasons. In fact, in this type of surgery, the fenestration of the cyst itself induces a redistribution of the CSF fluid. Moreover, blood collection in the surgical field is often present during the procedure. Both of these elements can clearly lead to a considerable shift of brain structures, making pre-operative films almost useless [35]. Of utmost relevance is that this landmark shift happens during the earliest phases of the procedure, as many surgeons prefer to pierce the cyst before performing the very cyst fenestration [61]. The result is that the so-called neuronavigation system do not really perform its main goal, acting more on the contrary as an "approach imaging" tool [55]. For these reasons, in our opinion, the wider implementation for AC surgery of a well-known tool, namely, the intraoperative endoscopic ultrasonography (US), may result in promising future improvements in AC therapeutic management.

Pioneered by general surgeons for tracking the changes in position of soft tissues, this image-guided surgery instrument can be very helpful in solving the intraoperative problems related to "brain-shift" AC surgery [6, 28]. Despite the enormous development that intraoperative endoscopic US technique has shown in many neighboring disciplines over the last decades, this image-guiding instrument has been a little bit overlooked. According to Klaus et al., this is a consequence mostly of the excellent results in visualization achieved with other tools, like CT and MRI, based on both intraoperative and pre- and post-operative films. However, these powerful systems are far from perfection, presenting many limitations that make them less suitable for AC image-guided surgery. First of all, they still lack in real-time information, configuring them as "approach imaging" techniques, more than navigation ones [55]. In addition, this surgery assistance tools significantly interrupt the surgical workflow, showing troubles in repeated intraoperative scanning and prolonging the surgical time. Moreover, they are very costly machines, not affordable to every center, especially concerning the intraoperative MRI. This issue makes it available only in a small proportion of hospitals, also because its usage requires specialized non-ferromagnetic instruments. Finally, intraoperative CT presents an additional disadvantage, which consists of the exposure to ionizing radiation of both the operators and the patient. This latter aspect is of particular importance in AC pathology, considering its preponderance in affecting pediatric population [50].

Keeping in mind the limits of these more widely used tools and with the aim to overcome them, we want to stress that endoscopic US technique, with some technical implementations, may be the only one available for navigation systems which could offer interesting improvements in a future perspective. This visualization tool, indeed, is characterized by being low cost and by the absence of logistical troubles, making it easily available to most neurosurgical centers and configuring itself as a cost-effective option [30, 55]. Furthermore, it is the only available navigation tool that is able to provide intraoperative real-time image guidance, improving AC surgery precision and efficacy, especially in cases of absent landmarks or displacement, allowing neurosurgeons to manage AC's surgery in a safer and more precise manner. It would be interesting to see how better-designed probes may contribute, especially in critical scenarios, in the near future. One example of criticism is the necessity of fenestrating a very thick basal cyst wall. This is a critical situation because the thickness configures a situation of reduced visibility through the cyst wall. The result is an increased risk of damaging the anatomical structures caudal to the cyst [66]. In this situation, endoscopic US can bring a great contribution in improving safety, also considering that a thicker membrane makes the operator more confident in applying the probe on the cystic wall. The result is a more efficient definition of the anatomical structures, converting a critical issue into a strength.

Obviously, in the actual state, although presenting promising advantages, endoscopic US is not free from important limitations. It is indeed characterized by a low-definition visualization quality. Moreover, it is a user-dependent instrument that requires a long learning curve which can be discouraging for younger neurosurgeons. Finally, this visualization technique is still bound to the necessity of physical contact to the surface of the structure that it is required to visualize. This could be dangerous since it may increase the risk of intraoperative blood collections and CSF fistula.

Noteworthy, these issues are mainly related to the probe's technical advance, and, for this reason, we are confident that they may be overcome in the near future, leading endoscopic US to play a key role in improving the efficacy of the surgical approach to ACs.

In conclusion, ultrasound should not be considered as an MRI/CT competitor, but it can surely fix many problems that are not fixed otherwise. Moreover, further implementations in image-guided processes may allow for more precise path planning and placement of the endoscope in AC surgery, improving the efficacy of endoscopic fenestrations and minimizing collateral damage.

3.3 Robotic Surgery for AC Treatment: Are We Ready for the (Robo)Revolution?

Speaking of future strategies for the treatment of neurosurgical pathologies (like ACs), it seems impossible to not consider a relatively new therapeutic option which is showing a rapid spreading all over the different fields of surgery: robotics. This appears even more true for neurosurgery, considering that this fascinating surgical branch firmly consists of high-tech accuracy-demanding procedures. It is not the first time that neurosurgery changes radically its shape by drawing from new technological inventions being maybe the most technology-intensive surgical discipline. Already recognized milestones in the path to the modern neurosurgery are, for example, the introduction of microsurgery, by Yasargil and the Donagh group in 1970 [40, 47], which broadly changed the neurosurgical approach to intracranial pathologies; later, the application of endoscopy to neurosurgery, by Jho et al. in 1997, Guiot et al. in the 1960s, and M. Apuzzo in 1977, expanding the neurosurgical horizon by allowing the eyes of the surgeon to arrive inside the surgical field [3, 11, 26, 33]; and finally the implementation of intraoperative image guidance [43]. Nowadays, it seems more and more evident that we are progressively witnessing a new technical breakthrough in the neurosurgical operating room: the "robo-revolution," consisting in the introduction of robotics in neurosurgical procedures to overcome the human kind limits, for the purpose of bringing a better surgical management to the patient.

Despite first reporting of robotic usage in neurosurgery that dates back to 1985, robotic is not to be considered as a suggestion or something abstract and nebulous [37]. On the contrary, it already is a reality in many operating rooms all over the world, affirming itself as the physical branch of artificial intelligence [29]. It presents many potential uses in medicine, comprising surgeon assistance during operations. In this scenario, it offers many features that undoubtedly turn out to be very precious, especially in the neurosurgical field [58]. Enhanced precision and steadiness, tremor filtration, high-resolution and better visualization of the operative field (thanks to the three-dimensional interface), motion scaling, wider wrist motion freedom, improved ergonomics, and the opportunity of introducing more instruments and tools in narrowed spaces are only the worthiest of note, from a wide range of advantages that are continuously growing [32, 58]. Thus, considering the great potential contribution that robotics may bring to minimally invasive surgery, it seems obvious that also surgical management of ACs may have plenty of benefits from this new opportunity, perfectly matching the list of improvements necessary to meliorate AC surgical treatment.

Unfortunately, although being already a reality in some fields of neurosurgery, like deep brain stimulation, brain biopsy, and pedicle screw fixation, efforts are continuing to be made with the scope to integrate it into the domain of minimally invasive keyhole surgery, both endoscopic and microscopic [5, 18, 20, 64]. This may be due, in part, to the fact that the neurosurgical community has reached a comfort zone, made of advanced imaging, surgical navigation, and microsurgical technique that they don't want to abandon. In our opinion, we firmly believe that the time is ripe to start debating the actual effort that robotics can carry to the surgical AC management.

However, in introducing a new instrumentation or a new technique, careful evaluations must be made especially in considering if a real needing for changing is present and how this innovation will impact on actual know-how, carrying tangible new benefits to the patient. In this regard, it is important to consider that, although numerous types of surgical robotic systems have been designed and developed for various purposes, only a few of them reached commercial or clinical use, because the others didn't really offer satisfactory advantages to clinical practice. Particularly explicative in this sense is the story of the first robot introduced in neurosurgery, the PUMA (Programmable Universal Machine for Assembly, Advance Research and Robotic, Oxford, Connecticut). It was an industrial robotic arm with six degrees of freedom, which has been used for biopsy needle insertion into the brain in 1985 and for the successful resection of thalamic astrocytoma in six children [19, 37]. Since this device didn't lead to a clear advantage over the existing methods of performing surgery and carried safety concerns, its further development was dismissed [60]. Keeping this in mind, it is important to underline which are the issues present in AC treatments to focalize which are the ones that may benefit from robotic implementation.

AC is a pathology which requires very high-precision surgery, considering the risks related to cyst fenestration, such as cauterizing or cutting eloquent structures, causing neurological deficits to the patient. According to Tamburrini et al., microscopic treatment of these cysts is associated with the risk of focal motor and cranial nerve deficits and death as well. Moreover, neuroendoscopic cyst fenestration is limited by the difficulties faced in visualizing small cysts, especially for middle fossa ones which are often covered by the temporal lobe [67]. It's also to consider that in this type of surgery it is necessary to maneuver the endoscope in narrowed spaces, a thing that is not simple for a human surgeon [63]. Furthermore, having a secure path for reaching the cyst and having the ability to follow it in an impeccable way are mandatory, especially with very deeply placed ACs. In some cases of ACs of large dimensions (Fig. 4), it is possible to lose any reference point in guiding the choice of the fenestration, since the inner face of the cyst wall has the same appearance in all its

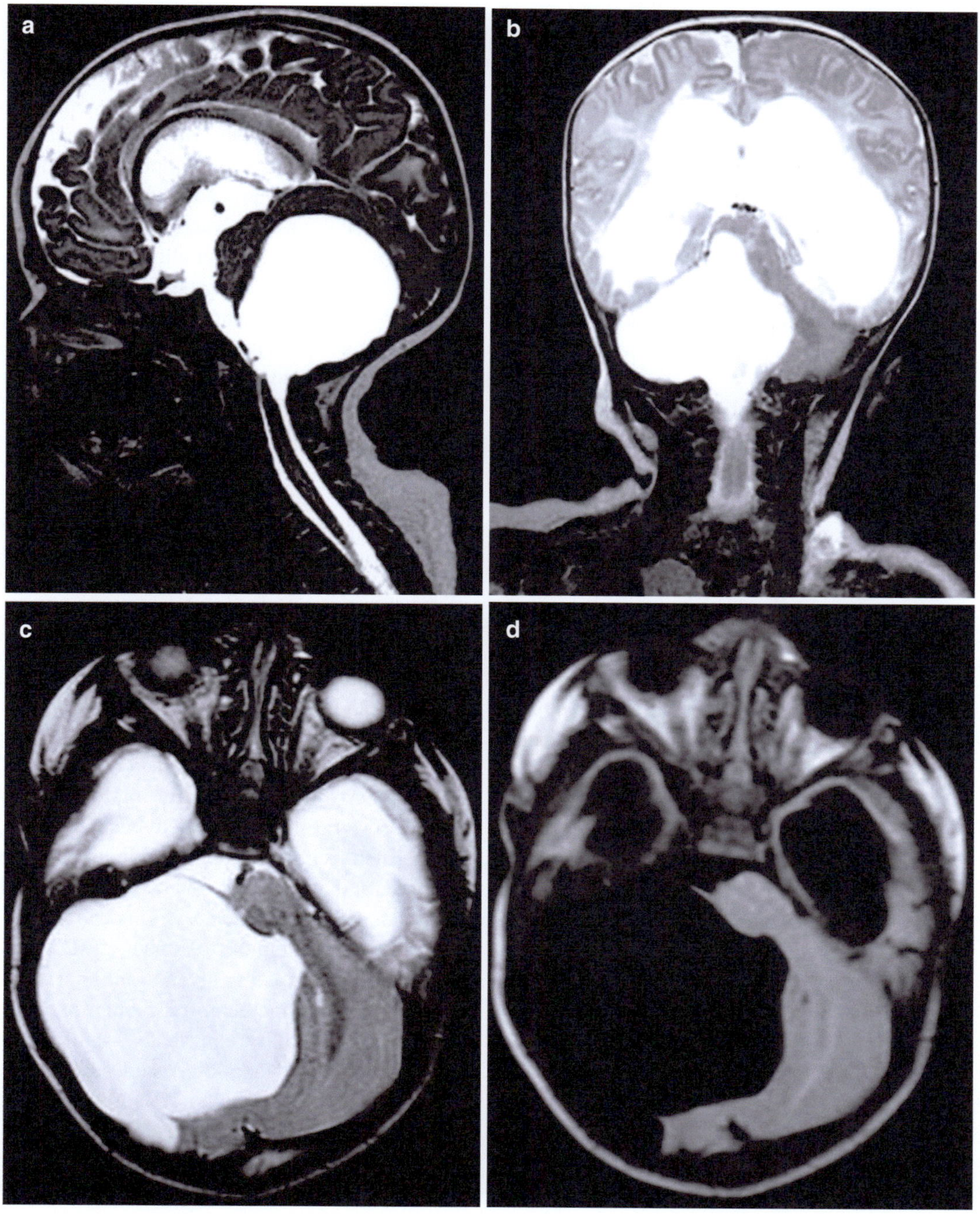

Fig. 4 MRI sequences of a huge right latero-cerebellar AC in an infant, causing intracranial hypertension. (**a**) Sagittal T2w MRI sequences showing the massive cerebellum dislocation. (**b**) Coronal T2w sequence of the same cyst. It's possible to better appreciate the pathologically increased volume of lateral ventricles. (**c**, **d**) Axial sequences, T2w and T1w, respectively, showing the axial profile of the cyst. It is also possible to appreciate the pathological expansion of the temporal horns of lateral ventricles

parts. In addition, during this type of surgery and in particular in the cases where the endoscopic approach has been preferred, visualization can often become difficult due to blood collected in the surgical field, which represents the main reason for switching to an open microscopic approach. This is related to another well-known limit of endoscopic surgery, namely, the possibility of introducing just one instrument at the time, which is disadvantageous in the case of profuse bleeding. These are, in our opinion, the main limitations that the neurosurgeon may face in surgical treating an AC.

In this scenario, robotics can offer interesting improvements for all the mentioned issues. First of all, surgical robots filter and attenuate physiologic tremor. According to what was reported by Nathoo et al., robots are indeed able to reduce human hand tremors from 40 micrometers to around 4 micrometers, due to built-in dexterity enhancement techniques [49]. This is obviously particularly useful in surgical treatment of such delicate lesions such as the arachnoid-made cysts. Moreover, surgical robots enable motion scaling and wrist movements. All these elements lead to a more safe surgery, reducing risks of neurological deficits, subdural collections, and death. Furthermore, it is worthy to say that this dexterity improvement, coupled with the possibility of placing pivot points very near to the cyst, with improving the surgical degree of freedom, contributes to an expansion of AC surgical indications, making cysts that were impossible to fenestrate previously now safely reachable [10]. Another interesting aspect related to robotics in neurosurgery is the opportunity for improving visualization and orientation, providing 3D-HD vision and haptic feedback. This is of the utmost importance in the microsurgical treatment of ACs, considering that visualization is a big issue during these procedures. One of the latest improvements in the field of robotic surgical visualization is the implementation of flexible cameras, which allow careful analysis of no flat plane areas, especially curved ones, like a cyst's walls. Another big plus of these devices is the opportunity to program the surgical trajectory based on radiological imaging. This is a big improvement for different reasons: not only does it allow one to find a safe trajectory for reaching the cysts, based on the reliability of artificial intelligence algorithms, but it also allows the surgeon to free himself from the visual feedback. This has a twofold beneficial implication: allowing completion of the procedure when visualization is difficult, such as when blood collects in the surgical field, but also for allowing the secure placement of the cyst fenestration at the correct location, even when anatomical landmarks are absent. This ability is possible because the radiological and mathematical calculations become the very surgical guide. Interestingly, J. Plonsker et al. report that they routinely use the ROSA device (Medtech SAS, Montpellier, France, now under Zimmer Biomet USA), which is a device for robotic stereotaxis, for guiding endoscopic third ventriculostomy placement. Precisely, they adopted this strategy as a way to solve the occasional difficulty in identifying anatomical landmarks. In this way, they have orchestrated an improvement in the ETV success rate [53]. Regarding the problem of blood collection, it is appropriate to report that robotics also offers the opportunity for introducing a major number of tools into a narrowed space, allowing for suctioning in cases of difficultly located ACs. Currently, multi-armed robotic systems include separate instruments that converge on the surgical field from wide angles of trajectory. This can be particularly convenient in the treatment of ACs, with particular attention being given to intraoperative complication management. Last but not least, surgeon comfortability contributes significantly to the adoption of robotic-assisted surgery. As reported by Little et al., up to 77% of endoscopic sinus surgeons reported experiencing discomfort attributable to surgery [41]. Robotics may be helpful in resolving this issue. In the case of any hesitancy regarding the use of robotics in AC treatment because this is mainly a pediatric pathology, it is important to realize that the first neurosurgical robot has been safely used in treating pediatric tumors without causing serious damage. The PUMA has already been used in the past for the resection of thalamic astrocytomas in six children, before being disregarded [56].

Since robotic surgery started in neurosurgery in the mid-1980s, numerous surgical robotic systems have been implemented over the last 30 years. Now there are numerous different applications in this discipline, many of which are slowly becoming or are already established in some subsets of neurosurgical procedures. In a recent literature review on robotics in neurosurgery, there are more than 17 different models of robots described [11], many of which not all suitable for AC surgery application. These devices can be utilized in different subgroups, depending on the surgical procedure in which they are involved. In our opinion, the ideal robotic device that can really improve the outcome of AC patients comes from the robotics for stereotaxis subgroup. From this group, the ROSA device (Medtech SAS, Montpellier, France, now under Zimmer Biomet USA) is undoubtedly the most promising technological advancement for AC's future treatment. It is the latest generation of neurosurgical robot that has been gaining acceptance in frameless stereotactic neurosurgical procedures. This system consists of both a supervisory-control and a shared-control robotic devices simultaneously, showing a manipulator with six degrees of freedom and control software for planning, registration, and guidance, already accounting for over 70 installations worldwide and over 4000 surgical interventions [60]. It has been used for tumor biopsies, DBS electrode placement, and laser ablation procedures [9, 12, 25, 39, 65]. Considering the wide range of indications where this tool has already proven its utility, the implementation in AC surgery seems just to be a matter of time. An interesting experience was reported in 2021 by Taboure et al. for treating for the first time a brain abscess patient with multiple recurrences using this amazing technology [62]. Considering that abscess perforation and aspiration can present some similarities, from a technical perspective to AC treatment, namely, the necessity to create an interruption in the cyst wall and the need for draining the inner cyst collection, and also noting that the ROSA platform offers the ability to introduce an endoscope into the surgical field, we are confident in proposing that the use of this technology in AC surgery will be a reality in the near future [53].

4 Conclusion

Although being well-known and described neoformations of the nervous system, AC treatment is still an evolving area, which lends itself to many additional possibilities. Despite AC's long history, future implementation is necessary and guideline development, for intraoperative endoscopic US and robotic systems adoption.

References

1. Al-Holou WN, Terman S, Kilburg C, Garton HJ, Muraszko KM, Maher CO. Prevalence and natural history of arachnoid cysts in adults. J Neurosurg. 2013;118:222–31. https://doi.org/10.3171/2012.10.JNS12548.
2. Al-Holou WN, Yew AY, Boomsaad ZE, Garton HJ, Muraszko KM, Maher CO. Prevalence and natural history of arachnoid cysts in children. J Neurosurg Pediatr. 2010;5:578–85. https://doi.org/10.3171/2010.2.PEDS09464.
3. Apuzzo ML, Heifetz MD, Weiss MH, Kurze T. Neurosurgical endoscopy using the side-viewing telescope. J Neurosurg. 1977;46:398–400. https://doi.org/10.3171/jns.1977.46.3.0398.
4. Azagury DE, Dua MM, Barrese JC, Henderson JM, Buchs NC, Ris F, Cloyd JM, Martinie JB, Razzaque S, Nicolau S, Soler L, Marescaux J, Visser BC. Image-guided surgery. Curr Probl Surg. 2015;52:476–520. https://doi.org/10.1067/j.cpsurg.2015.10.001.
5. Bagga V, Bhattacharyya D. Robotics in neurosurgery. Ann R Coll Surg Engl. 2018;100:23–6. https://doi.org/10.1308/rcsann.supp1.19.
6. Beller S, Hünerbein M, Eulenstein S, Lange T, Schlag PM. Feasibility of navigated resection of liver tumors using multiplanar visualization of intraoperative 3-dimensional ultrasound data. Ann Surg. 2007;246:288–94. https://doi.org/10.1097/01.sla.0000264233.48306.99.
7. Brisht R. Serous cysts of the arachnoid. Reports of medial cases, vol. 2. part 1. London: Lonamans; 1831.
8. Caemaert J, Abdullah J, Calliauw L, Carton D, Dhooge C, van Coster R. Endoscopic treatment of suprasellar arachnoid cysts. Acta Neurochir. 1992;119:68–73. https://doi.org/10.1007/BF01541784.
9. Calisto A, Dorfmüller G, Fohlen M, Bulteau C, Conti A, Delalande O. Endoscopic disconnection of hypothalamic hamartomas: safety and feasibility of robot-assisted, thulium laser-based procedures. J Neurosurg Pediatr. 2014;14:563–72. https://doi.org/10.3171/2014.8.PEDS13586.
10. Campbell RG. Robotic surgery of the anterior skull base. Int Forum Allergy Rhinol. 2019;9:1508–14. https://doi.org/10.1002/alr.22435.
11. Cavallo LM, Somma T, Solari D, Iannuzzo G, Frio F, Baiano C, Cappabianca P. Endoscopic endona-

sal transsphenoidal surgery: history and evolution. World Neurosurg. 2019;127:686–94. https://doi.org/10.1016/j.wneu.2019.03.048.
12. Chan AY, Tran DK, Gill AS, Hsu FP, Vadera S. Stereotactic robot-assisted MRI-guided laser thermal ablation of radiation necrosis in the posterior cranial fossa: technical note. Neurosurg Focus. 2016;41:E5. https://doi.org/10.3171/2016.4.FOCUS1622.
13. Chen Y, Fang HJ, Li ZF, Yu SY, Li CZ, Wu ZB, Zhang YZ. Treatment of middle cranial fossa arachnoid cysts: a systematic review and meta-analysis. World Neurosurg. 2016;92:480–490.e482. https://doi.org/10.1016/j.wneu.2016.06.046.
14. Choi JW, Lee JY, Phi JH, Kim SK, Wang KC. Stricter indications are recommended for fenestration surgery in intracranial arachnoid cysts of children. Childs Nerv Syst. 2015;31:77–86. https://doi.org/10.1007/s00381-014-2525-1.
15. Cincu R, Agrawal A, Eiras J. Intracranial arachnoid cysts: current concepts and treatment alternatives. Clin Neurol Neurosurg. 2007;109:837–43. https://doi.org/10.1016/j.clineuro.2007.07.013.
16. Czyż M, Tabakow P, Lechowicz-Głogowska B, Jarmundowicz W. Prospective study on the efficacy of low-field intraoperative magnetic resonance imaging in neurosurgical operations. Neurol Neurochir Pol. 2011;45:226–34. https://doi.org/10.1016/s0028-3843(14)60075-x.
17. Deopujari CE, Shaikh ST, Karmarkar VS, Sudke AY, Mohanty CB, Biyani NK. Experience with management of intracranial arachnoid cysts. J Neurol Surg A Cent Eur Neurosurg. 2021;82:43–52. https://doi.org/10.1055/s-0040-1718522.
18. Doulgeris JJ, Gonzalez-Blohm SA, Filis AK, Shea TM, Aghayev K, Vrionis FD. Robotics in neurosurgery: evolution, current challenges, and compromises. Cancer Control. 2015;22:352–9. https://doi.org/10.1177/107327481502200314.
19. Drake JM, Joy M, Goldenberg A, Kreindler D. Computer- and robot-assisted resection of thalamic astrocytomas in children. Neurosurgery. 1991;29:27–33. https://doi.org/10.1097/00006123-199107000-00005.
20. Faraji AH, Kokkinos V, Sweat JC, Crammond DJ, Richardson RM. Robotic-assisted stereotaxy for deep brain stimulation lead implantation in awake patients. Oper Neurosurg. 2020;19:444–52. https://doi.org/10.1093/ons/opaa029.
21. Fernández Molina G. Neuroendoscopic management of middle fossa arachnoid cysts. World Neurosurg. 2013;79:S19–23. https://doi.org/10.1016/j.wneu.2012.02.012.
22. Fewel ME, Levy ML, McComb JG. Surgical treatment of 95 children with 102 intracranial arachnoid cysts. Pediatr Neurosurg. 1996;25:165–73. https://doi.org/10.1159/000121119.
23. Gangemi M, Maiuri F, Cappabianca P, Alafaci C, de Divitiis O, Tomasello F, de Divitiis E. Endoscopic fenestration of symptomatic septum pellucidum cysts: three case reports with discussion on the approaches and technique. Minim Invasive Neurosurg. 2002;45:105–8.
24. Geissinger JD, Kohler WC, Robinson BW, Davis FM. Arachnoid cysts of the middle cranial fossa: surgical considerations. Surg Neurol. 1978;10:27–33.
25. González-Martínez J, Bulacio J, Thompson S, Gale J, Smithason S, Najm I, Bingaman W. Technique, results, and complications related to robot-assisted stereoelectroencephalography. Neurosurgery. 2016;78:169–80. https://doi.org/10.1227/NEU.0000000000001034.
26. Guiot G, Rougerie J, Fourestier M, Fournier A, Comoy C, Vulmiere J, Gronz R. A new endoscopic technique. Endoscopic intracranial explorations. Presse Med. 1963;72:1225–31.
27. Hayes MJ, TerMaath SC, Crook TR, Killeffer JA. A review on the effectiveness of surgical intervention for symptomatic intracranial arachnoid cysts in adults. World Neurosurg. 2019;123:e259–72. https://doi.org/10.1016/j.wneu.2018.11.149.
28. Herline AJ, Stefansic JD, Debelak JP, Hartmann SL, Pinson CW, Galloway RL, Chapman WC. Image-guided surgery: preliminary feasibility studies of frameless stereotactic liver surgery. Arch Surg. 1999;134:644–9; discussion 649-650. https://doi.org/10.1001/archsurg.134.6.644.
29. Holmes JH, Sacchi L, Bellazzi R, Peek N. Artificial intelligence in medicine AIME 2015. Artif Intell Med. 2017;81:1–2. https://doi.org/10.1016/j.artmed.2017.06.011.
30. Ishikawa M, Ota Y, Naritaka H, Katoh S. Endoscopic ultrasound imaging with high flow mode for endonasal transsphenoidal pituitary surgery. J Clin Neurosci. 2021;89:329–35. https://doi.org/10.1016/j.jocn.2021.05.024.
31. Jafrani R, Raskin JS, Kaufman A, Lam S. Intracranial arachnoid cysts: pediatric neurosurgery update. Surg Neurol Int. 2019;10:15. https://doi.org/10.4103/sni.sni_320_18.
32. Jara RD, Guerrón AD, Portenier D. Complications of robotic surgery. Surg Clin N Am. 2020;100:461–8. https://doi.org/10.1016/j.suc.2019.12.008.
33. Jho HD, Carrau RL. Endoscopic endonasal transsphenoidal surgery: experience with 50 patients. J Neurosurg. 1997;87:44–51. https://doi.org/10.3171/jns.1997.87.1.0044.
34. Karabagli H, Etus V. Success of pure neuroendoscopic technique in the treatment of Sylvian arachnoid cysts in children. Childs Nerv Syst. 2012;28:445–52. https://doi.org/10.1007/s00381-011-1632-5.
35. Karabatsou K, Hayhurst C, Buxton N, O'Brien DF, Mallucci CL. Endoscopic management of arachnoid cysts: an advancing technique. J Neurosurg. 2007;106:455–62. https://doi.org/10.3171/ped.2007.106.6.455.
36. Kim MH. The role of endoscopic fenestration procedures for cerebral arachnoid cysts. J Korean Med Sci. 1999;14:443–7. https://doi.org/10.3346/jkms.1999.14.4.443.
37. Kwoh YS, Hou J, Jonckheere EA, Hayati S. A robot with improved absolute positioning accu-

racy for CT guided stereotactic brain surgery. IEEE Trans Biomed Eng. 1988;35:153–60. https://doi.org/10.1109/10.1354.
38. LaCour F, Trevor R, Carey M. Arachnoid cyst and associated subdural hematoma. Observations on conventional roentgenographic and computerized tomographic diagnosis. Arch Neurol. 1978;35:84–9. https://doi.org/10.1001/archneur.1978.00500260022004.
39. Lefranc M, Capel C, Pruvot-Occean AS, Fichten A, Desenclos C, Toussaint P, Le Gars D, Peltier J. Frameless robotic stereotactic biopsies: a consecutive series of 100 cases. J Neurosurg. 2015;122:342–52. https://doi.org/10.3171/2014.9.JNS14107.
40. Link TE, Bisson E, Horgan MA, Tranmer BI. Raymond M. P. Donaghy: a pioneer in microneurosurgery. J Neurosurg. 2010;112:1176–81. https://doi.org/10.3171/2009.6.JNS09539.
41. Little RM, Deal AM, Zanation AM, McKinney K, Senior BA, Ebert CS Jr. Occupational hazards of endoscopic surgery. Int Forum Allergy Rhinol. 2012;2:212–6. https://doi.org/10.1002/alr.20108.
42. Ma G, Li X, Qiao N, Zhang B, Li C, Zhang Y, Zhao P, Gui SB. Suprasellar arachnoid cysts in adults: clinical presentations, radiological features, and treatment outcomes. Neurosurg Rev. 2021;44:1645–53. https://doi.org/10.1007/s10143-020-01358-4.
43. Marcus HJ, Payne CJ. Neurosurgical robotics. Cham: Springer; 2021.
44. Martínez-Lage JF, Pérez-Espejo MA, Almagro MJ, López-Guerrero AL. Hydrocephalus and arachnoid cysts. Childs Nerv Syst. 2011;27:1643–52. https://doi.org/10.1007/s00381-011-1481-2.
45. Masoudi M, Yousefi O, Azami P. Results of surgical treatment in patients with intracranial arachnoid cyst during last 5 years in a referral center in a developing country: Shiraz, Iran. World Neurosurg. 2021;150:e420–6. https://doi.org/10.1016/j.wneu.2021.03.038.
46. Mattox A, Choi JD, Leith-Gray L, Grant GA, Adamson DC. Guidelines for the management of obstructive hydrocephalus from suprasellar-prepontine arachnoid cysts using endoscopic third ventriculocystocisternostomy. Surg Innov. 2010;17:206–16. https://doi.org/10.1177/1553350610377212.
47. Mavrogenis AF, Markatos K, Saranteas T, Ignatiadis I, Spyridonos S, Bumbasirevic M, Georgescu AV, Beris A, Soucacos PN. The history of microsurgery. Eur J Orthop Surg Traumatol. 2019;29:247–54. https://doi.org/10.1007/s00590-019-02378-7.
48. Mustansir F, Bashir S, Darbar A. Management of arachnoid cysts: a comprehensive review. Cureus. 2018;10:e2458. https://doi.org/10.7759/cureus.2458.
49. Nathoo N, Cavuşoğlu MC, Vogelbaum MA, Barnett GH. In touch with robotics: neurosurgery for the future. Neurosurgery. 2005;56:421–33; discussion 421-433. https://doi.org/10.1227/01.neu.0000153929.68024.cf.
50. Nimsky C, von Keller B, Ganslandt O, Fahlbusch R. Intraoperative high-field magnetic resonance imaging in transsphenoidal surgery of hormonally inactive pituitary macroadenomas. Neurosurgery. 2006;59:105–14; discussion 105-114. https://doi.org/10.1227/01.NEU.0000219198.38423.1E.
51. Oertel J, Linsler S, Wagner W, Gaab M, Schroeder H, Rediker J. Endoscopic treatment of intracranial arachnoid cysts: a retrospective analysis of a 25-year experience. Oper Neurosurg. 2020;20:32–44. https://doi.org/10.1093/ons/opaa292.
52. Oertel JM, Wagner W, Mondorf Y, Baldauf J, Schroeder HW, Gaab MR. Endoscopic treatment of arachnoid cysts: a detailed account of surgical techniques and results. Neurosurgery. 2010;67:824–36. https://doi.org/10.1227/01.NEU.0000377852.75544.E4.
53. Plonsker J, Gonda D. Robot-assisted endoscopic third ventriculostomy. New York: Springer; 2021. p. 125–34. https://doi.org/10.1007/978-1-0716-0993-4_9.
54. Pradilla G, Jallo G. Arachnoid cysts: case series and review of the literature. Neurosurg Focus. 2007;22:E7. https://doi.org/10.3171/foc.2007.22.2.7.
55. Resch KD. Endoneurosonography: technique and equipment, anatomy and imaging, and clinical application. Neurosurgery. 2008;63:E1209; author reply E1209. https://doi.org/10.1227/01.NEU.0000315867.11459.89.
56. Saedi B, Aghili M, Motiee M, Valadkhani S, Niazi AB, Safavi A. Surgical outcomes of malignant sinonasal tumours: open versus endoscopic surgical approaches. J Laryngol Otol. 2014;128:784–90. https://doi.org/10.1017/s0022215114001583.
57. Schroeder HW, Gaab MR, Niendorf WR. Neuroendoscopic approach to arachnoid cysts. J Neurosurg. 1996;85:293–8. https://doi.org/10.3171/jns.1996.85.2.0293.
58. Soldozy S, Young S, Yağmurlu K, Norat P, Sokolowski J, Park MS, Jane JA, Syed HR. Transsphenoidal surgery using robotics to approach the sella turcica: integrative use of artificial intelligence, realistic motion tracking and telesurgery. Clin Neurol Neurosurg. 2020;197:106152. https://doi.org/10.1016/j.clineuro.2020.106152.
59. Sprau AC, McCrea HJ. Intracranial arachnoid cysts in an infant: a technical note on the innovative use of navigation and flexible endoscopy for cyst fenestration. Surg Neurol Int. 2021;12:160. https://doi.org/10.25259/SNI_81_2021.
60. Sugiyama T, Lama S, Hoshyarmanesh H, Baghdadi A, Sutherland GR. Early developments, current systems, and future directions. In: Marcus HJ, Payne CJ, editors. Neurosurgical robotics. New York: Springer; 2021. p. 193–227. https://doi.org/10.1007/978-1-0716-0993-4_15.
61. Tabakow P, Weiser A, Chmielak K, Blauciak P, Bladowska J, Czyz M. Navigated neuroendoscopy combined with intraoperative magnetic resonance cysternography for treatment of arachnoid cysts. Neurosurg Rev. 2020;43:1151–61. https://doi.org/10.1007/s10143-019-01136-x.
62. Tabourel G, Le Turnier P, Buffenoir K, Roualdes V. Robot-assisted stereotactic multiple brain abscesses' puncture: technical case report.

Acta Neurochir. 2021. https://doi.org/10.1007/s00701-021-04955-4.
63. Tamburrini G, Dal Fabbro M, Del Fabbro M, Di Rocco C. Sylvian fissure arachnoid cysts: a survey on their diagnostic workout and practical management. Childs Nerv Syst. 2008;24:593–604. https://doi.org/10.1007/s00381-008-0585-9.
64. Terrier L, Gilard V, Marguet F, Fontanilles M, Derrey S. Stereotactic brain biopsy: evaluation of robot-assisted procedure in 60 patients. Acta Neurochir. 2019;161:545–52. https://doi.org/10.1007/s00701-019-03808-5.
65. Vadera S, Chan A, Lo T, Gill A, Morenkova A, Phielipp NM, Hermanowicz N, Hsu FP. Frameless stereotactic robot-assisted subthalamic nucleus deep brain stimulation: case report. World Neurosurg. 2017;97:762.e711–4. https://doi.org/10.1016/j.wneu.2015.11.009.
66. Van Beijnum J, Hanlo PW, Han KS, Van Der Pol WL, Verdaasdonk RM, Van Nieuwenhuizen O. Navigated laser-assisted endoscopic fenestration of a suprasellar arachnoid cyst in a 2-year-old child with bobble-head doll syndrome: case report. J Neurosurg. 2006;104:348–51. https://doi.org/10.3171/ped.2006.104.5.348.
67. Wester K, Svendsen F, Hugdahl K. Intracranial arachnoidal cysts–localization, gender and sidedness. Tidsskr Nor Laegeforen. 1999;119:4162–4.

Medicolegal Aspects of Arachnoid Cysts

Mehmet Turgut

1 Introduction

Arachnoid cysts (ACs), cerebrospinal fluid (CSF)-filled congenital space-occupying benign lesions, are relatively common, with an incidence on imaging of 2% [2, 3, 19, 24, 51, 53, 54]. These lesions develop as a result of the abnormal separation of the arachnoid membrane during embryogenesis [53]. It is well-known that they are more common in males in several anatomical locations along the craniospinal axis, primarily in the middle cranial fossa, most often on the left side, and in the retrocerebellar cistern [2, 3, 19, 20, 24, 28, 37, 45, 54]. Rarely, spinal ACs are located in the anterior or posterior thoracic region of the spinal canal presenting with backache and fluctuating leg weakness [16, 40, 54].

As covered in detail in other parts of the book, the vast majority of the ACs located both in the intracranial and intraspinal compartments do not change substantially over time, although they may infrequently show spontaneous enlargement, resolution (either partial or complete), or a fluctuation in size [2, 3, 33, 45, 50]. Therefore, the natural course of the ACs is highly variable, although these cysts are usually asymptomatic in most cases, and there are common incidental imaging findings reported in the current literature [3, 19, 39, 47]. However, regarding the natural course of the AC, it is also important to realize that symptomatic subdural hygromas or hemorrhage may rarely develop from ACs, possibly due to spontaneous, iatrogenic, or traumatic rupture of the outer cyst lining [1, 12–14, 34, 38, 46, 54].

Clinically, when the patient is sent to a referral center, the typical presentation of the individual with a symptomatic intracranial AC frequently includes one or more unrelated "nonspecific" neurological symptoms, such as headache, nausea, dizziness, unsteadiness, disequilibrium, vertigo, macrocephaly, and neurocognitive or neuropsychiatric disturbances, possibly due to the mass effect on the brain or secondary to their rupture [6, 12, 17, 19, 23, 24, 27, 30, 45, 47, 49, 54, 55]. Among the nonspecific neurological complaints, the most commonly observed symptom is headache (80%), which varies in intensity, global or lateralized, and may also have asymptomatic periods followed by episodes of severe pain [19, 24]. In patients with intracranial ACs, however, only 10% present with subjective complaints related to deficits of cognitive functions involving verbal memory capacity, auditory attention, visual, and spatial tasks, which can only be demonstrated through detailed neuropsychological testing [6, 17, 23, 24, 27, 49, 52]. Recently, some authors have suggested that cognitive impairment may be due to hypoperfusion of the cortical areas next to the AC [11, 23, 32,

M. Turgut (✉)
Department of Neurosurgery, Aydın Adnan Menderes University School of Medicine, Aydın, Turkey

Department of Histology and Embryology, Aydın Adnan Menderes University Health Sciences, Aydin, Turkey

M. Turgut et al. (eds.), *Arachnoid Cysts*, https://doi.org/10.1007/978-3-031-22701-1_34

42, 49]. Furthermore, some patients with ACs have various neuropsychiatric disturbances that include anxiety, phobias, personality disorder, depression, and psychosis [6, 55]. Moreover, patients may present occasionally with "specific" neurologic signs or symptoms, motor or sensory function loss, cranial nerve palsies, or epileptic seizures [19, 54].

Radiographically, craniospinal ACs have a thin wall without contrast enhancement, and the fluid within the AC demonstrates fluid density and fluid intensities on computed tomography (CT) and magnetic resonance imaging (MRI), respectively, which are the imaging modalities of choice for evaluating their anatomical location, size, and any surrounding structures involved [45, 51, 53, 54]. On MRI, ACs display the signal intensity of CSF on T1, T2 spin-echo, T2-FLAIR, and diffusion-weighted imaging, although there may be slight signal differences between the fluid in the AC and the normal CSF on MRI sequences due to CSF pulsations [54]. CT or MRI cisternography and phase-contrast MRI may be used to confirm the diagnosis of an AC and to further evaluate a patient with an AC [51, 54]. In addition, the radiologist should assess the imaging finding of mass effect on a cranial nerve caused by the AC, hydrocephalus, or cyst rupture causing subdural hygroma or hematoma formation [38, 45, 54]. In such cases of the ACs with significant mass effect, it is also important for the radiologist to urgently inform the referring clinician, either neurologist or neurosurgeon [54].

Most authors suggest that, as a rule, intracranial ACs should not be treated surgically, if they are asymptomatic [24, 30, 45, 54]. The ACs may be very large or very small, and some authors have suggested that size alone does not correlate with either symptoms or the need for surgery [24, 30], although some other authors have reported that larger cysts are more likely to be symptomatic and hence require surgery more often than do smaller ones [54]. It is widely accepted that cases of ACs should be treated surgically if they are responsible for significant neurologic symptoms or they cause hydrocephalus as a result of obstruction of CSF pathways, regardless of the cyst size, as often occurs within the suprasellar location [14, 15, 24, 25, 29, 30, 45, 54]. Considering that ACs are common and their natural history is usually benign, the majority of neurosurgeons believe that evidence of mass effect on imaging is not an adequate criterion alone for selection of patients for surgical intervention in cases with an intracranial AC [30, 54]. These neurosurgeons believe that surgical treatment should be avoided except in rare instances in which an AC is definitely responsible for the presence of specific symptoms that are associated with the potential risk of neurologic morbidity or mortality [28, 30, 43–46, 54]. In recent years, some neurosurgeons have reported that nonspecific symptoms such as headache, dizziness, and cognitive impairment, affecting the quality of the life in patients with intracranial ACs, have also resolved following any kind of surgical intervention [24, 48]. Therefore, it is apparent that the indications for surgical treatment of these lesions should be carefully considered by clinicians, neurologists, and neurosurgeons.

Only in rare situations where a symptomatic intracranial AC present with significant mass effect impairing quality of the life, regardless of whether the symptoms present are specific or nonspecific, and surgical intervention for decompression of the AC is indicated [24, 35, 45, 54]. Currently, there are primarily four different surgical techniques used for this purpose: (1) craniotomy approach for microsurgical fenestration of the AC into the basal cisterns, (2) neuroendoscopic approach for fenestration of the cyst cavity into the basal subarachnoid cisterns with/without marsupialization, (3) internal (cystosubdural or cystoventricular) shunting of the AC into another CSF compartment within the cranium, and (4) external (cystoperitoneal) shunting of the AC into an extracranial compartment, such as the peritoneum [8, 10, 19, 22, 24, 41, 45, 54]. The craniotomy approach under general anesthesia for the excision of the parietal membrane of the AC under the dura mater allows for drainage of the cyst fluid into the subarachnoid space. The visceral membrane of the AC which is covering the brain surface and basal structures such as blood vessels and cranial nerves is fenestrated, to provide a communication between the cavity of the AC and the basal cisterns. Endoscopic approach under local anesthesia for fenestration of the cyst cavity into the basal subarachnoid cisterns with/without marsupialization is a minimally invasive procedure [8, 10, 19, 22, 24, 41, 54]. Internal (cystosubdural or cystoventricular) shunting through a burr hole is a minimally invasive procedure [20, 24]. External (cystoperitoneal) shunting under general anesthesia requires insertion of the proximal drainage catheter into the cyst cavity [9, 19, 24]. Presently, clinicians should be familiar that surgical decompression as a life-saving procedure or for improving the quality-of-life procedure is indicated in some patients affected by a symptomatic intracranial AC, presenting with significant mass effect with/without an intracystic and/or a subdural hematoma, although there is still controversy about the best option for the surgical management of ACs [21, 24, 54].

In the vast majority of patients, surgery is curative, and there is improvement of the preoperative complaints, such as headache and dizziness, in the postoperative period, although recurrence after surgery has been reported in some cases with the ACs [36]. Based on their retrospective study, Hall et al. reported that the reoperation rate was similar for those that underwent different treatment options, although the endoscopic and shunted groups had a shorter length of hospital stay compared to the microsurgical group [19]. They also found that all three treatment modalities had a very similar reduction in the cyst volume following surgical intervention [19]. Perfusion studies have also demonstrated that the preoperative areas of hypoperfusion in the cortex adjacent to the AC returned to the normal values after surgical decompression that was consistent with the postoperative cognitive function improvement that occurred [11, 32, 42, 49]. However, it is important to be aware that there is a small decrease in fluid volume in most patients, but that there is no correlation between the reduction of the cyst volume and the resolution of neurological symptoms following surgery [10, 24, 52]. Interestingly, it should also be kept in mind that neurological symptoms will frequently still persist in the early postoperative period in such cases [12, 28].

In this chapter, a summary of some common myths and facts about the management of the AC is first provided, and then various case scenarios of malpractice claims on these topics are discussed, including those with a delayed or inaccurate diagnosis and/or treatment. As described below with examples, the usual cases with negligence include a delay in diagnosis and treatment of the AC, a delay in obtaining diagnostic CT or MRI studies, or inadequate management of the AC.

2 Myths and Facts Regarding the Management of an Arachnoid Cyst

Even today, controversy still exists regarding some aspects of the clinical and surgical treatment of intracranial ACs. Some common misunderstandings and evidence-based scientific facts related to their management are as follows:

2.1 Indications for Surgical Treatment

Myth: No surgical treatment is necessary because they are relatively common, benign, and asymptomatic lesions, with the exception being only those life-threatening cases with specific symptoms, because such invasive procedures may be dangerous and risky with a high risk for neurologic morbidity or mortality.

Fact: Today, the indications for surgical treatment are not limited to life-threatening lesions and are also intended to improve the quality of life in symptomatic cases due to the AC causing significant mass effect, including nonspecific symptoms such as headache and cognitive dysfunction [24, 35, 54].

2.2 Relationship Between Clinical Symptoms and the Size of the AC

Myth: The severity of clinical symptoms including headache is directly proportional to the size of the AC.

Fact: There is no correlation between the volume of the AC and the severity of the symptoms, because the symptom intensity is more likely related to the intracystic pressure than to the size of the AC [20, 24, 30, 35].

2.3 Relationship Between the Location of Headache and the Side of the AC

Myth: The headache is usually located on the same side of the intracranial compartment as the AC; if it is lateralized to the right or left, it is not global.

Fact: The headache is not necessary on the side of the cyst in the cranial cavity [24, 54].

2.4 Resolution of Neurological Symptoms in the Early Postoperative Period

Myth: Decompressive surgery is always curative and is associated with a reduction of the AC volume and the subsequent resolution of the neurological symptoms.

Fact: Neurological symptoms such as headache and nausea are frequently still apparent in the immediate postoperative period, and there is no correlation between the reduction of the cyst volume and the resolution of neurological symptoms [10, 24, 52].

3 Case Scenarios of Malpractice due to the Negligent Management of the Arachnoid Cyst

The case scenarios of malpractice due to the negligent management of an AC that are described below provide useful guidelines regarding the correct diagnosis and appropriate management of physicians from various disciplines that include primary care or family physicians, pediatricians, radiologists, neurologists, and neurosurgeons in their future professional life.

3.1 Missed or Delayed Diagnosis and Treatment of an Arachnoid Cyst

Case 1: A claim was settled against a primary care physician and a neurosurgeon for a "delayed diagnosis" of an AC leading to severe disability.

A brief case scenario may be as follows: *A tragic situation involved the failure to diagnose in a child an intracranial AC, which is not malignant but benign, compressing the brain. In this unfortunate case, the AC presented clinically with blockage of the flow of CSF as a result of compression of the ventricle.... Initially, he visited the office of his primary care physician on numerous occasions reporting worrisome clinical complaints only to be managed by the physician's assistant who did not order a CT scan of the brain on an urgent basis. Afterward, he went to the local hospital, when the clinical symptoms became severe.... Subsequently, he was admitted to this hospital, and a neurosurgeon was called for the urgent management of an AC, which was demonstrated by the CT scan.... He required an urgent neurosurgical intervention, but the neurosurgeon never came to the hospital to manage the patient. During that night, the patient's brain herniated before he/she could have surgery to remove the AC.... Unfortunately, he was left with severe impairments that changed her life and that of his family....*

In this case scenario, there was a failure to diagnose the AC and to manage it properly. As expected, the expert will confirm negligence in the failure to identify the AC on the CT scan. Most likely, the child would have recovered without a neurological deficit, if these failures had not occurred. Medicolegally, it is evident that these failures led to the severe neurological impairment of the patient.

Case 2: A claim was settled against the radiologist for the "misdiagnosis" of an AC of the patient as an isolated agenesis of the corpus callosum leading to brain damage.

A brief case scenario may be as follows: *A woman was in her early 30s when she started to notice headache and memory loss, which she reported to her primary care physician.... A radiologist interpreted her brain CT scan as showing an isolated agenesis of the corpus callosum (CC) and reported that it was a congenital variant. The woman's headache and memory continued to deteriorate over the next 3 years, until finally a neurologist ordered a brain MRI, which identified an interhemispheric AC. The cyst was drained by a neurosurgeon.... Unfortunately, however, surgical intervention caused permanent damage to the surrounding cerebral structures.... Consequently, the woman suffered from seizures....*

In this case scenario, there was a "misdiagnosis" of an AC of the patient as agenesis of the CC on CT scan, leading to brain damage. The brain MRI revealed an interhemispheric AC in this patient. As anticipated, the expert report from a consultant radiologist will confirm negligence regarding the radiological evaluation of the patient that falls below the conventional standard of care. In accordance with the standard management algorithm for craniospinal ACs, it is crucial to perform decompressive surgery rather than observing the patient with an expanding intracranial lesion causing neurological symptoms that may lead to an undesirable outcome. Medicolegally, it is evident that these errors caused a failure to carry out urgent neurosurgical treatment to avoid her further neurological deterioration.

3.2 Failure in the Diagnosis of Shunt Failure in a Child with Hydrocephalus Caused by an Arachnoid Cyst

Case 1: A claim was settled against a family physician for the "failure to diagnose shunt failure" in a hydrocephalic child caused by an AC.

A brief case scenario may be as follows: *A boy who presented with complaints of headache, nausea, vomiting, and lethargy was diagnosed with severe hydrocephalus caused by a suprasellar AC, as a result of blockage in the flow of CSF, based on his imaging studies 4 months ago.... A ventriculoperitoneal shunt device was urgently inserted by a neurosurgeon in a tertiary care hospital to prevent the development of irreversible white matter damage and brain herniation.... Two years later, when complaints of headaches, nausea, vomiting, and impaired balance appeared, he was given analgesics and antiemetic drugs by his family physician... when his complaints did not improve; however, his family physician referred the patient to the department of neurosurgery at a local hospital, and he was admitted to the neurosurgeon.... An emergency brain CT scan was obtained because his neurological examination revealed papilledema, and ventriculomegaly was detected and shunt failure was diagnosed on CT.... Thus, surgical intervention was necessary to revise the shunt system....*

In this case scenario, there was a "failure to diagnose shunt failure" in a hydrocephalic child caused by an AC. As anticipated, the expert report from a consultant neurosurgeon or neurologist will confirm the presence of negligence regarding the management of the patient as a "failure in the diagnosis of shunt failure" in a child with hydrocephalus caused by an AC. It is expected that a family physician may be able to diagnose shunt failure when a brain CT scan revealed ventriculomegaly and the ophthalmoscopic examination revealed papilledema.

3.3 Shunt Placement in an Asymptomatic Arachnoid Cyst

Case 1: A claim was settled against a neurosurgeon and a medical center for shunt placement in an "asymptomatic" AC.

A brief case scenario may be as follows: *A man had a CT scan of his brain and was diagnosed with a large intracranial AC, but he was asymptomatic, and therefore his physicians advised him that his AC did not require surgical intervention. Two months later, the man experienced severe pain and went to a medical center's emergency room..., and a physician in the center referred him to a neurosurgeon who diagnosed him with a "symptomatic" AC and recommended surgical intervention...and anti-edema drugs to decrease the increased intracranial pressure (IICP)...afterward the neurosurgeon explained in detail to the man why surgical intervention is necessary for him…then the neurosurgeon placed a cystoperitoneal shunt to relieve the IICP caused by the AC…. About 2 weeks following the shunting procedure, his primary care physician noted that the man had clinical symptoms such as vision loss, disturbance of gait, and dizziness…. Two months after the shunting, the man was hospitalized with same complaints, and a CT scan disclosed that he had a shunt catheter within the AC. …his primary care physician noted that a neurologist recommended to remove the shunt device because the size of the AC had not decreased…, About 10 months after the shunting procedure, the patient and his two children sued the neurosurgeon and the medical center where the cystoperitoneal shunting procedure was undertaken. They claimed that the neurosurgeon did not inform them adequately about the risks associated with the shunting procedure before obtaining his consent and that the neurosurgeon engaged in a medical malpractice act…. The alleged malpractice concerned the decision for surgery for the AC, i.e., medical indication, not the professional qualification of the neurosurgeon's surgical technique…the complaint also contended that the medical center was eventually liable for the neurosurgeon's conduct….*

In this case scenario, the neurosurgeon recommended surgical intervention for a "symptomatic" AC to decrease the IICP, and then he/she informed the patient about the natural history of the AC and possible risks of the planned surgical intervention, i.e., cystoperitoneal shunting procedure. As anticipated, the expert will not confirm any negligence regarding the management of the AC in this patient. Medicolegally, it is important to note that the legal clock for the man's malpractice claim began shortly after his first clinical complaints began following the surgical intervention. And, the man's statement that he was unable to obtain informed consent accrued when he learned that he was experiencing clinical complaints. The man's requests for informed consent were unsuccessful because the neurosurgeon did not violate his duty to inform the man about the natural history and risks of the planned surgical procedure.

3.4 Failure in the Management of an Arachnoid Cyst by a Neurologist

Case 1: A claim was settled against a neurologist for a "failure of management" of a patient with intense headaches caused by an intracranial AC.

A brief case scenario may be as follows: *A 44-year-old man presented with a 6-year history of intermittent headaches, starting in the forehead and then generalizing but located predominantly on the right side, progressively increasing in frequency and intensity. There was no relief with analgesics and non-steroidal anti-inflammatory drugs, and his family physician referred him to the department of neurology in a secondary care clinic…. Because of the increase in the severity and frequency of his headaches in the following months, however, the neurologist asked for a CT scan of the brain, which disclosed a small middle fossa AC on the right side, and advised the patient that there was no indication for surgical intervention…. Afterward, his family physician referred him to the department of neurosurgery in the regional tertiary hospital, since the severity and frequency of his headaches had progressively increased…. Neurosurgeon indicated a surgical intervention was necessary because the quality of life had deteriorated due to excruciating headache, and a neurosurgical intervention composed of craniotomy with fenestration of the cyst into the basal subarachnoid space was performed…. His headaches dramatically resolved in the postoperative period, despite a transient increase in his headaches in the early postoperative period, …then, control CT scan of the brain showed the brain tissue had expanded and the AC disappeared completely…he remained without any complaints to date….*

In this case scenario, it is clear that the surgical treatment of the patient was delayed because of the failure of the neurologist's medical knowledge that intracranial ACs can cause headaches decreasing the quality of life and thus requiring surgical intervention. Therefore as anticipated, the expert report from a consultant neurologist or neurosurgeon will confirm negligence concerning the treatment of the patient by delaying the surgical treatment. It is expected that the neurologist treating such a patient should refer him/her to a neurosurgeon for surgical treatment. Otherwise, it may be a subject of a lawsuit against a neurologist for a malpractice claim by the patient and his/her relatives.

3.5 Misdiagnosis of a Spinal Arachnoid Cyst as Motor Neurone Disease Causing Delayed Treatment

Case 1: A claim was settled against a neurologist for "misdiagnosis" and delayed treatment of a patient with a lower cervical intradural AC as motor neuron disease.

A brief case scenario may be as follows: *A 53-year-old man was diagnosed with motor neurone disease (MND) 8 years ago. The patient had noted his symptoms were progressive, for about 3 years when he was referred to a neurologist.... His clinical presentation at that time already comprised objective weakness and atrophy in the lower and upper limb muscles, along with extremely brisk tendon reflexes. No sensory deficit was documented at that time. Electromyography (EMG) showed abnormal spontaneous activity in the left deltoid muscle, abductor pollicis brevis, and palmar interossei muscles and signs of bilateral chronic denervation in the upper limb. MRI of the brain was normal...he was diagnosed with MND by several neurologists.... At the time of admission to our clinic, neurological examination revealed that the cranial nerves were normal and there were no signs of bulbar dysfunction and no fasciculations or weakness of facial, tongue, or neck muscles.... Muscle atrophy along with mild fasciculations of the upper limbs with left-sided...was noted, ...motor strength of deltoid and biceps muscles, and the finger extensors was reduced to 2–3/5 in the upper limbs.... Motor strength was 3/5 for foot extensors in the lower limbs...although no obvious atrophy or fasciculations were found.... Furthermore, gait ataxia, reduced vibration and proprioception of all limbs, and hyper- and dysesthesia of the shoulders and proximal arms were found, while deep tendon reflexes were symmetric, Babinski's signs were absent, and superficial abdominal reflexes were preserved. Although he reported neck pain and numbness and clumsiness of both upper limbs, there were no symptoms of bladder or bowel dysfunction.... Proximal muscle atrophy in the upper limbs together with sensory dysfunction and pain suggested a new spinal pathology, and MRI of the cervical spine revealed a cyst in the lower cervical region. The lesion displaced the cervical spinal cord ventrally, and myelopathy was noted...the patient presented to the neurosurgeon for surgical treatment of the cyst localized in the intradural space in the lower cervical region. A C5–C7 hemilaminectomy on the left side was performed, and an increased pressure within the cyst was noted.... The cyst was incompletely removed with fenestration of the remaining parts.... Histopathological examination confirmed the lesion as an AC.... Postoperatively, the patient reported complete relief of her neck pain and regained strength in his upper limbs.... Two years later, minimal motor and sensory dysfunctions were found on his neurological examination...any acute denervation was not recorded on EMG....*

In this case scenario, there was a "misdiagnosis" of a lower cervical AC in the patient as MND leading to delayed management because of the progressive fasciculations along with brisk tendon reflexes and electrophysiological signs of acute and chronic denervation, in spite of the presence of fluctuating neurological symptoms. After a long follow-up, the spinal MRI clearly revealed an intraspinal cyst in this patient. Therefore as anticipated, the expert report from a consultant neurologist or neurosurgeon will confirm negligence concerning the correct diagnosis of the patient by delaying the surgical treatment. Based on the neurological examination and imaging findings, it is expected that the neurologists treating such a patient should be able to make the differential diagnosis between a spinal AC and MND and then refer him/her to a neurosurgeon for surgical treatment. Otherwise, it may be the subject of a lawsuit against a neurologist for a malpractice claim by the patient.

4 Comment Upon Case Scenarios

Today, it is well-known that craniospinal ACs may present with variable clinical signs and symptoms as well as neuroimaging appearances which depend principally on the anatomic locations, cyst sizes, etiological forms, and the patient's age. Unfortunately, neuroimaging features of the ACs are neither uniform nor pathognomonic; therefore, these cysts may be confused with many normal anatomic variants, as described above in a case with an isolated agenesis of the CC, and intracranial cysts of different etiologies. As a result, the differential diagnosis is very important, because all of these diagnoses can interfere with the correct management of the patients.

As can be seen very clearly in the case scenarios presented above, most malpractice related to the negligent management of AC includes misdiagnosis or delayed diagnosis and/or mistakes in the treatment of the patients by physicians that include primary care or family physicians, radiologists, neurologists, and neurosurgeons. In fact, the case scenarios highlight the importance of misconceptions regarding management of the ACs that surgery is not indicated in patients with AC, unless there is a life-threatening condition caused by the presence of ACs. This misinformation is most likely based on a myth in textbooks that originates from the master-apprentice relationship [24]. Today, however, in addition to eliminating the life-threatening condition, improving the quality of life is accepted as an indication for surgical treatment in such patients with an AC [24]. As a rule, the decision for treatment depends on whether there is a clinical symptom and/or any deterioration in the quality of life of the patient affected by the AC, as in the case scenarios described above.

"Medical malpractice" has been defined as "damage caused by the physician not performing the standard, up-to-date practice during treatment, lack of skills or not giving the treatment to the patient" by the World Medical Association (WMA) [4, 7, 18, 26]. From the legal point of view, for a medical malpractice claim to be appropriate, it must include an injury that resulted in significant damages to the patient that were caused by the omission or negligence and a violation of the medical treatment accepted as the standard of care by a medical center, physician, or other healthcare professionals, as a result of mistakes in diagnosis, treatment, and aftercare health management, as stated by the American Board of Professional Liability Attorneys (ABPLA) [5, 31]. In clinical practice, hitherto unpublished reports show that it is possible to encounter a large number of examples of negligence that might result in a lawsuit, some of which are demonstrated in the above case scenarios: disregarding or not taking an appropriate history from the patient, failure to order the proper testing for making a correct diagnosis, failure to recognize the symptoms of the patient, misreading or ignoring laboratory results, failure to diagnose or misdiagnose, unnecessary surgical intervention, various surgical errors, application of improper medication or dosage, poor follow-up of the patient, and premature discharge of the patient from hospital.

Undoubtedly, the physician is not medicolegally responsible for the failure to achieve the desired result while fulfilling the obligation to treat the patient according to the authority of the physician contract, although he/she is responsible for the damages arising from the lack of care in his/her efforts, actions, and behaviors to reach this result [5, 18, 26, 31]. More importantly, the physician should act carefully and be responsible for even the slightest error [26]. In cases that cause uncertainty, therefore, the physician is obligated to conduct investigations to eradicate the uncertainty, even at a minimum level, and to take preventive measures in the meantime [18, 26]. As a legitimate request, the patient has the right to expect from his/her physician, who is a healthcare professional, to show meticulousness and alertness at every stage of the treatment.

In the case scenarios presented under the five headings listed above, situations such as delay in diagnosis and inadequacy in radiological and clinical management by the radiologist and the neurologist, respectively, as a result of failure regarding medical knowledge that intracranial

ACs can cause headaches diminish the quality of life and thus require surgical intervention. As a precaution, both neurologists and neurosurgeons should at least be warned about proper management of these patients. In fact, in many nations worldwide, including the United States, it is possible that such cases may be the subject of a lawsuit against physicians for a malpractice claim. It should never be forgotten that the physician's duty is not to act with the guarantee of healing the patient completely, but the physician has to continue the follow-up treatment of his/her patient with the utmost care and attention. Lastly, it also should be emphasized that the patient and his/her relatives should be informed about the potential risks and benefits of surgical intervention.

5 Conclusion

Even today, an AC might be mistreated because of the high frequency of underlying medical myths regarding its diagnosis and treatment, leading to delayed surgery. Decompressive surgery should be undertaken for any symptomatic craniospinal AC, regardless of size or location, presenting with significant mass effect and impairing the quality of life, even if it is not life-threatening. In clinical practice, therefore, cases of malpractice regarding the management of an AC with delayed surgical treatment are frequently encountered. In terms of forensic medicine, it is important that every physician realizes that any negligence, carelessness, and carelessness at any of these stages will lead to serious medical malpractice in the management of cases affected by AC.

References

1. Albuquerque FC, Giannotta SL. Arachnoid cyst rupture producing subdural hygroma and intracranial hypertension: case reports. Neurosurgery. 1997;41(4):951–5; discussion 955–956.
2. Al-Holou WN, Terman S, Kilburg C, Garton HJ, Muraszko KM, Maher CO. Prevalence and natural history of arachnoid cysts in adults. J Neurosurg. 2013;118(2):222–31.
3. Al-Holou WN, Yew AY, Boomsaad ZE, Garton HJ, Muraszko KM, Maher CO. Prevalence and natural history of arachnoid cysts in children. J Neurosurg Pediatr. 2010;5(6):578–85.
4. Arıkan M, Kalkan E, Erdi F, Deniz M, İzci E. The distinction between cases and malpractice-complications in medical law: the perspectives of the senior students of the faculty of medicine and the faculty of law, problems and suggestiosn for solution (in Turkish). Türk Nöroşir. 2016;26:40–8.
5. Bal BS. An introduction to medical malpractice in the United States. Clin Orthop Relat Res. 2009;467(2):339–47.
6. Bechter K, Wittek R, Seitz K, Antoniadis G. Personality disorders improved after arachnoid cyst neurosurgery, then rediagnosed as 'minor' organic personality disorders. Psychiatry Res. 2010;184:196–200.
7. Birtek F. Complication-malpractice distinction in terms of medical interventions (in Turkish). İstanbul Barosu Dergisi. 2007;81:1997–2007.
8. Choi JU, Kim DS, Huh R. Endoscopic approach to arachnoid cyst. Childs Nerv Syst. 1999;15:285–91.
9. Ciricillo SF, Cogen PH, Harsh GR, Edwards MS. Intracranial arachnoid cysts in children. A comparison of the effects of fenestration and shunting. J Neurosurg. 1991;74:230–5.
10. Couvreur T, Hallaert G, Van Der Heggen T, Baert E, Dewaele F, Okito JPK, Vanhauwaert D, Deruytter M, Roost DV, Caemaert J. Endoscopic treatment of temporal arachnoid cysts in 34 patients. World Neurosurg. 2015;84:734–40.
11. De Volder AG, Michel C, Thauvoy C, Willems G, Ferrière G. Brain glucose utilisation in acquired childhood aphasia associated with a sylvian arachnoid cyst: recovery after shunting as demonstrated by PET. J Neurol Neurosurg Psychiatry. 1994;57:296–300.
12. Di Rocco C. Sylvian fissure arachnoid cysts: we do operate on them but should it be done? Childs Nerv Syst. 2010;26(2):173–5.
13. Domenicucci M, Russo N, Giugni E, Pierallini A. Relationship between supratentorial arachnoid cyst and chronic subdural hematoma: neuroradiological evidence and surgical treatment. J Neurosurg. 2009;110(6):1250–5.
14. Fewel ME, Levy ML, McComb JG. Surgical treatment of 95 children with 102 intracranial arachnoid cysts. Pediatr Neurosurg. 1996;25(4):165–73.
15. Gangemi M, Seneca V, Colella G, Cioffi V, Imperato A, Maiuri F. Endoscopy versus microsurgical cyst excision and shunting for treating intracranial arachnoid cysts. J Neurosurg Pediatr. 2011;8(2):158–64.
16. Garg K, Borkar SA, Kale SS, Sharma BS. Spinal arachnoid cysts - our experience and review of literature. Br J Neurosurg. 2017;31(2):172–8.
17. Gjerde B, Schmid M, Hammar A, Wester K. Intracranial arachnoid cysts: impairment of higher cognitive functions and postoperative improvement. J Neurodev Disord. 2013;5:21.

18. Hakeri H. Distiction between malpractice and complication in medical law (in Turkish). Toraks Cerrahisi Bülteni. 2014;1:23–8.
19. Hall S, Smedley A, Rae S, Mathad N, Waters R, Chakraborty A, Sparrow O, Tsitouras V. Clinical and radiological outcomes following surgical treatment for intra-cranial arachnoid cysts. Clin Neurol Neurosurg. 2019;177:42–6.
20. Helland CA, Lund-Johansen M, Wester K. Location, sidedness, and sex distribution of intracranial arachnoid cysts in a population-based sample. J Neurosurg. 2010;113(5):934–9.
21. Helland CA, Wester K. How often do extra-cerebral haematomas occur in patients with intracranial arachnoid cysts? J Neurol Neurosurg Psychiatry. 2008;79:72–5.
22. Hopf NJ, Perneczky A. Endoscopic neurosurgery and endoscope-assisted microneurosurgery for the treatment of intracranial cysts. Neurosurgery. 1998;43:1330–6.
23. Horiguchi T, Takeshita K. Cognitive function and language of a child with an arachnoid cyst in the left frontal fossa. World J Biol Psychiatry. 2000;1:159–63.
24. Johnston JC, Wester K, Sartwelle TP. Neurological fallacies leading to malpractice: a case studies approach. Neurol Clin. 2016;34(3):747–73.
25. Kang JK, Lee KS, Lee IW, Jeun SS, Son BC, Jung CK, Park YS, Lee SW. Shunt-independent surgical treatment of middle cranial fossa arachnoid cysts in children. Childs Nerv Syst. 2000;16(2):111–6.
26. Kök N. Malpractice and complication distinction. In: Kalkan E, Serel TA, Yılmaz EN, editors. Legal guide for physicians, Turkish neurosurgery academy publications no: 1. Ankara: Sage Publishing; 2018. p. 109–39.
27. Lebowitz BK, Schefft BK, Testa SM, Patton JA, Yeh HS. Neurocognitive sequelae of a giant arachnoid cyst: case study. Neurocase. 2006;12:339–45.
28. Levy ML, Wang M, Aryan HE, Yoo K, Meltzer H. Microsurgical keyhole approach for middle fossa arachnoid cyst fenestration. Neurosurgery. 2003;53(5):1138–44; discussion 1144–1145.
29. Maher CO, Goumnerova L. The effectiveness of ventriculocystocisternostomy for suprasellar arachnoid cysts. J Neurosurg Pediatr. 2011;7(1):64–72.
30. Maher CO, Piatt JH Jr. Section on Neurologic Surgery, American Academy of Pediatrics. Incidental findings on brain and spine imaging in children. Pediatrics. 2015;135(4):e1084–96.
31. Marcus P. Book review of medical malpractice law: a comparative law study of civil responsibility arising from medical care. Hastings Int Comparat Law Rev. 1981;5:235–43.
32. Martinez-Lage JF, Valenti JA, Piqueras C, Ruiz-Espejo AM, Román F, Nuño de la Rosa JA. Functional assessment of intracranial arachnoid cysts with TC99 m-HMPAO SPECT: a preliminary report. Childs Nerv Syst. 2006;22:1091–7.
33. Moorthy S, Garg K, Aggarwal A, Kale SS, Sharma BS, Mahapatra AK. Spontaneous resolution of a spinal arachnoid cyst. Neurology. 2017;65(6):1416–7.
34. Mori K, Yamamoto T, Horinaka N, Maeda M. Arachnoid cyst is a risk factor for chronic subdural hematoma in juveniles: twelve cases of chronic subdural hematoma associated with arachnoid cyst. J Neurotrauma. 2002;19(9):1017–27.
35. Moss T, Helland CA, Mørkve SH, Wester K. Surgical decompression of arachnoid cysts leads to improved quality of life: a prospective study-long-term follow-up. Acta Neurochir. 2019;161(11):2253–63.
36. Nakahashi M, Uei H, Tokuhashi Y. Recurrence of a symptomatic spinal intradural arachnoid cyst 29 years after fenestration. J Int Med Res. 2019;47(9):4530–6.
37. Oberbauer RW, Haase J, Pucher R. Arachnoid cysts in children: a European co-operative study. Childs Nerv Syst. 1992;8(5):281–6.
38. Parsch CS, Krauss J, Hofmann E, Meixensberger J, Roosen K. Arachnoid cysts associated with subdural hematomas and hygromas: analysis of 16 cases, long-term follow-up, and review of the literature. Neurosurgery. 1997;40(3):483–90.
39. Pradilla G, Jallo G. Arachnoid cysts: case series and review of the literature. Neurosurg Focus. 2007;22(2):E7.
40. Sämann PG, Himmerich H, Merl T, Erös C, Müller MB, Tonn JC, Buchwald B. Cervicothoracic intradural arachnoid cyst misdiagnosed as motor neuron disease. Case Rep Med. 2010;2010:261657. https://doi.org/10.1155/2010/261657.
41. Schroeder HW, Gaab MR, Niendorf WR. Neuroendoscopic approach to arachnoid cysts. J Neurosurg. 1996;85:293–8.
42. Sgouros S, Chapman S. Congenital middle fossa arachnoid cysts may cause global brain ischaemia: a study with 99Tc-hexamethylpropyleneamineoxime single photon emission computerised tomography scans. Pediatr Neurosurg. 2001;35:188–94.
43. Shim KW, Lee YH, Park EK, Park YS, Choi JU, Kim DS. Treatment option for arachnoid cysts. Childs Nerv Syst. 2009;25(11):1459–66.
44. Spacca B, Kandasamy J, Mallucci CL, Genitori L. Endoscopic treatment of middle fossa arachnoid cysts: a series of 40 patients treated endoscopically in two centres. Childs Nerv Syst. 2010;26(2):163–72.
45. Takeshige N, Eto T, Nakashima S, Sakata K, Uchikado H, Abe T, Motohiro MM. Rare case of a rapidly enlarging symptomatic arachnoid cyst of the posterior fossa in an infant: a case report and review of the literature. Surg Neurol Int. 2018;9:57.
46. Tamburrini G, Caldarelli M, Massimi L, Santini P, Di Rocco C. Subdural hygroma: an unwanted result of Sylvian arachnoid cyst marsupialization. Childs Nerv Syst. 2003;19(3):159–65.
47. Tamburrini G, Dal Fabbro M, Di Rocco C. Sylvian fissure arachnoid cysts: a survey on their diagnostic

workout and practical management. Childs Nerv Syst. 2008;24(5):593–604.

48. Torgersen J, Helland C, Flaatten H, Wester K. Reversible dyscognition in patients with a unilateral, middle fossa arachnoid cyst revealed by using a laptop based neuropsychological test battery (CANTAB). J Neurol. 2010;257(11):1909–16.
49. Tsurushima H, Harakuni T, Saito A, Tominaga D, Hyodo A, Yoshii Y. Symptomatic arachnoid cyst of the left frontal convexity presenting with memory disturbance–case report. Neurol Med Chir. 2000;40:339–41.
50. Turgut M. Complete spontaneous resolution of an intra-axial cystic lesion in the cerebellum: a case report. Curr Pediatr Res. 2002;6:33–4.
51. Vernooij MW, Ikram MA, Tanghe HL, Vincent AJPE, Hofman A, Krestin GP, Niessen WJ, Breteler MMB, van der Lugt A. Incidental findings on brain MRI in the general population. N Engl J Med. 2007;357(18):1821–8.
52. Wang Y, Wang F, Yu M, Wang W. Clinical and radiological outcomes of surgical treatment for symptomatic arachnoid cysts in adults. J Clin Neurosci. 2015;22:1456–61.
53. Weber F, Knopf H. Incidental findings in magnetic resonance imaging of the brains of healthy young men. J Neurol Sci. 2006;240(1–2):81–4.
54. White ML, Das M, J. Arachnoid cysts. In: StatPearls. Treasure Island: StatPearls Publishing; 2021. Available from https://www.ncbi.nlm.nih.gov/books/NBK563272/.
55. Yang C, Zhang J, Zhang X, Feng N, Hao L, Gaonkar S. Anxiety, phobia, and depression in patients with temporal arachnoid cyst–a case report. MOJ Clin Med Case Rep. 2020;10:119–21.

Index

M. Turgut et al. (eds.), *Arachnoid Cysts*, https://doi.org/10.1007/978-3-031-22701-1

MIX
Papier aus verantwortungsvollen Quellen
Paper from responsible sources
FSC® C105338

If you have any concerns about our products,
you can contact us on
ProductSafety@springernature.com

In case Publisher is established outside the EU,
the EU authorized representative is:
Springer Nature Customer Service Center GmbH
Europaplatz 3, 69115 Heidelberg, Germany

Printed by Libri Plureos GmbH
in Hamburg, Germany